Mosby's EMT–Intermediate Textbook

CONTRIBUTING AUTHORS

DALE A. BARKHURST, EMT-P
EMS Coordinator
The Cleveland Clinic Foundation
Cleveland, Ohio

ELLEN COREY, MD, FACEP
Emergency Physician
Fairview Health Systems
Cleveland, Ohio

JOHN A. KUBINCANEK, EMT-P
Clinical Coordinator of EMS
Division of Allied Health and Nursing
Lorain County Community College
Elyria, Ohio

WILLIAM RAYNOVICH, MPH, NREMT-P
Senior Program Director
EMS Academy, University of New Mexico
Albuquerque, New Mexico

MICK J. SANDERS, EMT-P, MSA
Training Specialist
St. Charles, Missouri

Mosby's EMT–Intermediate Textbook

BRUCE SHADE, EMT-P
Commissioner of EMS
City of Cleveland, Ohio
Immediate Past President
National Association of Emergency Medical Technicians
Cleveland, Ohio

MIKEL A. ROTHENBERG, MD
Emergency Care Educator
North Olmstead, Ohio

ELIZABETH WERTZ, RN, BSN, MPM, EMT-P, PHRN
Executive Director
U.S. Heart and Vascular
Pittsburgh, Pennsylvania

SHIRLEY JONES, MS Ed, MHA, EMT-P
Program Director, EMS Education
Methodist Hospital
Indianapolis, Indiana

with 615 illustrations

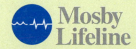

St. Louis Baltimore Boston Carlsbad Chicago Naples New York Philadelphia Portland
London Madrid Mexico City Singapore Sydney Tokyo Toronto Wiesbaden

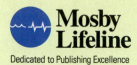

Mosby Lifeline

Dedicated to Publishing Excellence

A Times Mirror
Company

Publisher: David Dusthimer
Editor in Chief: Claire Merrick
Editor: Rina Steinhauer
Senior Assistant Editors: John Goucher, Melissa Blair
Editorial Assistants: Marilyn Boyd, Kathy Davidson
Project Manager: Chris Baumle
Production Editor: Susie Coladonato
Manufacturing Supervisor: Bill Winneberger
Design Manager: Nancy McDonald
Cover Design: GW Graphics

A NOTE TO THE READER:
The author and publisher have made every attempt to ensure that the drug
dosages and patient care procedures presented in this textbook are accurate and
represent accepted practices in the United States. They are not provided as a
standard of care. EMT–Intermediates perform advanced life support procedures
under the authority of a licensed physician. It is the reader's responsibility to
follow patient care protocols established by a medical direction physician and to
remain current in the delivery of emergency care.

Library of Congress Cataloging in Publication Data

Mosby's EMT–Intermediate textbook / Bruce Shade . . . [et al.] ;
    contributing authors, Dale A. Barkhurst, Ellen Correy, John A.
    Kubincanek.
        p.   cm.
    ISBN 0-8151-8022-5
    1. Emergency medicine.   2. Emergency medical technicians.
    [DNLM: 1. Emergencies.   2. Emergency Medical Services.
    3. Emergency Medical Technicians.   WB 105 M894 1997]
    RC86.7.M675 1997
    616.02`5--dc20
    DNLM/DLC
    for Library of Congress   96-41315
                                                         CIP

97 98 99 00 01/9 8 7 6 5 4 3 2 1

This book is dedicated to my wife Cheri and our children, Katie and Christopher. Their sacrifice allowed me to spend the countless hours needed to bring this book to print. Throughout the years their love and support have allowed me to continue my efforts to make learning easier and more complete for out-of-hospital providers, who in turn are able to provide better patient care to those in need.

Bruce Shade, EMT-P

To Diane, Kara, and Marc with all my love . . . without you, all my work would be in vain.

Mikel A. Rothenberg, MD

To my colleagues in emergency care: Thanks for sharing and teaching me. Don't lose sight of your goals even though the days may be long and you may not always feel appreciated— you do make a difference.

Elizabeth Wertz, RN, BSN, MPM, EMT-P, PHRN

To Melissa Blair and John Goucher for their dedication and commitment to this project.

Shirley Jones, MS Ed, MHA, EMT-P

Although many would consider emergency medical services to be in its adolescence, the field has recently experienced more change and growth than ever before. The healthcare revolution has been placed on the national agenda, and much discussion about healthcare took place in Congress and in corporate board rooms. It seemed that current practices were not cost effective. Unfortunately, what was best for the patient was often ignored or forgotten.

What was referred to as the "healthcare revolution" was really not a revolution at all, but an evolution. Attempts to change by revolution were just not successful. Healthcare is too massive and cumbersome, and occupies too much of our economy and life to be overhauled quickly. However, an evolution dictated by societal changes, needs, and technology seems to be taking hold. No one argues that there is not a need to change the way we deliver healthcare and to more closely realign our incentives. How we go about doing that is the challenge that lies ahead.

Two national milestone projects, the *National EMS Education and Practice Blueprint,* and *The EMS Agenda for the Future* attempt to give structure to the changing picture of EMS and out-of-hospital care. The *Blueprint* helps to define and standardize levels of out-of-hospital care and the associated knowledge and skills for each. The *EMS Agenda* attempts to determine the most important directions for future EMS development, to "paint" a picture of the future. As we proceed through this evolution, as we paint the picture of the future, we are and will continue to see tremendous change.

Our human resources, particularly our out-of-hospital providers, become pivotal as we evolve to respond to the health needs of society and our EMS systems. Our resources for these providers are essential. The Emergency Medical Technician–Intermediate represents that bridge to the future. There are more "levels" and descriptions of Intermediates than there are patches for them! This situation creates some real challenges for those who try to educate EMT–Intermediate students. As the DOT goes through the long process of revising the various levels of EMT–National Standard Curricula, there must be stability in the educational process. **Mosby's EMT–Intermediate Textbook** provides that platform in the most variable of all the curricula. For those educational programs that choose to take a more traditional educational approach, this text provides that traditional information in a clear, precise, and easily read format. It assumes that the reader is an EMS professional and provides the opportunity to reach for more. For those programs that are helping to "paint the picture of the future," **Mosby's EMT–Intermediate Textbook** provides much of what EMT–Is will likely be doing in the future. It recognizes the move toward integrated health services, and uses "Case Histories" and "Street Wise" sidebars that embrace the changing picture of the way we do business. The format uses "Key Terms," "Learning Objectives," and "Clinical Notes" that help the student capture important concepts and information. The Pharmacology, Intravenous Cannulation, and Assessment and Management of Shock chapters are the critical areas that create the bridge between the EMT–Basic and the EMT–Paramedic. These chapters are thorough, progressive, and allow significant adaptation to various EMS systems. **Mosby's EMT–Intermediate Textbook** provides a quality, flexible resource for educators and students alike, and furnishes an essential tool to help move EMS into the future.

John L. Chew, Jr., President
EMSSTAR Group, LLC

The goal of this text is to bridge the "educational gap" between EMT–Basic training and Paramedic training according to the US DOT National Standard Curricula. The approach of this textbook is simple: Each objective contained in the National Standard Curriculum for the EMT–Intermediates is addressed, focusing the student on the most critical content. In addition, we have purposely exceeded the DOT objectives for EMT–Intermediate training in many areas to provide a more comprehensive and advanced-level textbook. By addressing a broad scope of information, **Mosby's EMT–Intermediate Textbook** offers a complete training package for a wide audience of educators and students.

Mosby's EMT–Intermediate Textbook contains 18 chapters, separated into three divisions. The first division, "Introduction," addresses preparatory information, including chapters on Roles and Responsibilities, Documentation, and Medical/Legal Considerations. The "Essentials" division is the crux of EMT–Intermediate training. It contains chapters on Airway Management, Assessment and Management of Shock, and Intravenous Cannulation. The "Enrichment" division discusses topics that may go beyond the scope of the EMT–I National Standard Curriculum, in such chapters as Trauma Emergencies and Obstetric and Gynecologic Emergencies.

Each chapter contains a number of learning devices that have been designed to enhance the reader's comprehension and application of the material.

Each chapter opens with a brief **content outline,** which provides the reader with a quick overview of the organization and content of the chapter. A **case history** places the chapter content in a prehospital or clinical context. A **follow-up** to each case history is found at the end of the chapter. Chapter **objectives,** identified by the apple icon appear next. The objectives also appear in boxes in the chapter text, just above the section in which the objective is contained. **Key terms** relating to the chapter are then listed. These terms also appear throughout the chapter, above the section in which they are discussed. These boxes are identified by the key symbol . Each chapter concludes with a **summary,** which highlights the major points discussed in the chapter.

Three types of supplemental learning material appear in the chapter text. **Street Wise** boxes call attention to the information that will help the EMT–Intermediate become more efficient in delivering emergency field care. **Helpful Hint** boxes identify background, "nice-to-know" information, giving the reader a deeper understanding of concepts and skills. **Clinical Notes** boxes provide the reader with background information from a clinical perspective.

The authors and publishers are confident that instructors and students will find that this progressive textbook facilitates an effective and enjoyable learning experience. The best of luck to you, the student, in your endeavors in advanced prehospital emergency care.

AUTHOR ACKNOWLEDGMENTS

As we reach the end of developing this exciting new textbook, I want to thank those people who helped make it a reality. First, my thanks and love goes to my mother Lucille Shade, who was an aspiring author; she encouraged me to put pen to paper. Also, to my father, Elmer Shade, Jr., who taught me the value of a hard day's work and to continually strive for what I believe in.

This textbook came to life during a discussion Claire Merrick and I had over dinner in Bethesda, Maryland. Claire's vision and willingness to take a chance on a new market resulted in the textbook proposal moving from ideas to print on pages.

Next came the editorial people who helped to drive the project along as it chugged, and even stalled a few times. Rina Steinhauer, with her dry humor and "get it done or else" attitude, John Goucher with his relentless encouragement and constant reminders that we were past our deadline, and Melissa Blair who filled in the gaps on pushing to get chapters done, all made this project happen. We also enjoyed the support of wonderful reviewers (listed on the next page) who helped shape the chapters into a more readable and usable text. Particular thanks to Mick Sanders, who went that extra mile (or two).

Then there were the "artists." Tom Page, one of the best photographers and nicest people I ever met, created phenomenal work and showed extraordinary patience. The illustrations were done by a wonderful artist named Kim Battista, who I almost drove crazy with change after change and who delivered images that are among the best in the business.

Last comes Susie Coladonato, who had the hardest job of all. Not only did she have to put all of the text and pictures into final form, she had to put up with my frequent and ongoing last minute changes. The beauty of this textbook speaks of her excellence.

Bruce Shade, EMT-P

My writing and teaching over the years has been significantly influenced by several close friends and colleagues. Thanks to Dick Clinchy for believing in me when I needed it the most . . . And to Dale Dubin for being a true friend and gentleman, as well as my inspiration for "plain English" education—his encouragement has had an everlasting effect on my life. To Harold Cohen, truly a rising star in EMS . . . his "ADDitions" to our profession are a true inspiration. Sincere thanks to Bruce Shade for asking me to become involved with this project initially. It's really nice to have someone else "run the show" for once. Last, and never least . . . thanks to Jim Page— little did either of us know what a profound effect "Roy and Johnny" would have on my career. Without "Emergency," I would have just been another doctor . . . . Your inspiration has allowed me to become a well-respected writer, teacher, and speaker. Thank you, Jim, for opening the door . . . .

Mikel A. Rothenberg, MD

Thanks to my parents, Helen and Bill Hodgson (who I call Mom and Dad), for giving me the opportunity to pursue my dreams and for picking me up when the road got bumpy. To my husband, Pat, for his never-ending love and support and for first introducing me to this incredible life of EMS. On that first day he said, "Let's just stop by the base for a few minutes." Those few minutes turned into a lifetime of love for EMS.

Thanks to my wonderful children: Patrick, Amanda, and Ashley. Thank you for trying to understand why Mom spent so much time on the computer writing when you wanted to do something else. This is all for you—to educate people to make a better and safer world for you.

And lastly, my thanks to God for giving me the ability and creativity to care for people in need and to educate others who do the same.

Elizabeth Wertz, RN, BSN, MPM, EMT-P, PHRN

PUBLISHER ACKNOWLEDGMENTS

The editors wish to acknowledge and thank the many reviewers of this book, who devoted countless hours to intensive review. Their comments were invaluable in helping develop and fine-tune this manuscript.

Barbara Ahlert, RN
Director, EMS Education
Samaritan Health System
Phoenix, AZ

Jerry L. Bardwell, NREMT-P, I/C
American Medical Response
Brockton, MA

Shelley Cohen, RNCEN/EMT
Tennessee Christian Medical Center
Springfield, TN

Randy C. Krantz, RN, JD
Commonwealth's Attorney
Bedford, VA

Randall Likens, EMT-P, I/C
Training–Safety Officer
Franklin County Emergency Services
Louisburg, NC

Sal Marini
ALS Coordinator, EMS Degree Program
The George Washington University
Washington, DC

Tim McQuade, MBA, EMT-P, I/C
Instructor, Department of Health, Physical
Education, and Recreation
Erie Community College
Buffalo, NY

Dwight A. Polk, MSW, NREMT-P
Paramedic Program Coordinator
University of Maryland, Baltimore County
Baltimore, MD

William Raynovich, MPH, NREMT-P
Senior Program Director
EMS Academy, University of New Mexico
Albuquerque, NM

Stuart Redfearn, NREMT-P
EMS Educator, Redfearn Enterprises, Inc.
Metairie, LA

Mick J. Sanders, EMT-P, MSA
Training Specialist
St. Charles, MO

Andrew W. Stern, MPA, MA, NREMT-P
Senior Paramedic
Town of Colonie Emergency Medical Services
Colonie, NY

Bernice D. Stiansen, RN, BscN
Instructor
Grant MacEwan Community College
Edmonton, Alberta, Canada

Mary Alice Witzel, RN, CEN
AREA Coordinator
Good Samaritan Regional Medical Center
Phoenix, AZ

CONTENTS

17 Pediatric Emergencies

18 Substance Abuse and Behavioral Emergencies

Mosby's EMT–Intermediate Textbook

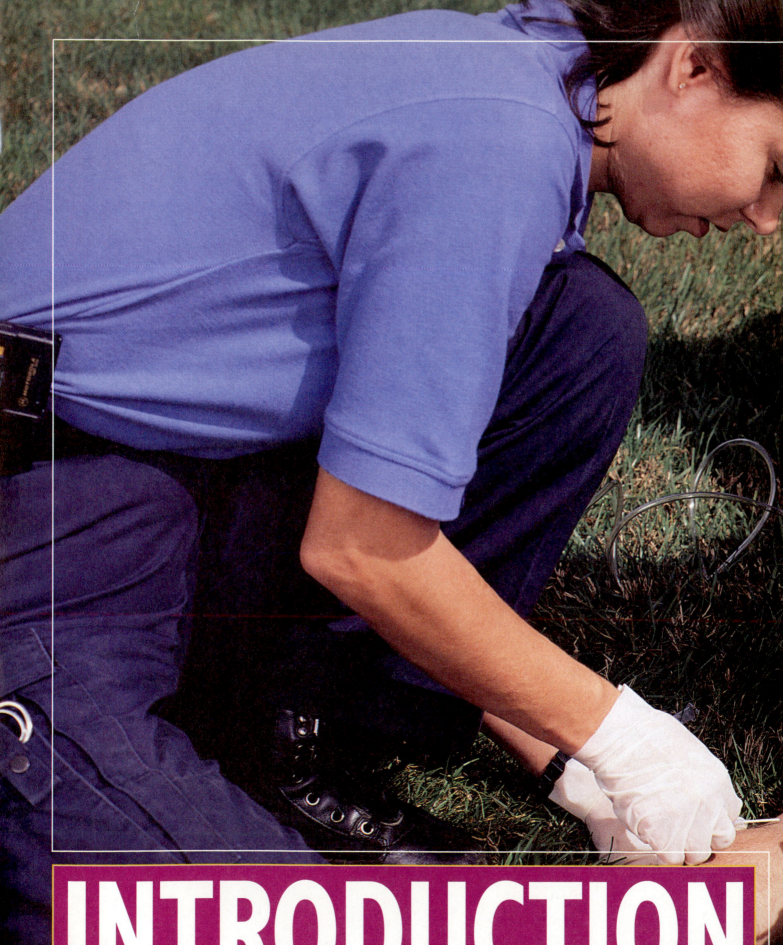

INTRODUCTION

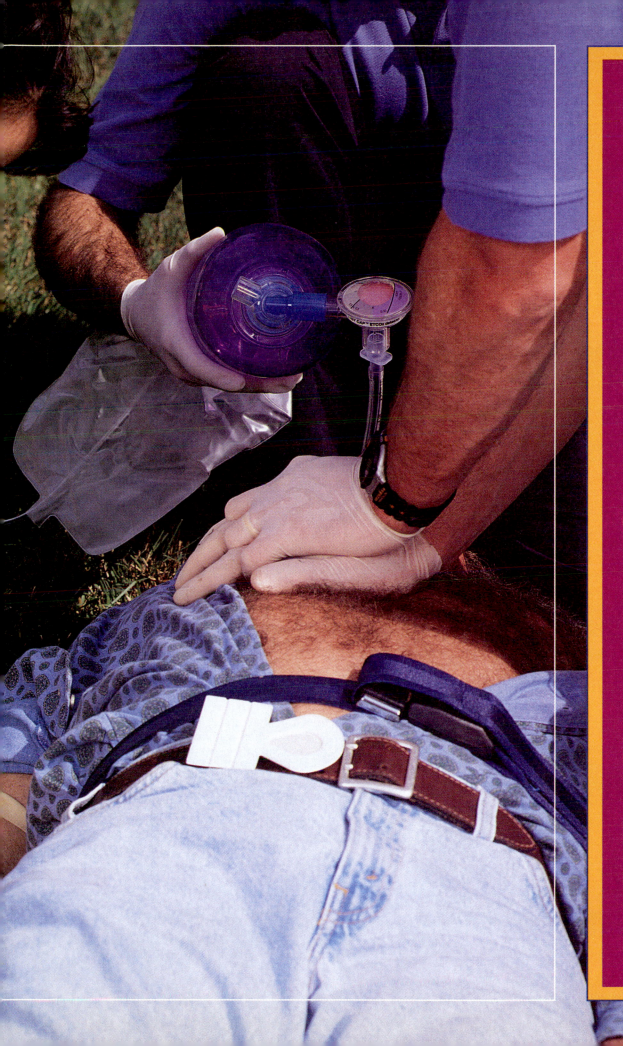

DIVISION ONE

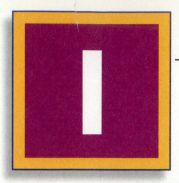

ROLES AND RESPONSIBILITIES OF THE EMT–INTERMEDIATE

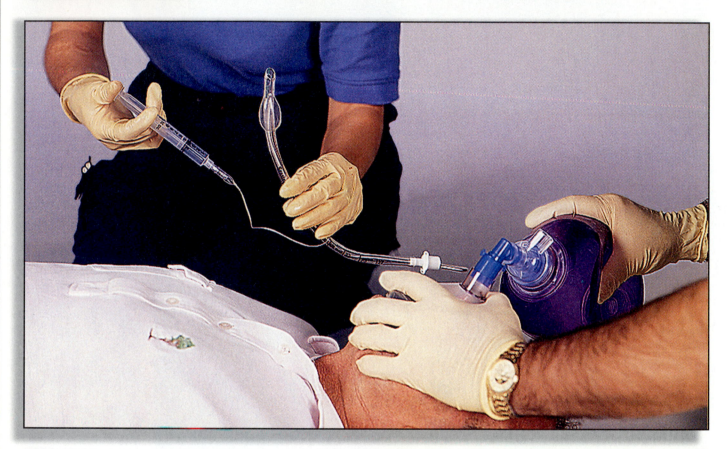

CASE HISTORY

Williams and Brown, EMTs at Station 17, report to work 5 minutes prior to the start of the scheduled day shift, to discover that the unit is returning from a trauma call.

Both of their uniforms are clean, pressed, and starched, and their steel-toe leather shoes are polished. They both check the bulletin board for personnel memos and traffic notices, and then sit down for a cup of coffee.

Medic 17 arrives approximately 5 minutes later; the EMTs begin checking the unit while the night shift crew gives their report. The crew reports that the Streets department is working on a water main break at 16th and Walnut, and that 4 amps of naloxone and two prefilled syringes of lidocaine will expire next month. Both Williams and Brown make a note to avoid the road work area. While EMT-I Williams assesses all of the vehicle supplies

Case History, continued

and equipment, EMT-I Brown checks the vehicle fluid levels, radios, tires, and batteries.

The two EMTs respond to two calls before lunch: one for a 63-year-old man with chest pain, and the second for a 13-year-old patient with asthma. Then, the EMTs stop at a local diner for lunch on the way back to the station.

LEARNING OBJECTIVES

Upon completion of this chapter, the EMT–Intermediate should be able to:

- DIFFERENTIATE between the levels of EMT–Basic, EMT–Intermediate (EMT–I), and EMT–Paramedic.
- RELATE the roles and responsibilities of the EMT–I.
- DEFINE the terms *certification* and *licensure.*
- STATE the role of the National Registry of Emergency Medical Technicians.
- RELATE the meaning of *EMT–Intermediate certification.*
- DISCUSS the reason why it is important to keep one's EMT–Intermediate certification or licensure current.
- LIST three reasons why continuing education is important to the EMT–I.
- RECALL the benefits of subscribing to professional journals.
- IDENTIFY the benefits of EMT–I teaching in the community.
- DEFINE the terms *ethics* and *professionalism.*
- LIST those behaviors on the part of the EMT–I that are considered professional.
- DESCRIBE appropriate appearance of an EMT–I.
- IDENTIFY five attributes of ethical conduct by the EMT–I.
- STATE the major purposes of a National Association of EMTs.

KEY TERMS

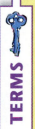

CERTIFICATION

EMERGENCY MEDICAL SERVICES (EMS) SYSTEM

EMERGENCY MEDICAL TECHNICIAN (EMT)

EMT–BASIC

EMT–INTERMEDIATE

EMT–PARAMEDIC

ETHICS

FIRST RESPONDER

LICENSURE

PROFESSIONAL

PROTOCOLS

RECIPROCITY

RUN CRITIQUES

INTRODUCTION

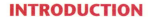

EMT–INTERMEDIATE: An EMT who has completed training beyond the EMT–Basic level; the degree of training and skills practiced varies widely between states and EMS systems.

Approach

This text presents the knowledge and skills needed by an **EMT–Intermediate (EMT–I)** to function in a professional, medically appropriate, and efficient manner. Basic and advanced principles are presented, which serve as building blocks for the provision of quality patient care. This chapter describes the roles and responsibilities of the EMT–I.

EMS SYSTEM: An organized approach to providing emergency care to the sick and injured.

A young profession

The classification of EMT–I is little more than 15 years old. It follows the evolution of the Emergency Medical Technician (EMT) over the past century from stretcher-bearer and ambulance driver to today's healthcare professional. In the early years there were no curricula or textbooks available to teach the principles of prehospital care, and the equipment used was largely drawn from the hospital setting. Clearly though, the controlled hospital setting differed vastly from the field environment. For this reason, the practice of the EMT has evolved into a profession with its own specific equipment and training.

Along with the EMT has come the development of an increasingly sophisticated **Emergency Medical Services (EMS) system.** EMS systems serve as a bridge between the community and the medical facilities that provide definitive healthcare.

WHAT IS AN EMT–INTERMEDIATE?

An EMT–I is a person trained in advanced care of the acutely sick or injured. Most EMT–Is function in the prehospital care environment and serve as early links in the provision of emergency care. Some EMT–Is are paid, whereas others volunteer their services.

Actions taken by EMT–Is can make the difference between life and death. Proper handling and care of patients at the scene can minimize suffering, prevent further injury, and reduce recuperation time.

Few professions offer the excitement and adventure that one experiences working as a prehospital care provider. One morning the EMT–I may be delivering a baby, that afternoon treating a patient who has abdominal pain, and the next day extricating a trauma patient from the wreckage of an overturned automobile on the freeway.

A career as an EMT–I can be exciting, but it also can be one that challenges the safety, composure, and humanity of the provider. It can be disheartening for the EMT–I to perform cardiopulmonary resuscitation (CPR) for 20 minutes on a patient suffering cardiac arrest, carry the patient down three flights of stairs, and deliver chest compressions while off-balance in the back of a moving ambulance, only to have the patient succumb to the cardiac condition in the hospital emergency department. It can be almost as frustrating to rush to the scene of a reported serious emergency only to find that someone has called in a false alarm or greatly exaggerated the situation to get help there sooner.

Often, EMT–Is perform their duties in uncontrolled and volatile circumstances, and under considerable physical and emotional stress. EMT–Is often place their lives at risk to ensure the safety and well-being of the communities they are sworn to serve. Long work hours, heavy workloads, lifting injuries, stress, violence, drugs, gangs, exposure to bloodborne pathogens and hazardous materials, as well as other dangers, challenge the EMT–I's ability to remain in the field setting until retirement.

To survive as a prehospital care provider, the EMT–I must be realistic about the job. It is not all glory and excitement, nor is it mundane. With some cases it is necessary to use all the skills the EMT–I has been trained to perform, whereas in other situations, simply holding the patient's hand or offering comfort during transport to the hospital is what is needed. To help deal with the stress inherent in the job, the EMT–I must maintain an appropriate sense of compassion and humor.

LEVELS OF EMT CERTIFICATION

 Differentiate between the levels of EMT–Basic, EMT–Intermediate, and EMT–Paramedic.

EMERGENCY MEDICAL TECHNICIAN (EMT): A person trained according to criteria established by the Department of Transportation in the care of the acutely sick or injured person.

Since the early 1980s, the United States Department of Transportation (DOT) has recognized three levels of **Emergency Medical Technician (EMT)** certification: EMT–Basic (EMT–B), EMT–Intermediate (EMT–I), and EMT–Paramedic (EMT–P). An additional level, EMT–Defibrillation, was developed by the American Heart Association in 1990 to provide for a state- or nationally-certified EMT–B who has completed additional training in the use of cardiac defibrillators. More recently, the National EMS Education and Practice Blueprint, a consensus document issued in September, 1993, recommended that there be four levels of prehospital providers: first responder, EMT–B, EMT–I, and EMT–P.

FIRST RESPONDER: A trained person who provides initial care until other EMS providers arrive on the scene.

First responder

The **first responder** uses a limited amount of equipment to perform early assessment and intervention. This level of prehospital care provider is often thought of as an "independent practice" role because care is provided at a very basic level. First responders typically possess the knowledge and skills needed to deliver care and do not require on-line medical direction to make treatment decisions.

First responders serve a vital role in shortening the time it takes to begin patient care because they can provide life-sustaining care until other EMS units arrive. The extra time gained by having trained first responders at the scene before the arrival of the EMS system can make a big difference in a patient's outcome.

First responders may be fire department personnel, police officers, construction safety crews, industry first-aid teams, athletic trainers, or other trained personnel. The first responder receives 40 hours of DOT approved training in basic prehospital care including the recognition of emergencies, CPR, bleeding control, and how to assist the EMT.

EMT–BASIC: AN EMT who has completed the primary level of EMT–Basic training, including completion of a minimum 110-hour EMT–B training program meeting DOT standards.

EMT–Basic

The **EMT–basic (EMT–B)** possesses the knowledge and skills of the first responder but also is qualified to staff an ambulance. The EMT–B receives at least 110 hours of training based on the 1994 DOT Emergency Medical Technician–Basic Curriculum. The EMT–B provides basic prehospital care during emergency and nonemergency situations. This care may be as simple as transporting a patient from home to the hospital for evaluation or as complex as caring for a patient experiencing multisystem trauma or cardiac arrest. In addition to basic skills, EMT–Bs in many communities perform advanced level skills. These skills can include assisting patients with medication administration, employing automatic external defibrillation, and performing endotracheal intubation. For this reason on-line/off-line medical direction is a necessary element at the basic level.

EMT–B certification is a prerequisite for entering training programs for advanced-level EMS providers.

EMT–Intermediate

The EMT–Intermediate fills the void between the levels of EMT–Basic and EMT–Paramedic. There are many different levels of EMT–Is throughout the nation. Some of these include EMT–II, EMT–Advanced, EMT–Cardiac, EMT–Special Skills, and Cardiac Rescue Technician (CRT).

The EMT–I possesses both basic skills and key advanced-care skills, including additional patient assessment skills, use of the pneumatic antishock garment (PASG), advanced airway adjuncts, intravenous therapy, and defibrillation. Some EMT–Is also are trained to monitor and interpret basic cardiac dysrhythmias as well as administer some medications including: epinephrine, 50% dextrose, naloxone, aerosol bronchodilators, and first-round cardiac drugs such as atropine and lidocaine (Fig. 1-1).

In addition to keeping the emergency vehicle adequately equipped, supplied, and maintained, EMT–Is are responsible for checking the expiration dates on intravenous solutions and medications, as well as testing the PASG and esophageal airway/endotracheal devices for proper function.

Because of the advanced level of care provided, many states require EMT–Is to work under medical direction.

 EMT–PARAMEDIC: An EMT who has advanced training in patient assessment, medical emergencies, pharmacology, trauma, obstetrics, rescue, behavioral emergencies, and other EMS activities.

EMT–Paramedic

The most advanced level of prehospital care provider is the **EMT–Paramedic (EMT–P).** Training for EMT–Ps is based on the DOT Emergency Medical Technician–Paramedic curriculum. The training for the EMT–P generally includes 300 to 1600 hours beyond the EMT–B level training. Many colleges and universities offer 2- or 4-year programs in EMS that include EMT–P certification.

The EMT–P has advanced training in patient assessment, dysrhythmia recognition, defibrillation and synchronized cardioversion, drug therapy, definitive airway management (endotracheal intubation),

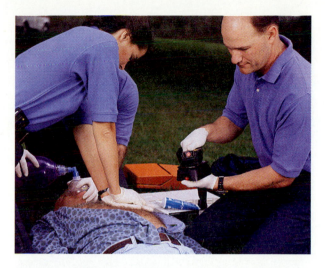

Fig. 1-1 **EMT–Intermediates providing advanced-level patient care.**

and techniques for managing tension pneumothorax. Because advanced life-support providers often treat patients under standing orders, a significant portion of the instruction is devoted to assessment skills and dealing with as many additional potential emergency situations as possible.

Because of the increased complexity of the advanced treatments provided, a "partnership role" exists between EMT–Ps and physicians who provide medical direction via radio/cellular telephone or standing orders.

ROLES AND RESPONSIBILITIES OF THE EMT–INTERMEDIATE

> Relate the roles and responsibilities of the EMT–I.

Role

The role of the EMT–I is to provide basic and advanced care to persons experiencing medical and traumatic emergencies.

Responsibilities

The foremost responsibility of the EMT–I is to ensure his or her own safety and the safety of fellow workers. Duties the EMT–I is typically expected to perform include:

- Driving the emergency vehicle to the scene in a safe, timely, and lawful manner while exercising due regard for others.
- Using protective equipment in hazardous or dangerous situations including employing body substance isolation precautions.
- Interacting with first responders who are already on the scene providing care.

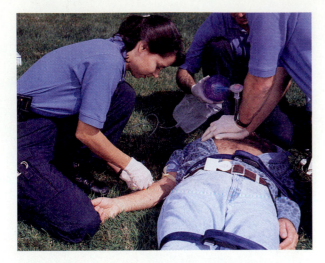

Fig. 1-2 Intravenous therapy is an important aspect of the EMT–I's care for the patient.

- Initially controlling the scene, ensuring safety, and regulating access to potentially harmful situations. Police or other emergency personnel often assume these duties on their arrival at the scene.
- Determining the needs of those involved in the incident and communicating that information to the dispatch center, including requesting the response of and coordinating with supportive agencies as needed.
- Using basic tools and procedures to gain access to and extricate entrapped patients.
- Establishing rapport with patients, maintaining their confidentiality, and shielding them from onlookers.
- Treating patients with the appropriate dignity, compassion, and respect.
- Rapidly assessing and managing life-threatening illnesses and injuries.
- Performing a careful patient assessment, recognizing the nature and seriousness of illnesses or injuries, and determining the requirements for emergency medical care.

PROTOCOLS: Written instructions listing guidelines for the care of patients with specific conditions, illnesses, or injuries.

- Within the confines of given **protocols,** providing prompt and efficient care for illnesses or injuries (Fig. 1-2).
- Assessing the effects of treatment.
- Establishing communications with medical direction, including physician consultation, when needed.
- Recognizing when the limits of field care have been reached and when prompt transportation to the appropriate medical facility is needed.

- Lifting, moving, positioning, and handling patients in such a way as to minimize discomfort and further injury, including spinal immobilization, splinting fractures, and proper lifting and carrying techniques.
- Transporting patients safely and expeditiously to an appropriate medical facility. The EMT–I must know what resources are available and be familiar with local protocols involving patient transportation. These resources include specialty referral care for trauma, pediatrics, or burns. The EMT–I also may be responsible for making arrangements for other forms of transportation such as aeromedical evacuation of a critically injured motor vehicle accident victim.
- Transferring care of patients to the emergency department staff (usually the emergency department nurse) in an orderly and efficient manner.
- Properly completing the run sheet (run report) used by the EMS system. The EMS run report is the legal record of the events that occurred. It gives the hospital staff important information about the incident and patient history.
- Preparing for the next incident. The EMT–I is responsible for cleaning and maintaining equipment in proper working order, which ensures that quality patient care can be provided.
- Recognizing when patient transport is not warranted and following established protocols for handling such situations.

Growing employment opportunities
EMT–Intermediates are no longer limited to working on an ambulance or rescue squad. There is a wide range of jobs in which the EMT–I can practice his or her profession. Some of these jobs offer a salary whereas others are on a volunteer basis. In addition to working in the field setting, EMT–Is are finding employment in hospital emergency departments, as well as in industrial and corporate settings. Many are becoming educators and administrators in EMS systems.

THE CERTIFICATION PROCESS

 Define the terms *certification* **and** *licensure.*

To practice as an EMT–I in most states, one must attend a recognized EMT–Intermediate course, successfully complete a written and practical examination, and become certified or licensed.

EMT–Intermediate training
The EMT–Intermediate curriculum is based on the first portion of the DOT EMT–Paramedic curriculum. This curriculum includes:

- Roles and responsibilities
- EMS systems

- Medical/legal considerations
- Medical terminology
- EMS communications
- General patient assessment and initial management
- Airway management and ventilation
- Assessment and management of shock
- Defibrillation

The number of hours required for EMT–Intermediate training differs widely from state to state. It may include more than 300 hours of classroom, practical skills, and clinical training.

Knowledge and skill examinations
At the completion of the training, most states require EMT–I students to successfully complete written and skill examinations to demonstrate their knowledge and skills. Some states use their own testing process for EMT–Is whereas others use the National Registry of Emergency Medical Technicians (NREMT) EMT–Intermediate Examination.

 State the role of the National Registry of Emergency Medical Technicians.

The NREMT is a private, nonprofit agency formed to provide testing and registration of EMTs on a nationwide basis. To meet the NREMT requirements for certification the candidate must:

- Successfully complete an EMT–I training program that meets DOT standards.
- Successfully pass the EMT–I written examination and practical skills testing of the NREMT.

In states in which national registration is not required, EMT–Is should view becoming nationally registered as a demonstration of their commitment to excellence. To remain nationally registered, the EMT–I must recertify at 2-year intervals. This recertification is done by attending a structured refresher program or obtaining the required continuing education during the certification period.

CERTIFICATION: Action by which an agency or association grants recognition to an individual who has met its qualifications.
LICENSURE: Process by which a governmental agency grants permission to an individual to engage in a given occupation on finding that the applicant has attained the minimal degree of competency necessary.

Credentialing
Following successful completion of the required training and testing, the candidate must undergo a credentialing process. The objective of credentialing is to protect the public from incompetence and provide for professional identification. **Certification** and **licensure** are common forms of credentialing used for today's prehospital care providers.

The process of credentialing varies from state to state. In some states, after meeting the necessary testing and training requirements the process may be as simple as filling out a form that is signed by the training program medical advisor and submitted to the state EMS office. The state EMS office issues a certification card that can be carried in the EMT–I's wallet. In other states, EMT–I certification or licensure is administered through the State Department of Health, Board of Medical Examiners, or other state agency.

 Relate the meaning of *EMT–Intermediate certification.*

Meaning of EMT–Intermediate certification
It is important to understand what certification represents. Certification implies that the EMT–I has demonstrated the minimum written and practical proficiency in the subject matter. Certification does not give the EMT–I the right to function as an EMT–I or to be selected for employment. Both volunteer and paid EMS systems may add other requirements, including examinations, internships, or other demonstrations of proficiency before the EMT–I is able to function in the field setting.

 RECIPROCITY: Mutual exchange of privileges or licenses by two certifying agencies.

Reciprocity
It is not uncommon for EMT–Is who are certified in one state to relocate to another. Rather than requiring those individuals to repeat the EMT–I training, most states have a process in place called **reciprocity** that allows the transfer of certification or licensure. In some states reciprocity is automatic, especially if the EMT–I is nationally registered.

RECERTIFICATION AND CONTINUING EDUCATION

 Discuss the reason why it is important to keep one's EMT–I certification or licensure current.

To maintain the right to function as an EMT–I, most states require recertification every 1 to 4 years (the average being 2 years). In most states it is legally necessary to maintain certification or licensure as long as one practices as an EMT–I.

In some states, recertification involves participating in a refresher course, whereas in other states, EMT–Is are required to obtain a specific amount of continuing education each year. Some jurisdictions require successful completion of written and/or skill testing to become recertified as an EMT–I.

 List three reasons why continuing education is important to the EMT–I.

Benefits of continuing education

The public and medical community need to be continually assured that quality patient care is being delivered in the prehospital setting. Many of the skills and much of the knowledge learned in the EMT–I course may not be used frequently, and skill decay can occur rapidly. Continuing education helps reduce the erosion of knowledge and skills. It also keeps the EMT–I current on new procedures and treatments, allows a sharing of real-life experiences with other prehospital care providers, and encourages further professional development.

RUN CRITIQUES: Sessions in which prehospital care providers and medical direction physicians (typically in a group setting) review run reports and/or case histories to identify positive and negative aspects of care and documentation provided by EMT–Is in given cases.

Continuing education for the EMT–Intermediate

There are countless continuing education opportunities available for the EMT–I. On a local level, EMS systems, EMS associations, and hospitals often provide in-service training programs, seminars, and **run critiques.** On a state and national level a variety of conferences are held annually. These conferences expose the EMT–I to a wide range of nationally recognized experts in EMS relaying the most current information (research updates, newest equipment, new techniques) in EMS.

Another common type of continuing education activity is the 1- or 2-day training program. Prehospital Trauma Life Support (PHTLS), developed by the National Association of EMTs in conjunction with the American College of Surgeons Committee on Trauma, is one example of such a program (Fig. 1-3). In this PHTLS course, students are exposed to basic and advanced concepts in managing trauma patients. Brief, information-packed courses such as this require only a modest time commitment on the part of the EMT–I while providing enormous knowledge, skill learning, and remediation.

Alternatively, there are many excellent continuing education programs that can be conveniently reviewed while at home or on the job. These programs can be found in EMS-related textbooks, magazines, subscription videos, and computer programs.

 Recall the benefits of subscribing to professional journals.

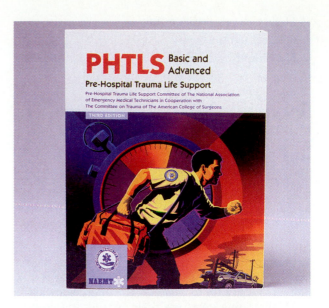

Fig. 1-3 PHTLS, 3 edition, by The National Association for Emergency Medical Technicians.

EMS-related reading

EMS-related publishing companies have had a strong influence on the evolution of the EMS profession. A variety of EMS–related textbooks and magazines are available to the EMT–I. EMS magazines help keep the EMT–I aware of the latest changes in a constantly evolving industry and provide excellent sources of continuing education to sharpen knowledge and skills. EMS magazines also list employment opportunities, EMS seminars, and conferences; provide details about new products and equipment; highlight tips that can be used on the job; and review various EMS–related books, videos, and films. An additional benefit of EMS magazines is that the EMT–I can write articles, communicating important information to other EMS professionals. Listed below are several of the primary EMS–related magazines. Many offer student subscription rates.

Emergency Magazine
(Journal of Emergency Services)
Hare Publications

Emergency Medical Services Magazine
(Journal of Emergency Care and Transportation)
Creative Age Publications, Inc.

JEMS Magazine
(Journal of Emergency Medical Services)
JEMS Communications, Inc.

Rescue Magazine
JEMS Communications, Inc.

9-1-1 Magazine
Official Publications, Inc.

Identify the benefits of the EMT–I teaching in the community.

Serving as an instructor

Serving as an instructor in CPR, first aid, or EMT courses or as a preceptor in EMT–B or EMT–I field internships is another way to keep one's skills current. Teaching can serve as a source of continuing education credit. Serving as an educator also establishes the EMT–I as a leader and a reliable resource in the community.

PROFESSIONALISM, ETHICS, AND CONFIDENTIALITY

 Define the terms *ethics* and *professionalism*.

 PROFESSIONAL: A person who has certain special skills and knowledge in a specific area and conforms to the standards of conduct and performance in that area. The EMT–I does not need to be paid to be a professional.

Professionalism

Despite the differences in training, all EMTs have two things in common: they are all basic EMTs, and they all are **professionals.** Professionalism is necessary to promote quality patient care, instill pride in the prehospital environment, promote high standards, and earn the respect of other members of the healthcare team.

 List those behaviors on the part of the EMT–I that are considered professional.

People who are involved in emergencies usually experience pain, fear, and great anxiety. Sick and injured patients feel vulnerable and helpless when depending on strangers for assistance. The EMT–I's attitude and professionalism can positively influence a patient's judgment of the EMS system. Patients made to feel at ease by the actions of caring, confident, and well-trained EMT–Is may show both psychologic and physical improvement. Some attributes of professional conduct include:

- *A professional manner*—The EMT–I should be courteous, be in control of his or her emotions, avoid inappropriate conversation, and appear confident. The EMT–I should not eat, drink, or smoke while caring for patients.

Describe the appropriate appearance of an EMT–I.

- *Appearance*—The EMT–I should be well groomed and wear an appropriate uniform and personal protection apparel.

- *General conduct*—The EMT–I should show interest and pride in his or her service. In striving to provide the best quality patient care, the EMT–I also has a responsibility to be nondiscriminatory and nonjudgmental in dealing with patients. The EMT–I should work well as a member of the prehospital team, share equally in the workload, and communicate effectively with the patients, bystanders, partner(s), fellow workers, and other safety professionals.

- *Concern for the patient*—The EMT–I should place all his or her efforts toward the patient's welfare. Concern also means safety, reassurance, and prevention of patient embarrassment.

- *Treating others with respect*—The EMT–I should call patients by their proper name (*eg*, Mr. Smith) not "pops," "gramps," "bub," etc. Avoid making negative comments about a person's gender, race, sexual orientation, ethnicity, religion, physical appearance, profession, social status, or disability.

- *Personal improvement*—The EMT–I must strive to be the best he or she can be. Attending continuing education, practicing skills, reading EMS-related literature, and participating in quality improvement activities are all characteristic of a professional.

 STREET WISE

To become proficient, the EMT–I must be able to use all equipment and carry out procedures without having to think about it; in other words, it must be "second nature." One way to accomplish this goal is to practice frequently with the equipment and rehearse all necessary skills. Handling equipment gives the EMT–I a feel for each device, making it easier to use under less than ideal conditions, such as when the lighting is poor or one is in a hurry.

During the training program, the EMT–I student should visit the local EMS station from time to time to observe how equipment is stored, maintained, and used. If the student builds a positive relationship with the crew(s), the crew may be willing to allow the EMT–I student to practice with the equipment during visits.

Ethics in prehospital care

ETHICS: The discipline dealing with what is good and bad.

Meaning of ethics

The word **ethics** is derived from the Greek word meaning "character." Ethics set standards for the rightness and wrongness of human behavior. Ethics govern one's conduct as a practicing EMT–I. They deal with the EMT–I's relationship with his or her peers, patients, the patient's family, and society in general.

When faced with situations that call for a choice of behavior, the EMT–I must act ethically. For example, it is unethical and/or illegal to:

- Make a statement to a patient about a fellow healthcare worker's perceived faults

- Solicit a patient for a date

- Give an attorney's business card to the victim of a motor vehicle accident

- Discourage a patient from going to the hospital because he or she has no insurance

- Fail to maintain patient confidentiality

Working as an EMT–I, one is likely to be confronted with various ethical issues. These issues might include having to decide if attempts should be made to preserve a terminally ill patient's life, meeting the needs of patients who are unable to pay, or requesting medical help from others when needed. If the EMT–I places the patient's well-being above all else when providing care and always does what is in the patient's best interest, there is rarely a need to worry about committing an unethical act.

 Identify five attributes of ethical conduct by the EMT–I.

Code of ethics

Many health professions publish written codes of ethics to help guide their members who face difficult ethical decisions. A code of ethics provides a model of ideal conduct. In January 1978, a Code of Ethics for Emergency Medical Technicians was issued by the National Association of EMTs. The Code states:

Professional status as an Emergency Medical Technician is maintained and enriched by the willingness of the individual practitioner to accept and fulfill obligations to society, other medical professionals, and the profession of Emergency Medical Technician. As an Emergency Medical Technician, I solemnly pledge myself to the following code of professional ethics:

A fundamental responsibility of the Emergency Medical Technician is to conserve life, to alleviate suffering, to promote health, to do no harm, and to encourage the quality and equal availability of emergency medical care.

The Emergency Medical Technician provides services based on human need, with respect for human dignity, unrestricted by considerations of nationality, race, creed, color or status.

The Emergency Medical Technician does not use professional knowledge and skills in any enterprise detrimental to the public well being.

The Emergency Medical Technician respects and holds in confidence all information of a confidential nature obtained in the course of professional work unless required by law to divulge such information.

The Emergency Medical Technician, as a citizen, understands and upholds the law and performs the duties of citizenship; as a professional the Emergency Medical Technician has the never-ending responsibility to work with concerned citizens and other health care professionals in promoting a high standard of emergency medical care to all people.

The Emergency Medical Technician shall maintain professional competence and demonstrate concern for the competence of other members of the Emergency Medical Services health care team.

An Emergency Medical Technician assumes responsibility in defining and upholding standards of professional practice and education.

The Emergency Medical Technician assumes responsibility for individual professional actions and judgment, both in dependent and independent emergency functions, and knows and upholds the laws which affect the practice of the Emergency Medical Technician.

An Emergency Medical Technician has the responsibility to be aware of and participate in, matters of legislation affecting the Emergency Medical Technician and the Emergency Medical Services System.

The Emergency Medical Technician adheres to standards of personal ethics which reflect credit upon the profession.

Emergency Medical Technicians, or groups of Emergency Medical Technicians, who advertise professional services, do so in conformity with the dignity of the profession.

The Emergency Medical Technician has an obligation to protect the public by not delegating to a person less qualified any service which requires the professional competence of an Emergency Medical Technician.

The Emergency Medical Technician will work harmoniously with, and sustain confidence in, Emergency Medical Technician associates, the nurse, the physician, and other members of the Emergency Medical Services health care team.

The Emergency Medical Technician refuses to participate in unethical procedures, and assumes the responsibility to expose incompetence or unethical conduct of others to the appropriate authority in a proper and professional manner.

—The National Association of Emergency Medical Technicians

This code stems from the premise that all EMTs should be concerned with the welfare of others. It is a moral, rather than legal, standard of behavior.

Patient confidentiality

EMTs must hold patient care in strict confidence. It is unethical for the EMT–I to divulge patients' names, details of their illness or care, or any other aspect of their care to anyone except designated EMS systems and law enforcement personnel. Telling friends or family about patients could result in a leak of confidential information. The EMT–I cannot reveal information about a patient to anyone, including his or her own family, without the patient's permission. An exception to this rule exists if the patient is a minor or is legally certified as incompetent.

Violation of patient confidentiality may be met with civil or administrative penalties.

EMS ORGANIZATIONS

Benefits of belonging

Across the country, a variety of local and state EMS associations exist for the EMT–I. These organizations provide an assortment of membership benefits including educational opportunities, newsletters, and representation on issues that affect local legislation. State associations serve not only as a clearinghouse for EMS news and training information but also as a strong, collective voice for EMT–Is when key issues are being lobbied before the state legislature.

 State the major purposes of a National Association of EMTs.

National Association of EMTs

On a national level, the EMT–I can join the National Association of EMTs (NAEMT). NAEMT was formed in 1975 by a group of nationally registered EMTs from existing state EMT organizations, national EMS leaders, and the NREMT. The association's goals are to serve the needs of EMTs throughout the country, promote the professional status of the EMT, encourage the constant upgrading of the education and abilities of the EMT, and strive for a national standard of recognition for the skills and abilities of the EMT. The association has over 4000 members in 26 affiliated EMT associations. The NAEMT sponsors continuing education programs on a national, regional, and local level, and provides a variety of membership programs and services.

Belonging to a professional organization allows the EMT–I to be aware of the latest emergency medical technologies. It also allows communication with members from other parts of the country (or world) to share ideas with people of similar backgrounds. Additionally, EMS associations that have large memberships carry a great deal of political influence. This clout enhances the prehospital care professionals' chances of obtaining favorable EMS-related positions/legislation and/or funding.

Key national EMS-related organizations include:
- American Ambulance Association (AAA)
- American College of Emergency Physicians (ACEP)
- International Association of Firefighters (IAFF)
- National Association of Flight Paramedics (NAFP)
- National Association of Emergency Medical Technicians (NAEMT)
- National Association of EMS Physicians (NAEMSP)
- National Association of Search and Rescue (NASAR)
- National Association of State EMS Directors (NASEMSD)
- National Council of State EMS Training Coordinators (NCSEMSTC)

CASE HISTORY FOLLOW-UP

EMT-I Brown's supervisor pages him to call the station as he is waiting for his lunch order. He calls the unit from the cellular telephone and asks, "What's up?"

"We have a group of students from Lincoln Elementary coming in at 1:30 this afternoon. I'll place your unit on back-up; I want you to come in and show them your unit and answer their questions. OK?"

"That's great, I really enjoy the kids. I hope we don't miss anything good," Brown says. He walks back to the table and says to Williams, "We've got a show and tell this afternoon."

EMTs Williams and Brown know all of the questions, and have all of the answers because they have both done public presentations for many years: "What's it like to be an EMT-I?" "What do you do when someone isn't breathing?" "What's the worst thing you've ever seen?"

Both realize they can't tell the children about the worst thing they have ever seen—there are too many incidents to speak of.

SUMMARY

EMT–Is are advanced prehospital care providers. The EMT–I certification process involves completion of DOT requirements and the demonstration of skills on both practical and written examinations. Specific training requirements for EMT–I certification vary widely from state to state.

The first rule of prehospital care is "Do no harm." The EMT–I must ensure the safety of himself or herself and fellow EMT–Is. The EMT–I has a responsibility to provide competent care in a professional, ethical, and caring manner.

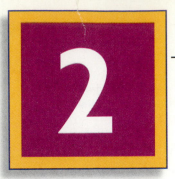

EMS SYSTEMS

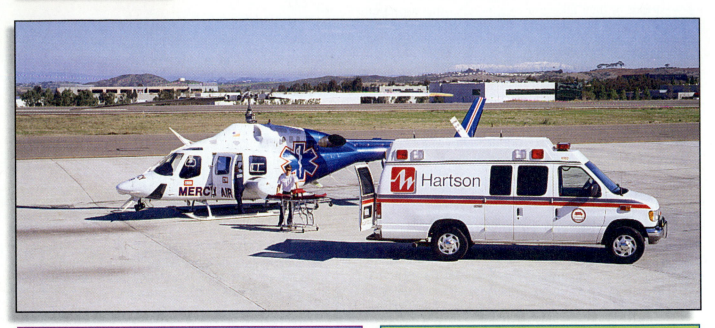

CASE HISTORY

The year is 1964. At 3:00 AM, a 52-year-old man awakens from his sleep with a crushing chest pain. He gets out of bed and attempts to "walk off the pain," but it doesn't go away. He begins to worry, gets a little short of breath, and feels cool and sweaty. He wakes his wife and tells her he must go to the hospital.

Afraid that he's having a heart attack, she convinces him to let her call an ambulance. She knows there is one in town, but cannot remember the name of the ambulance company. She had always planned to write the number down by the phone but never had. While he is sitting by the door waiting, she grabs the phone book and frantically searches for the telephone number. There it is: Callahan's mortuary and 24-hour ambulance service. She makes the call and waits with her husband by the door.

Twenty-five minutes later, they are still waiting for the ambulance to arrive. His pain is worse, and he is beginning to feel lightheaded. In his heart of hearts, he is aware that he is going to die. Finally, the red ambulance light illuminates the street outside their home. Hurriedly, the mortuary owner and his teenage daughter run to the man's side. They tell him and his wife to try and relax as they rush the man to the hospital. They help the man walk to the back of the hearse-style ambulance, and place him on a stretcher. The teenage girl

Case History, continued

holds a black rubber oxygen mask to the man's face and tells him to breathe deeply. His wife is in the front seat of the car with the mortuary owner, pleading with him to drive faster. The last thing the man remembers is that the light and sirens are overwhelming.

It's 4:30 AM when the man and his wife arrive at the hospital emergency room. He is unresponsive and in cardiac arrest. Attempts by the emergency room staff to revive him are unsuccessful. How would a modern EMS system change this scenario?

LEARNING OBJECTIVES

Upon completion of this chapter, the EMT–Intermediate should be able to:

- RELATE to prehospital care as an extension of hospital care.
- DIFFERENTIATE between situations in which the EMT–Intermediate should attempt to stabilize the patient on scene and situations that require rapid and immediate transportation of the patient to the hospital.
- DESCRIBE the integration of prehospital care into the continuum of total patient care with the emergency phase of hospital care.
- DISCUSS citizen access and the various mechanisms of obtaining it.
- LIST the members of the EMS team.
- IDENTIFY typical components of an EMS system.
- RECALL the KKK Ambulance standards and the American College of Surgeons Essential Equipment List.
- DISCUSS the replacement of supplies and equipment.
- DEFINE and DESCRIBE medical direction.
- DISCUSS the role of the medical community in overseeing prehospital care.
- DEFINE protocols and standing orders.
- DESCRIBE the relationship between the physician on the radio and the EMT–I at the scene.
- DESCRIBE physician responsibility for medical direction.
- DESCRIBE retrospective evaluation of patient care, including run report review, continuing education, skill practice, and skill deterioration.

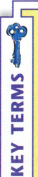

KEY TERMS

EMERGENCY MEDICAL DISPATCHER

MEDICAL DIRECTION

PREARRIVAL INSTRUCTIONS

PROTOCOLS

QUALITY IMPROVEMENT

RESEARCH

STANDING ORDERS

THE WHITE PAPER

HISTORICAL BACKGROUND

Wars—the origin of early EMS systems

The battlefield was the birthplace of organized care for the sick and injured. Napoleon's surgeons developed the first special army ambulance corps, which consisted of a horse-drawn covered cart. Battle victims were loaded in back and taken to rear lines for treatment. The first air ambulance originated in 1870 when a hot-air balloon was used to transport injured soldiers from Paris during the Prussian siege.

In the United States, the Civil War brought attention to the need for an ambulance transportation system. The military medical service proved inadequate for the transportation of the great number of battlefield casualties to field hospitals. Wounded soldiers were cared for in a haphazard fashion. In 1862, the Union Army formed an ambulance corps to more rapidly move casualties from the field to treatment areas.

Improved battlefield care during subsequent military conflicts resulted in lower casualty rates. The Korean War initiated the use of "field" hospitals as the standard of care for initiating treatment in war time. During the Vietnam War, "physician extenders" or "medics" initiated treatment prior to evacuating the injured to a field hospital.

Significant progress in aeromedical patient transport occurred during World War II, the Korean conflict, and in Vietnam. Currently, helicopter and fixed-wing services provide sophisticated on-scene care and transportation of patients to medical facilities.

Early civilian systems

Prior to the 1970s, prehospital care in the United States was crude. In the early twentieth century, ambulance service was provided mostly by funeral homes. Fire department or hospital-based services were the exception. Until the mid-twentieth century, most ambulances were manned simply by a driver whose mission was to collect patients and rapidly transport them to the hospital. These "ambulance drivers" had little formal training and carried only minimal medical equipment.

Hospital emergency care at this time was also unorganized. Early emergency departments were called "accident rooms," had irregular hours, and were staffed by physicians or medical students with little or no formal training in emergency medicine.

In the 1960s, fire departments began equipping their vehicles with oxygen mask systems. These systems were met with widespread public acceptance of prehospital treatment and were instrumental in setting the stage for the development of public agency emergency medical response vehicles.

In 1966, a landmark report was published by the National Academy of Sciences entitled *Accidental Death and Disability, The Neglected Disease of Modern Society*. This report, often referred to as **The White Paper**, declared "injury" as the most neglected disease in America and documented the inadequate emergency medical care patients received in the United States. The report emphasized the need for a concerted effort to develop a group of health professionals to care for prehospital emergencies.

THE WHITE PAPER: A 1966 report published by the National Academy of Sciences entitled *Accidental Death and Disability, The Neglected Disease of Modern Society.* This report was responsible for emphasizing the need for organized prehospital patient care.

Evolution of modern EMS systems

Modern EMS had its early beginnings in Belfast, Northern Ireland. It was there that Dr. J. Frank Pantridge of the Royal Victoria Hospital pioneered the concept of "mobile coronary care"—a system whereby medical and nursing personnel drove from the hospital to remote locations to treat heart attack victims.

About the same time, Dr. James V. Warren at Ohio State University was researching the possibility of implementing mobile coronary care in Columbus, OH. Using grant monies, the Columbus "Heartmobile" went on duty in 1969, staffed on each shift by one cardiologist and three off-duty Columbus Fire Department rescue squad members.

These early years also saw Dr. Eugene Nagel of the University of Miami School of Medicine train firefighters as paramedics in Florida (Fig. 2-1). In Seattle, WA, Dr. Leonard Cobb launched the famous "Medic I" project in cooperation with the Seattle Fire Department while Dr. J. Michael Criley trained firefighters to be paramedics in Los Angeles.

Emergency

In the early 1970s, the television program *Emergency,* based on the Los Angeles County Fire Department paramedic service, brought prehospital emergency care into the living rooms of Americans. Johnny Gage and Roy DeSoto (Fig. 2-2) were clean-cut firefighter/paramedics who responded promptly, had a solution for every situation that confronted them, and remained calm even in the most stressful situations. This show is credited with the rapid acceptance of the need for paramedics in communities throughout the United States. *Emergency* also set the first standard for the professional paramedic.

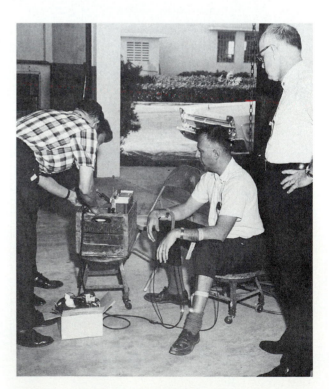

Fig. 2-1 Dr. Eugene Nagel hooked up to first telemetry transmitter.

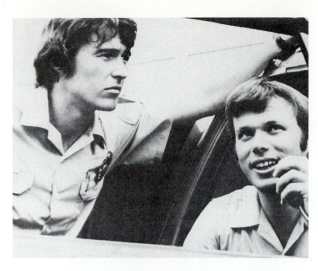

Fig. 2-2 Johnny Gage and Roy DeSoto.

Emergency Medical Services Act of 1973

In 1973, Congress passed the Emergency Medical Services Act of 1973 (Public Law 93-154). This federal legislation paved the way for improvements in the level of care for victims of trauma and acute illness by providing federal monies to establish EMS systems throughout the United States. The Department of Transportation (DOT) established minimum training standards for EMTs and equipment standards for ambulances. During the 1970s and early 1980s federal legislation provided additional grant monies for communities to start or upgrade their EMS systems.

> **HELPFUL HINT**
> The original 1973 legislation outlined 15 areas that had to be addressed for EMS systems to receive federal funding: manpower, training, communications, transportation, emergency facilities, critical care units, public safety agencies, consumer participation, access to care, patient transfer, standardized record-keeping, public information and education, system review and evaluation, disaster, and mutual aid.

Individual states and local communities began to create EMS systems. The major developments within these EMS systems were state EMS offices, certification mechanisms for EMTs, development of specialty care centers (trauma, pediatric, burn, and neonatal), transportation, communication (9-1-1), and management systems. Technologic advances in equipment facilitated the mobility of patient care initiated in the field.

Decreasing federal funds

During the 1980s federal money allocated for EMS systems decreased. Many different systems emerged, and many organizations came to participate in the management and delivery of EMS systems. Funding for EMS systems now comes mostly from local and state taxes, revenue generated from patient transportation fees or contributions, and fund-raisers.

In 1986, the *White Paper Revised* declared that despite federal investment in the development of EMS systems, injury continued to be the cause of many years of lost productivity to Americans.

In 1990, the Trauma Systems Development Act appropriated federal dollars to developing and implementing "trauma" systems.

The introduction of the TV series *Rescue 911* once again brought the actions of EMS systems to the public's attention and further expanded the level of expectations that citizens have when they call for help.

THE EMERGENCY CALL

Emergency calls, regardless of the nature, follow a similar evolution that often includes the following (Fig. 2-3):

- Incident occurrence
- Recognition
- System access and dispatch
- Prehospital care
- Patient stabilization and transport
- Delivery to hospital
- Preparation for the next event

Incident occurrence and recognition

The emergency call begins with the onset of illness or injury such as the sudden onset of acute myocardial infarction, an asthma attack, a motor vehicle crash, or a shooting incident. The incident is then recognized by the victims themselves, family members, friends, coworkers, or bystanders. Once the emergency is identified, the victim may receive care from bystanders before arrival of the EMS system. Bystander care may include such procedures as

- relief of airway obstruction due to a foreign body
- cardiopulmonary resuscitation (CPR)
- bleeding control
- comfort and reassurance

System access and dispatch

Next, a decision is made to seek medical assistance. The EMS system is then accessed, usually by phone.

> **Discuss citizen access and the various mechanisms of obtaining it.**

EMS systems receive calls for help into the dispatch center. Callers in many communities reach the EMS dispatch center by dialing 9-1-1. Other

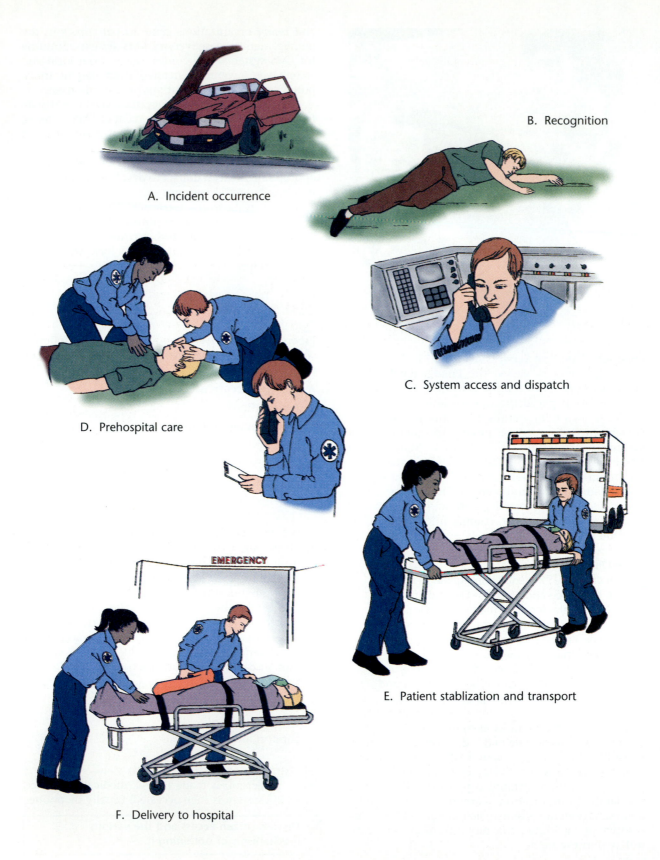

A. Incident occurrence

B. Recognition

C. System access and dispatch

D. Prehospital care

E. Patient stablization and transport

F. Delivery to hospital

Fig. 2-3 **Phases of emergency medical care.**

communities may access EMS via the local sheriff, police, or fire department dispatcher. In some communities people contact private ambulance services or volunteer systems directly rather than contacting a municipal service.

Universal emergency number

Much of the United States is served by the "universal" emergency phone number 9-1-1. This number eliminates the need for separate phone numbers for fire, police, and EMS as well as different access numbers for each community. As a result, help can be accessed more quickly.

 EMERGENCY MEDICAL DISPATCHER: A specially trained person who receives calls for emergency assistance and ensures proper EMS response.

Many dispatch centers are staffed with **Emergency Medical Dispatchers (EMDs)** (Fig. 2-4). The EMD's duties go beyond answering phones and dispatching ambulances. Often, the EMD also receives extensive training in computer-aided dispatch, priority dispatch, prearrival instructions, and system status management.

Once the emergency call is processed, the EMD must select the most appropriate ambulance to dispatch to the scene. This decision usually is based on the distance to the call, the time of day, and the level of care needed to handle the emergency.

Prehospital care

 Relate to prehospital care as an extension of hospital care.

The treatment a patient receives before arrival at the hospital is referred to as *prehospital care* (Fig. 2-5). Prehospital care is essentially an extension of hospital care. Lifesaving treatments, performed only by physicians just a couple of decades ago, are now delivered by prehospital care providers. Although EMTs (EMT–Basics, EMT–Intermediates, EMT–Paramedics) are delivering the care, the legal responsibility for providing advanced management skills still falls on the medical direction physician.

 Differentiate between situations in which the EMT–I should attempt to stabilize the patient on scene and situations that require immediate transportation of the patient to the hospital.

 STREET WISE
The first rule of patient care is "Do no harm."

Serious and life-threatening conditions require that definitive prehospital care must be provided as soon as possible. For many patients this care can be started, and to a great measure, completed in the field. However, trauma patients who require blood replacement and hemorrhage control can only be stabilized in the operating room. For these patients, resuscitation must be initiated in the field or during rapid transport to the appropriate hospital (preferably a trauma center). The ability of the EMT–I to differentiate between patients who can be stabilized on-scene and those requiring transport to the hospital is critical for increasing long-term survival and reducing complications and patient disability.

In some cases, patient transport to the hospital may not be necessary. The call may be a false alarm, the patient may have gone to the hospital on his or her own by the time the ambulance arrives on scene, or the patient may refuse treatment and/or transport. Also, some EMS systems permit their EMT–Is to decide when patient transport to the hospital is not warranted. Referral to another means of transport is then provided.

Fig. 2-4   **EMDs in computerized dispatch center.**

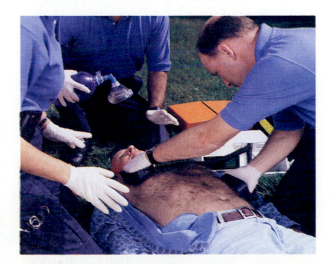

Fig. 2-5   **EMT–Is providing prehospital care.**

Hospital emergency care and recuperation

 Describe the integration of prehospital care into the continuum of total patient care with the emergency phase of hospital care.

On arrival at the hospital the patient receives additional treatment in the emergency department. If required, the patient is admitted to the hospital for further care and recuperation. After release from the hospital, the patient may need follow-up treatment and/or physical therapy as part of his or her rehabilitation.

The emergency department
The EMS team extends to the hospital emergency department, which includes physicians, nurses, and specialized technicians.

Emergency department physicians
Emergency department physicians are licensed physicians who have special training and experience in emergency medicine. These physicians spend 3 to 4 years beyond medical school concentrating on care for the emergency patient.

Over the years, organizations such as the American College of Emergency Physicians (ACEP) and the National Association of EMS Physicians (NAEMSP) have encouraged emergency physicians to take an active role in EMS systems as medical administrators, EMS advisers, and emergency medicine instructors to help ensure that EMTs provide quality patient care.

Emergency department nurses
Emergency department nurses provide special experience and expertise in emergency nursing. Emergency department nurses assess the patient on arrival at the emergency department (a process commonly known as *triage*) and determine the need for emergency care.

Prehospital providers likely have more direct contact with emergency department nurses than any other hospital employee. Besides caring for patients, many emergency department nurses are actively involved in EMS training, case review, and administrative situations.

Other healthcare professionals
Other healthcare professionals are part of the EMS system. These professionals include respiratory therapists, radiology (x-ray) technicians, rehabilitation specialists, and other technical and administrative personnel. Many of these professionals work in a hospital setting.

EMT–Is in the emergency department
In some hospitals, EMT–Is are hired to work in the emergency department. These EMT–Is typically perform nursing assistant duties, which may include obtaining patient vital signs, documenting patient information, transporting patients to radiology or to hospital floors, cleaning and bandaging wounds, delivering CPR, restocking supplies, splinting minor fractures, drawing blood, placing intravenous lines, and sometimes performing endotracheal intubation.

THE EMS SYSTEM

The primary responsibilities of an EMS system are to respond to requests for medical assistance, to provide life-saving or stabilizing treatment, and to transport patients to definitive medical care. All other components of the system indirectly involved in the response, treatment, or transport of patients are considered support services. These support services are vital to the overall operation of the EMS system.

 Identify the typical components of an EMS system.

Components of today's EMS systems, large or small, private or municipal, paid or volunteer, include some or all of the following elements:
Manpower
Communications
Administration
Transportation
Equipment/supplies procurement and inventory
Facilities
Funding
Consumer information and education
Medical direction
Medical record keeping
Quality improvement
Research
Training
Critical care units
Public safety agencies
Disaster linkage
Mutual aid

Manpower

 List the members of the EMS team.

The EMS system is dependent on a variety of team members to ensure adequate delivery of quality patient care. Most persons are involved in day-to-day prehospital patient care, whereas others tend to the administrative aspects of EMS.

As described in Chapter 1, "Roles and Responsibilities of the EMT–Intermediate," the four key levels of prehospital care providers include the first responder, EMT–Basic (EMT–B), EMT–Intermediate (EMT–I), and EMT–Paramedic (EMT–P) (Fig. 2-6).

The levels of EMTs and their interaction with one another are determined by the EMS system. Many use first responders to lessen the time it takes for a patient to receive definitive care. Some EMS systems pair EMTs and EMT–Is or EMT–Ps on the same unit, whereas others employ a tiered response system. With a tiered response system, EMT–Bs are sent as the initial response to all calls. Advanced providers are only dispatched to a call if the patient needs advanced-level care.

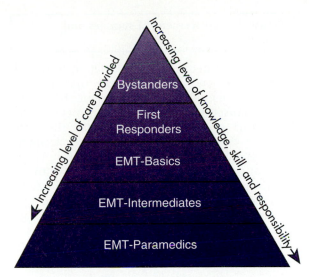

Fig. 2-6   Pyramid of care.

Communications

The function of EMS communications is to receive emergency calls, provide prearrival instructions, dispatch ambulances, deploy units, and provide ongoing communication throughout the EMS system. EMS communications are discussed in more depth in Chapter 4, "EMS Communications."

Modern EMS systems use sophisticated procedures and equipment to effectively manage EMS communications. Such procedures and equipment include computer-aided dispatch, priority dispatch, prearrival instructions, and system status management.

Computer-aided dispatch ensures the most rapid system access from the initial call throughout the EMS response. Priority dispatch is a method used to determine the type of response necessary (*eg,* emergency versus nonemergency, EMT–B versus paramedic response).

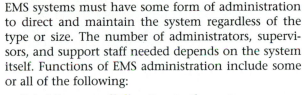

PREARRIVAL INSTRUCTIONS: Instructions for initial care of the patient, often provided by the emergency medical dispatcher, to a person who calls for EMS assistance.

Prearrival instructions are used by EMDs to direct callers in delivering care to patients before EMS arrives. Instructions are based on a standardized set of questions asked of the caller and may include such activities as having the caller, family members, or friends gather medications, stop severe bleeding, or begin CPR. The primary benefit of prearrival instructions is that time to treatment can be significantly reduced.

System status management is a process that manages EMS resources from the time a patient is delivered to the hospital until the next call is received. System status management anticipates coverage needs and positions emergency units to provide rapid response to the community it serves.

Administration

EMS systems must have some form of administration to direct and maintain the system regardless of the type or size. The number of administrators, supervisors, and support staff needed depends on the system itself. Functions of EMS administration include some or all of the following:

- Providing overall direction to the system
- Developing and administering policies
- Promoting ongoing development of the system
- Preparing budgets, monitoring expenditures, and recommending adjustments to accommodate for over- or underexpenditures
- Hiring and promoting employees
- Completing employee payroll records
- Investigating complaints from the public, the hospital, and fellow EMTs
- Conducting hearings, issuing discipline, and hearing and processing grievances
- Communicating with news media, issuing news releases, conducting interviews, conveying positive elements of EMS systems, and developing flyers, brochures, and media campaigns to build a positive relationship with the community
- Filing documents, retrieving information, scheduling appointments, and typing letters, reports, and documents
- Preparing employee work schedules and allocating vacation and benefit time
- Preparing equipment specifications and orders, inventorying and issuing equipment, and establishing supply exchange programs with local hospitals
- Providing medical direction, developing patient care protocols, monitoring system performance, and evaluating patient care and run report documentation
- Providing direct on-line supervision of day-to-day EMS activities
- Generating and sending bills to patients for transportation and supplies used, submitting claims to insurance companies, and processing and accounting for money received

Given the diversity of the future work force and the movement toward total quality improvement, today's EMS administrators must possess strong managerial and leadership skills. To function efficiently, local EMS systems must coordinate their efforts with regional and state EMS systems. Input by local EMS administrations into the development of national standards and guidelines also is important in the shaping of future EMS.

Transportation

 KKK AMBULANCE STANDARDS: In 1974, the General Services Administration of the Federal Government devised a set of standards for emergency vehicles that were to be purchased by the Federal Government. These standards were designated the KKK-A-1822-A Standards; the initials KKK have no particular significance.

Recall the KKK Ambulance standards and the American College of Surgeons Essential Equipment List.

EMS systems need a mode of transportation to deliver prehospital care providers to patients and to transport patients to the hospital. In addition to ambulances, EMS systems may use a variety of other vehicles such as staff or supervisory cars, equipment trucks, rescue trucks, all-terrain vehicles, boats, and, in some systems, fixed-wing aircrafts or helicopters.

EMS vehicles require a substantial capital investment for any EMS organization. For this reason many EMS systems have a fleet management program. Important functions of such programs include developing specifications for new vehicles, conducting routine repair work and repairs on vehicles damaged from accidents, and conducting preventative maintenance. At a minimum, ambulances should meet current KKK Ambulance standards.

Equipment/supplies procurement and inventory

EMS systems use a host of supplies and equipment. Minimally, the required stock should match that listed on the American College of Surgeons' Committee on Trauma Essential Equipment List. Advanced equipment includes esophageal obturator airways (EOA)/EGTA, endotracheal tubes, laryngoscope handles and blades, syringes, stylets, and intravenous (IV) therapy equipment including solutions, administration sets, extension sets, IV catheters, needles, alcohol wipes, and tape. Depending on the community, additional equipment may be needed to deal with environmental, rescue, geographic, and special service needs.

A comprehensive but functional procurement and inventory control process is necessary to safeguard the system. The EMS system must ensure that it can afford the supplies and equipment being purchased, that items purchased fulfill the needs of the service, and that items ordered and paid for arrive at the facility.

 Discuss the replacement of supplies and equipment.

Some EMS systems maintain relationships with hospital emergency departments that provide supply and equipment replacement for those patients transported to their emergency departments. This practice helps minimize the costs incurred by the EMS system for supply replacement. Many hospital emergency departments also play an important role in securing equipment left with the patient when the ambulance crew returns to service. Ideally, after removal from the patient, the EMS equipment is stored in a secured cabinet or storage area in the hospital until the EMS crew retrieves it. Typical items include long backboards, pneumatic antishock garments (PASGs), and splints.

Facilities

A variety of facilities are necessary to support the 24-hour-a-day, 7-day-a-week operations of an EMS system. These facilities include base stations, headquarters, communication centers, and training facilities. The EMS system may have its own facilities or share housing in fire stations, police stations, or hospitals.

Funding

Delivering EMS to the public is expensive. EMS systems must be financially supported whether from taxes, direct billing of patients, subscriptions for service, donations, or grants. Items that typically require funding include personnel salaries, fuel, insurance, vehicle purchase and maintenance, quality improvement, training programs, expendable supplies, capital equipment, and housing—to name a few. To deliver optimal services, it is critical that the system be operated efficiently. Efficient operation requires an in-depth analysis of needs, patient flow, population served, level of EMS provision, and hours of operation to make accurate judgments as to how the service should operate. In large measure, the efficiency of the EMS organization acts to control the cost.

Consumer information and education

The ability to recognize a serious medical emergency and activate the system may mean the difference between patient survival and death. Effective consumer information and education programs are needed to prepare the public to respond appropriately to medical emergencies. These programs should teach consumers how to

- recognize the signs and symptoms of serious illnesses or injuries

- access EMS

- provide lifesaving interventions such as CPR, relief of airway obstruction, and hemorrhage control

Consumer information and education campaigns also can be used to prevent disease, reduce unnecessary use of precious EMS resources, and recruit future employees or volunteers into the EMS system.

Many EMS systems are becoming increasingly aware of the need to boost their images in their communities and to promote themselves through aggressive marketing. Some systems use off-duty personnel to offer classes or deliver speeches to schools and civic organizations (Fig. 2-7). Others find it beneficial to align themselves with other healthcare organizations such as hospitals or other provider agencies to demonstrate a team effort in providing quality care.

Medical direction

 Define and describe *medical direction.*

Discuss the role of the medical community in overseeing prehospital care.

Describe physician responsibility for medical direction.

MEDICAL DIRECTION: Medical supervision of an EMS system and the field performance of EMTs.

The care provided by an EMT–I in the field is an extension of hospital and physician services. As such, accepted standards of medical practice must be met. **Medical direction** ensures that an EMT is providing the appropriate high-quality care. Although the system's medical director is ultimately responsible for all the medical care provided by his or her service, many duties may be delegated to other qualified colleagues.

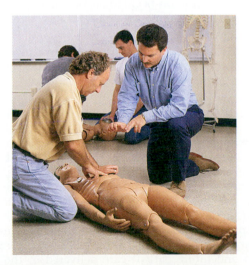

Fig. 2-7 CPR courses prepare the public to respond appropriately in a cardiac emergency situation.

 Describe the relationship between the physician on the radio and the EMT–I at the scene.

The day-to-day activities of the EMT–I are guided by two types of medical direction. Direct medical direction, sometimes called *on-line medical direction,* is care rendered under direct orders, usually over the radio or telephone. Direct medical direction is provided when the EMT–I sees a patient and contacts medical direction for instruction before rendering certain care. Direct medical direction is often provided by the hospital emergency department.

 Define protocols and standing orders.

PROTOCOLS: A set of written policies and procedures.

Indirect medical direction, or *off-line medical direction,* includes the development of a set of written instructions, known as **protocols.** EMTs are expected to be familiar with their EMS system's protocols. When encountering a patient with a particular illness or injury, EMTs should initiate patient care based on the provisions of the protocol for that particular emergency.

EMS physician involvement in indirect medical direction has been divided into three phases: prospective, immediate, and retrospective.

- *Prospective phase*—Primarily administrative in nature. Duties include training, protocol development, and system design.

- *Immediate phase*—Consists of both clinical and administrative responsibilities. The physician provides patient care, predominantly in the emergency department but sometimes in the field as well. The EMS physician participates in prehospital research studies. In addition, he or she performs concurrent review of the EMT's activities. This on-going review process may take place in the field or the emergency department. Finally, radio direction (direct medical direction) may be given by the EMS physician.

- *Retrospective phase*—Physician reviews previous EMT performance, including run report review, quality control, and risk management, in an attempt to improve future care.

STANDING ORDERS: EMT–I field interventions that are completed before contacting medical direction.

EMS systems usually are influenced by a combination of direct and indirect medical direction. Commonly, protocols are followed for initial care of life-threatening problems, such as cardiac arrest, severe bleeding, major trauma, and shock. Once care has been provided to a certain point, the EMT–I is required to contact the medical director for further instructions. Portions of the protocols that are completed before the EMT–I is required to contact medical direction are referred to as **standing orders.**

All EMTs function under some sort of medical direction, regardless of a state's policy. In some states, EMTs operate under direction of a physician adviser. In others, the use of a medical adviser or director is only recommended, not required. Most systems, however, require active medical direction.

Medical record keeping

Accurate and thorough documentation of patient information and treatment is an essential ingredient in maintaining the overall quality of the EMS system. Documentation provides a record of what has taken place and conveys vital information about the patient and his or her emergency situation to other healthcare providers. Documentation also serves as a key element in quality improvement activities designed to make the EMS system better.

From a system standpoint, documentation involves the EMT–I's accurate and thorough documentation at the time of the patient contact (or shortly thereafter if the situation dictates), including retrieving the run reports or electronic data, processing it to obtain the necessary information for each case, and storing it for later retrieval when indicated. Documentation is discussed in more depth in Chapter 5, "Documentation."

Quality improvement

 Describe retrospective evaluation of patient care, including run report review, continuing education, skill practice, and skill deterioration.

QUALITY IMPROVEMENT: An evaluation of services provided and the results achieved as compared with accepted standards.

The quality of an EMS system is reflected in the daily performance of its EMTs and operational efficiency. On-going quality improvement processes should be in place to monitor and evaluate the delivery of care. **Quality improvement** is considered an essential component of modern EMS systems.

Simply stated, quality improvement is the evaluation of EMS performance for the purpose of identifying areas of needed improvement and implementing necessary corrections. This evaluation is based on a comparison of the care delivered with the accepted standards. These evaluations are most often completed by management personnel and physicians responsible for system oversight. The quality improvement process reveals problems that might not otherwise be recognized by looking at the EMS

system from the surface. It can propel changes in treatment protocols and help support the EMS system to acquire additional resources at budget time. It also allows the EMS system's management and medical direction to evaluate the performance of individual EMTs and the delivery of care throughout the system.

A primary component of any quality improvement program is documentation. Patient care reports are checked for completeness, accuracy of charting and assessment, adherence to system treatment protocols, and patterns of error or system-related problems.

Another element used to determine levels of performance is the direct observation of patient care provided by the EMTs. This evaluation is usually done by riding with the EMTs as they respond to emergency calls and provide patient care.

Response time data can be used to reveal operational efficiency and can show the need for relocation of units or the acquisition of additional units. Other data that are evaluated include dispatch tapes, prehospital care data, incident reports, and emergency department and in-patient records, to name a few.

Corrective action must be taken when improper care is revealed. Likewise, proper or exceptional performance must be communicated to the EMTs to help reinforce the behavior. Most importantly, quality improvement must be linked with ongoing professional education.

Research

Until recently, treatment protocols often were drawn directly from the hospital setting, despite marked differences between the prehospital and hospital environments. Many protocols and procedures that are in use today evolved without clinical evidence of their usefulness, safety, or benefit to the patient. EMS providers must now begin to prove which patient care protocols and techniques are useful and beneficial.

RESEARCH: The scientific study, investigation, and experimentation conducted to establish facts and determine their significance.

Prehospital **research** can help eliminate much of the uncertainty associated with prehospital care. Questions such as, "Why do we treat patients this way in the field?" "Does this treatment benefit many patients?" "Does it harm some?" must be asked to continually justify EMS practices and protocols.

A number of benefits can be derived from conducting prehospital research. Most importantly, prehospital research has the immediate potential of saving lives or limiting morbidity by improving current and future patient care delivered in the field. Research also can prove that prehospital care makes a difference and is valuable. This is particularly important in times of recession and slow growth, when budget cuts are seen in every area of medicine and public service.

Training

Quality training is needed to develop and maintain each healthcare provider's ability to deliver the necessary interventions in the prehospital environment. Functions of an EMS system training program include such things as conducting basic and advanced training for new and current employees, developing and providing ongoing education to EMTs (Fig. 2-8), maintaining continuing education records, and preparing and submitting paperwork for recertification or relicensure to local or state offices. Some EMS systems maintain their own training programs, whereas others contract with hospitals, colleges, or other educational centers for their training needs.

Critical care units

Critical care interfacility transport is a sophisticated area of prehospital care. This type of transport typically involves the provision of advanced or highly specialized care to patients with complicated illnesses or injuries who are being transported from one healthcare facility to another. The emphasis of patient care is on the delivery of sophisticated treatment while en route.

The objectives of critical care transport are much the same as those for EMS—rapid response time, high-quality medical care, rapid transport to the appropriate facility, safe operation, cost-efficiency, accurate reporting, and continuous quality improvement based on performance review.

Many of today's critical care transport services are managed by hospitals or private ambulance transport systems. These units are usually staffed by paramedics, nurses, and/or physicians and carry sophisticated clinical equipment that allows them to provide complicated treatments to their patients during transport. These units may be specialty ground units, helicopters, or fixed-wing air medical transport units (Fig. 2-9).

Public safety agencies

EMS systems do not operate in the public safety arena alone. Other services are often simultaneously needed to address the many complex situations people face. A call for a person injured in a fight should prompt the response of EMS for medical care and police for protection or filing of a complaint against the assailant. A person injured in a motor vehicle accident may require EMS, the fire department for extrication or gasoline wash-down, police for reports/traffic control and public utilities to handle downed wires or broken water or gas lines.

These interactions require the various public agencies to communicate with each other. For this reason policies are needed to define the roles and responsibilities of each organization and how each interrelates with the others. In some cases, the difference in purpose can create conflicts at the scene. An example

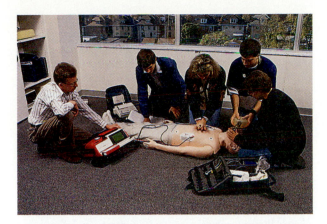

Fig. 2-8   Continuing education activities.

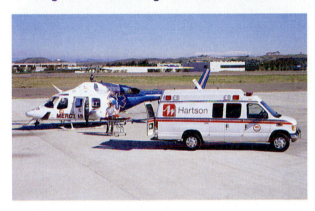

Fig. 2-9   Helicopter and ground critical care transport units.

of public agency cooperation is the patient who is transported to a trauma center rather than the nearest hospital. It makes perfect sense for the patient and the EMS system but not to the police officer who must then travel to a more distant hospital to fill out the accident report. For this reason, each organization must actively work to address concerns and mediate solutions at all levels.

Mutual aid

To provide EMS in the face of personnel or funding shortages, many EMS systems establish mutual aid agreements with adjacent communities. These agreements call for provider services to cross geographic boundaries when needed to provide patient care. These arrangements should be formal agreements and should be on a reciprocal basis when necessary.

Disaster linkage

Mass casualty incidents (MCIs) and disasters can overburden even the biggest EMS system. Most EMS systems have arrangements with nearby communities to provide assistance in the event of such catastrophes. These arrangements may be managed by local, regional, or statewide emergency management centers that coordinate the response to these types of emergencies.

Regardless of who provides coordination in these types of situations, the responsible agency should ensure that a comprehensive plan exists for its service area. This plan should address coordinated central management, integration of all EMS system components, and communications during disasters. These plans should be rehearsed to assess performance and correct deficiencies when identified.

Types of systems

EMS systems evolve due to geographic, political, demographic, and economic pressures that are unique to each community. Consequently, vast differences are found in EMS systems from area to area. Although many different types of EMS systems exist around the country today, no one type is superior to another. Each system offers its own unique advantages and disadvantages.

EMS systems are organized or structured in several different ways including fire service–based, third service, private ambulance companies, hospital-based, and volunteer systems. Additionally, some EMS systems are configured as public utilities or housed within law enforcement agencies.

Fire service

Fire departments have been a mainstay provider of EMS since its inception. More EMS systems operate in the fire department than in any other type of service including private third service or hospital-based systems. Fire departments make excellent bases for EMS operations. Their geographically based vehicles and personnel and availability make the fire service a natural location to base EMS services. Whether as the primary providers of patient care delivery or as first responders, the members of the fire service are capable of providing excellent initial patient care.

Fire departments generally provide EMS in one of three configurations: cross-trained firefighter/EMTs who work in both fire suppression and EMS, firefighter/EMTs who work only on the ambulance, and civilian/EMTs who only work on the ambulance. Probably the most versatile of the three is the cross-trained firefighter/EMT. These employees function in both areas and can transfer back and forth between EMS and fire suppression when they become "burned out" or need a change of pace.

Fire departments maintain highly structured methods of training and advancement with regular continuing education. Furthermore, firefighter/EMTs are usually trained in all facets of rescue work including search and rescue, vehicle extrication, rope and above-ground rescue, water rescue, and confined-space entry.

Third service

Third services are EMS systems that function on an equal level to other safety forces such as police and fire departments. EMTs working for third services enjoy the benefit of having a specific focus in their work rather than having to undergo training and work in areas they do not necessarily enjoy. Third-service EMS also tends to maintain highly structured methods of training and advancement, with regular continuing education. EMTs working in third services may work 8-, 10-, 12-, or 24-hour shifts.

Private services

Private ambulance services are one of the oldest providers of EMS in the United States. Originating in the funeral homes in the 1950s, these systems have evolved to provide highly efficient EMS delivery. In prior years, private ambulance companies provided mostly routine transfer services, moving patients between the hospital and home or nursing facilities. Today, many private services serve as the primary emergency provider, whereas others work in combination with their local fire department or EMS system to provide patient transport to the hospital.

Hospital-based systems

Hospitals serve as another common provider of EMS systems by hiring and training EMS personnel and administrators, purchasing equipment, and contracting with medical direction personnel. Some hospital-based systems are privately owned, much like the private ownership of hospital-based air ambulance systems. Other hospital-based systems are an extension of public hospital authorities. These systems are public entities that direct public monies and actions on the behalf of certain geographic, tax-based locations. The hospital-based systems generally are managed in a fashion typical to hospital environments, with administrators assigned to report to the hospital administration. These systems are financially bound to the hospital. An advantage of hospital-based EMS is that its EMS personnel are often exposed to sophisticated assessments and emergency care procedures. They may even work as emergency department staff members when not handling emergency calls. These experiences help build on the training of the EMTs and can help make them excellent healthcare providers.

Volunteer systems

Volunteer systems provide a significant portion of the EMS coverage around the country. Many of these systems are based in volunteer fire departments. These systems usually provide coverage to small communities. However, a number of large communities also are served by volunteer departments. Volunteer systems are configured in a variety of ways. Some systems operate purely on the basis of donations from the community, whereas others receive support from taxes or fees for service. The biggest challenge facing volunteer services is staffing the ambulance(s) 24 hours a day. Much of the activity in volunteer systems centers around the recruiting and training of EMTs.

CASE HISTORY FOLLOW-UP

The case history at the beginning of the chapter would have read much differently had it taken place in today's modern EMS system. In fact, let's rewrite it.

A man awakens at 3:00 AM with a crushing chest pain. He realizes that it must be a heart attack. He and his wife were trained in CPR at the local hospital and learned to recognize the warning signs and symptoms. He also knows that it is important to act quickly. He wakes his wife and tells her to activate the EMS system by dialing 9-1-1. The Emergency Medical Dispatcher instructs the wife to tell her husband to sit quietly until EMS arrives.

Within minutes, a pumper truck, an ambulance, and a police car arrive at the home. EMT–Is Randall and Emerson rush in carrying a jump kit, oxygen, and a cardiac monitor/defibrillator. Working under established protocols, the EMT–Is place the man on oxygen and obtain a brief history of the event. As an initial assessment is performed, electrocardiogram (ECG) electrodes are applied and an IV established. EMT–I Emerson contacts on-line medical directions and gives the emergency department physician a brief patient report. Using telemetry, the ECG is transmitted to the hospital for evaluation. Because the man's chest pain is still present and his vital signs are stable, the physician instructs EMT–I Emerson to place a nitroglycerin tablet under the man's tongue. He has some relief from the pain, and feels confident that he is receiving good patient care. The man is placed gently on a stretcher and rolled to the ambulance for transport to the emergency department. EMT–I Randall tells the wife that lights and sirens are not being used in an effort to make her husband less anxious. En route to the hospital, EMT–I Emerson performs an ongoing assessment of the man's pain and physical condition.

The man is delivered to the emergency department within 30 minutes of his wife's initial 9-1-1 call. The emergency department nurse and physician continue the man's care and assessment. His suspicions about heart attack are substantiated by diagnostic tests. Thrombolytics are administered in the emergency department, and the man is transferred to the coronary intensive care unit for monitoring and recuperation. The doctors advise him that he has an excellent chance of full recovery.

SUMMARY

Emergency medical systems have evolved from battlefield care to sophisticated prehospital patient care for acute illness and accidents. The Emergency Medical Services Act of 1973 was an important legal basis for the development of training and equipment standards by the Department of Transportation.

The EMT–I is a member of the EMS team. The EMS system is usually accessed, and the team set into action, by a phone call. The dispatcher may use one of several techniques to send help. Once the EMTs have arrived on the scene and provided initial care, the patient is transported to the hospital emergency department where necessary care is continued.

Not all states require that EMS systems have medical direction. Medical direction, however, is provided for all levels of prehospital care either via protocols (off-line direction), direct voice direction (on-line direction), or a combination of the two. EMS physicians and emergency department nurses are often actively involved in EMS training, medical direction, and quality assurance and are part of the EMS team.

Evaluation and research are critical to the EMS chain, because it is by evaluating the job we do that we learn how to make it better. Research and evaluation deal with the compilation and evaluation of data on the present, past, and future emergency needs of the public and the resources of the various system components for meeting those needs. It also entails the identification of needed improvements and updates for emergency services and the determination of the system's effectiveness.

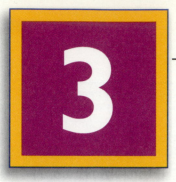

3

MEDICAL/LEGAL CONSIDERATIONS

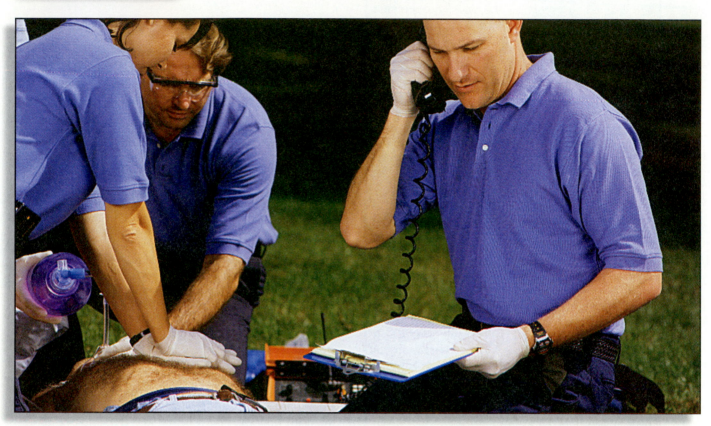

CASE HISTORY

EMT–I Reynolds is attending the annual State EMS conference and is taking a break after sitting in on a talk about Medical-Legal Issues in EMS. She pours a ginger ale and sits down in the lobby to think about the complex issues that the lawyer spoke of.

Several groups of people are in the lobby having lively discussions about personal medical liability, assault charges stemming from invasive field interventions, and false imprisonment for using hard restraints. One group is discussing a charge against an EMT-Intermediate training institute for violating the American Disabilities Act because they failed to accommodate a hearing-impaired student.

EMT–I Reynolds wants a few quiet minutes to herself, when she overhears EMT-Thomas, who works at her service, saying, "I heard Tom Reilly from platoon B is HIV-positive."

EMT–I Reynolds stands and walks away, disgusted with Thomas' gossiping.

LEARNING OBJECTIVES

Upon completion of this chapter, the EMT–Intermediate should be able to:

- DEFINE the term *tort.*
- DISCUSS the significance and scope of the following in relationship to EMT–I practice:
  - State Medical Practice Act
  - Good Samaritan Act/Civil Immunity
  - State EMS statutes
  - State motor vehicle codes
  - State and local guidelines for "Do Not Resuscitate" orders
- IDENTIFY those situations that require the EMT–I to report incidents to appropriate authorities.
- DEFINE the terms *negligence, medical liability,* and *duty to act.*
- DESCRIBE the four elements that must be present to prove negligence.
- DEFINE the terms *consent, expressed consent, informed consent,* and *implied consent.*
- DESCRIBE the significance of obtaining expressed and informed consent.
- DEFINE the terms *abandonment, assault, battery, false imprisonment, slander,* and *libel.*
- DESCRIBE the significance of knowing state laws relating to the use of force and restraint to protect the EMT–I, the patient, and any third party.
- DESCRIBE the provisions of COBRA that relate to the EMT–I and the transfer of patients.
- DESCRIBE the significance of accurate documentation and record keeping in substantiating an incident.

KEY TERMS

ABANDONMENT	IMPLIED CONSENT
ASSAULT	INFORMED CONSENT
BATTERY	LIBEL
CONSENT	NEGLIGENCE
DO NOT RESUSCITATE ORDER	ORDINARY NEGLIGENCE
DUTY TO ACT	SCOPE OF PRACTICE
EXPRESSED CONSENT	SLANDER
FALSE IMPRISONMENT	STANDARD OF CARE
GOOD SAMARITAN LAWS	TORT
GROSS NEGLIGENCE	TORT LAW

INTRODUCTION

Legal issues are an important aspect of patient care for the EMT–I. It is helpful for an EMT–I to understand some basic legal concepts and to have a working knowledge of applicable state laws and regulations. The information in this chapter should not be substituted for legal advice. Laws vary widely from state to state. Consult an experienced attorney or your local EMS authority for interpretation of specific rules and regulations as they pertain to your EMS system. Remember, ignorance of the law is rarely, if ever, an acceptable excuse or defense.

ESSENTIAL PRINCIPLES

Prevention of legal problems

In dealing with legal issues, prevention of problems is the cardinal rule. Appropriate emergency medical care and accurate call documentation are the best protection in the case of medical-legal questions. Successful suits against most healthcare providers involve failure to adhere to one or more of three practices:

- Caring for patients as if each is a family member. Many malpractice claims against healthcare providers stem not from what the provider did but how he or she did it.

- Following state and local guidelines and protocols concerning prehospital care, including appropriate use of on- and off-line medical direction. Do not perform procedures that you are not certified to perform or allowed to do within protocol guidelines. *Know your department's policies and procedures and always follow them!*

- Keeping proper, thorough, and accurate patient care documentation as required by your EMS system. It is important that your handwriting is legible. Because legal proceedings can take place years after the original event, ensure run reports can be easily read for years after an incident.

CLASSIFICATION OF LAWS

 Define the term *tort*.

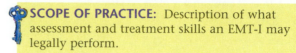 **TORT LAW**: Law that covers a private or public wrong or injury that occurs due to a breach, or break, of a legal duty or obligation.

Criminal laws prohibit the performance of any act that is considered damaging to the public. Violations of these laws result in crimes and violators may be prosecuted in a criminal proceeding—a trial before a judge and sometimes a jury in which evidence is heard and a verdict of "guilty" or "not guilty" is reached. If a guilty verdict is reached, a fine, imprisonment, or both may result. Typical criminal acts include robbery, assault, and murder.

A **tort** is the breach of a legal duty or obligation resulting in an injury, either physical, mental, or financial. **Tort law** (also called *civil law)* is different from criminal law—under tort law, the plaintiff, or injured person, files a lawsuit, or legal action, against the defendant, or person accused of committing the breach of duty. If the plaintiff successfully proves that the defendant caused harm by violating a legal duty, the plaintiff may collect damages, monetary compensation awarded by the court. Injuries include medical bills, loss of employment, pain, suffering, and loss of ability to be with others (loss of consortium).

 Discuss the significance and scope of the following in relationship to EMT–I practice:
- State Medical Practice Act
- Good Samaritan Act/Civil Immunity
- State EMS statutes
- State motor vehicle codes
- State and local guidelines for "Do Not Resuscitate" orders

State legislation
Medical Practice Act
Each state has a set of laws called the Medical Practice Act that govern the practice of medicine within that state. These laws, although different from state to state, define the limits for **scope of practice,** which are those patient assessment and treatment skills that medical direction physicians allow EMT–Is to perform. EMT–Is must be familiar with the appropriate state act that defines the scope of practice.

 SCOPE OF PRACTICE: Description of what assessment and treatment skills an EMT-I may legally perform.

State EMS statutes
State EMS statutes are the actual rules and regulations governing the practice of EMS providers. These laws differ widely from state to state. In general, state EMS statutes cover the following areas:

- *Scope of practice*—Defines what assessment and treatment skills an EMT–I may legally perform.

- *Licensure, regulations, and certification*—Defines the requirements that a person must fulfill in order to practice as an EMT–I in that state; also states the rules that an EMT–I must follow while practicing.

- *Medical direction*—Defines the requirements for a medical director to delegate practice to the EMT–I.

- *Protocols and communications*—Specifies the need for protocols for EMS, as well as the types of radio and phone systems that must be in place.

State motor vehicle codes
State motor vehicle codes vary considerably from state to state. Many areas, for example, require that a person possess a chauffeur's license to drive an emergency vehicle. Thus, an EMT–I must be familiar with appropriate statutes regarding the operation of emergency vehicles in his or her state, paying particular attention to sections dealing with speeding, right-of-way, and use of lights and siren.

Identify those situations that require the EMT–I to report incidents to appropriate authorities.

In addition to specific EMS legislation and motor vehicle laws, the EMT-I also should be aware of state laws regarding three other important areas:

1. *Obligation to report certain injuries to appropriate officials*—Examples include suspected abuse or neglect of the elderly, suspected abuse or neglect of children, alleged rape, gunshot wounds, and animal bites. Generally, these laws provide immunity from lawsuits for providers who report these problems in good faith. Exactly which incidents are mandatory to report differs from state to state—follow your state laws and local protocols.

2. *Specific privileges and responsibilities*—These govern the use of restraints, the degree of force allowed

when managing a violent or uncooperative patient, access to restricted areas, and obtaining blood samples for alcohol or drug testing. Laws regulating the use of force and restraints vary widely—EMT–Is should know those laws that apply where they practice.

3. *Interfacing with other agencies*—These laws or agreements determine who is in charge of a scene. These laws also outline the appropriate interrelationships between the EMT–I and law enforcement personnel, firefighters, search and rescue agencies, and the military.

Right to die, living wills, and Do Not Resuscitate orders

Another form of legislation, recently enacted in many states, that affects prehospital care is right to die or Do Not Resuscitate legislation.

> **DO NOT RESUSCITATE ORDER:** A physician's order indicating that a patient is not to be resuscitated in the event of a cardiac arrest.

Right to die legislation

In general, cardiopulmonary resuscitation (CPR) should be started on all patients who are without a pulse and respirations unless there is evidence of decomposition, decapitation, incineration, or massive injury incompatible with life. Do not stop CPR once it is begun unless patient care is transferred to a higher level provider (such as the hospital emergency department) or unless instructed to do so by medical direction.

Living wills and related documents

Certain patients do not wish to be resuscitated if they suffer a cardiac arrest. Often, this desire is expressed in terms of a written document entitled a *living will*, *healthcare proxy*, or *advance directive*. The wording of such documents varies widely, but the intention is that the patient wishes no measures taken to resuscitate him or her in the event of cardiac arrest.

State and local guidelines for Do Not Resuscitate orders

A similar situation may arise when a patient's personal physician writes a **Do Not Resuscitate (DNR) order** (Fig. 3-1). This order may be in the form of a legal document but more commonly is simply written in a letter or on a prescription pad.

On arrival at a scene, the EMT–I may be presented with either a living will or a DNR order by a friend or family member. The legality of accepting living wills or DNR orders varies from state to state. Some states require that the EMT–I comply with the provisions in a living will or DNR order. Other states have not addressed the issue at all. It is important for the EMT–I to be familiar with the specific

local legislation, policies, and protocols concerning DNR orders.

Although a lawsuit conceivably could be brought against an EMT–I for attempting to resuscitate a patient with a living will or DNR order, family members at the scene may not be in total agreement as to the best course of action. The safest course of action is to proceed with care unless it is certain that the patient's or physician's intentions are *clearly and legibly documented*.

If the rare instance arises in which someone physically obstructs patient care, police officers may be helpful in managing the situation. All pertinent facts must be documented concisely on the written run report.

STANDARD OF CARE

Legally, the **standard of care** is defined as the degree of medical care and skill that is expected of a reasonably competent EMT–I acting in the same or similar circumstances. This standard is based on community practice; federal, state, and local laws; scientific literature; and EMS system standards. Some of these standards are applicable to all EMS systems, whereas others pertain to specific areas.

IMMUNITIES

> **GOOD SAMARITAN LAWS:** Laws that may provide immunity from prosecution or civil suit for people who render care at the scene of an emergency.

Good Samaritan laws

Most states have **Good Samaritan laws** in place to protect persons who provide assistance at emergency scenes. These laws may apply to lay persons or medical personnel.

> **NEGLIGENCE:** Professional conduct that falls below the standard of care; also known as medical liability.
> **ORDINARY NEGLIGENCE:** Acts or omissions that occur in the attempt to deliver proper care.
> **GROSS NEGLIGENCE:** The willful and reckless giving of care that causes injury to the patient.

Although Good Samaritan laws are not equal from state to state in scope of their coverage or requirements, under certain circumstances, the EMT–I may be immune from being successfully sued for **negligence.** A trial or hearing may be required to determine if the EMT–I's actions place him or her within the scope of the particular state's Good Samaritan law.

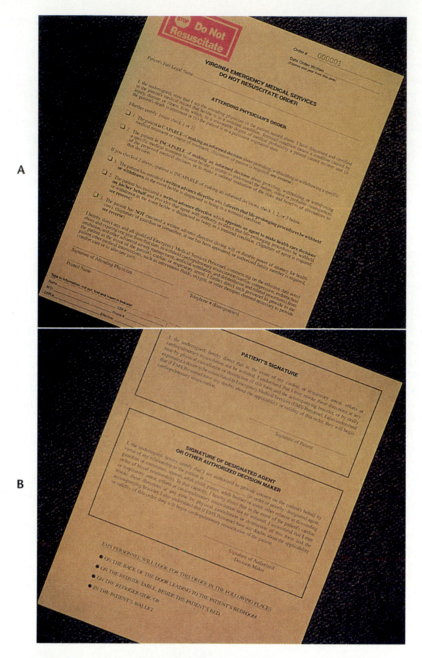

Fig. 3-1 A sample Do Not Resuscitate form. A, Front. B, Back.

Good Samaritan laws typically have the following three conditions:

- Immunity usually covers charges of **ordinary negligence** but not charges of **gross negligence.** Proving gross negligence may be difficult in a court of law.

- The provider must give care without charging a fee for service.

- The provider must only give care that is appropriate for his or her certification level.

Good Samaritan laws have not been well tested in the courts. Therefore, many attorneys caution their EMS clients not to rely heavily on these laws for protection. These laws do NOT prevent an EMT–I from being sued in the first place—in the United States, anyone is free to file a lawsuit against anyone for anything! Whether or not the EMT–I is ultimately held responsible is another question, and

Good Samaritan laws may prevent the EMT–I from being successfully sued.

Many questions remain to be answered in regard to Good Samaritan laws. These include concerns as to vagueness in the laws and the true definition of "fee for service" (*ie,* career versus volunteer EMT) prehospital care.

Civil immunity

Civil immunity means that an EMS service may be protected from a charge of negligence because it is a designated government agency. These laws vary from area to area. As with Good Samaritan laws, do not rely on civil immunity statutes to protect you.

MEDICAL NEGLIGENCE

 Define the terms *negligence, medical liability,* and *duty to act.*

Negligence, or medical liability, is conduct that falls below the standard of care. This conduct may entail either *doing something that should not have been done or failing to do something that should have been done.* For example, defibrillating a resonsive patient in normal sinus rhythm is doing something that should not have been done. Failure to defibrillate an arrested person in ventricular fibrillation, however, would be considered failing to do something that should have been done. In either of these two cases the care rendered the patient would be considered negligent because it falls below the standard of care. Although the EMT–I may violate the standard of care, a legal finding of professional negligence is not as simple.

 STREET WISE
Giving either the wrong care or substandard care is considered to be negligent, or below the standard of care.

The requirements for professional negligence to be proven

 Describe the four elements that must be present to prove negligence.

For the EMT–I to be found negligent, the following four distinct requirements must be met (Fig. 3-2):

- The act or omission must have been within the EMT–I's duty to act.
- The act or omission must have been below the standard of care.
- An injury must have occurred to the patient.
- The act or omission must have been the proximate (direct) cause of injury.

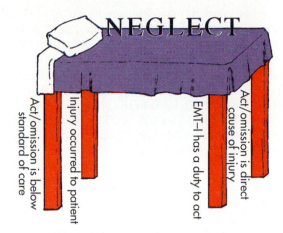

Fig. 3-2   The four elements of negligence.

Duty to act
Duty to act means that the EMT–I has an obligation to provide care. Generally, just by being dispatched and responding to a scene, the EMT–I has incurred a duty to act. This duty applies to both paid and volunteer EMS systems.

Act or omission below the standard of care
An act or omission below the standard of care may include providing improper care, performing skills the EMT–I is not certified to perform, violation of rules and regulations set forth by the EMT–I's EMS system, or failure of equipment to work properly. In court, violation of the standard of care is usually established by testimony from expert witnesses, as well as from various rules, regulations, and protocols that may be presented.

An expert witness is an individual who has special knowledge, not normally possessed by the average person, about a subject; *eg,* a physician may serve as an expert witness in medical negligence cases.

Injury to the patient
Generally, for the EMT–I to be found negligent, the injury to the patient must have resulted in damages that can be estimated in financial terms. It is not necessary, however, for the damages to merely represent absolute monetary losses. Pain, suffering, and loss of companionship often are successfully claimed as damages in professional negligence lawsuits.

Proximate cause
Proximate cause means that something was directly responsible for damage. Within reasonable medical probability, the error of the EMT–I must be the direct cause of the patient's injuries. The patient may claim to have suffered a new injury or worsening of his or her original problem due to the EMT–I's negligence.

Whether or not the EMT–I is familiar with the intricacies of the legal system, he or she should remember two important facts:

- Excellent patient care, appropriate use of medical direction, professional behavior, and good judgment are the best ways to avoid legal problems.

- The EMT–I should immediately consult with a supervisor if he or she receives any kind of legal notice or subpoena, or is requested to sign any legal documents related to his or her work as an EMT–I. The EMT–I should consider consulting an attorney as well if he or she has any questions or receives a subpoena.

The anatomy of a malpractice suit

EMT–Is Jones and Smith are called to the home of Mr. Reid, an accountant aged 60 years, who is in cardiac arrest. Mr. Reid's adopted son, Mr. Law, is performing one-person CPR. EMT–I Jones joins Mr. Law in performing two-person CPR, while EMT–I Smith calls for ALS back-up. After EMT–I Smith discovers that the ambulance radio will not work, he takes the oxygen tank and bag-valve-mask equipment from the ambulance and joins EMT–I Jones. Between the EMT–Is and Mr. Law, CPR is performed for 5 minutes. Mr. Reid does not respond. At that time, EMT–I Jones notices that the oxygen tank was empty and runs back to the ambulance to get another one.

The three men again perform CPR, using a new oxygen tank, for another 5 minutes. When there is no response, EMT–Is Smith and Jones decide to transport Mr. Reid to the nearest hospital, which is 10 minutes away.

On arrival at the hospital emergency department, the emergency physician notes that Mr. Reid is in a cardiac rhythm known as *ventricular fibrillation*, a chaotic quivering of the heart that results in the absence of cardiac output. She administers an electrical shock, or defibrillation, to Mr. Reid, resulting in normal cardiac contraction.

After other advanced life-support therapy, Mr. Reid's heart is again beating normally and he is breathing on his own. He remains unresponsive, however—in fact, Mr. Reid never does wake up, although his other bodily functions are normal. He requires around-the-clock care in a nursing home for the rest of his life.

Mr. Law later files a lawsuit on behalf of Mr. Reid against EMT–Is Smith and Jones, the ambulance company, and the medical director of the ambulance service. He claims that the EMT–Is spent too much time performing CPR in the field. The lawsuit also questions whether or not EMT–Is Smith and Jones should have carried an automated external defibrillator on their unit and tried to use it on Mr. Reid. Combined with the fact that the first oxygen tank was empty and that their radio was broken, Mr. Law's attorney states that Mr. Reid's brain was deprived of sufficient oxygen to allow for him to recover responsiveness, even though the heart problem was reversed at the hospital.

The suit claims:

1. A duty to act existed because EMT–Is Smith and Jones were dispatched and responded to the call for help.

2. An act below the standard of care occurred because EMT–Is Smith and Jones performed CPR for too long before taking Mr. Reid to the hospital. The suit also states that the EMT–Is should have ensured that the first oxygen tank was full prior to using it. The ambulance service's protocols require that oxygen tanks be checked before and after each run. A review of the checklist for that day revealed that EMT–Is Smith and Jones had failed to check their oxygen supply properly. Substandard care also may have occurred because EMT–Is Smith and Jones failed to attempt defibrillation.

3. An injury occurred to the patient because Mr. Reid never regained responsiveness despite the fact that the emergency department physician was able to treat the heart problem. The suit claims compensable damages for the cost of nursing home care for the rest of Mr. Reid's expected life, as well as loss of wages because he is now unable to work as an accountant.

4. The failure of EMT-Is Smith and Jones to ensure an adequate oxygen supply during CPR, provide early defibrillation, as well as to transport Mr. Reid as soon as possible to the hospital directly caused the brain injuries that prevented the patient from regaining responsiveness.

What happens when a lawsuit is filed?
Complaint filing
When people feel they have been injured due to malpractice, they seek the advice of an attorney. After investigating the facts and agreeing that the case has merit, the attorney will file a complaint for the individual in the appropriate court. The complaint states the reasons for the charge of negligence and asks for damages. The person who files the complaint, along with his or her attorney, is known as the *plaintiff*.

When a complaint is received, the court issues a subpoena to the defendant, the individual charged with the negligence. The defendant has a certain number of days to file an answer to the complaint with the court.

Discovery
At this stage, the defendant's attorney investigates the facts and prepares an answer to the complaint. Once the answer has been filed, both sides begin a process known as *discovery*. During the discovery phase, each side tries to find out as much as possible about the opposition's case. Both sides usually will have expert witnesses, who will testify in support of either the plaintiff's or defendant's case.

Much of the discovery process consists of the taking of depositions. A deposition is a sworn statement, usually taken in an attorney's office. Although the setting for a deposition is informal, the testimony offered is recorded by a court reporter. Anything said in a deposition may ultimately be used in a trial, if one occurs.

Deposition

The plaintiff's attorney will almost always take a deposition from both the plaintiff and the defendant, trying to ascertain both sides of the story. Both sides will depose each others' expert witnesses. Attorneys for both sides are always present at the deposition and may cross-examine the person being questioned.

Settlement

After preliminary information is obtained through the discovery process, both sides will reevaluate their case. At this stage, the involved parties, including the malpractice insurance company, usually try to reach some type of agreement, or settlement. This process is known as a *settlement conference*. The court reporter is not usually present during these meetings.

Trial

If an out-of-court settlement is not reached, a trial date is set. A trial is the presentation of both sides of the case in a court, and may take place several years after the alleged incident occurred. In most cases, a jury will decide whether or not the defendant is guilty; however, in some cases, the case is heard only by a judge. If the judge or jury finds the defendant liable, they will state what damages should be paid to the plaintiff.

Appeal

The liable party may pay at this stage or file an appeal. An appeal is a complaint filed with a higher level court stating that something was done improperly during the trial. The side filing the appeal usually believes that an error during the trial wrongly led to a verdict against them. The appellate court will decide whether to let the decision of the lower level court stand, to change the decision, or to order a new trial.

The lawsuit process may take years. A lawsuit may not even be filed until years after the event has occurred. The maximum period from the occurrence of an alleged injury to the ultimate filing of a lawsuit is called the *statute of limitations*. This period varies from state to state but is usually no greater than 2 or 3 years.

CONSENT

Elements of consent

 Define the terms *consent, expressed consent, informed consent,* and *implied consent.*

Describe the significance of obtaining expressed and informed consent.

Consent

Consent means agreement for approval. Responsive and mentally competent adult patients have the right to accept or refuse any examination, care, or transportation offered by the EMT–I. The EMT–I who performs any of these actions without appropriate patient consent risks legal action.

There are two types of valid consent in prehospital care: expressed consent and implied consent. Some situations may involve consent from minors or mentally incompetent patients.

Expressed consent

Expressed consent is given when the patient provides verbal or written consent for the EMT–I to examine, care for, and transport the patient to an appropriate medical facility. Expressed consent may be withdrawn at any time by the patient. Consent also can be expressed by gestures. A patient's presentation of an injury to the EMT–I usually expresses consent.

Implied consent

Implied consent concerns the patient who is unresponsive or in a state in which he or she is unable to respond to the EMT–I. Implied consent means that the EMT–I assumes that a patient who is severely ill or injured would want care if he or she were able to respond. Legally, one is asking the question, "What would a responsible person want done under similar circumstances?" In these instances, it is implied that a patient who is severely ill or injured would want care.

Informed consent and informed refusal of care

Informed consent means that the patient consents to care only after receiving all the information necessary to understand his or her condition, the risks and benefits of care, and the risks and benefits of refusal of care. Similarly, a patient armed with the same information may make an informed refusal of care. In either case, the patient must be given the following information so that he or she may make an informed decision:

- The EMT-I's assessment of the situation based on his or her field impression
- What care is being considered and why
- An explanation of the benefits and possible risks (including potential side effects) of accepting or refusing either examination, care, or transportation

The degree to which the EMT–I must explain things to a patient varies, especially when faced with an urgent situation. In nonurgent situations, and especially when a competent patient wishes to refuse care, explain all of the information previously mentioned and document the event carefully.

Minors

Persons under 18 years of age are minors and cannot legally consent to or refuse medical care. If the parent or legal guardian cannot be contacted for consent, emergency care can be provided under the implied consent standard. Emancipated minors have been legally freed of the need for parental consent; most often this occurs if a minor becomes married. Eman-cipated minors are able to give their own consent. Most states also do not require parental consent for treatment of sexually transmitted diseases, pregnancy, or pregnancy-related conditions in minors.

The mentally incompetent patient

A patient who has been legally determined mentally incompetent cannot give actual consent for care. In these cases, consent usually is given by a legal guardian. It may be very difficult to make this determination in the prehospital setting. Often, others who are present at the scene, such as caretakers or friends, can be helpful. If the legally responsible party is not available, the patient can receive care under the implied consent standard.

Ambigious legal issues may develop when a patient who is temporarily unable to make rational decisions refuses care. If the patient is experiencing alcohol or substance intoxication, emotional (psychiatric) problems, or certain medical conditions, he or she may be temporarily unable to make rational decisions. Usually this patient can be treated under the implied consent standard. It is always better to err on the side of caring for patients who appear to be mentally incompetent, regardless of the reason. Serious medical problems, such as poisoning and hypothermia, may produce symptoms similar to those of intoxication. A patient who appears to be intoxicated may actually have a serious medical problem, which, if left untreated, may result in serious harm to the patient.

Some states have laws that permit police officers, mental health professionals, or physicians to place apparently mentally incompetent persons into custody for the patient's own protection. It is essential that EMT-Is are aware of local laws that make provisions for mentally incompetent persons to be treated when no one is available to give consent for them.

The patient who refuses care

Perhaps one of the most stressful situations for the EMT-I is the patient who needs care but refuses it. Responsive adult patients have the absolute right to refuse examination, care, and transportation by EMS.

An EMT-I dealing with this situation should attempt to convince the patient to allow care. In many cases, a careful explanation of the possible consequences of refusing care may change the patient's mind. Occasionally a family member, friend, or medical direction physician may be able to assist in convincing the patient to consent.

In a situation in which a patient refuses care, the EMT-I should:

- Explain the consequences of the refusal of care to the patient and remember that, like consent, refusal should be based on an informed decision.

- Provide an explanation of the consequences of refusal of care and attempt to ensure patient understanding prior to allowing the patient to sign a refusal of care form.

- Be certain that the patient is competent to understand the consequences of refusal. If the EMT-I does not believe that the patient is mentally competent to refuse care, he or she should consider use of any local laws that permit persons to be taken into custody for their own protection.

Always respect the patient's beliefs. If all reasonable methods to encourage consent fail, the EMT-I may not legally be able to provide care. Patients may refuse care for many reasons: religious beliefs, denial of the severity of their symptoms, or simply because of their priorities. The EMT-I should not view this as a personal rejection. No matter how frustrating the situation might be, all EMS providers must maintain a high standard of professionalism.

It is extremely important to accurately and thoroughly document a patient's refusal of care. Obtain a written refusal from the patient on a standardized form (Fig. 3-3), and, when possible, have the refusal witnessed by a family member, police officer, or firefighter. If a patient refuses to sign the form, record the details in narrative fashion on the run report.

REFUSAL OF SERVICES

I hereby refuse the emergency medical services and/or transportation offered and advised by the above named service provider and its emergency personnel, _____ hospital, and the emergency medical and nursing personnel from said hospital giving directions to the service provider. I understand that my refusal may jeopardize the health of the patient, and hereby release the above named parties from any and all claims of liability in connection with my refusal.

_____
Signature of Patient or Legally Authorized Representative

_____
Signature of EMT/Field RN

_____
Witness   Date

Fig. 3-3 A "Release from Liability" form.

Obtaining a signed refusal form may not completely clear the EMT–I from responsibility. A patient could later claim that stress, injury, or other factors led to the uninformed signing of a refusal form. For this reason, the patient's refusal of care should always be documented on the run report sheet as well. In addition to vital signs and other pertinent physical observations, the EMT–I should carefully note the patient's mental condition and establish that the patient appeared mentally competent *at the time* to make a decision to refuse care. It is also important to document that the patient received an explanation of the consequences of refusing treatment and understood or acknowledged these consequences.

General rules concerning consent

These general rules should be followed when dealing with the issue of consent:

- When in doubt, care for the patient.

- Obtain police assistance, particularly if a patient appears to be emotionally disturbed or is making an obviously irrational decision due to an altered level of awareness.

- If available, use the EMS communications system to obtain physician direction. Some EMS systems require that an EMT–I contact medical direction prior to accepting a refusal of care by the patient. In some instances, the physician may be able to talk the patient into accepting needed care.

AREAS OF POTENTIAL MEDICAL LIABILITY

 Define the terms *abandonment, assault, battery, false imprisonment, slander,* and *libel.*

Abandonment

Abandonment is a form of negligence that occurs when the relationship between the EMT–I and the patient is terminated by the EMT–I without ensuring continuity of care for the patient. Once patient care is begun, remain with the patient until one of the following situations occurs:

- Care is continued by equally- or more highly-trained personnel.

- The patient is delivered to an appropriate care facility and it is certain that transfer has been accepted. Initial transfer is done by verbal report to the emergency department physician or nurse. This verbal report is followed by the appropriate written documentation.

- The patient makes an informed decision to sign a refusal statement. Remember—a signed refusal form alone may not absolve providers from charges of abandonment.

Abandonment also may be implied if equipment does not function properly or if the appropriate care supplies are lacking.

> **ASSAULT:** Creation of the fear of immediate bodily harm in a person, without his or her consent; does not require physical contact by the perpetrator.
> **BATTERY:** Criminal offense of inflicting bodily injury on another.
> **FALSE IMPRISONMENT:** Intentional and unjustifiable detention of a person against his or her will.

Assault and battery

Assault occurs when a patient fears that the EMT–I will cause him or her immediate bodily harm without his or her consent. The EMT–I does *not* need to touch the patient to be accused of assault. Charges of assault may be brought under either criminal or tort law.

Battery occurs when the EMT–I actually touches the patient without his or her consent, causing the patient physical harm. As with assault, battery may be either a criminal or a tort charge. Charges against EMT–Is for assault and/or battery are extremely unusual. When they are made, it is usually because the patient claims that he or she did not give consent for a procedure, such as spinal immobilization or starting an IV line. The best way to avoid accusations of assault and/or battery is to obtain expressed consent from the patient.

 Describe the significance of knowing state laws relating to the use of force and restraint to protect the EMT, the patient, and any third party.

False imprisonment

False imprisonment is the intentional and unjustifiable detention of a person against his or her will. When this charge is made, the case often involves a patient with psychiatric problems, a patient who has abused alcohol or drugs, or a suicidal patient. Depending on state or local laws, the patient's circumstances may justify the detention. Expressed consent to the detention should be obtained if at all possible. If the EMT is unable to obtain consent and detention is medically necessary, he or she must be certain to carefully document the need for as well as the method of detention. Local law enforcement officials may provide assistance under these circumstances.

Libel and slander

Libel is the injury of a person's character, name, or reputation by false and malicious writings. An EMT–I can be sued for writing something in a run report that could be considered harmful to a patient. Thus, the written record must be accurate and confidential.

- Avoid slang terms—do not write, "Patient is high as a kite." Instead, write, "Patient appears to be intoxicated."

- Avoid labels when describing behavior—do not write, "Patient walked like a drunken slob." Instead, write, "Patient's gait was unsteady."

Slander is the utterance of false statements that defame and damage another's reputation. Limit oral reporting to appropriate personnel. Again, avoid slang terms—describe the patient's behavior, not an "editorial" opinion of his or her condition. An EMT–I may be sued for slander if he or she says something false or malicious about a patient that injures a patient's character, name, or reputation.

Remember that all written and verbal information regarding patient encounters and care is confidential. This information should not be shared with friends or relatives, even if names are not mentioned. Patient information belongs only to the EMT–I, the patient, and medical professionals who need the information to provide proper patient care.

PATIENT TRANSFER LAWS— COBRA

 Describe the provisions of COBRA that relate to the EMT-I and the transfer of patients.

EMT–Is often are involved in transferring patients between healthcare facilities (hospital to hospital, hospital to nursing home, etc.). Emergency department physicians and hospitals are now subject to the provisions of the Consolidated Omnibus Budget Reconciliation Act of 1985 (COBRA). COBRA specifies several responsibilities of the emergency department that must be met prior to transferring a patient.

The significance of COBRA for EMT–Is

Because EMT–Is perform many patient transfers, it is essential to be aware of COBRA's patient transfer provisions. These provisions are meant to prevent unstable emergency patients from being transferred between care facilities solely for economic reasons. Any patient transferred should satisfy COBRA requirements. If the patient's condition deteriorates in transit, it may be because he or she was not adequately stabilized prior to transfer. In addition, COBRA provisions apply to hospital-owned ambulance services. Once the patient is within the ambulance, he or she is legally considered to have "come to the hospital." Therefore, the EMT–I and the hospital are potentially liable under COBRA if a patient is not appropriately transported to the hospital.

The provisions of COBRA

Failure to properly transfer a patient subjects the hospital and physician to significant penalties. These penalties include a fine of up to $50,000 per violation and the loss of the hospital's Medicare privileges. The provisions of COBRA are:

1. All persons who present to an emergency department must undergo a medical examination, which may be performed by either a nurse or a physician. The purpose of this examination is to determine whether the patient is suffering from an emergency medical condition or is in active labor.

2. All persons who present to an emergency department must be treated alike, regardless of their ability to pay for services.

3. Unstable patients (or those in active labor) are not to be transferred unless the patient or representative so requests, or if appropriate treatment facilities are not available at the initial institution.

4. Prior to transfer, all patients must first be stabilized unless the risk of waiting to attempt stabilization outweighs the potential benefit of transferring the patient to a more specialized facility.

5. The treatment given at the transferring facility must be documented.

SPECIAL SITUATIONS

Situations involving child abuse, crime, motor vehicle accidents, or a physician already at the scene require special, well-defined EMS system protocols that EMT–Is must follow. The following are suggestions for dealing with these protocols.

 Describe the significance of accurate documentation and record keeping in substantiating an incident.

Crime and accident scenes

The EMT–I's first responsibility is to maintain his or her own safety. Never enter the scene of a known violent crime until it has been secured by law enforcement personnel.

Police investigation of crimes or motor vehicle accidents can be seriously hindered by emergency personnel who inadvertently disturb or destroy evidence at the scene. The role of the EMT–I is to provide good patient care and, at the same time, to preserve evidence. Consider virtually everything at the scene to be of potential use to investigators.

When working crime and accident scenes it is essential that unauthorized persons be kept off the premises. Do not touch, kick, or move anything (including vehicles or debris) unless absolutely necessary to provide patient care (Fig. 3-4). If it becomes necessary to move vehicles at the scene of a motor vehicle accident, mark their original position on the pavement with a large piece of chalk or crayon. Both patient care and preservation of evidence can be accomplished, but patient care is your first priority.

Make mental notes of what is observed—the position of a weapon, overturned furniture, pooled blood, or the position and location of a victim. It may be helpful to investigators if a diagram is drawn in the run report. Relay any findings to the investigating officer as soon as possible after the necessary patient care is provided.

Child abuse

Child abuse is defined as the physical, sexual, or emotional maltreatment of a child. The EMT–I may be the only medical care provider who sees an abused child in both the home and the clinical context; therefore, the EMT–I may be the only provider who can allow the legal system to come to the aid of such a child. It is extremely important that hospital personnel are alerted when child abuse is suspected. The EMT–I may be legally obligated to report suspected child abuse—follow all local laws and protocols. Additionally, document and report any suspicious findings to the appropriate authorities. An EMT–I could be subjected to fines, imprisonment, and loss of state certification to practice for failing to report suspected child abuse.

All states have laws that protect healthcare professionals from liability for reporting, in good faith, suspected child abuse. It is important to note that the law does not require *proof* of abuse, only suspicion. On the other hand, do not speculate on the run report—state only factual information.

It is very helpful to have a specific protocol within an EMS system for dealing with this difficult situation. Most importantly, do not delay care of the sick or injured child to pursue any suspicion of child abuse. Handle these matters *after* transporting the child to the hospital.

Physicians at the scene of patient encounters

Occasionally, a person on-scene may claim to be a physician. Usually, these individuals are bona fide physicians who truly are interested in providing assistance. In rare instances, EMT–Is may be confronted with a citizen who claims to be a physician but who actually is not. It usually is impossible to tell whether the person is really a physician simply because he or she claims to be one. Thus, the EMT–I must follow an established protocol when dealing with a physician on the scene.

Legally, the initial responsibility for patient care rests with the on-line medical direction physician. If an on-scene physician can document his or her licensure and ability to deal with the situation, some medical direction facilities will allow him or her to take over, provided the physician is willing to accompany the patient to the hospital. Therefore, the EMT–I should contact medical direction when dealing with an on-scene physician. A physician on the scene should not be allowed to assume control of patient care against the advice of the on-line medical direction physician. If the individual continues

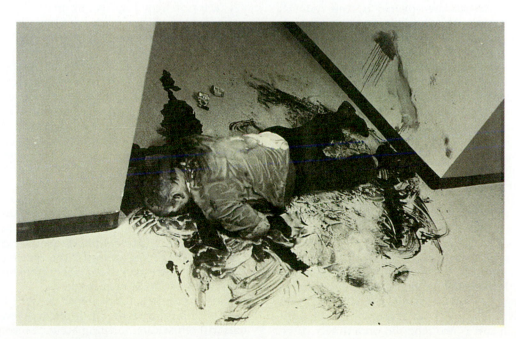

Fig. 3-4   It is important to preserve a crime scene as much as possible when delivering patient care.

to interfere with patient care, immediately seek police assistance.

Some EMS systems do not have the ability to contact on-line medical direction. Those systems should have written protocols for dealing with on-scene physicians. These protocols should require that if a licensed bystander physician wishes to take control, he or she MUST:

1. Ride in the ambulance with the patient to the hospital.
2. Sign all necessary care forms, including the run report.

The EMT–I must record the name, place of practice, and medical license number of the physician on the run sheet.

MEDICAL LIABILITY PROTECTION

The sophistication of EMS has created the obligation and expectation to provide quality patient care. Many EMT–Is are not covered by Good Samaritan laws, and, as a result, more EMT–Is are being named as defendants in malpractice suits. For these reasons, many EMS systems and individual EMT–Is have purchased malpractice insurance. Some of the larger EMS systems are self-insured, meaning they have the money available to cover possible claims without outside companies.

Although most EMS systems carry some types of insurance, this insurance may or may not provide adequate protection for the individual provider. Check with your own EMS system to clarify the extent to which you are covered by the system's malpractice insurance. Separate (individual) malpractice insurance is recommended for career EMT–Is and those whose EMS system lacks adequate coverage. The specific dollar amounts of insurance necessary differ from area to area. Talk to colleagues, insurance agents, attorneys, supervisors, and risk management or continuous quality improvement personnel for suggestions regarding individual malpractice insurance.

Service-supplied malpractice insurance alone may be very limited in coverage and it may not cover any medical care administered while off duty. On the other hand, individual medical liability insurance is written for each EMT–I's specific needs. The insurer then acts as an advocate for the EMT-I, not for the EMS service.

Regardless of who provides malpractice coverage, the EMT–I should understand the contract. Be familiar with reporting requirements. Some insurers require that the EMT–I report any incident, no matter how small, that may develop into a lawsuit. If a potential suit is not reported on a timely basis, the insurer may refuse to provide coverage if a suit actually occurs.

CASE HISTORY FOLLOW-UP

EMT–I Reynolds reports to work a few minutes early Tuesday morning after the conference, hoping to talk with EMT–I Thomas about his gossip.

"Hi, Tony. Can I have a word with you?" she asks.

"Sure, Stacy. What's up? Great conference, huh?"

"Yeah, fine, Tony. Listen, I unintentionally overheard you saying to a group of people that Tom's HIV-positive."

"I didn't say that. I said I *heard* that he's positive," Thomas answers.

Reynolds reminds him, "Do you realize that even if he really has tested positive for HIV, that it's illegal, criminally and civilly, to disclose that information? And, if he hasn't tested positive, you've committed slander?"

"Hey, we were just talking. I really wasn't thinking about it all that much. I just heard someone say it once. That's all. No big deal, right?"

EMT–I Reynolds returns, "I think it's a big deal, and I'd rather not hear anything like that said again. I'm going to mention the incident to Tom, just to let him know what's been said. I think he'll be okay to let it drop—but maybe he won't. Is everything OK on the vehicle?"

SUMMARY

The EMT–I, like any healthcare professional, is subject to charges of professional negligence. Proper care of patients, adherence to established guidelines, and maintaining complete, legible documentation are key factors in avoiding legal troubles.

Encounters with patients who have living wills or physician-generated Do Not Resuscitate orders may still require the EMT–I to attempt resuscitation during cardiac arrest unless very specific requirements are met. The EMT–I should be aware of how the laws of his or her state deal with these issues.

Good Samaritan laws exist in most states, and they may or may not apply to the EMT–I. To a large extent, these laws have not been challenged in court. Thus, the EMT–I is best served by assuming that Good Samaritan legislation will not necessarily provide protection against a lawsuit.

Legally, the EMT–I is held to a certain standard of care. For a negligence action to be successful, it must be proven that four elements exist: a duty to act, negligent care that fell below the standard of care, damages, and proximate cause of the damages by the EMT–I's negligence. Patient abandonment may be considered a form of negligence.

Most patients will give their consent to receive care, whether expressed or implied. A few individuals will refuse care. Keeping accurate records of any patient who refuses care may help avoid later charges of patient abandonment or negligence. If in doubt, it is generally better to attempt care of a patient rather than to not provide care. The patient should be informed, whenever possible, with adequate information to determine the benefits and risks of his or her decision.

Numerous provisions contained in the Consolidated Omnibus Budget Reconciliation Act of 1985 (COBRA) affect the transfer of patients from hospitals. These provisions were enacted to prevent the transfer of an unstable patient for purely financial reasons. The majority of regulations apply directly to physicians and hospitals, but the EMT–I should be aware of the major provisions of this legislation, especially regarding hospital-owned ambulance services. Good communication between all levels of emergency providers should prevent problems related to COBRA.

Crime and accident scenes require that the EMT–I pay special attention to the preservation of evidence. Police should always be present prior to an EMT–I attempting to enter the scene of a violent crime. Child abuse laws may require that all healthcare providers report suspected abuse to local authorities.

Physicians who are bystanders at the scene of an emergency may be helpful or may be a hindrance to emergency care. It is ultimately the decision of the on-line medical direction physician as to whether or not the on-scene physician may assume the patient's care. Written protocols to deal with the situation are helpful. Police assistance should be enlisted if prompt cooperation is not offered by the on-scene physician.

It is advisable for individual EMT–Is to consider carrying some type of malpractice insurance, as not all jurisdictions are covered by Good Samaritan laws.

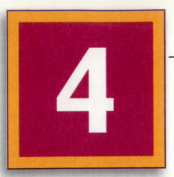

4

EMS COMMUNICATIONS

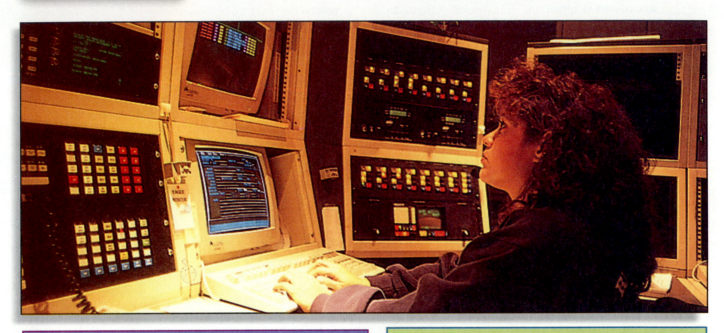

CASE HISTORY

EMT–I Walters has just received a phone call from an attorney representing his ambulance service. It seems as though an emergency response handled by Walters and a previous partner has become part of a lawsuit against his EMS service and his medical direction hospital. EMT–I Walters has no immediate recall of the incident, because it happened several years ago. The attorney briefly describes it for him, based on the patient's hospital records.

The call occurred 2 years ago on September 5, at 0445. EMT–I Walters and his partner were dispatched to a motor vehicle accident where a driver had struck a utility post head-on. Walters begins to remember the incident. It was a rainy morning and the end of a busy shift. He pulled up on the scene to find a group of bystanders surrounding the patient, who was lying face down on the pavement next to the car. The bystanders said that they had been with the patient at a party and were following him back to his apartment. They were concerned that he was "too drunk to drive." As EMT–I Walters secured the patient's head and neck to place him supine, he heard the group say that they pulled their friend from the car after the crash and moved him to the pavement. The patient was breathing, smelled of alcohol, and had vomitus on his face

Case History, continued

and neck. The EMT–Is maintained cervical spinal immobilization, suctioned the patient's airway, and administered high-concentration oxygen.

The patient was disoriented, but could follow simple commands. He had a laceration on his forehead from striking the windshield, but there were no other obvious signs of injury. During the physical examination, EMT–I Walters noted that the patient could not move his lower extremities. He appeared to have no sensation below the level of his umbilicus, and EMT–I Walters marked the area on the patient's skin where the sensation stopped. The EMT–Is secured the patient's neck and spine to a long backboard and prepared him for transport. En route, EMT–I Walters contacted medical direction and gave the following report:

"We are en route to your facility with a 24-year-old male who was involved in a head-on collision. He was removed from the car by friends and placed prone on the pavement prior to our arrival. We immobilized his spine and placed him in a supine position. He has a laceration on his forehead from striking the windshield. He is disoriented but able to follow simple commands. He is unable to move his lower extremities and has no sensation or movement below the level of his umbilicus. Strength and motion in the upper extremities are within normal range. Vital signs are stable. Friends state that the patient has been drinking. He has vomited once. The patient's airway was suctioned, and he was placed on high-flow oxygen. He is fully immobilized on a long backboard. Our ETA is 8 minutes."

After delivering the patient to the emergency department, EMT–I Walters carefully documented the specifics of the call on the prehospital care report and returned to service. Later that week, he heard that the patient suffered a complete cord lesion and was permanently paralyzed.

LEARNING OBJECTIVES

Upon completion of this chapter, the EMT–Intermediate should be able to:

- NAME the typical components of an EMS communication system and explain the function of each.
- IDENTIFY the advantage of a repeater system over a nonrepeater system.
- DESCRIBE the proper use of a digital encoder.
- LIST basic functions and responsibilities of the Federal Communications Commission (FCC).
- IDENTIFY the phases of communications necessary to complete a typical EMS event.
- DESCRIBE the responsibilities of an EMS dispatcher.
- NAME the information that must be gathered from a caller by the dispatcher.
- DESCRIBE two purposes for verbally communicating patient information to the hospital.
- LIST the patient assessment information that should be verbally reported to the physician.
- ORGANIZE a list of patient assessment information in the correct order for radio transmission to the physician according to the format used locally.
- DESCRIBE three communication techniques that influence the clarity of radio transmission.
- RECALL how to properly use mobile and portable radios to receive and transmit information.
- DESCRIBE the position of the antenna on a portable radio that will deliver maximum coverage.

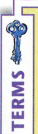

KEY TERMS

BIOTELEMETRY

EMERGENCY MEDICAL DISPATCHER (EMD)

ENCODER/DECODER

DEDICATED LAND LINES

ENHANCED 9-1-1

FEDERAL COMMUNICATIONS COMMISSION (FCC)

OSCILLOSCOPE

REPEATER SYSTEMS

TRANSCEIVERS

TRUNKING

INTRODUCTION

Effective communication is an essential component of all EMS systems. Each system must have a coordinated communication system that allows information to flow internally and externally, in both routine and emergency modes. The communication system must provide for communication between:

- Callers and the dispatch center
  - Requests for help
  - Verification of addresses/locations
  - Updates on patient or scene status
- The dispatch center and EMT–Is

- Dispatch information and response to emergency calls and nonemergency calls
- Updates to and reports from responding teams (hazards, patient information, directions for accessing the scene)
- Requests for backup units and/or rescue, fire, law enforcement specialty teams
- Resolving communication difficulties between the field and the emergency department
- EMT–Is and backup units
  - Communicating equipment needs
  - Scene and patient updates
  - Advice on what routes should be used to best access the scene
- EMT–Is who are working together on the ambulance
  - Ensures safety of team members when they are apart (such as the use of portable radios)
  - Communication between team members and the dispatch center in multiple-patient incidents
- EMT–Is and the emergency department
  - Medical direction and advice
  - Information about patients being transported to their facility
- EMT–Is in the field and EMS system administration
  - Sending and receiving messages
  - Routine activities such as sending the unit to the ambulance repair facility for vehicle maintenance
- The dispatch center and public safety units (fire, police, and other EMS units), as well as other community agencies
- The EMS system and public in general
  - Public relations
  - Media coverage
  - Evacuation information, storm or hazard warnings
- The dispatch center and disaster networks
  - Personnel, resource, and equipment needs
  - Number of patients distributed to area hospitals
- Emergency departments
  - Relaying patient information
  - Announcing bed and resource availability
  - Announcing availability of air and ground ambulance units

COMMUNICATION EQUIPMENT

Typical components
When setting up a communication system, the EMS service must consider the unique nature of

its resources, geography, and funding. Modern EMS communication systems have specific equipment needs. The typical configuration includes telephones, radios, repeater systems, and recording equipment.

 Name the typical components of an EMS communication system and explain the function of each.

Telephones

ENHANCED 9-1-1: Emergency phone number that includes a visual system that displays the caller's phone number and address.

The widespread availability of the telephone makes it an excellent communication link for EMS systems. In fact, the telephone is one of the most common devices the public uses to reach the EMS system. **Enhanced 9-1-1** is the recommended access number for EMS systems.

DEDICATED LAND LINES: Telephone lines with continuous direct connection from one geographical location to another.

The telephone also allows EMS systems to communicate internally as well as externally for routine and emergency situations. **Dedicated land lines** often are used by dispatchers to notify EMS personnel of emergency calls and are a reliable method of communicating with receiving hospitals, medical direction facilities, remote radio communication receivers, communication consoles, and police and fire dispatch centers. Dedicated land lines eliminate the need for the dispatcher to go through a switchboard, dial a phone number, or confront busy signals. Their biggest benefit is in saving time.

Cellular phones
Cellular phones are another time-saving way for the public to access EMS systems, particularly in the case of motor vehicle accidents and other emergencies that motorists might encounter. They also are popular for use in the prehospital setting due to their ease of use and decreasing cost.

Cellular communication allows for excellent reception and better continuity in transmission than that achieved with typical radio systems. The geographic area served by a cellular telephone network is divided into regions called *cells,* each with its own base station and antenna that interconnects the mobile units and the telephone network. When the transmission falls out of one cell's range, it is immediately picked up by another cell. Most major metropolitan and many rural areas are now covered by cellular systems, and the network is growing.

Cellular phones can be used by EMS systems for dispatch, on-scene communications, and scene-to-hospital communication. In addition to voice communication, cellular telephones allow EMT–Is to transmit 12-lead electrocardiograms (ECGs) (using a phone patch with a modem tone), faxes, and computer data to the dispatch center and the hospital. Communications between the EMT–I and the hospital must be conducted over a telephone line that is dedicated to this purpose. Otherwise, there is a risk that the EMT–I may get a busy signal when attempting to establish communications with the hospital.

One drawback to relying on cellular telephones is that available cells can become tied up with public communication. This is often the case during disasters, when cellular systems are tied up with a large volume of calls made by private citizens and the news media.

Radios

Radios are the primary means of communications between the dispatch center and EMS teams. Radios allow communication between:

- The EMS team and the base station or dispatch center
- EMT–Is on the EMS team (using portable radios)
- The EMS team and other responding or on-scene units
- The EMS team and receiving hospitals or facility(s) providing medical direction
- The EMS team and other public agencies (police, fire)

The radio system consists of three primary components: the base station, mobile two-way radios, and portable radios.

Base station

The base station is the most powerful radio in the system, with a typical power output of 45 to 275 watts. It may be controlled by a remote console. Usually, the base station is located in a dispatch center that serves as the communication network for the EMS system. In some communities, one dispatch center is responsible for all fire, police, and EMS communications. Many base stations are multiple-channel systems, but often the dispatch center only communicates on one channel at a time.

Mobile radios

Mobile two-way radios are mounted in vehicles such as ambulances, rescue units, and supervisory vehicles. With a typical power output of 40 to 100 watts, they allow communication to take place between the base station and the EMT–Is on the road. The characteristic transmission range is 10 to 15 miles over average terrain. This range is diminished in mountainous areas, where dense foliage is present, and in cities with large buildings. Mobile radios often have multiple channels.

Portable radios

Portable radios allow EMT–Is to communicate while away from the ambulance. These radios are hand-held devices with a typical power output of 1 to 5 watts. This low-power output significantly limits the range of the radios. Like mobile radios, portable radios can be equipped with multiple channels. Some EMS systems equip each EMS team with one portable radio, whereas other systems provide a portable radio for each EMT on duty.

> **STREET WISE**
> Each EMT–I should be equipped with a portable radio. This provides for greater safety. When one EMT–I is temporarily separated from his or her partner, the EMT–I is still able to communicate with his or her base station or partner if trouble develops or additional equipment or resources are needed.

Radio system characteristics

Each radio component serves as both a transmitter and receiver. As such, they are referred to as **transceivers**. Transceivers operate in a simplex, duplex, or multiplex mode.

Simplex mode

As the name suggests, simplex mode is the least complicated type of transmission. In this mode, communication can occur in only one direction at a time. In other words, while the EMT–I is transmitting a message, he or she cannot receive one. Simplex operation requires adherence to proper radio etiquette, meaning that the EMT–I must avoid starting any communication until all other communications have ended.

Duplex system

In the duplex mode, two separate frequencies are paired together to allow simultaneous transmission and reception to take place. This mode is much the same as talking on a telephone.

Multiplex system

A multiplex system is one that has the ability to transmit simultaneously two or more different types of information (*eg*, voice and telemetry) in either or both directions over the same frequency. Many base station hospitals that provide on-line medical direction use multiplex systems.

Radio frequencies

Radio frequencies are designated by cycles per second called *megahertz* (MHz). Radios used for EMS communications employ one of four major frequency bands. These are:

- VHF (very high frequency) low band
- VHF high band
- UHF (ultra high frequencies)
- 800-MHz band

Each of the radio frequencies has characteristics that make it useful for certain types of applications. The frequencies within these bands are assigned by the Federal Communications Commission (FCC).

VHF low band
VHF low band, operating between 32 to 50 MHz, offers the greatest distance. It is excellent for forested or open areas. Radio transmissions in this range are able to bend and follow the curvature of the earth, allowing transmission to stations over the horizon. However, weather disturbances, buildings, electrical equipment, and mountains can interrupt these transmissions. This poor penetration makes VHF low band less effective for use in metropolitan areas. Under certain circumstances, VHF low band transmissions skip, bouncing off atmospheric layers, and are received hundreds of miles away, interrupting local transmission. This band is limited to voice communications because it is against FCC regulations to transmit telemetry on VHF low band frequencies.

VHF high band
The VHF high band is the medium range frequency, operating between 150 to 174 MHz. Signals at this range are transmitted in a straight line and do not follow the curvature of the earth. The VHF high band is less susceptible to electrical disturbances and skip phenomena, but it is vulnerable to interference by solid structures, such as buildings and expressway overpasses. This makes transmissions inside concrete buildings difficult. The VHF high band is better for communications in metropolitan areas than VHF low band and provides reliable coverage for dispatcher-to-unit and EMT–I-to-hospital communication over a relatively large area. Base station antennas usually are located on high sites to increase the area of coverage.

Both low and high VHF bands operate in the simplex mode.

UHF band
UHF is the frequency band operating between 450 to 470 MHz. UHF signals transmit in a straight line but have excellent penetration. Of the three bands, the UHF band is least susceptible to electrical interference and skip phenomena. Because of straight line transmission characteristics, UHF is not normally used for long-distance transmission but is better suited to large metropolitan areas where there are large obstructions such as buildings. The FCC has designated 10 (1 through 10) frequencies of the UHF band for EMS communications. Eight frequencies are used for medical communications and telemetry, and two frequencies are available for EMS dispatch. UHF frequencies are often paired to allow duplex operations.

800-MHz frequency
Current technology also offers a frequency range within the 800-MHz spectrum. This spectrum has excellent penetration of buildings, minimal interference, and reduced channel noise; requires only a short channel; and has characteristics that make it ideal for use in major metropolitan operations. A unique feature of this band is **trunking**, which allows multiple agencies or systems to share frequencies. Sharing permits more effective utilization of the assigned frequencies and can facilitate interagency communications. Frequencies in the 800-MHz range also can be tied to a computer system that can send voiceless communications to a computer in the vehicle.

Additional communication equipment
Recording equipment
Today, most EMS systems use recording equipment to maintain an active record of the radio and phone communications taking place within the system. Communications that take place between the EMT–Is and medical direction also are recorded. Therefore, EMT–Is should be mindful that their radio and phone communications may be replayed for a variety of reasons, including (but not limited to) media broadcasts, educational activities, disciplinary hearings, and litigation. Professionalism in all communications within the EMS system is of paramount importance.

 Identify the advantage of a repeater system over a nonrepeater system.

Repeater systems
Portable radios allow the EMT–I to communicate from the patient's side or from remote locations. Unfortunately, using portable radios to communicate directly with hospitals or the dispatch center is sometimes impossible due to their short range. This drawback is due to their small size, low power output, and short antenna height. Poor output is sometimes a problem with mobile radios as well. To overcome this dilemma, some EMS systems use repeater systems to increase the range of their portable and mobile radios. **Repeater systems** are devices that receive transmissions from relatively low-wattage transmitters on one frequency and retransmit them at a higher power on another frequency, increasing the range of the transmissions. Some repeater units are mounted on the vehicle, whereas others are mounted on towers (Fig. 4-1).

 Describe the proper use of a digital encoder.

Encoders and decoders
When a number of base stations are on one frequency, the ongoing radio traffic can be distracting. This is particularly true of radios that are located in the hospital emergency department for the purpose of receiving patient information. The hospital staff may tend to turn the radio volume down or off to decrease or eliminate disruptive radio communication. Encoder/

decoder devices block out radio traffic that is not directed at the specific base station (Fig. 4-2).

An **encoder** looks like a telephone key pad. Each base station is assigned a numeric code, transmitted as a set of tones. To transmit a message to a specific base station, the user punches that station's code into the encoder. The station's **decoder** recognizes the code and allows the signal to be received.

HELPFUL HINT

How to use a digital encoder:

1. Turn the unit on.
2. Adjust the squelch.
3. Listen to be sure the airways are free of other communications.
4. Select the address code to be dialed and dial the number.
5. Hold the microphone at a proper distance from the mouth.
6. Push the transmit button and pause before speaking.
7. Call the unit dialed using the assigned identification numbers.
8. On termination of communication, state that you are clear on the channel so other users may transmit.

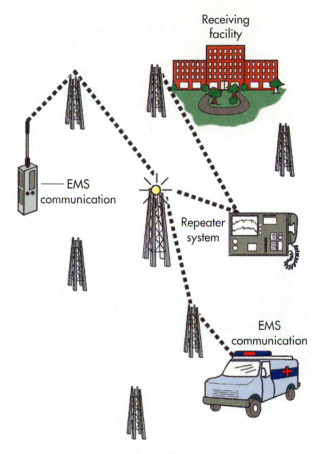

Fig. 4-1 Repeater systems allow EMS systems to overcome poor output capabilities of portable radios.

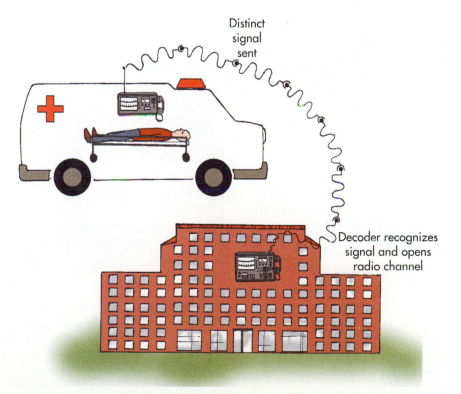

Fig. 4-2 An encoder/decoder device in a hospital accepts only calls directed specifically to it. All other radio traffic is blocked out.

> **BIOTELEMETRY:** The process of transmitting physiologic data, such as an ECG, over distance, usually by radio.
>
> **OSCILLOSCOPE:** Television-like screen that displays an electrical current, such as the impulse that travels through the heart's conduction system.

Biotelemetry

Biotelemetry has been used in the prehospital setting for almost three decades. The electrical activity (voltage changes) in a patient's heart picked up by an ECG is converted into audio tones, which are transmitted to the hospital. The receiver at the hospital converts the audio signal back into measurable voltage changes, which can be traced on an **oscilloscope** and/or onto an ECG tape.

Interference is a problem that can occur during telemetry transmission. It is caused by loose ECG electrodes, muscle tremors, 60-MHz noise, fluctuations in transmitter power, and interference of the actual radio transmission.

Mobile communication units

Some EMS systems have special mobile communication vehicles available for their use. Typically, these vehicles are large, bus-type units equipped with radio consoles, cellular telephones, and video monitoring equipment. They often are built with a space within the vehicle that is large enough to serve as a meeting area. Some vehicles even have restroom and kitchen facilities, which allows the vehicle to be used in disaster and multicasualty situations in which EMS personnel are required to stay on-site for long periods of time.

Microwave communication

Some large rural regions use microwave communications instead of dedicated telephone lines for relaying transmissions from remote radios. Microwaves travel in a straight line, are unidirectional, and follow a very narrow path for long distances along a line of sight. However, microwave communication requires multiple transmitters. To -offset the high cost of the transmitters, EMS systems often rent or share equipment with other users.

Rapid changes in both the communication needs of the EMS community and the available equipment require continual monitoring, upgrading, and training.

THE FEDERAL COMMUNICATIONS COMMISSION

 List basic functions and responsibilities of the Federal Communications Commission (FCC).

The **Federal Communications Commission (FCC)** is the federal agency established to control and regulate all radio communications in the United States. The FCC's primary functions include licensing and allocating radio frequencies, establishing technical standards for radio equipment, and establishing and enforcing rules and regulations for radio equipment operation. The FCC also is responsible for monitoring frequencies for appropriate usage and spot checking base stations and dispatch centers for appropriate licensing and records.

State and local governments may have additional requirements for radio operations. In some communities regional plans are used to ensure cooperation of all radio users. In other areas there are minimum equipment standards for ambulance licensure that specify the type of radio equipment to be used.

TYPES OF COMMUNICATIONS

EMS communications can be broken down into three types: routine, emergency response, and patient care or medical related.

Routine communications

Much of the communication that takes place in the EMS system is routine in nature. This communication occurs over the phone, on the ambulance radio, using portable radios, or by written or electronic means. Routine communication could be advising the dispatch center when the EMS team is taking time to eat lunch, picking up supplies or equipment, or when en route to have vehicle maintenance performed. It also may include messages from the dispatch center to the crew.

> **STREET WISE**
> Example of routine radio communication:
> "Unit 2 to dispatch."
> "Dispatch, go ahead Unit 2."
> "Unit 2 to dispatch, we are en route to headquarters to pick up medical supplies."
> "Dispatch to Unit 2, that's affirmative at 2122."
> "Unit 2 to dispatch, we are arriving at headquarters. We will remain in-service on the air."
> "Dispatch to Unit 2, that's affirmative at 2129."

Emergency communications

Emergency communications include all exchanges of information that occur from the beginning until the end of an emergency call.

 Identify the phases of communications necessary to complete a typical EMS event.

The steps in the progression of a typical EMS event include:

- Incident occurrence
- Recognition
- System access and dispatch
- Prehospital care
- Patient stabilization and transport
- Delivery to hospital
- Preparation for the next event

A variety of communication links in the EMS chain are necessary to accomplish these seven steps.

The call for help

Communication between the person requesting help and the dispatcher typically occurs via the public telephone system, ideally 9-1-1 or some other widely publicized emergency number. Many 9-1-1 systems display the address and phone number of a call's origin. This is referred to as enhanced or E 9-1-1. If the caller is incoherent or unsure of his or her location, E 9-1-1 is invaluable and potentially life-saving. Calls for help also may come into the communication center from other emergency agencies such as police or fire departments via nonpublic telephone or radio. Public agencies such as school districts, regional transit authority, or housing authorities may place calls for assistance as well.

> **Describe the responsibilities of an EMS dispatcher.**
>
> **Name the information that must be gathered from a caller by the dispatcher.**

Emergency Medical Dispatcher

The person with whom the caller comes into initial contact is typically the **Emergency Medical Dispatcher (EMD)**. The EMD plays an essential role in prehospital EMS systems (Fig. 4-3). The EMD must:

- Obtain, in a rapid and controlled manner, as much information about the emergency from the caller as possible.

- Direct the appropriate emergency response unit(s) to the scene.

- Provide prearrival medical instructions by telephone for the caller to follow until emergency care arrives.

- Monitor and oversee communications between EMS and other public safety personnel.

- Help to ensure the safety of the providers on scene (call for police, fire, hazardous materials team, or additional EMS units, if needed)

- Assist with the resolution of communication difficulties.

- Secure and maintain written records.

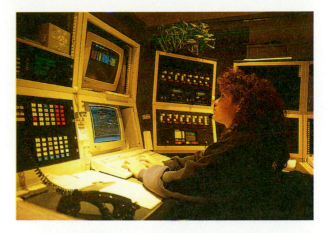

Fig. 4-3   An EMD is a critical part of the EMS chain of communication.

The EMD must gather key pieces of information from the caller including the:

- Location and nature of the emergency (the ambulance can be dispatched as soon as these are known)

- Call-back number (in case of accidental telephone disconnection)

- Specific information that will help in determining the resources needed to handle the case (*eg,* seriousness of the emergency, entrapment of victim(s), fire hazards on scene, etc.)

Once this essential information has been gathered, the EMD may find it necessary to provide prearrival telephone medical instructions to the caller. The provision of prearrival instructions may continue throughout the time the ambulance is being dispatched and responding to the scene. This instruction allows for the delivery of emergency care until the first responding unit arrives.

Next, the EMD must make appropriate decisions regarding which response vehicles to send to a scene. As such, the EMD must:

- Know the location of all units

- Know the capabilities (basic or advanced life support, specialty equipment, etc.) of the various units

- Determine if any support services are necessary

Initial dispatch communication

The initial communication between the EMD and the EMT–I often involves the EMD alerting the response team of an emergency call and directing them to the scene. This communication may be done through telephone notification, voice or digital radio communication, radio paging, tone-alert systems, and/or mobile data terminals. Initial dispatch communication usually includes the address, age, sex, and type of emergency to which the EMT–Is are to respond. Next, the EMT–Is typically recite the call information back to the EMD, confirming that the information has been communicated without error. While the EMS team is en route to the scene, the dispatch center may update them with additional information regarding the scene or patient.

Run times

From the time the call is received by the unit until it is back in quarters, a variety of communication takes place. At a minimum, the EMT–I calls the dispatch center when the unit is:

- En route to the scene
- On scene
- En route to the hospital
- Arriving at the hospital
- In service and returning to quarters
- Off the air at quarters

Some systems use mobile data terminals in the ambulance to transmit this information to the dispatch center. Sending the information may be as simple as pushing a button for each event time.

With each communication between the dispatch center and EMT–Is, the EMD will usually announce the time. For the purpose of clarity, military time (the 24-hour clock) is used.

Calling on scene

Next, the unit calls "on scene," advising the dispatch center of their arrival. Communications that immediately follow this call may include a scene survey or report from the EMT–Is of any hazards present. Additionally, assistance may be requested based on the number of patients found or the severity of the patient's condition.

Medical communications

If the patient's condition warrants, the next radio communication is between the EMT–Is and medical direction. The EMS team contacts medical direction for advice or to pass patient information to the receiving hospital. This communication can be done either on scene or en route to the hospital.

Calling en route to the hospital, on arrival, and "returning to service"

The EMT–Is call dispatch en route to the hospital and also on arrival at the hospital. Finally, the EMT–Is advise the dispatcher that they are "returning to service" when leaving the hospital.

If a call is completed without any patient being transported to the hospital, the EMT–Is advise the dispatcher of the reason, eg, "the patient refused transport" or "the patient was gone on our arrival."

Medical communications

 Describe two purposes of verbally communicating patient information to the hospital.

The EMT–I can bridge the gap between the prehospital setting and the emergency department by communicating findings and treatments provided to the medical direction physician or the receiving hospital. Depending on local, regional, or state requirements, this communication may be mandated by law or protocol. Most EMS systems have guidelines for when EMT–Is are to communicate patient or medical information. These communications may occur via radio, cellular telephone, or land line.

Purpose of medical communications

One of the most important purposes of medical communications is to obtain orders for patient care in the field. The EMS team also can solicit advice from medical direction when uncertain of the course of action to take with a given patient. Medical communication also provides the hospital with information regarding the patient's condition so the hospital can begin preparing to provide care. Communication with medical direction also can aid the EMT–I when dealing with obviously ill patients who are refusing care. A medical direction physician may be able to convince the patient of his or her need for treatment and/or hospital care. Medical direction also can resolve uncertainty as to the continuation or termination of resuscitation (eg, questionable "do not resuscitate" cases) and assist in resolving difficulties with non-EMS physicians who are interfering at the scene. Lastly, EMT–Is may find it useful to consult with a physician when patient transport is deemed unnecessary.

 List the patient assessment information that should be verbally reported to the physician.

Organize a list of patient assessment information in the correct order for radio transmission to the physician according to the format used locally.

The oral report

When communicating with the medical direction physician or the receiving hospital, an oral report should be given. EMT–Is must paint a clear picture of what they find on scene, remembering that they are the eyes and ears of the physician. A standard format should be employed to permit efficient use of radio time and allow the physician to quickly receive and assimilate information regarding the patient's condition (Fig. 4-4). Useful elements of the report, in the order they are given, include:

- Identification number and level of training of the provider
- Description of the scene
- Patient's age and sex
- Chief complaint
- Associated signs and symptoms
- Brief, pertinent history of the present illness

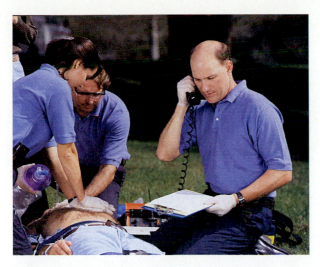

Fig. 4-4 A standard list of patient information allows the emergency department to receive and assume care of a patient quickly.

- Pertinent past medical history, medications, and allergies
- Physical examination findings, including:
  - Level of responsiveness
  - Vital signs
  - General appearance and degree of distress
  - Trauma index or Glasgow coma scale (if applicable)
  - Pertinent findings of the physical examination
- Treatment given so far
- Response to treatment
- Advanced life support given on standing orders
- Orders being requested
- Name of private physician
- Estimated time of arrival at the hospital

When communicating from the field, EMT–Is must provide the physician with a complete and accurate report. EMT-Is also must be prepared to provide additional information when requested.

Treatment instructions

Good communication skills are necessary if the patient is to receive appropriate treatment. Any treatment orders given by the physician should be repeated back by the EMT–I to prevent mistakes. The EMT–I also must be prepared to question orders that do not seem appropriate for the patient's condition, that are unclear, or the EMT–I is not authorized to perform. Once the orders have been carried out, the EMT–I should report the patient's response to treatment back to medical direction. The patient's vital signs should be reported to the medical direction physician with each medication administration.

Changes in the patient's condition also should be reported. These changes can be relayed to the hospital directly or through the communication center. The patient's privacy must be protected throughout all medical communications.

Notifying the receiving hospital

Hospitals must be notified of patients they will soon receive. This notification is an important element in the overall provision of care. If the emergency department knows of the patient's problem before his or her arrival at the hospital, they can mobilize resources, determine bed availability, and prepare teams within the hospital to deal with the patient's problems.

COMMUNICATIONS BASICS

 Describe three communication techniques that influence the clarity of radio transmission.

Recall how to properly use mobile and portable radios to receive and transmit information.

Proper radio use results in efficient and effective communications. However, there is more to proper radio use than picking up the microphone and speaking. Transmissions must be clear, and content must be concise and professional. When using the radio, the EMT–I should comply with the following rules (Fig. 4-5):

- Before beginning to talk, always listen to the frequency to be sure no one is transmitting.
- Press the transmission button on the microphone and wait 1 second before speaking.
- Keep the microphone approximately 2 to 3 inches from the mouth.
- Speak slowly and clearly, pronouncing each word distinctly.
- Speak in a normal pitch, keeping your voice free of emotion.
- Keep the transmission brief. If longer transmissions are needed, pause for a few seconds after every 30 seconds or so to allow other units to transmit information if needed.
- Give the name of the unit or number from which the call is originating. Next, address the unit being called (*eg*, "Dispatch center to Unit 5.").
- The unit being called should signal that they are ready to receive the communication by saying, "Go ahead." A response of, "Stand by," indicates that the unit is not ready to receive the communication.
- Always get confirmation that the message was received.
- Use proper unit numbers, hospital numbers, names, and titles.
- Do not use slang or profanity over the air.

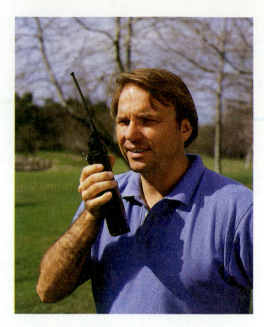

Fig. 4-5   Clear and concise messages given over the radio allow for better communication and patient care.

- Avoid using codes and abbreviations unless they are part of your system and everyone understands them.

- When transmitting a number that might be confused, give the number and then the individual digits.

- Receive the full message from the sender. Do not attempt to cut that person off so you can speak.

- Do not use a person's name or divulge confidential information that is not essential to the radio report.

- Because EMT–Is rarely act alone, use "we" instead of "I."

- Avoid words that are difficult to hear like "yes" or "no." Use "affirmative" and "negative."

- Use a standard format for transmitting information.

- Use EMS frequencies only for EMS communication.

- Before transmitting, reduce the background noise as much as possible by closing the window, or turning the volume down on other radios.

- When the medical direction physician gives treatment orders, they should be "echoed" (repeated back) to the physician.

 Describe the position of the antenna on a portable radio that will deliver maximum coverage.

- Hold portable radios in an upright (vertical) position to achieve maximum radio coverage.

It is important to understand that the air waves are public and that scanners are popular. EMS communications can be overheard by more than just the EMS community, and inappropriate language is subject to fines and penalties by the FCC. Additionally, unprofessional communication creates a bad public image. It can lead to a loss of credibility with colleagues in prehospital and hospital settings and in the EMT–Is own agency.

 STREET WISE
Portable radios carried on the belt are hard to hear in a large crowd or loud environment (eg, sporting events, civil disorders, construction sites, industrial plants). This problem can be overcome by equipping the portable radio with a remote microphone/ speaker. The microphone can then be attached to the shirt or coat pocket, collar, or epaulette so that the EMT-I can hear and be heard despite other noise. Alternatively, an ear piece is useful when the EMT-I does not want the radio to be heard.

SYSTEM MAINTENANCE

Communication equipment is costly and breakable. Dropping it, submerging it in water, or exposing it to harsh environments can cause damage. Additionally, beverages spilled onto radio equipment surfaces can harm the internal parts. Careful handling is essential.

 HELPFUL HINTS
Here are two simple precautions that, if followed, will significantly reduce the incidence of damage to radio equipment: 1) always carry your portable radio in a radio case and 2) never set soft drinks or coffee on radio consoles.

Radios are less likely to be dropped when carried in a case on your belt. If the radio is accidentally dropped, the case offers some protection, particularly if it is made of leather.

Soft drinks or coffee set on a radio console are likely to be spilled onto the radio. These liquids seep into the radio interior and damage the delicate internal radio parts. Far too many radios have been severely damaged this way.

Radios must be checked on an ongoing basis to ensure that they are working properly. Malfunctioning radio equipment should be repaired only by qualified individuals. Portable radio batteries should be recharged according to the manufacturer's instructions. Spare batteries should always be available.

Regular cleaning of radio equipment will improve its physical appearance. Exterior surfaces should be wiped with a moist cloth and mild detergent. Harsh cleaning agents should be avoided.

COMMUNICATIONS WITH THE PUBLIC

The EMS system continually interacts with the general public, which is responsible for funding the system. Public relations programs and the news media help make the public aware of the resources that the EMS system offers and helps teach the public about how and when to use the EMS system. Blood pressure screenings, demonstrations, open houses, extrication/disaster drills, short news spots, and programs on the dangers of drinking and driving all contribute to public awareness of the EMS system.

The news media also is valuable when vital information must be distributed quickly and/or to large communities. Evacuations due to weather or other disasters fall into this category.

Perhaps the least costly and most effective communication program is everyday contact with patients, family, and bystanders. Each run has the potential for wide public interaction, and serious events draw media coverage. Media involvement should be positive and productive; far-reaching damage can be inflicted to systems that disregard or antagonize these communications specialists.

Dealing with the press

EMS systems and their personnel are being increasingly thrust into positions of interaction with the news media (Fig. 4-6). These interactions can either boost public confidence or cause widespread public mistrust. In all situations, however, the patient comes first, and care cannot be delayed in favor of talking to a reporter.

Many EMS systems designate a public information officer (PIO) to design and implement public information programs and to respond to questions from the media.

Even when there is a PIO in your service, news reporters often want to get as close to the story as possible. This means they may request interviews with the EMT–Is who were on the scene or who directly experienced the topic of their story. As such, you may be called on to represent your service in a television, radio, or newspaper interview. Be sure to obtain permission from your agency before participating in an interview, because some EMS systems may prohibit such activities or require prior permission.

When giving an interview, remember the following:

- Relax and be yourself. Make your EMS system appear human.
- Know your system's policy on what kind of information can be released to the media.
- Use simple terms and explain information in such a way that a layperson can understand. Most

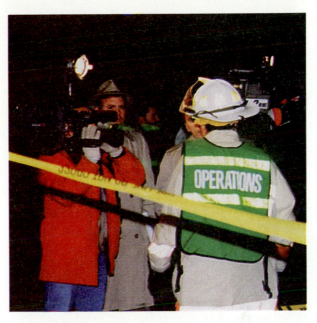

Fig. 4-6   The news media are often found at large-scale emergency scenes. Be prepared to interact accurately and professionally.

people won't understand work-related jargon, even though the reporter may.

- Brief yourself by reviewing the appropriate material beforehand (EMS run report, reference materials, etc.)
- Know what information is a matter of public record.
- Maintain patient confidentiality at all times.
- Speak clearly and be brief. Answer questions directly. Don't beat around the bush. Don't give more than you are asked.
- Give only the facts. If you don't have an answer to a question, don't speculate or guess.
- Take a few seconds to think of the appropriate response to questions you are asked. If uncertain, ask for clarification.
- After you answer a question, some reporters will say nothing, hoping you'll feel compelled to say more. Do not volunteer information. Instead, ask for the next question.
- If a reporter says, "Would you say . . . ," and then adds a quote for you to agree to, don't. Always make your own statement.
- Don't be fooled when reporters close their notebooks and say, "I know the official position, but just between us, how do you feel about it?" Nine times out of 10, they'll use the quote.
- Don't respond to "what if" questions. When you guess, what you say could return to haunt you.

- Some reporters will ask you two questions at once. Answer the first question and then ask the reporter to repeat the second question.

- Always anticipate other issues for which the reporter may be looking for answers. If you are unprepared for the question, take a few seconds to think of the appropriate answer. Don't be afraid to say, "I don't know" or "I don't have any comment on that issue."

Although the EMS team's top priorities are safety and patient care, news reporters may not recognize the importance of these two duties. If a reporter is hampering the EMT–I's ability to provide care, the EMT–I should first suggest that the reporter speak to someone else, then request that the reporter allow the crew to attend to the tasks at hand. If, after reasonable requests for cooperation, the reporter persists, the EMT–I should get assistance from the local police. However, the EMT–I must be certain that patient care, not his or her pride, is being compromised prior to soliciting police intervention.

Although the EMS system cannot expect the news media to be a cheerleader for them, they can expect to be treated fairly (especially if a good relationship already exists). To establish a positive working relationship with local media, try being responsive to their needs and honest when responding to inquiries.

STREET WISE
The lights of a video camera can be extremely useful when you are trying to provide patient care in a darkened area.

COMMUNICATIONS IN DISASTER SITUATIONS

Any number of problems can hinder communications during a disaster, including:

- Overloaded radio frequencies

- Incompatible frequencies between agencies

- Damage to the communications infrastructure

- General equipment failure

In disaster situations, the EMS communication system is a key component of a meaningful and organized response. EMS services must cooperate with other agencies in establishing guidelines for radio use in mass casualty or disaster events. A disaster plan should be in place to allow communications with other agencies and hospitals as well as emergency response and coordinating personnel. The plan must anticipate and provide for the breakdown of any component of the communication system and specify alternate means of communication. For example, during a disaster, telephone lines might not be available or may be overloaded. Guidelines must be in place for overriding the existing communication system components and

restricting nonessential communications. Emergency radios should be available in the event of landline failure, and alternate radio frequencies must be designated in case the usual channels become overloaded. It is important that all responders use a common language so that all "players" can understand each other. Avoid the use of codes that some responders may not understand.

In multicasualty incidents (MCIs), it is crucial that patients be dispersed to various hospitals without overloading a single emergency department. Tracking patients from the scene of the event to the destination is important. This requires a predetermined format designated to provide information and status of victims treated in the field by EMS personnel or designated first-aid areas. EMS personnel should design and test disaster communication procedures well in advance so that resources can be coordinated reliably under stress.

CASE HISTORY FOLLOW-UP

According to the attorney, EMT–I Walters' previous partner has a different memory of the event. In fact, he remembers applying a Kendrick extrication device and removing the patient from the wrecked car. He has no recollection of the patient's paralysis. Lucky for EMT–I Walters, his partner, the EMS service, and the hospital, the patient's contention that his paralysis resulted from inappropriate handling at the scene and at the emergency department can be dispelled.

EMS communications provide for an orderly and safe emergency response, allow for state-of-the-art prehospital patient care, and may sometimes help to protect the EMT–I and other members of the healthcare team from litigation. Had it not been for the clear and concise radio report taped by the hospital and the carefully documented prehospital care report, this case scenario may have had a much different outcome.

SUMMARY

A working knowledge of EMS communications is important for all prehospital care providers. Access to the system begins with the citizen and does not end until the patient is delivered to the hospital and the run report is completed. Effective and concise communication is required among all involved parties for the system to work.

Modern EMS communication systems have specific equipment needs. The typical configuration includes telephones, radios, repeater systems, and recording equipment. The most powerful radio in the system is the base station, with a typical power output of 45 to 275 watts.

The ambulance is equipped with mobile two-way radios and/or cellular communications to allow communication between:

- The EMS team and base station

- Other responding or on-scene units

- The EMS team and receiving hospitals or facility(s) providing medical direction

- Other public agencies (police and fire)

Portable radios are hand-held devices with a typical power output of 1 to 5 watts. Portable radios allow communications to take place while EMT–Is are away from the ambulance.

Poor output is sometimes a problem with mobile and portable radios. Repeater systems may be used to increase the range of these devices. Repeater systems are devices that receive transmissions from relatively low-wattage transmitters on one frequency and retransmit them at a higher power on another frequency. This increases the range of the transmissions.

Communication equipment is costly and breakable. Dropping it, submerging it in water, or exposing it to harsh environments can cause damage. Regular cleaning of the radio equipment will improve its physical appearance. Exterior surfaces should be wiped with a moist cloth and mild detergent.

The Federal Communications Commission (FCC) is the federal agency established to control and regulate all radio communications in the United States.

EMS communications can be broken down into three types: routine, emergency response, and patient care or medical related.

Skill and knowledge on the part of all parties (EMT–Is, EMDs) are required to communicate well on the radio. Transmissions must be clear, and the content must be concise and professional.

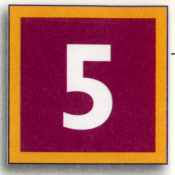

5 DOCUMENTATION

NARRATIVE	68 Y/O ♀ C/O CHEST PAIN/DISCOMFORT, IN MODERATE DISTRESS.

(HPI) PT. STATED THAT THE ONSET OF THE PAIN WAS WHILE WALKING. NO CHANGE IN PAIN ON PALPATION OR RESPIRATION. PT. DENIES RADIATION OF PAIN. ALSO DENIES SHORTNESS OF BREATH, NAUSEA OR VOMITING. PT. DESCRIBES THE PAIN AS CRUSHING IN NATURE. SEVERITY OF PAIN RATED AS A 6 ON A 1-10 SCALE. PT. STATED THAT THE PAIN BEGAN 1 HOUR PRIOR TO EMS ARRIVAL NOTIFICATION. (PMH) HIGH BLOOD PRESSURE, ANGINA. (MEDS) NTG, LANOXIN 0.125 mg. & TENORMIN 10mg NKDA (PE) PT. CAOX3 ASSESSMENT OF CHEST UNREMARKABLE. LUNGS CLEAR & (=). ABDOMEN SOFT, NON-TENDER. SKIN PINK, WARM & DRY. GOOD PULSES, SENSATION & MOTOR FUNCTION ALL EXTREMITIES. ⊖ SACRAL OR PERIPHERAL EDEMA. VITAL SIGNS AS NOTED BELOW. (RX) PT. WAS ALLOWED TO STAY IN A POSITION OF COMFORT. INITIAL ASSESSMENT COMPLETED. OXYGEN ADMINISTERED @ 15 LPM VIA NON-REBREATHER. FOCUSED HISTORY AND PHYSICAL EXAM COMPLETED. DR. JOHNSON @ COMMUNITY CONSULTED. ORDERS FOR ↑ SL NTG TABLET. PT. PLACED ON STRETCHER INTO AMBULANCE. ASSISTED WITH THE ADMINISTRATION OF NTG. PT. STATED THAT PAIN WAS RELIEVED. V/S REASSESSED. TRANSPORTED TO COMMUNITY HOSPITAL c̄ ONGOING ASSESSMENTS EN ROUTE.

● Narrative 1 of __1__

CASE HISTORY

EMT-I Johnson reports to work at 7:00 AM on Monday, ready for a typical EMS week of shootings, stabbings, and heart attacks. His supervisor hands him a subpoena to appear for a deposition the coming Wednesday morning and a manila envelope with a prehospital report from the call.

Johnson opens the envelope and begins to study the report. The call occurred just 2 weeks after he received his EMT–Intermediate certification. The report states that the call occurred on November 5th, at 2035, at 425 Miami Lane. The patient was Natalie Browning, age 23 years. Johnson wrote that her chief complaint was SOB and that she was combative and intoxicated on alcohol. Johnson recorded that he had to restrain her with hard restraints and that her behavior was obnoxious.

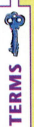

Upon completion of this chapter, the EMT–Intermediate should be able to:

- LIST the reasons for patient care documentation.
- RATIONALIZE the need for the EMS system to gather data.
- IDENTIFY the components of the written report and list the information that should be included on the written report.
- DESCRIBE what should be done when mistakes are made.
- DEFINE special considerations that must be exercised with a patient refusal.

LEARNING OBJECTIVES

KEY TERMS

ANATOMIC FIGURE

CHIEF COMPLAINT

DEMOGRAPHIC INFORMATION

DOCUMENTATION

HISTORY OF PRESENT ILLNESS/INJURY

NARRATIVE

PAST MEDICAL HISTORY

PERTINENT NEGATIVE

PERTINENT POSITIVE

RESPONSE TO TREATMENT

INTRODUCTION

The EMT–I has an obligation and a responsibility to accurately document each emergency response. Proper **documentation** should describe:

- A record of the scene
- The patient's chief complaint
- The patient's condition
- The nature and extent of emergency care given
- Changes in the patient's condition

In addition, documentation should include patient information such as name, address, age, and sex, as well as administrative information such as disposition of the call.

 List the reasons for patient care documentation.

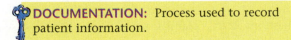 **DOCUMENTATION:** Process used to record patient information.

Reasons for patient care documentation

The EMS run report facilitates the continuation of care from the prehospital setting to the hospital setting by supplying vital information to the emergency department staff. It can point out improvement ("the patient became alert and oriented following the administration of 50% dextrose") or deterioration ("the patient's blood pressure dropped to 80/60 en route") in the patient's condition. The run report lists treatments administered, thus avoiding duplication of care in the emergency department. The report contains some information that would otherwise be unavailable to hospital staff after the EMT–I leaves, such as a description of the damage to an accident victim's car. A bent steering wheel or spider-webbed windshield can alert the hospital staff to look for injuries that might otherwise go unnoticed.

Medical direction performs quality improvement audits to monitor a system's compliance with standing orders. EMT–Is practice, at least with regard to invasive procedures, under the auspices of a licensed physician. The EMT–I's documentation provides a record of these procedures, not only for the EMT–I, but also for the medical director and the EMS system as a whole. Proper documentation demonstrates that the EMT–I adheres to appropriate protocols and that his or her care is in compliance with the law and meets the standard of care.

 Rationalize the need for the EMS system to gather data.

System need for EMS documentation

EMS run reports are a key source for data collection. The data from run reports guide system improvements, training programs, revenue collection, and research. Operational statistics, such as the times calls were received, the distances traveled, and the times ambulances arrived on the scene, properly correlated with geographic and definitive care considerations can help determine the most appropriate locations for stationing ambulances and other equipment. Patient care statistics can show which EMT–Is need additional training, such as continuing education and skill practice. Properly written run reports also can be used as training tools by illustrating how to keep good records or how to handle unusual or uncommon cases.

Permanent record

Once in the hospital, the run report usually becomes a permanent part of the patient's medical record. The length of time the medical record (including the run report) is kept by the hospital depends on statutes of limitations, accreditation, licensure, and other regulatory requirements. These requirements vary from state to state. Run reports concerning minors must be kept until the minor reaches legal age, plus any additional period of time as defined by statute or other requirements. Fear of lawsuits also influences the length of time a run report is kept. In some cases, lawsuits are filed years after the situation occurs. At some time during an EMT–I's career, he or she may be called on to explain the content of a run report in a deposition or in a courtroom, even if the case does not involve the EMT–I directly. Although many of today's lawsuits involve personal injury or product liability, the majority of cases against EMTs relate to improper care. Additionally, the run report may be used as part of a criminal investigation. The EMT–I may have seen and recorded something that can reveal a person's innocence or guilt. In any circumstance, for all those involved, the best protection is a thorough and accurate run report.

TYPES OF RUN REPORTS

Present types
There are many types of run reports in use today (Fig. 5-1 A, B). The run report may be referred to as the *prehospital report, ambulance call report, EMS sheet, trip ticket, trip sheet,* or any number of other names. The more traditional written form includes check boxes and sections for narrative. Some forms have an anatomic figure for labeling patient injuries or physical assessment findings. Scannable run reports, now used in many states, list treatments, assessment findings, past medical conditions, and so forth. To fill out a scannable run report, the EMT–I darkens in circles or boxes to show which items apply to each case. Most scannable run reports also have a narrative section where the EMT–I can further elaborate on the specifics of each case.

A run report form usually consists of an original and two or three copies. At least one copy is left at the emergency department, while the other copy and the original are used for EMS billing, quality assurance, or record-keeping purposes. Many systems use noncarbon reproduction (NCR) paper to keep expenses down and for its ease of use.

HELPFUL HINT
For legal purposes, the original copy of the run report usually is kept by the EMS system. A copy is then provided to the hospital.

Although run reports may be different in design and length, the basic data are generally the same. The content of the run report includes both administrative and clinical data.

The future
New technology has given us hand-held data entry computers, so-called "electronic clipboards." Electronic clipboards allow wireless transfer of patient information to the hospital before the patient even arrives (Fig. 5-2).

RULES FOR DOCUMENTING

STREET WISE
The golden rules of documentation: If it isn't documented, it will be assumed that it was not done, and if you didn't do it, don't document it.

Be objective
When documenting any aspect of the emergency case, the EMT–I must be objective, accurately describing what is seen. The EMT–I must be careful to avoid making assumptions about what has taken place.

Be specific
Generalizations, such as: "The patient was uncooperative," should be avoided. How was the patient unco-operative? Did the patient refuse care? Was he or she abusive toward the EMT–I or his or her partner(s)? Describe the patient's behavior as specifically as possible; for example, "Patient refused to be carried, insisting on walking to the ambulance."

Examples of general versus specific statements:	
Generalizations	**Specifics**
Patient looks sick	Patient has a grayish color to his skin.
Patient is intoxicated	Patient has slurred speech, staggering gait, etc.
Patient refused care	Patient refused to allow us to take his blood pressure or administer oxygen.

Special attention should be given to calls involving domestic violence, suspected abuse, or other situations that the EMT–I may be obligated to report to law enforcement agencies.

Write legibly
An illegible run report breaks down the continuity of patient care; if physicians and nurses cannot glean important information from it, it is of no value. Write legibly, clearly, and concisely. Printed writing is often more readable than cursive writing. Additionally, the EMT–I can be placed in an embarrassing situation if seated in a courtroom responding to questions from a plaintiff's attorney and the documentation is illegible.

Illinois • Emergency Medical Services NARRATIVE

SERVICE NAME	SERVICE #	TODAY'S DATE
INCIDENT LOCATION	HOSPITAL DESTINATION	

PATIENT INFO						
PATIENT LAST NAME	FIRST	M.I.	HOME PHONE #	AGE	DATE OF BIRTH
STREET ADDRESS					
CITY	STATE	ZIP CODE	LEGAL GUARDIAN		

ALLERGIES (MEDS) ◯ NONE KNOWN

CURRENT MEDICATIONS ◯ NONE KNOWN ◯ BROUGHT W/PT.

CHIEF COMPLAINT

NARRATIVE

NARRATIVE 1 OF ____

TIME	P	R	B/P	TEMP	BS	RHYTHM	TREATMENT	DOSE	ROUTE	02 SAT.	COMMENTS

LEFT	LUNG SOUNDS	RIGHT
Ⓘ Ⓛ	CLEAR	Ⓘ Ⓛ
Ⓘ Ⓛ	RHONCHI	Ⓘ Ⓛ
Ⓘ Ⓛ	RALES	Ⓘ Ⓛ
Ⓘ Ⓛ	WHEEZES	Ⓘ Ⓛ
Ⓘ Ⓛ	DIMINISHED	Ⓘ Ⓛ
Ⓘ Ⓛ	ABSENT	Ⓘ Ⓛ

SKIN TEMP			SKIN MOISTURE			SKIN COLOR			ABDOMEN		
Initial		Last	Initial		Last	Initial		Last	Initial		Last
☐	NORMAL	☐	☐	NORMAL	☐	☐	NORMAL	☐	☐	NORMAL	☐
☐	COOL	☐	☐	MOIST	☐	☐	PALE	☐	☐	SOFT	☐
☐	COLD	☐	☐	DRY	☐	☐	CYANOTIC	☐	☐	RIGID	☐
☐	HOT	☐	☐	WET	☐	☐	FLUSHED	☐	☐	DISTENDED	☐
☐	WARM	☐				☐	JAUNDICED	☐	☐	TENDER	☐
						☐	MOTTLED	☐			
						☐	ASHENED	☐			

SIGNATURE OF PERSON RECEIVING PATIENT

X ______________________

514313

CREW SIGNATURES DRIVER COMPLETED REPORT

CREW MEMBER 1 ______________ Ⓓ Ⓡ

CREW MEMBER 2 ______________ Ⓓ Ⓡ

CREW MEMBER 3 ______________ Ⓓ Ⓡ

CREW MEMBER 4 ______________ Ⓓ Ⓡ

(Signatures should correspond with license numbers on back of data sheet.)

Service/Provider Copy

Fig. 5-1A Many different types of run reports are used in EMS.

(Continued)

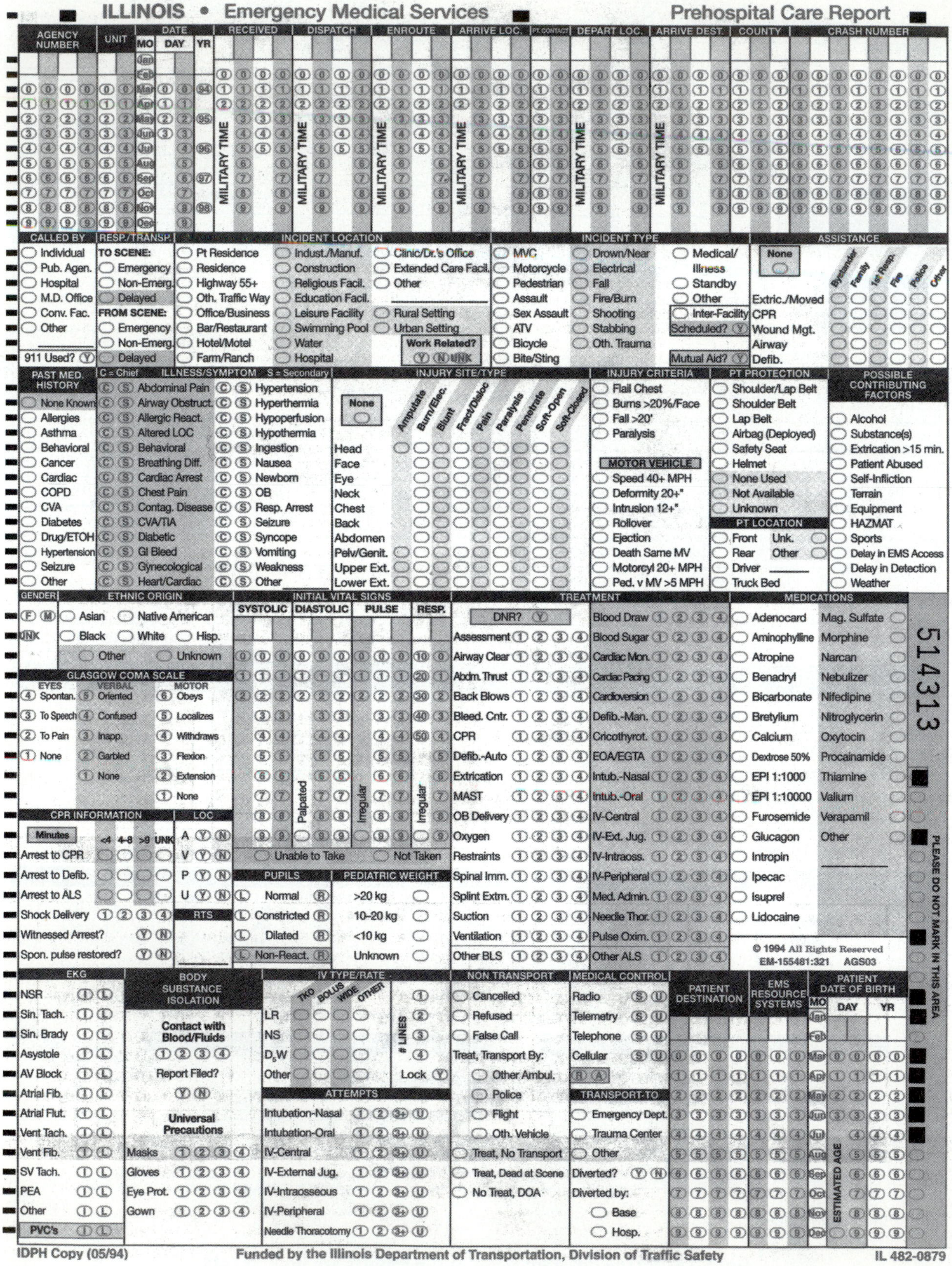

Fig. 5-1B Many different types of run reports are used in EMS.

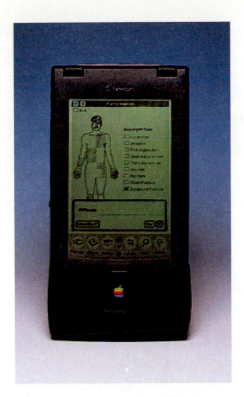

Fig. 5-2 Computer-based reporting systems allow EMT–Is to transfer patient information to the receiving facility using wireless technology.

Use a ball-point pen

To make the record permanent, the run report should be filled out using a ball-point pen. This makes it difficult to tamper with or erase information on the run report and results in the second and third copies of the report being more legible.

 HELPFUL HINT
Felt-tip pens are impractical for use in the prehospital care setting. They don't press through NCR type reports and tend to look sloppy, particularly if they get wet from rain or snow.

Use correct spelling

The EMT–I's run report is the first impression he or she makes on hospital staff and other personnel. Misspelled words (especially medical words) reflect poorly on the EMT–I's professionalism. If you do not know how to spell a word, find out, or use another word. You may find it helpful to carry a small dictionary or stow one in the ambulance.

Avoid soiling the report with blood, body fluids, or other liquids

In addition to looking bad, a soiled run report poses some health risks to people who handle it. Take appropriate measures to prevent the run report from being contaminated with blood, body fluids, or other liquids. Avoid filling out the run report while still wearing gloves that were used to treat the patient. Also, do not place the run report close to where patient care is occurring.

Coffee, rain, and other liquids also can render a run report illegible. Again, take precautionary measures to prevent the report from getting wet. Many run report clipboards have a storage compartment that keeps completed forms dry and protected.

Use abbreviations with care

Use of medical abbreviations can increase the amount of information the EMT–I can include on the run report and can allow information to be written down more quickly. However, because abbreviations can have multiple meanings, only use those that are approved by your EMS system. Many EMS systems maintain a list of acceptable medical abbreviations that can be used as part of the documentation.

Promptly record information

The longer you wait before writing down the patient care information, the less likely you are to remember it, especially if you respond to one call right after another. However, patient care should not be delayed or compromised in order to fill out the run report.

 STREET WISE
Sometimes, essential information such as vital signs can be written down on a piece of tape or other medium for later transcription.

 HELPFUL HINT
When the EMT–I only has a precious few minutes to get the patient to the ambulance, or when ongoing care must be provided *(ie,* in situations such as shootings or cardiac arrest), filling out the run report should wait until after arrival at the hospital.

Once at the hospital, the run report should be completed and copies left with the emergency department staff.

Be consistent

The run report must be consistent and accurate. If the patient's left arm is injured, care must be taken to avoid citing his right arm as the location of injury elsewhere in the report.

Be professional

Professional documentation is an obligation of the prehospital care provider. Remember that your run report can be subject to scrutiny by a variety of individuals, including hospital personnel, quality assurance personnel, supervisors, the court system, and the news media. Also, the patient or patient's family may request a copy of the run report. For these reasons the EMT–I must avoid making entries on the run report using street slang, flippant or derogatory remarks, such as the patient is "faking it," or is "a drunk." These types of remarks can come back to haunt you and your service. Likewise, complaints about being overworked, a lack of police protection, an unpleasant emergency department staff, and so forth have no place on the run report. These are best documented on an incident or complaint form issued for use within the EMS system.

Practice the skills

You can avoid pitfalls, enhance the delivery of patient care, reduce the risk of litigation, and promote the image of the EMT–I if you refine a few basic abilities such as grammar, spelling, and conciseness. It is often helpful to solicit feedback on the thoroughness and appearance of the run report from other members on the call before it is turned in. Review of run reports is an important part of the quality improvement process.

INFORMATION INCLUDED ON THE RUN REPORT

 Identify the components of the written report and list the information that should be included on the written report.

This section lists the general information usually requested on a run report. Your service will teach you how to fill out the specific run report you will be using (Fig. 5-3).

Dispatch information

The first block of information on the run report is the information received from the dispatcher. This information includes the address, nature of the call, priority level, run number, and time of dispatch. This information usually is recorded while the EMT–I is taking the call. In some EMS systems, this information is recorded via mobile data terminals in the ambulance.

If the patient's condition is relatively stable, one EMT–I can do the patient assessment while the other fills out the run report. This way, important information is immediately captured. This also improves the legibility of the report and improves the EMT–I's ability to provide care.

Care being provided before arrival

In some cases, the EMT–I arrives on the scene to find care being provided by first responders or bystanders. The delivery of this care must be documented by the EMT–I, by the first responder unit, or by both. Many first responder agencies use a specific form to record assessment findings and treatments provided to patients prior to arrival of the EMT–I. Two copies of

this report should be given to the EMT–I. One of these copies should be attached to the run report, and the other should go to the emergency department staff. In some states, this information is used to study the need for public education in CPR or first aid.

 CHIEF COMPLAINT: Brief statement describing the reason why the patient is seeking medical attention.

Chief complaint

The **chief complaint** is the medical problem that prompted the patient, family member, friend, or bystander to call for EMS assistance. When the chief complaint comes directly from the patient, it is considered *subjective* information. When listing the patient's complaint, use the patient's own words, if possible, using quotation marks:

- Patient states, "My chest hurts."
- Patient states, "I can't catch my breath."
- Patient states, "I felt dizzy and fell to the floor."
- Patient states, "I feel sick to my stomach."
- Patient states, "My head is killing me and I can't bend my neck."

If the patient is unresponsive or in cardiac arrest, the chief complaint should be reported as that. Obviously, this type of reporting is *objective* because the EMT–I can directly observe these conditions.

Important observations

Important observations that must be recorded might include child or elderly abuse or the presence of a suicide note, weapon, or mechanism of injury. If foul play is suspected, the surroundings must be examined more closely because the scene can change before law enforcement personnel arrive. If a parent states, "My son fell off the swing in our back yard," the EMT–I's partner should check the back yard for a swing. If there is no swing, this information should be noted. Note the location where the injury occurred, such as on a roadway, sidewalk, and so forth. Some run reports also ask whether the patient was wearing or using safety equipment such as a helmet or seat belt. Whenever information is of a sensitive nature, note the source of that information.

When the patient refuses treatment or transport, you must thoroughly document the situation, assessment findings (vital signs, physical examination, and so forth) and treatments provided. Clearly state the patient's reason for refusing treatment or transport. Also, record your explanation to the patient of the possible consequences of refusing treatment or transfer. The number of times the patient was advised of the need to be transported also should be noted and the names of the persons who witnessed the refusal should be listed.

Use Blue/Black Ink - Press Firmly

| SERVICE NAME COMMUNITY AMBULANCE | SERVICE # 02165 | INCIDENT # 95-1379 | TODAY'S DATE 03 16 96 |

INCIDENT LOCATION 123 MAIN STREET

PATIENT INFO

| PATIENT LAST NAME SMITH | FIRST JANE | M.I. C. | PHONE 555-1212 | AGE 68 | DATE OF BIRTH 02 04 27 | SEX F |

STREET ADDRESS 123 MAIN STREET

SOCIAL SECURITY NUMBER 1 2 3 - 4 5 - 6 7 8 9   MEMBERSHIP ● Yes Ⓝ No

| CITY ANYTOWN | STATE PA | ZIP CODE 15123 | INSURANCE CODE # | | MILEAGE |

PRIVATE PHYSICIAN DR. MARTINEZ   MEDICAID #   OUT 24652

○ BILL TO (COMPANY or NAME)   PHONE   MEDICARE #   SCENE 24656

ADDRESS N/A   STREET   GROUP INSURANCE #   DEST 24666

CITY   STATE   ZIP CODE   OTHER INSURANCE #   IN 24678

CHIEF COMPLAINT CHEST PAIN/DISCOMFORT

CURRENT MEDICATIONS ○ NONE KNOWN   NTG, LANOXIN 0-125 MG., TENORNIM

ALLERGIES (MEDS) ● NONE KNOWN   NKDA

PAST MEDICAL HISTORY ○ MI ○ CHF ○ COPD ● ↑BP ○ DIABETES ○ CANCER ○ NONE KNOWN ● OTHER ANGINA

NARRATIVE 68 Y/O ♀ C/O CHEST PAIN/DISCOMFORT, IN MODERATE DISTRESS.
(HPI) PT. STATED THAT THE ONSET OF THE PAIN WAS WHILE WALKING. NO
CHANGE IN PAIN ON PALPATION OR RESPIRATION. PT. DENIES RADIATION
OF PAIN. ALSO DENIES SHORTNESS OF BREATH, NAUSEA OR VOMITING.
PT. DESCRIBES THE PAIN AS CRUSHING IN NATURE. SEVERITY OF PAIN
RATED AS A 6 ON A 1-10 SCALE. PT. STATED THAT THE PAIN BEGAN 1 HOUR
PRIOR TO EMS NOTIFICATION. (PMH) HIGH BLOOD PRESSURE, ANGINA. (MEDS) NTG,
LANOXIN 0.125 mg. & TENORNIM 10mg. NKDA (PE) PT. CAOx3, ASSESSMENT OF
CHEST UNREMARKABLE. LUNGS CLEAR & Ⓔ. ABDOMEN SOFT, NON-TENDER.
SKIN PINK, WARM & DRY. GOOD PULSES, SENSATION & MOTOR FUNCTION ALL
EXTREMITIES. ⊖ SACRAC OR PERIPHERAL EDEMA. VITAL SIGNS AS NOTED BELOW.
(RX) PT. WAS ALLOWED TO STAY IN A POSITION OF COMFORT. INITIAL ASSESSMENT
COMPLETED. OXYGEN ADMINISTERED @ 15 LPM VIA NON-REBREATHER. FOCUSED
HISTORY AND PHYSICAL EXAM COMPLETED. DR. JOHNSON @ COMMUNITY CONSULTED.
ORDERS FOR ↑ SL NTG TABLET. PT. PLACED ON STRETCHER INTO AMBULANCE.
ASSISTED WITH THE ADMINISTRATION OF NTG. PT. STATED THAT PAIN WAS
RELIEVED. V/S REASSESSED. TRANSPORTED TO COMMUNITY HOSPITAL
c̄ ON GOING ASSESSMENTS EN ROUTE.

● Narrative 1 of 1

TIME	P	R	B/P	RHYTHM	TREATMENT	PROVIDER ID #	RESPONSE/COMMENTS
1000					ASSESSMENT, O₂	067133	15 LPM VIA NON-REBREATHER
1005	88	18	128/76		FOCUSED Hx, P.E. VITALS	062247	
1008					STRETCHER	CREW	POSITION OF COMFORT
1010	88	16	128/76		VITALS/CONSULT	067133	ORDERS = ↑ SL NTG
1012					ASSISTED NTG	062247	PT. FELT RELIEF
1014	86	16	120/70		VITALS	062247	
1019	86	16	122/74		VITALS	062247	PT. PAIN FREE NOW

Signature of Person Receiving Patient *[signature]*   Time

Command Physician DR. JOHNSON   1234   ID#

Crew Signatures:
A#1 *[signature]*
A#2
A#3 *[signature]*
A#4

Service Copy

Fig. 5-3 A completed run report.

Present medical history

Next, the EMT–I must document the patient's **history of present illness/injury**. This history should be recorded in chronologic order and should include the time of onset, frequency, location, quality, character of the problem, setting, and anything that aggravates or alleviates the problem. An EMT–I recording the history of a patient with chest pain may write, "The patient states his chest pain started approximately 1 hour ago while he was watching his granddaughter roller skate. He reports it as a constant pain beneath his breastbone, that radiates to his left arm. The patient described it as an aching pain that is unrelieved with nitroglycerin, which he reports to have taken 10 minutes ago." **Pertinent positives** and **pertinent negatives** should also be recorded.

Past medical history

After recording the patient's present history, the EMT–I should document any significant **past medical history,** including surgeries, hospitalizations, illnesses, injuries, allergies, current medications the patient is taking, and the last meal the patient ingested. The name of the patient's physician also should be listed.

Physical assessment findings

Next, the EMT–I should record the physical assessment findings. The EMT–I should begin by reporting how the patient was found on arrival; *eg,* "Patient found sitting on edge of bed," "patient ambulatory," or "patient greeted us at his front door." This assessment includes the patient's vital signs, level of responsiveness, respiratory rate and character, pulse rate and character, blood pressure, skin color and temperature, capillary refill (if appropriate), and the findings of the secondary examination. Repeat vital signs provide important information regarding changes in the patient's condition over time and must be documented on the run report. The vital signs section usually includes space to record multiple sets of vital signs and the time each was taken. This information is particularly important in situations in which the patient is seriously ill or injured or his or her condition is changing for the better or worse. Pertinent positives or negatives, such as "the patient denies shortness of breath and nausea" also should be noted.

Treatments provided

Following documentation of the physical findings, the EMT–I should record the treatment provided to the patient. Many treatments can be noted by checking a box, but others must be described in the **narrative** section of the run report. This documentation should include what procedure was performed, who performed it, and at what time. Delivered treatments should be described in appropriate detail. Instead of only stating "oxygen was administered," identify the liter flow rate, device used, and time initiated, *eg,* "15 L of oxygen administered via nonrebreather mask, started at 2215."

Documentation of invasive or advanced treatments should note whether the treatment was performed with permission of on- or off-line medical direction.

Examples of proper narrative reports:

- *IV of D5W, 18-gauge needle to right antecubital fossa, microdrip administration set, run TKO, established at 1805 according to standing orders.*

- *Proventil, 0.25 ML by inhalation, administered at 0804 per medical direction (MD1).*

When documenting orders from on-line medical direction, the identification number of the physician (or other medical professional) who authorized care to be given should be listed as well.

Treatments that are attempted without success and problems with delivering treatment should be noted on the run report. Include a brief description of the problem and your identification number or initials.

Response to treatment

The patient's **response to treatment** should be noted. Likewise note any other changes, both positive and negative, in the patient's condition. These changes can reveal important information about the patient's condition.

The following are examples of a patient's response to treatment:

- Chest pain or shortness of breath that subsides with oxygen administration
- Severe leg pain that disappears after application of a traction splint
- Chest pain that subsides after the patient takes a nitroglycerin tablet
- Patient who goes from having diminished level of responsiveness to being alert
- Patient who has trouble breathing when he or she is placed in a supine position

When completing the narrative portion of the run report, you can use a supplemental sheet if you are running out of room. Do not sacrifice clarity for brevity.

 DEMOGRAPHIC INFORMATION: Includes patient's name, address, age, phone number, and parent's name if the patient is a minor.

Demographic and billing information

Collect all patient **demographic information** such as name, age, sex, date of birth, address, and phone number. In some systems you also may be required to obtain billing information such as type of medical insurance. Some run reports even request the patient to sign his or her name as a means of expediting the billing process.

> **STREET WISE**
> When the patient's condition allows, document pertinent patient information such as name, address, age, medical insurance information, and present and past medical histories before transporting the patient to the hospital. It often is difficult to hear the patient or complete the narrative portion of the report while the ambulance is moving.

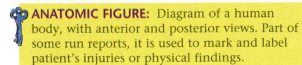 **ANATOMIC FIGURE:** Diagram of a human body, with anterior and posterior views. Part of some run reports, it is used to mark and label patient's injuries or physical findings.

Anatomic figure

If applicable and included in the run report, circle or shade in the areas of the **anatomic figure** to represent the affected area(s) of the patient's body. Do not limit this use of the diagram to injuries, because certain medical conditions or physical assessment findings can be highlighted using this type of chart.

Run times

In the administrative section of many EMS run reports, there is space to record your run times.

Times that are recorded include dispatch, en route to the call, arrival on scene, departure time from scene, arrival at the hospital, transfer of care, and back in-service (available for the next call). Some reports include a place to indicate when the EMT–I actually reaches the patient. This information helps show the actual time to treatment for each incident. These times are recorded using military times.

Military times		
00 hours	=	12:00 AM
0100 hours	=	1:00 AM
0200 hours	=	2:00 AM
0300 hours	=	3:00 AM
0400 hours	=	4:00 AM
0500 hours	=	5:00 AM
0600 hours	=	6:00 AM
0700 hours	=	7:00 AM
0800 hours	=	8:00 AM
0900 hours	=	9:00 AM
1000 hours	=	10:00 AM
1100 hours	=	11:00 AM
1200 hours	=	12:00 PM
1300 hours	=	1:00 PM
1400 hours	=	2:00 PM
1500 hours	=	3:00 PM
1600 hours	=	4:00 PM
1700 hours	=	5:00 PM
1800 hours	=	6:00 PM
1900 hours	=	7:00 PM
2000 hours	=	8:00 PM
2100 hours	=	9:00 PM
2200 hours	=	10:00 PM
2300 hours	=	11:00 PM

Run disposition

You must note the disposition of the call, including whether the patient is gone on your arrival, refuses transportation, or is handed over to another ambulance crew. When applicable, you also must note to which hospital the patient is transported. Some EMS systems use numbers to denote the hospital identification. Any direct radio or cellular telephone communication with the hospital or your medical direction facility should be indicated on the run report as well.

Signatures

Lastly, the run report is usually signed (or at least the names clearly printed) by all personnel responsible for the run. This signature includes the first initial, last name, and professional credentials. Signatures must be legible. Some EMS systems, however, only require that EMT—Is record their identification number.

WHEN A MISTAKE IS MADE

 Describe what should be done when mistakes are made.

Fixing mistakes

There is a right way and a wrong way to correct mistakes. Do not destroy the run report and start over again. Draw a single, horizontal line through the incorrect entry, so that it is still legible (Fig. 5-4). Indicate that the crossed-out entry is an error and initial it. The correct information should then be written beside it. You may want to document the reason for the correction and/or have it witnessed. Make every effort to ensure that your correction cannot be interpreted as tampering.

Documenting late entries

If an entry is added after a run report has been completed, the time and date of the entry, as well as an explanation for its lateness, should be written next to it. No attempt should be made to cover up the fact that it is a late entry.

Documenting deviations from protocol

If the normal protocol or standard of care is not followed, document the reason why and what steps were taken (if any) to correct the situation. Specify whether medical direction was notified of the problem. Also, document any delays or problems responding, gaining access, or transporting the patient. Include an explanation of the problem (eg, weather conditions, traffic congestion) and the length of the delay.

Alternatively, in some EMS systems, the EMT–Is do not make corrections directly on the run report. Rather, corrections are documented on a supplemental form and attached to the run report.

Documenting questionable medical direction

Occasionally, the EMT–I may be directed by medical direction to administer a medication or dose that seems to be inappropriate or inconsistent with established protocols. Record the facts of the incident and how it was handled.

Tampering with the run report

Tampering with the run report can cause serious trouble for the EMT–I. Changing or obliterating the run report can provide a plaintiff's attorney with information to use against the EMT–I, even though he or she may be completely innocent. Erasures, scratching or crossing out an entry, tearing or cutting off a portion of a report, using correction fluid or ink markers, or squeezing an entry between lines of a report may be interpreted as tampering, even if tampering was not the intent.

NARRATIVE 68 Y/O ♀ C/O CHEST PAIN / DISCOMFORT, IN MODERATE DISTRESS.
(HPI) PT. STATED THAT THE ONSET OF THE PAIN WAS WHILE WALKING. NO
CHANGE IN PAIN ON PALPATION OR RESPIRATION. PT. DENIES RADIATION
OF PAIN. ALSO DENIES SHORTNESS OF BREATH, NAUSEA OR VOMITING.
PT. DESCRIBES THE PAIN AS CRUSHING IN NATURE. SEVERITY OF PAIN
RATED AS A 6 ON A 1-10 SCALE. PT. STATED THAT THE PAIN BEGAN 1 HOUR
PRIOR TO EMS ~~ARRIVAL~~ NOTIFICATION. (PMH) HIGH BLOOD PRESSURE, ANGINA.
(MEDS) NTG, LANOXIN 0.125 mg. & TENORMIN 10 mg. NKDA (PE) PT. CAOX3 ASSESSMENT
OF CHEST UNREMARKABLE. LUNGS CLEAR & ⊜. ABDOMEN SOFT, NON-TENDER.
SKIN PINK, WARM & DRY. GOOD PULSES, SENSATION & MOTOR FUNCTION ALL
EXTREMITIES. ⊖ SACRAL OR PERIPHERAL EDEMA. VITAL SIGNS AS NOTED BELOW.
(RX) PT. WAS ALLOWED TO STAY IN A POSITION OF COMFORT. INITIAL ASSESSMENT
COMPLETED. OXYGEN ADMINISTERED @ 15 LPM VIA NON-REBREATHER. FOCUSED
HISTORY AND PHYSICAL EXAM COMPLETED. DR. JOHNSON @ COMMUNITY CONSULTED
ORDERS FOR ↑ SL NTG TABLET. PT. PLACED ON STRETCHER INTO AMBULANCE.
ASSISTED WITH THE ADMINISTRATION OF NTG. PT. STATED THAT PAIN WAS
RELIEVED. V/S REASSESSED. TRANSPORTED TO COMMUNITY HOSPITAL
c̄ ONGOING ASSESSMENTS EN ROUTE.

● Narrative 1 of __1__

Fig. 5-4 The proper way to correct a mistake on a run report.

Falsifying information

Falsification of information on the run report can have severe consequences. It can lead to suspension or revocation of your certification or license, and it increases the risk of poor patient care. Accurate care cannot be provided by paramedics or emergency department staff if they are working with inaccurate information. Remember, your run report can be compared with the hospital chart.

CONFIDENTIALITY

Maintaining patient confidentiality is a major responsibility of the EMT–I, one that must be taken very seriously. Information recorded on the run report is considered confidential. For this reason, care is used to prevent unauthorized persons from having access to its contents. EMS systems have a responsibility to properly educate their membership (employees) on the importance of patient confidentiality. Some states have laws and regulations concerning confidentiality of patient care records. Although the run report is a confidential document, it is routinely reviewed by multiple individuals. Whether being used for continuity of care, reimbursement, legal issues, education, research, quality assurance, or other significant requirements, the run report is constantly being evaluated. As such, great care must be taken to protect the patient's right to confidentiality while allowing for necessary use of data contained on the form. During quality improvement and training activities, the patient's name should be crossed out or blackened.

 Define special considerations that must be exercised with a patient refusal.

DOCUMENTATION OF PATIENT REFUSAL

Competent adult patients have the right to refuse treatment. However, before leaving the scene, the EMT–I should try to persuade the patient to go to a hospital. It is absolutely essential that the EMT–I ensures that the patient is able to make a rational, informed decision. Patients under the influence of alcohol or other drugs or who are experiencing diminished mental capacity due to illness or injury should not be asked to sign a refusal.

If the patient absolutely refuses care or transport (and is able to make a rational, competent decision), document any assessment findings and emergency medical care given, then have the patient sign a refusal form. Some EMS systems use a separate refusal form, whereas others include the refusal as part of the run report. Have a police officer or bystander sign the form as a witness. If the patient refuses to sign the refusal form, have a police officer or bystander sign the form verifying that the patient refused to sign. If no other witnesses are available, it may be necessary to ask a family member to sign as a witness. When obtaining signatures from witnesses, record the correct spelling of each name, along with an address and phone number (if available), as it may be difficult to read the witness's signature.

Both patient confidentiality and patient refusal are discussed further in Chapter 3, "Medical/Legal Considerations."

DOCUMENTATION OF MULTIPLE CASUALTY INCIDENTS

When treating more than one patient at a time, a run report must be completed for each patient. In the case of multiple casualty incidents, you may have to complete the documentation after delivering the patients to the hospital. The local multiple casualty incident plan typically tells the EMT–I how to temporarily record important medical information. The standard for completing the form in an MCI is not the same as for a typical call. Often, the EMT–I must do the best he or she can with the limited information available.

SPECIAL SITUATION REPORTS

Special situations include suspected child abuse or abuse of the elderly, equipment failure, and/or complaints about the EMT–I's care or demeanor. You may be obligated to report these or other situations to local authorities, and in some cases this requires a special report form. Other supplemental reports may include documentation of exposure to infectious disease, accident or injury reports, and hazardous materials reports.

Supplemental reports must be submitted in a timely manner, and must be accurate and objective. When completing this type of report the EMT–I should keep a copy for his or her own records. The report and other copies should be submitted to the authority specified by local protocol.

CASE HISTORY FOLLOW-UP

EMT-I Johnson becomes uneasy, then agitated, as he considers the documentation errors on the run report. He realizes that the errors in judgment could cost his employer thousands of dollars and possibly a great deal of negative publicity. They could also cost Johnson his job and ruin his chances for promotion. After 2 years of experience as an EMT–Intermediate and some distance from the call, the errors are obvious to Johnson.

First, when he recorded the patient's chief complaint as "SOB," Johnson didn't use an abbreviation approved by his service. Although SOB may mean "shortness of breath" to an EMT, it may mean something different—and demeaning—to a jury.

Second, Johnson reported that the patient was "intoxicated on alcohol." Facing deposition, Johnson is now aware that he had no way of knowing that the patient was intoxicated on alcohol because he hadn't seen her drinking any alcoholic beverages, nor did he have any confirming laboratory results.

Last, Johnson reported that the patient was "combative" and that he had to restrain her with "hard restraints." Although restraining her *was* necessary, there was no documentation that she required only hand restraints, nor that she attempted to bite him and his partner, nor that he requested police assistance. Now, Johnson realizes how hard it will be to justify to a jury restraining the patient with straps.

SUMMARY

Learning to write organized, efficient run reports is an integral part of being an EMT–I. The EMT–I must accurately document all the events of each case. The run report should be a positive reflection on the excellence of the EMT–I and the EMS system. The run report provides for a continuum of care by communicating how the patient was found on the EMT–I's arrival, what care was provided, and how the patient's condition changed over time. Proper documentation also helps to protect the EMT–I against unfounded lawsuits and serves as an important data source for quality improvement activities.

Although there are many different types of run reports in use today, they all at least include patient and administrative information. The run report usually consists of an original and one or two copies. One copy is left with the patient at the hospital to be entered into his or her patient record, supplying the hospital staff with information they might not otherwise be able to access.

The run report must be concise, accurate, and legible. When completing the report, use a ball-point pen, and avoid using abbreviations unless they are approved by the EMS system.

Key information includes the patient's demographic information (name, address, age, sex, phone number, etc.) and patient information (patient complaint, present history, past history, treatments delivered, etc.). Remember, if it wasn't written in the report, it wasn't done.

When an error or omission occurs, be sure to follow the appropriate procedure to correct the problem. The EMT–I must never allow false information to enter the patient record.

If a patient refuses care, document it appropriately and get signatures from both the patient and a witness. Patients experiencing diminished mental status must not be allowed to refuse care.

Be careful to document information carefully and professionally. Keep in mind that the run report becomes a part of patients' permanent medical record and may be viewed by many others both inside and outside the EMS system.

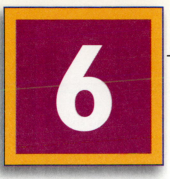

6

MEDICAL TERMINOLOGY

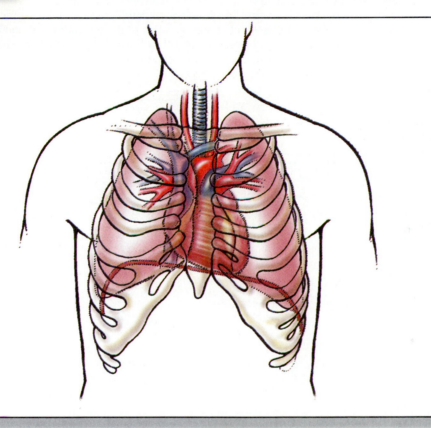

CASE HISTORY

EMT–I Douglas is working as an EMS preceptor today for a local training program. Julie, the student assigned to him, is young and energetic and he's been warned by her instructor that she tends to be a little "over enthusiastic." She has helped with the morning duties at the base and has just finished checking out the equipment in the rig. EMT–I Douglas and his partner are having a cup of coffee and talking with Julie about base operations when the alarm sounds. "Unit 4...Respond to 1354 Clark Street...Difficulty breathing...Time out 0833." En route, Dispatch advises that the patient is a man aged 60 years with a history of heart failure.

While responding to the scene, EMT–I Douglas and Julie discuss what her patient-care responsibilities will be on this call. Her initial duties will be to apply oxygen and attach the ECG electrodes. If the man is stable, EMT–I Douglas agrees to let Julie perform the physical examination, call in the radio report to the hospital, and start an IV line if needed.

Case History, continued

On arrival at the scene, EMT–I Douglas finds the patient sitting in a chair in his living room. He is anxious and in moderate respiratory distress. Oxygen is administered by mask, vital signs are assessed, and ECG electrodes are applied. Julie gathers a focused history from the patient and performs a detailed physical assessment. EMT–I Douglas and his partner stay in the background and evaluate Julie's patient-care skills. She seems confident and is doing a good job. The patient appears less anxious and his respirations are improved. Julie completes the assessment and contacts medical direction.

During her radio report, it becomes obvious that Julie is unfamiliar with communication protocols. The report is disorganized and difficult to follow, and she stumbles with the pronunciation of the patient's medications and previous medical history. The emergency department nurse taking the report is obviously frustrated and asks her to repeat much of the information. The IV request is denied, and the nurse advises Julie to "just transport the patient." En route to the hospital, EMT–I Douglas contacts medical direction and repeats the patient report. An authorization for the IV is obtained.

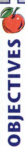

LEARNING OBJECTIVES

Upon completion of this chapter, the EMT–Intermediate should be able to:

- EXPLAIN the meaning of medical terminology.
- PROVIDE three examples of each of the following: word root, prefix, suffix, combining form, and combining vowel.
- EXPLAIN the importance of pronunciation and spelling of medical terms.
- IDENTIFY common medical abbreviations from a list.
- DESCRIBE the four planes of the human body.
- DESCRIBE the main directional terms for the human body.
- DESCRIBE the six normal body movements.
- DESCRIBE the anatomic postures of the body.

KEY TERMS

ABBREVIATIONS	MEDIAL
ANTERIOR	MIDSAGITTAL
CAUDAL	POSTERIOR
COMBINING FORM	PREFIX
COMBINING VOWEL	PROXIMAL
CRANIAL	SAGITTAL
DISTAL	SUFFIX
FRONTAL	SUPERIOR
INFERIOR	TRANSVERSE
LATERAL	WORD ROOT

MEDICAL TERMINOLOGY

 Explain the meaning of medical terminology.

Medical terminology differs from "plain English" in that it is a special vocabulary used in the medical field. Whenever an unfamiliar word is used, you must learn its meaning, spelling, pronunciation, and proper usage. Learning medical terminology is an ongoing process of vocabulary building. Consistent use of a medical dictionary is essential. Understanding medical terms will help you communicate with members of the healthcare team, such as doctors, nurses, paramedics, and other EMTs.

Medical terms often can seem complex in their spelling and pronunciation. They can be confusing and overwhelming unless you know how they came into being and what they mean. It is much easier to remember the meaning of a medical term if you know where it came from. Most medical terms come from Greek or Latin words. The original words and their meanings are interesting; *eg, muscle* comes from a Latin word for "mouse." It was thought that the movement of a muscle under the skin resembled the scampering of a mouse. The coccyx, the lower end of the spine, is named for the cuckoo because it was thought to resemble the cuckoo's bill.

 Provide three examples of each of the following: word root, prefix, suffix, combining form, and combining vowel.

Word building

Whenever you encounter a new word, try to break it up into its component parts. Some medical terms are very long, but they become less threatening when broken into smaller parts. If you can figure out the meaning of each part of a word and then combine the meanings, you will have the essential meaning of the word. Many medical words consist of two or three parts: the prefix (beginning), the word root (center), and the suffix (end) (Table 6-1).

Word roots

The foundation of a word is the **word root.** The word root establishes the basic meaning of the word and is the part to which the prefixes (before) and suffixes (after) are added. Some word roots are complete words, but not all. The same word root may have different meanings in different fields of study. You may have to consider the context of a word before assigning its meaning.

Suffix, prefix, affix, and fixation all have *fix* as their word root.

WORD ROOT: The foundation of a word; establishes the basic meaning of a word.

Some words contain more than one word root. Each word root retains its basic meaning in the word

(*see* Table 6-2 for some common word roots). These words are called *compounds*. Simple examples of compound words containing two word roots are *frostbite* and *bedpan*. A more complicated example is *osteoarthritis*. The combining form *osteo* comes from the word root *oste*, meaning bone. The word root *arthr* means joint or joints. The suffix *-itis* means inflammation. Therefore the combining word *osteoarthritis* means inflammation of the bone joints.

Prefixes

A **prefix** introduces another thought or explains the word root (Table 6-3). It is added before the word root and changes or adds to its meaning. For example, the prefix *sub-* in subcutaneous means below. The word *cutaneous* means skin, therefore subcutaneous is below the skin. Another word, *atypical*, which means not typical, can be easily understood when you know that it is formed by adding the prefix *a-*, meaning not, to *typical*, which is the word root.

Other examples of prefixes:

The word root *-pnea* means breath. If we add the prefix *a-*, meaning not, we have the new word *apnea*, meaning without breath.

The word root *-logy* means study of. If we add the prefix *bio-* we have the new word biology, meaning the study of life.

The word root *-cardia* means heart. If we add the prefix *brady-*, meaning slow, we have the new word *bradycardia*, meaning slow heart.

PREFIX: A sequence of letters that comes before the word root and often describes a variation of the norm.

Suffixes

SUFFIX: A sequence of letters that occurs at the end of the word, that often describes a condition of or act performed on the word root.

The **suffix** is added at the end of a word and changes or adds to its meaning (Table 6-4). For example, the suffix *-ase* indicates an enzyme. Lipase (*lip-*, meaning fat, plus *-ase*) is an enzyme that digests fats. Gastritis, meaning inflammation of the stomach, is a combination of the word root *gastr-*, meaning stomach, and the suffix, *-itis*, meaning inflammation.

Examples of suffixes:

The word root *neur-* means nerve. If we add the suffix *-algia*, meaning pain, we have the new word *neuralgia*, meaning pain along a nerve.

The word root *psych-* means the mind. If we add the suffix *-osis*, meaning condition, we have the new word *psychosis*, meaning condition of the mind.

The word root *hepato-* means liver. If we add the suffix *-megaly*, meaning enlargement, we have the new word *hepatomagaly*, meaning enlargement of the liver.

TABLE 6-1	Word Building

Pericardium

peri- is a prefix meaning *around.*

-cardi is a word root meaning *heart.*

Pericardium is a membrane around the heart.

(The pericardium is a sac that encloses the heart, holding in fluid.)

Pericarditis

peri- is a prefix meaning *around.*

-cardi is a word root meaning *heart.*

-itis is a suffix meaning *inflammation.*

Pericarditis means inflammation around the heart.

(In pericarditis, the pericardium becomes inflamed due to a microorganism or a variety of other causes.)

Myocardium

my/o is a combining form meaning *muscle.*

-cardi is a word root meaning *heart.*

Myocardium means heart muscle.

(The myocardium is the middle and thickest tissue of the heart, which is composed of cardiac muscle.)

Endotracheal

endo- is a prefix meaning *inside of.*

trache/o is a combining form for *trachea,* or the *windpipe.*

trache/al means pertaining to the *trachea.*

Endotracheal means pertaining to the inside of the trachea.

(In endotracheal intubation a tube is inserted through the mouth or nose into the trachea to open an airway.)

Pyromania

pyr/o- is a combining form meaning *fire.*

-mania is a suffix that means *excessive preoccupation.*

Pyromania is excessive preoccupation with fire.

(A mania is a type of psychosis characterized by inappropriate overactivity.)

Pyrophobia

pyr/o- is a combining form meaning *fire.*

-phobia is a suffix meaning *abnormal fear.*

Pyrophobia is abnormal fear of fire.

TABLE 6-2	Common Word Roots
WORD ROOT	**MEANING**
arthr-	joint
bucc-	cheek
cardi-	heart
cost-	rib
cyt-	cell
enter-	intestine
faci-	face
gastr-	stomach
gnath-	jaw
hist-	tissue
later-	side
mel-	limb
my-	muscle
nephr-	kidney
occipit-	back of head
ophthalm-	eye or eyes
pulm-	lungs
rhin-	nose
splen-	spleen

Combining forms

COMBINING FORM: A word root followed by a vowel.
COMBINING VOWEL: A vowel that is added to a word root before a suffix.

Some word roots cannot combine with other word roots and/or suffixes without help (Table 6-5). For example, *gastr-*, meaning stomach, cannot gracefully combine with *megaly*, meaning enlargement—gastrmegaly is an impossible word. The hyphen at the end (or beginning) of a **combining form** indicates that it is not a completed word. A combining form is a word root with an added vowel, known as a **combining vowel.** We solve this problem by adding a vowel at the end of the word root, in this case, an *o* at the end of *gastr*. The result, *gastro-*, is referred to as a combining form because it is used when combining the root with other roots or suffixes. *Gastr + o + megaly* makes gastromegaly, enlargement of the stomach. In this chapter, we will indicate word roots with combining vowels with a slash; *eg, gastr/o*.

Examples of combining forms and combining vowels:
cardi + o + logy = cardiology (study of the heart)
neur + o + logy = neurology (study of the nervous system)

USING A MEDICAL DICTIONARY

A medical dictionary is very useful during the EMT–I course, and it is indispensable to the EMT–Paramedic. When choosing a medical dictionary, look for one that includes abbreviations, symbols, and pronunciations.

Some medical dictionaries are generic to all medical specialties, whereas others are aimed at particular professions such as EMS, nursing, or allied health. Check with your course instructor or a local bookstore to see which dictionary would be best for you.

PRONUNCIATION AND SPELLING

Explain the importance of pronunciation and spelling of medical terms.

A useful way to familiarize yourself with each medical term is to say it aloud several times and learn to pronounce it correctly. Soon it will become part of your vocabulary.

It is also very important to consult a medical dictionary when you are unsure of a word's spelling. Some terms sound alike but are spelled differently. For example, *ileum* is part of the intestinal tract, but *ilium* is a pelvic bone. Misspellings can cause confusion and can even lead to misdiagnosis.

ABBREVIATIONS

Identify common medical abbreviations from a list.

ABBREVIATION: A shorter way of writing something.

Some **abbreviations** are standard and used universally, such as OH for Ohio and Dr. for Doctor. Some abbreviations are specific to organizations or professions; outside the medical profession MCI (multicasuality incident) is a long-distance company. Some abbreviations have found their way into our spoken language, such as ASAP.

Abbreviations in the medical field are fairly universal, but you should check with your local EMS provider or hospital for their approved list of abbreviations. When in doubt about whether to use an abbreviation, you should write out the term in full. Table 6-6 lists some of the most common medical abbreviations used by the EMT–I.

BODY ORIENTATION

For ease of description, the body is divided into imaginary planes (Fig. 6-1). Terminology is also given to

TABLE 6-3	Common Prefixes	
PREFIXES	**MEANINGS**	**EXAMPLES**
a-, an-	without, from	apnea (without breath); asepsis (without infection)
ab-	away from	abnormal (away from the normal)
ad-	toward, to, near	adhesion (something stuck to)
aden-	pertaining to gland	adenitis (inflammation of gland)
ana-	up, toward, apart	anastomosis (joining of two parts)
ante-	before, in front of, forward	antenatal (occurring or formed before birth)
anti-	against, opposing	antiseptic (against or preventing sepsis)
bi-	two, double, twice	bilateral (both sides)
circum-	around, about	circumoral (around the mouth)
contra-	opposed, against	contraindication (indication opposing usually indicated treatment)
derma-	skin	dermatitis (inflammation of the skin)
dia-	through, completely	diagnosis (knowing completely)
dys-	difficult, bad, painful	dyspnea (difficulty breathing)
ecto-	outer, outside	ectopic (out of place)
edem-	swelling	edema (swelling)
endo-	within, inner	endometrium (within the uterus)
ep-, epi-	upon, on, over	epidermis (on the skin)
erythro-	red	erythrocyte (red blood cell)
hemi-	half	hemiplegia (paralysis of one side of the body)
hyper-	excessive, above	hyperplasia (excessive formation)
hypo-	under, deficient	hypotension (low blood pressure)
infra-	below, beneath	infrascapular (below the scapular bone)
inter-	between	intercostal (between ribs)
intra-	within	intralobar (within the lobe)
macro-	large	macroblast (abnormally large cell)
micro-	small	microdrip (small drop)
my-	pertaining to muscle	myoma (muscle tumor)
para-	beside, beyond, after	parathyroids (along side of thyroid)
per-	through, excessive	perforation (a breaking through)
peri-	around	periosteum (covering of bone)
post-	after, behind	postpartum (after childbirth)
pre-	before, in front of	prediastolic (before diastole)
retro-	backward, behind	retroflexion (bending backward)
semi-	half	semilunar (half moon)
sub-	under, beneath	subdiaphragmatic (under the diaphragm)
supra-	above, superior, excess	supraventricular (above the ventricles)

TABLE 6-4 Common Suffixes

Suffixes	Meanings	Examples
-algia	pain	neuralgia (pain along a nerve)
-cyte	cell	leukocyte (white blood cell)
-ectomy	cutting out	tonsillectomy (cutting out of tonsils)
-emia	blood	anemia (lack of blood)
-esthesia	sensation	anesthesia (without sensation)
-genic	causing	carcinogenic (cancer causing)
-gram	record	angiogram (record or graph of)
-itis	inflammation	tonsillitis (inflammation of the tonsils)
-logy	science, study of	biology (study of life)
-ostomy	creation of an opening	gastrostomy (artificial opening of)
-oma	tumor	neuroma (nerve tumor)
-osis	condition of	psychosis (condition of the mind)
-paresis	weakness	hemiparesis (one-sided weakness)
-phagia	eating	polyphagia (excessive eating)
-plegia	paralysis	hemiplegia (one-sided paralysis)
-pnea	breathing	apnea (no breathing)
-phasia	speech	aphasia (inability to speak)
-phobia	fear	hydrophobia (fear of water)
-rhythmia	rhythm	arrhythmia (variation from normal rhythm)
-rrhea	flow or discharge	pyorrhea (discharge of pus)
-taxia	order, arrangement of	ataxia (without muscle coordination)
-uria	to do with urine	polyuria (excessive secretion of urine)

TABLE 6-5 Common Combining Forms

Combining Form	Meaning
brachi/o-	arm
carp/o-	wrist
cephal/o-	head
cervic/o-	neck
encephal/o-	brain
faci/o-	face
gloss/o-	tongue
nas/o-	nose
ot/o-	ear
pil/o-	hair
steth/o-	chest
thorac/o-	chest, thorax
thyr/o-	thyroid gland
trache/o-	trachea
ureter/o-	ureter
vas/o-	vessel
vesic/o-	bladder, blister
viscer/o-	viscera

directions and movements. Understanding these terms will help you in your description and documentation of patient complaints and injuries. It also will allow for better communication over the radio to the receiving hospital.

Planes

 Describe the four planes of the human body.

The **frontal** plane divides the body vertically, into a front and back portion. It passes through the body longitudinally from head to toe. The front portion of the body is referred to as the ventral or anterior aspect and the back as the dorsal or posterior aspect.

If you were to cut the body in two parts, vertically, into right and left portions, the imaginary cut would be referred to as the **sagittal** plane. The sagittal plane does not divide the body equally. A cut down the midline, or center, of the body separating it vertically equally into right and left halves is called the **midsagittal** plane.

The **transverse** plane runs horizontally through the body perpendicular to the frontal and sagittal

TABLE 6-6 Common Medical Abbreviations

Abbreviation	Meaning	Abbreviation	Meaning
a	before	IV	intravenous
ac	before meals	kg	kilogram(s)
ad lib	as much as needed, as desired	L	liter(s)
AIDS	acquired immune deficiency syndrome	lb	pound
		LLQ	left lower quadrant
A & P	auscultation and percussion	LUQ	left upper quadrant
AMI	acute myocardial infarction	mcg	microgram(s)
bid	twice a day	MCI	multicasualty incident
BM	bowel movement	mg	milligram(s)
BP	blood pressure	mmHg	millimeters of mercury
BSA	body surface area	MI	myocardial infarction
$\bar{c}$	with	mL	milliliter(s)
C	centigrade, Celsius	mm	millimeter(s)
Ca	cancer, calcium	NPO	nothing by mouth
CAD	coronary artery disease	NS	normal saline
CBC	complete blood count	O_2	oxygen
cc	cubic centimeter(s)	OB	obstetrics
CC	chief complaint	OR	operating room
CCU	cardiac care unit, coronary care unit, critical care unit	P	pulse, phosphorus
		$\bar{p}$	after
cm	centimeter(s)	pc	after meals
CNS	central nervous system	PDR	*Physician's Desk Reference*
CO	carbon monoxide	PE	physical examination, pulmonary embolus
CO_2	carbon dioxide		
CSF	cerebrospinal fluid	PMH	past medical history
CVA	cerebrovascular accident	PID	pelvic inflammatory disease
CVD	cerebrovascular disease	po	orally
Dx	diagnosis	prn	as needed, as desired, whenever necessary
ECG or EKG	electrocardiogram		
EC	emergency center	pt	patient
ED	emergency department	q	every
EEG	electroencephalogram	qd	every day
EMS	Emergency Medical Services	qh	every hour
ER	emergency room	q2h	every two hours
F	Fahrenheit	qid	four times a day
GB	gall bladder	qm	every morning
GI	gastrointestinal	qn	every night
gm or g	gram(s)	R	respiration, rectal
gr	grain(s)	RLQ	right lower quadrant
GSW	gunshot wound	RUQ	right upper quadrant
gtt	drop	Rx	drug, prescription, therapy
gtts	drops	$\bar{s}$	without
GU	genitourinary	SC, SQ	subcutaneously
Gyn	gynecologic	SOB	shortness of breath
hb, hgB	hemoglobin	stat	immediately
HPI	history of present illness	S & S	signs and symptoms
hs	hours of sleep	T	temperature
ICU	intensive care unit	Td	tetanus
IM	intramuscular	tid	three times a day

TABLE 6-6	Continued
ABBREVIATION	**MEANING**
TPR	temperature, pulse, and respirations
ULQ	upper left quadrant
URQ	upper right quadrant
USP	*US Pharmacopeia*
VC	vital capacity
VS	vital signs
wt	weight
x-ray	roentgen ray
SYMBOLS	
>	greater than
<	lesser than
♀	female
♂	male

plane. It divides the body into an upper (superior) part and a lower (inferior) part. There could be many cross sections, each of which would be on a transverse plane.

Directions

 Describe the main directional terms for the human body.

Just as medical terminology helps us understand the medical language, a number of terms have been devised to designate specific directions for the human body (Table 6-7). Using standard directional terms in both your written and verbal reports helps explain where the patient's injuries are located. These terms refer to the body in the anatomic position: upright with eyes directed straight ahead, arms hanging by the side, feet together and the palms of the hands facing forward (Fig. 6-2).

Superior means above or in a higher position. For example, the brain is superior to the heart, and

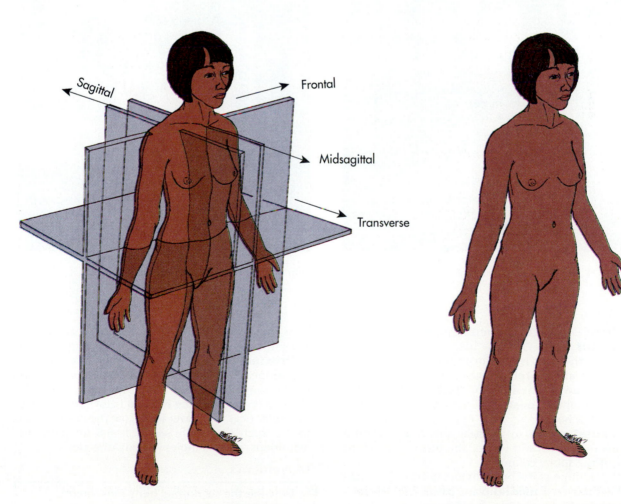

Fig. 6-1　**Planes of the body.**　　　　Fig. 6-2　**The anatomic position.**

TABLE 6-7	Planes of the Body
POSITION	**DEFINITION**
Frontal	Vertical line dividing the body into a front and back portion.
Sagittal	A vertical line dividing the body into right and left portions.
Midsagittal	A vertical line dividing the body into right and left halves; can be thought of as the same as the midline.
Transverse	A horizontal line dividing the body into an upper and lower portion.

A

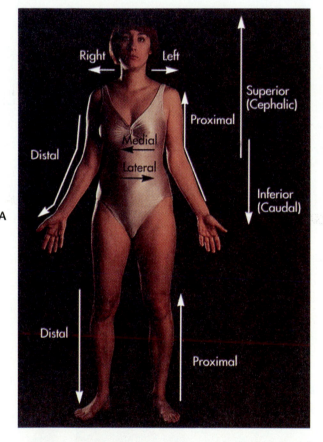

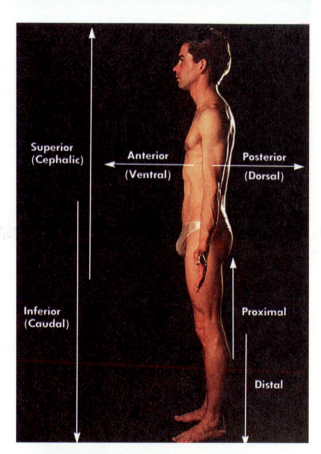

B

Fig. 6-3   A, B Directional terms for the human body.

the heart is superior to the intestine. The opposite term, **inferior,** means below or lower. For example, the neck is inferior to the mouth.

Ventral and **anterior** mean the same thing in humans: toward the front or "belly" surface of the body. Dorsal and **posterior** both mean toward the back of the body.

Cranial means in or near the head. **Caudal** means near the lower end of the torso, *ie,* near the base of the spinal column.

The midline of the body divides it into equal right and left halves. A **medial** plane passes near the midline of the body, dividing it into right and left por-

tions. **Lateral,** as opposite to medial, means farther away from the midline, or toward the side.

Proximal means nearest the origin of a structure. **Distal** means farthest from that point. For example, in the upper extremity (arm), the arm above the elbow is proximal to the forearm below. In the lower extremity (leg), the lower leg below the knee is distal to the thigh (Fig. 6-3). See Table 6-8 for positions, definitions, and examples of body directions.

Movements

🍒 **Describe the six normal body movements.**

TABLE 6-8 **Body Directions**

Position	Definition	Examples
Superior	Above, higher	The head is superior to the neck.
Inferior	Below, lower	The chest is inferior to the neck.
Anterior (ventral)	Toward the front	The nose is on the anterior, or ventral, surface of the head.
Posterior (dorsal)	Toward the back	The calf is on the posterior, or dorsal, surface of the leg.
Cranial	In or near the head	The brain is in the cranial cavity.
Caudal	Near the sacral region of the spinal column	The buttocks, the muscles on which we sit, are located at the caudal end of the body.
Medial	A vertical line that passes near the midline of the body	The nose is medial to the eyes.
Lateral	Toward the side, away from the midline	The ears are lateral to the nose.
Proximal	Nearest the origin of a structure	The part of your thumb where it joins your hand is its proximal region.
Distal	Farther from the origin of a structure	The tip of the thumb is the distal region compared with the part of your thumb where it joins your hand.

Most movements have to do with some kind of motion at a joint (Fig. 6-4). Flexion decreases the angle at a joint by bringing two parts closer together, whereas extension increases the angle by moving the parts further apart. For example, the movement of squatting causes flexion in the knees and hips, whereas standing up causes extension in the same joints. Abduction is the act of moving a part away from the midline of the body, whereas adduction means moving the part toward the midline.

Circumduction is the swinging of a body part in a circle. For example, drawing a circle in the sand with your foot would cause your leg to swing in a circle. Rotation means twisting or turning a part on its own axis. A lateral rotation of the arm twists the hand so that the thumb is turned outward, away from the midline of the body. A medial rotation turns the thumb inward, toward the midline.

Postures

 Describe the anatomic postures of the body.

Postures of the body describe the position in which the patient's body was found. The erect position is standing in an upright position. Supine is lying on the back, face up. A person lying on the dorsal surface of the body, or on the back, is supine. Prone is lying on the stomach, face down. A person lying on the ventral surface, or the front of the body, is prone. A person lying in the lateral recumbent position is lying on the right or left side (Fig. 6-5).

CASE HISTORY FOLLOW-UP

After leaving the emergency department, EMT–I Douglas tells Julie that her patient care skills are excellent and that the patient's condition improved because Julie was confident and well-educated to deliver emergency care. Julie thanks him but is obviously upset about the poor radio report and the fact that her IV request was denied because of it. Julie tells EMT–I Douglas that this was the first time she called in a "real" patient report to the hospital. Although she had practiced a little in class, she didn't realize how important it is to communicate effectively with the hospital and to "talk the talk" of the profession. She admits that she needs to do some work in communicating medical terminology, and she promises that she will not make the same mistake twice.

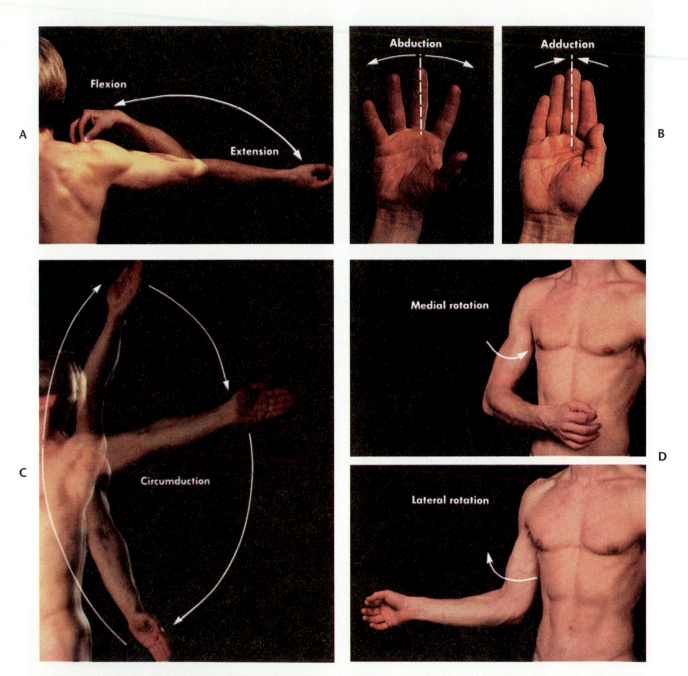

Fig. 6-4   A, Flexion and extension of the elbow. B, Abduction and adduction in the fingers. C, Circumduction of the shoulder. D, Medial and lateral rotation of the arm.

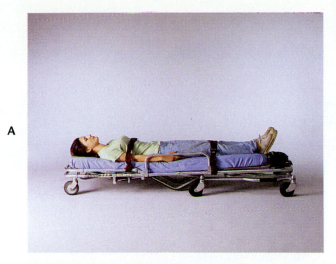
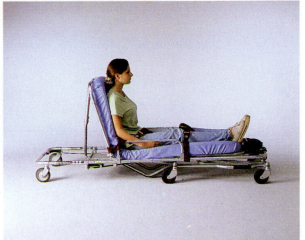
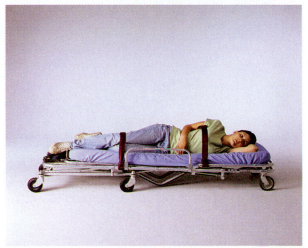
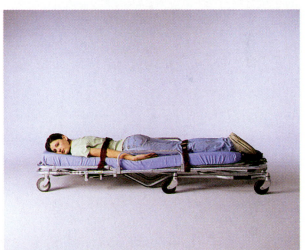

Fig. 6-5   A, Patient in the supine position. **B,** Patient in the sitting position. **C,** Patient in the left lateral recumbent position. **D,** Patient in the prone position.

CASE HISTORY FOLLOW-UP, continued

In class the next night, Julie tells her instructor and her classmates that a competent EMT is able to assess an ill or injured patient, provide good patient care, and communicate his or her findings to other members of the healthcare team. All agree that each of these abilities is equally important in the delivery of quality prehospital care.

SUMMARY

Medical terms are made up of combinations of word roots, prefixes, and suffixes. It is important to get into the habit of breaking down complex words into their separate parts when studying medical terminology. Because medical terms can sometimes be very long and complex, words are separated to help improve understanding of how they are put together.

As the EMT–I learns various word roots, prefixes and suffixes, he or she will better understand, interpret, and define new medical terms. In addition, the EMT–I should make a practice of looking up new terms in a glossary or dictionary when studying. Spelling and pronunciation are essential elements of effective communication with other health professionals; errors endanger the patient and the EMT–I's reputation. So much is involved in medical terminology that it can be regarded as a separate course of study in itself.

Understanding certain anatomic directions, planes, movements, and postures for orientation to the human body is essential for identifying and reporting location of injuries. A knowledge of medical terminology and body orientation will help make your communication and documentation of patient information much more precise.

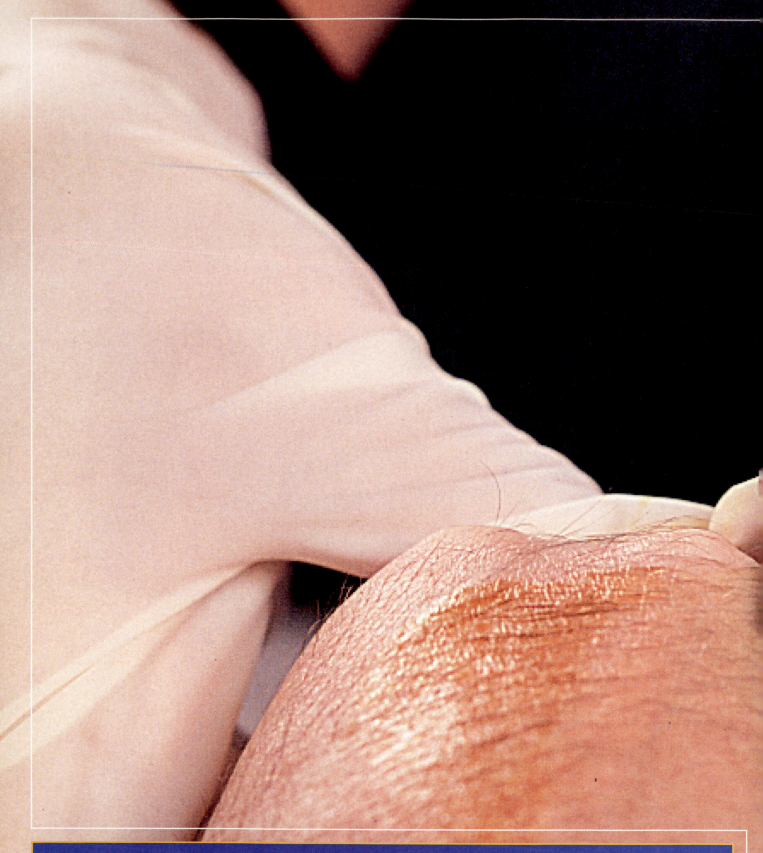

ESSENTIALS

DIVISION TWO

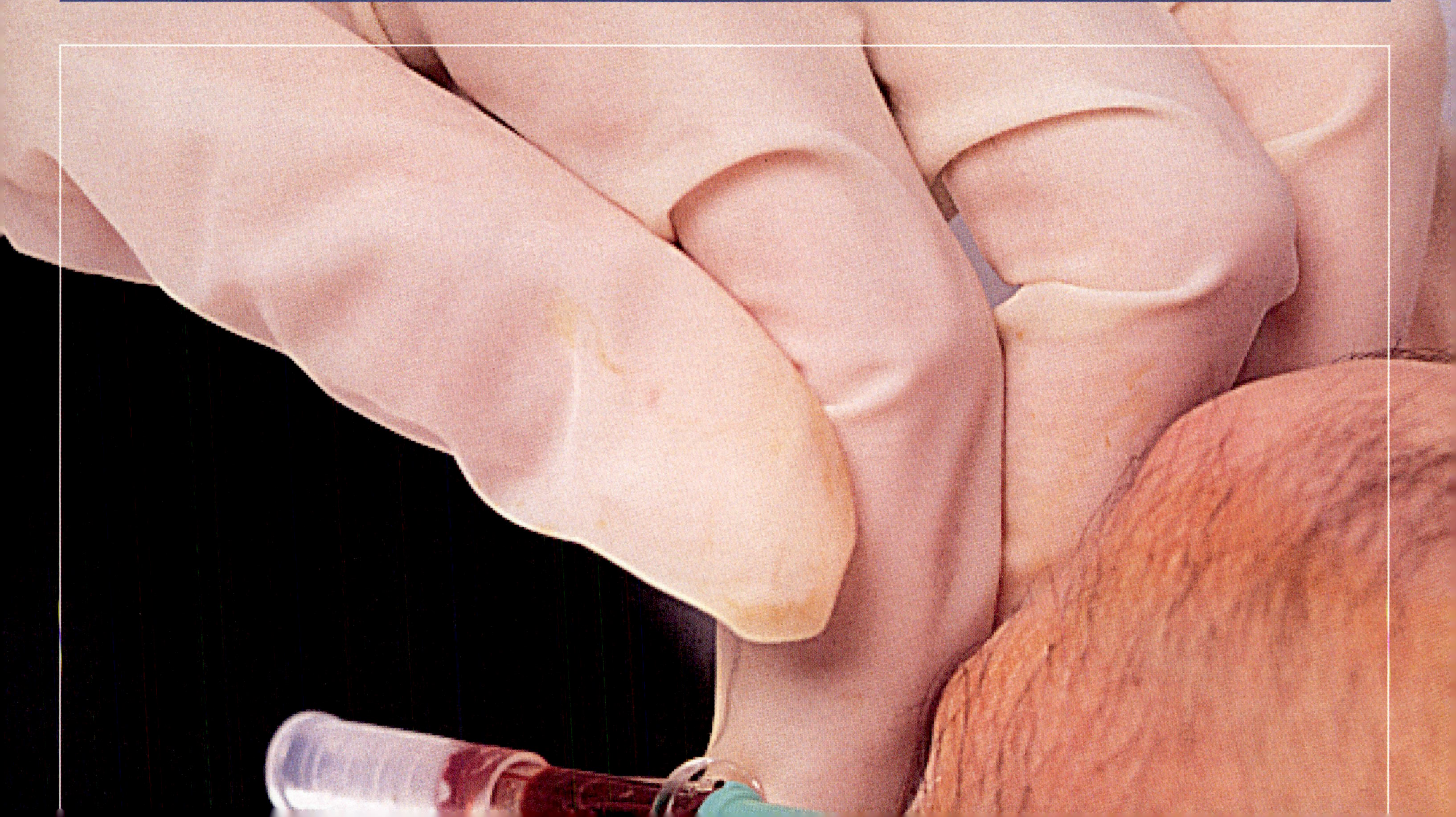

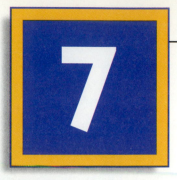

BODY SYSTEMS

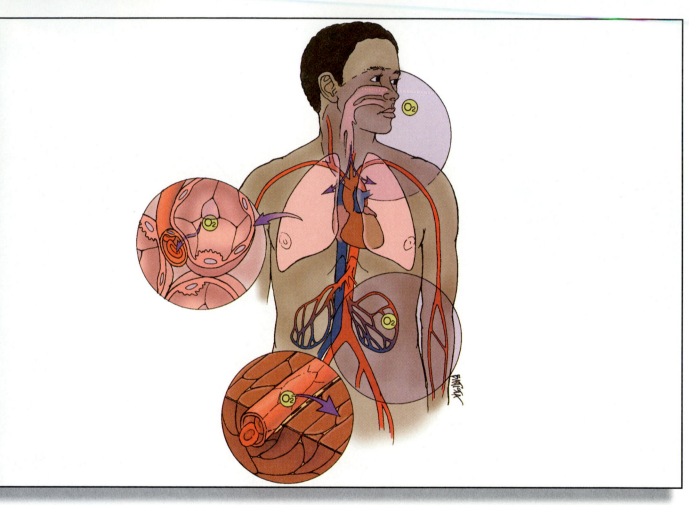

CASE HISTORY

EMT–I Jackson is precepting an EMT–Intermediate student who has just completed the anatomy and physiology portion of his class, when her unit is dispatched for a trauma call at an after-hours club. Jackson arrives on the scene in 8 minutes and is met by a police officer who tells her that a 20 year old has been stabbed. The suspect is in custody.

The patient is lying unconscious in a pool of blood as Jackson approaches him. Her initial assessment reveals five stab wounds: two in the chest, one in the abdomen, one in the left buttock, and one in the right thigh.

The crew ventilates the patient with 100% oxygen and a bag-valve-mask to assist his

Case History, continued

breathing and then starts two IVs, per protocol. EMT–I Jackson calls medical direction to report:

"We have a male, approximately 20 years of age, with five stab wounds. He is responding to painful stimuli only. We placed an OP airway, and we're assisting ventilations with 100% O_2. We loaded the patient and began transporting immediately, starting two IVs, LR wide open en route.

"Vital signs are: pulse 142 and weak; respirations 28 and labored with central cyanosis; BP is 92/68.

"The stab wounds are on the right anterior axillary line at T4, left midaxillary line at T6, left epigastric region, left mid-buttock, and right anterior midthigh. The right thigh is approximately 5 cm larger than the left, and there's no response to painful stimulation of the left leg.

"We've applied a porous dressing over the open chest wound and controlled open bleeding with dry, sterile dressings over all of the other wounds. We have an ETA to your facility of approximately 12 minutes. Do you have any further orders?"

LEARNING OBJECTIVES

Upon completion of this chapter, the EMT-Intermediate should be able to:

- DEFINE the term *connective tissue*.
- IDENTIFY the five body cavities.
- DEFINE the terms *joints*, *cartilage*, *ligaments*, and *tendons*.
- IDENTIFY the two major divisions of the skeletal system and describe their function.
- DESCRIBE the structure and function of the muscular system and identfy three types of muscle.
- DESCRIBE the structure and function of the circulatory system.
- DESCRIBE the structure and function of the respiratory system.
- DESCRIBE the structure and function of the nervous system.
- IDENTIFY the four quadrants of the abdomen.
- DESCRIBE the structure and function of the urinary system.
- DESCRIBE the structure and function of the male and female reproductive systems.
- DESCRIBE the structure and function of the immune system.
- DESCRIBE the structure and function of the endocrine system.

KEY TERMS

ANATOMY

AUTONOMIC NERVOUS SYSTEM

CARDIAC CONDUCTION SYSTEM

CARDIAC TAMPONADE

CARTILAGE

CENTRAL NERVOUS SYSTEM

CIRCULATORY SYSTEM

CONNECTIVE TISSUE

ENDOCRINE SYSTEM

GASTROINTESTINAL SYSTEM

IMMUNE SYSTEM

INTEGUMENTARY SYSTEM

JOINTS

LYMPHATIC SYSTEM

MUSCULAR SYSTEM

NERVOUS SYSTEM

OXYGENATION

PARASYMPATHETIC NERVOUS SYSTEM

PERIPHERAL NERVOUS SYSTEM

PHYSIOLOGY

ANATOMY: The study of structures and organs of the body.
PHYSIOLOGY: The study of the functions and processes undertaken by the body.

ANATOMY AND PHYSIOLOGY

Anatomy refers to the study of the structure of an organism and its parts. **Physiology** is the study of an organism's body functions (Fig. 7-1). By being familiar with the structure and function of the various body systems, you will be better able to assess a patient's signs and symptoms. For example, if a person hits the breastbone (sternum) hard against the steering wheel in a motor vehicle accident, damage would be suspected not only to the bones but also to the underlying structures—the heart, lungs, and major blood vessels.

ORGANIZATION OF THE HUMAN BODY

The Body's building blocks

The human body consists of increasingly sophisticated levels of organization (Fig. 7-2). Cells are the basic building blocks of all life. In less-advanced forms of life, such as bacteria, the entire organism consists of a single cell. The human body contains approximately 100 trillion cells, all specialized for particular functions. Red blood cells transport oxygen, for example, and are very different from bone cells, which are designed to support weight. Cells contain various components, known as organelles, which carry out the processes necessary for life within each cell. An example of an organelle is the nucleus, or nerve center, of the cell (Fig. 7-3).

 Define the term *connective tissue*.

Tissue is composed of groups of similar cells working together to accomplish a common function. There are four types of tissue: 1) Epithelial tissue covers

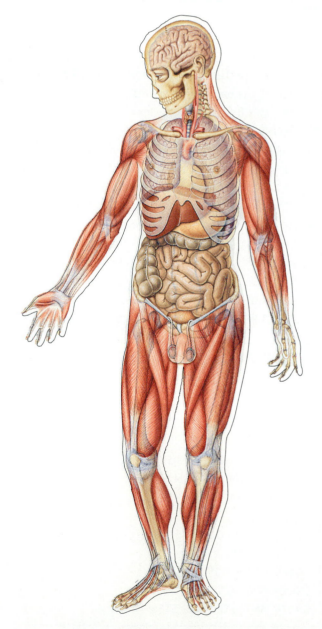

Fig. 7-1 Anatomy refers to the study of the structure of an organism; physiology refers to the function of these structures.

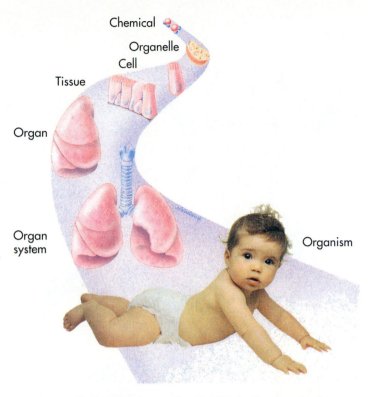

Chemical

Organelle

Cell

Tissue

Organ

Organ system

Organism

Fig. 7-2 **The levels of organization in the human body are: organelle, cell, tissue, organ, organ system, and organism.**

all external surfaces of the body and lines the hollow organs, such as the intestines and bronchi. It provides a protective barrier and aids in the absorption of food (in the intestines) and secretion of various body substances (in the sweat glands). 2) **Connective tissue** binds other types of tissue together. Types of connective tissue include bone, cartilage, and adipose (fat) tissue. 3) Muscle tissue contracts, leading to movement of body structures. The three types of muscle tissue are skeletal muscle, cardiac muscle, and smooth muscle. 4) Nerve tissue includes the brain, the spinal cord, and all the nerves that pass from these to various parts of the body. Nerves generate and transmit impulses throughout the body, controlling all bodily processes.

Organs are composed of different types of tissue. The heart, for example, contains muscle, nerves, and connective tissue. The skin, which also is composed of many different types of tissue, is the largest organ in the body.

An organ system, or simply system, is a group of organs that have a common function and purpose. Although often found in close anatomic proximity, the organs of a system may be scattered throughout the body. Organ systems include skeletal, muscular, circulatory, respiratory, nervous, gastrointestinal, urinary, reproductive, immune, endocrine, lymphatic, integumentary, and special sensory (Fig. 7-4).

Body cavities

 Identify the five body cavities.

Body cavities are hollow areas within the body that contain organs and systems (Fig. 7-5). The hollow portion of the skull, called the *cranial cavity*, has a domed top and a base composed of several bones. The cranial cavity houses the brain and is continuous with the spinal cavity, also known as the *spinal* or *vertebral canal*. The spinal cavity travels through the backbone, or vertebral column, and contains the spinal cord. Organs within the cranial and spinal cavities are part of the nervous and special sensory systems.

The thoracic cavity (thorax), between the base of the neck and the diaphragm, is formed by the roughly circular boundary of the rib cage. The major structures within the thoracic cavity belong to the cardiovascular and respiratory systems—the heart, major blood vessels, and lungs.

The space between the lungs is known as the mediastinum, which contains the heart, trachea (windpipe), mainstem bronchi, part of the esophagus, and large blood vessels.

The abdominal cavity is a single large cavity that extends from the diaphragm to the pelvic bones. It is

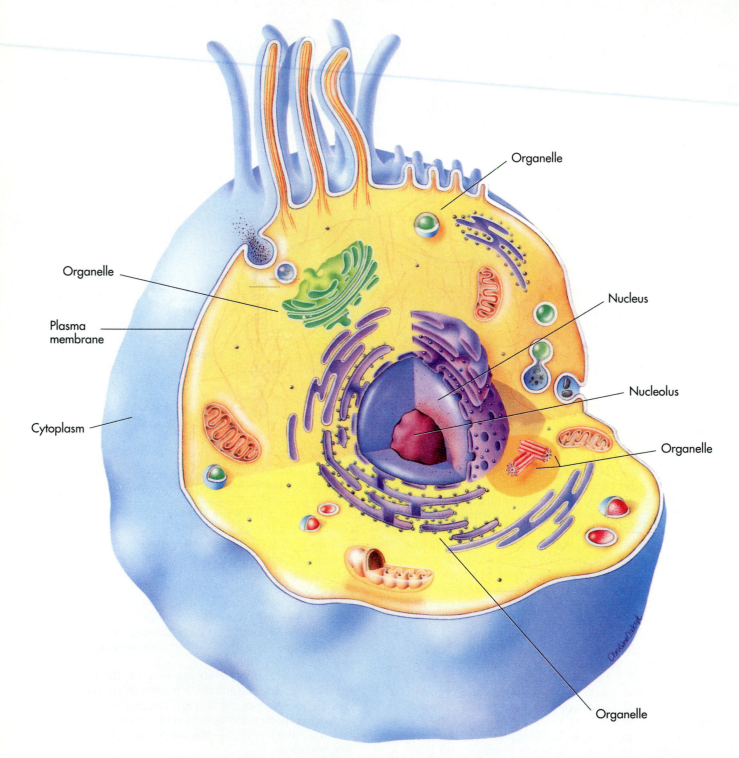

Organelle

Organelle

Plasma
membrane

Cytoplasm

Nucleus

Nucleolus

Organelle

Organelle

Fig. 7-3   **A typical cell in the human body.**

Organ Systems of the Body

SYSTEM	MAJOR COMPONENTS	FUNCTIONS
Integumentary	Skin, hair, nails, and sweat glands	Protects, regulates temperature, prevents water loss, and produces vitamin D precursors
Skeletal	Bones, associated cartilage, and joints	Protects, supports, and allows body movement, produces blood cells, and stores minerals
Muscular	Muscles attached to the skeleton	Produces body movement, maintains posture, and produces body heat
Nervous	Brain, spinal cord, nerves, and sensory receptors	A major regulatory system: detects sensation, controls movements, controls physiological and intellectual functions
Endocrine	Endocrine glands such as the pituitary, thyroid, and adrenal glands	A major regulatory system: participates in the regulation of metabolism, production, and many other functions
Circulatory	Heart, blood vessels, and blood	Transports nutrients, waste products, gases, and hormones throughout the body; plays a role in the immune response and the regulation of body temperature
Lymphatic	Lymph vessels, lymph nodes, and other lymph	Removes foreign substances, from the body and lymph, combats disease, maintains tissue fluid balance, and absorbs fats
Respiratory	Lungs and respiratory passages	Exchanges gases (oxygen and carbon dioxide) between the blood and the air and helps regulate blood pH
Gastrointestinal	Mouth, esophagus, stomach, intestines, and accessory structures	Performs the mechanical and chemical processes of digestion, absorption of nutrients, and elimination of wastes
Urinary	Kidneys, urinary bladder, and the ducts that carry urine	Removes waste products from the circulatory system; helps regulate blood pH, ion balance, and water balance
Reproductive	Gonads, accessory structures, and genitals of males and females	Performs the processes of reproduction and controls sexual function and behaviors

Fig. 7-4 Body systems.

(Continued)

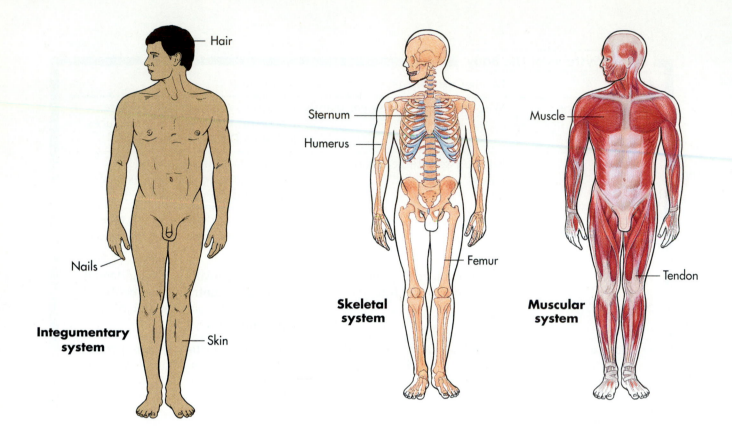

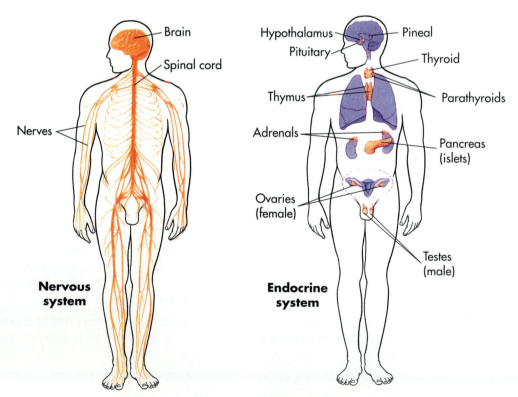

Fig. 7-4 **Body systems.** *(Continued)*

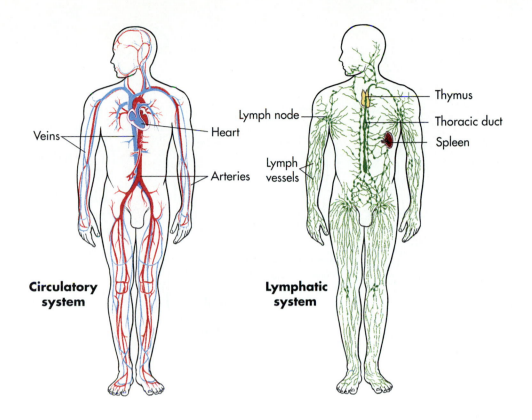

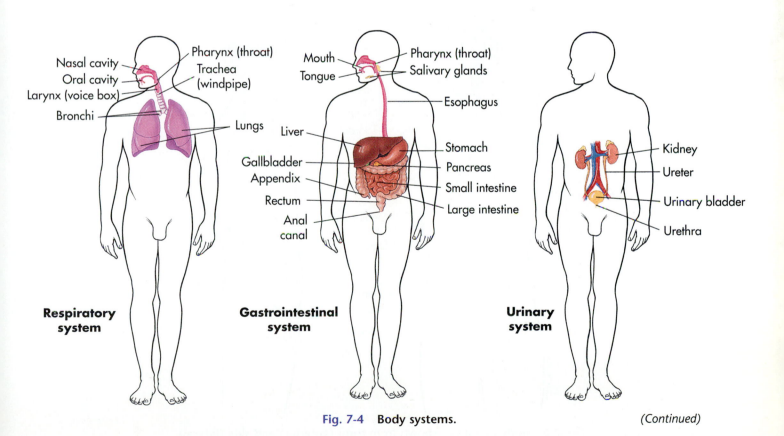

Fig. 7-4 **Body systems.**

(Continued)

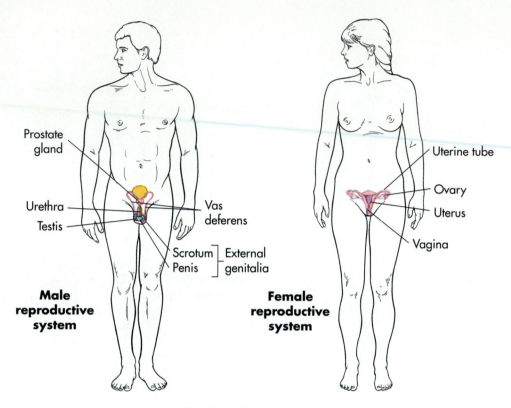

Prostate gland

Urethra

Testis

Vas deferens

Scrotum
Penis } External genitalia

Male reproductive system

Uterine tube

Ovary

Uterus

Vagina

Female reproductive system

Fig. 7-4   Body systems.

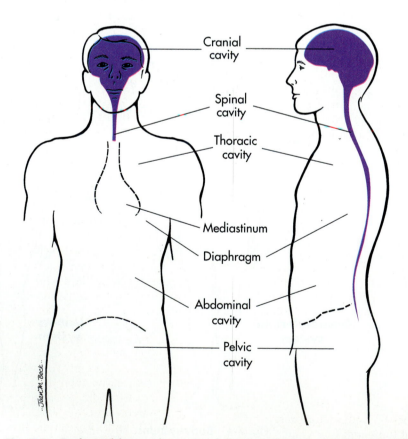

Cranial cavity

Spinal cavity

Thoracic cavity

Mediastinum

Diaphragm

Abdominal cavity

Pelvic cavity

Fig. 7-5   Body cavities as shown from front (anterior) and side (lateral).

The skeletal system

The **skeletal system,** composed of 206 bones, provides a framework for the human body (Fig. 7-8). Bones protect internal organs and, with muscles, assist in movement. Bones also serve as a storage site for minerals, particularly calcium, and have a role in the formation of certain blood cells. Many bones have an internal cavity that contains a substance known as bone marrow. It is within the bone marrow that most of our red blood cells (erythrocytes) and white blood cells (leukocytes) are manufactured (Fig. 7-9).

 Define the terms *joints, cartilage, ligaments, and tendons.*

 JOINTS: The convergence of two bones in the body.
CARTILAGE: Connective tissue found primarily in the joints that allows for movement.
LIGAMENTS: A fibrous tissue that attaches bones to cartilage.
TENDONS: White fibrous tissue that attaches muscles to bones.

Joints occur where two or more bones meet or articulate (Fig. 7-10). Movement at joints is aided by **cartilage.** Cartilages are plates of shiny connective tissue that enable bones to move freely. **Ligaments** are tough white bands of tissue that bind joints together, connecting bone and cartilage (Fig. 7-11). **Tendons** connect muscles to bones.

 Identify the two major divisions of the skeletal system and describe their function.

The skeletal system is divided into two major components: the axial skeleton and the appendicular skeleton. The axial skeleton consists of the entire torso. The appendicular skeleton consists of the extremities (the arms and legs), as well as the girdles, or bony belts that attach the limbs to the body. The shoulder girdle attaches the upper extremity, and the pelvic girdle attaches the lower extremity.

The axial skeleton

At the top of the axial skeleton is the skull, which consists of the cranium and the face (Fig. 7-12). Several individual bones fuse together to comprise the cranium and the face. The brain is contained within the cranium. The brain connects with the spinal cord through a large opening at the base of the skull called the *foramen magnum.*

The spine, which serves as the primary support structure of the body, consists of 33 bones called *vertebrae* and is divided into five sections (Fig. 7-13).

There are seven *cervical vertebrae* in the neck. The first vertebra directly beneath the skull is called the *atlas*, C1, and supports the head. The next vertebra, C2, is called the *axis*. The axis is the point at which

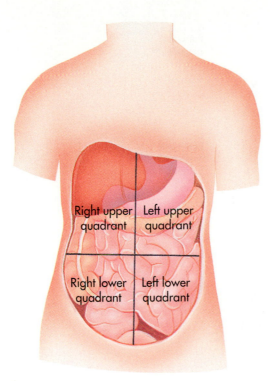

Fig. 7-6 **Four quadrants of the abdomen.**

bordered by the spine and the abdominal wall. The abdomen can be divided into quadrants by crossing the umbilicus (navel) with imaginary perpendicular lines. It is important for the EMT–I to know the four quadrants and the underlying anatomy of the abdomen when assessing patients (Fig. 7-6).

The abdominal cavity contains the organs of digestion and excretion, which comprise the gastrointestinal and urinary systems. The digestive organs are surrounded by the peritoneum, which is a double-layered smooth membrane of connective tissue. The kidneys and major blood vessels of the abdominal cavity are located in an area posterior to the digestive organs known as the retroperitoneal space (Fig. 7-7).

The pelvic cavity, comprising the lower portion of the abdominal cavity, contains the organs of the gastrointestinal, reproductive and urinary systems. The cavity is bounded by the pelvic girdle (pelvic bones): the ilium, ischium, pubis, sacrum, and coccyx. The strong pelvic bones provide protection for internal organs.

BODY SYSTEMS

 SKELETAL SYSTEM: The framework of the body comprised of bones that allows for protection and movement of the body.

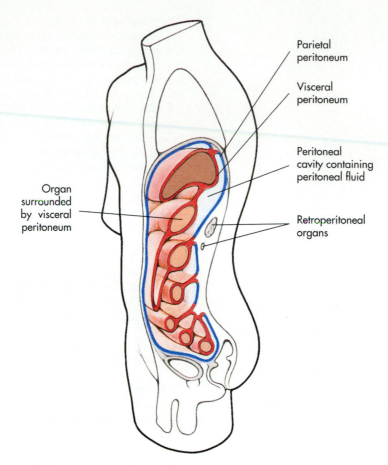

Parietal
peritoneum

Visceral
peritoneum

Peritoneal
cavity containing
peritoneal fluid

Organ
surrounded
by visceral
peritoneum

Retroperitoneal
organs

Fig. 7-7 **A lateral (side) view of the peritoneum in the human body.**

the head turns. The remainder of the cervical verte-brae are simply numbered, C3 through C7, and have no special names.

There are 12 thoracic vertebrae in the posterior chest. There are five lumbar vertebrae in the lower back and five sacral vertebrae, fused into a platelike bone, the sacrum, which forms the posterior portion of the pelvic bone. Four vertebrae are fused into the coccyx, or tailbone which is attached to the lower portion of the sacrum.

Attached to each thoracic vertebra is a pair of ribs. These 12 pairs of ribs form the ribcage. The upper 10 pairs attach directly to the sternum, or breastbone. The remaining two pair of ribs, called *floating ribs*, are held in place by cartilage (Fig. 7-14).

The appendicular skeleton

The shoulder girdle attaches the upper extremity to the body and consists of the scapula (shoulder blade) pos-teriorly and the clavicle (collarbone) anteriorly. The clavicle is attached to the sternum by ligaments. The upper extremities consist of the arms, forearms, wrists, hands, and fingers. Although the entire extremity is often called the *arm*, the arm in a pure anatomic sense actually extends only from the shoulder to the elbow. The humerus is the bone of the arm.

The forearm is that portion of the upper extremity from the elbow to the wrist. Two bones make up the forearm: the radius and the ulna. The radius is the bone on the thumb side. A group of irregularly shaped bones, called the *carpals*, comprise the wrist. Beyond the wrist are the metacarpal bones, which form the hand. Each finger is composed of a series of small bones called phalanges (Fig. 7-15).

The pelvic girdle attaches the lower extremity to the body. It consists of a ring of bones formed by the sacrum posteriorly and the coxae, or pelvic bones, on each side (Fig. 7-16). Each pelvic bone consists of three fused bones: the ilium, the ischium, and the pubis. The superior portion of the ilium is called the *iliac crest*. The ilium joins the sacrum to form the sacroiliac joint.

The lower extremities include the hips, thighs, knees, legs, ankles, feet, and toes. The thigh is that part of the lower extremity from the hip to the knee. The femur is the bone of the thigh and is the longest and strongest bone in the body. The femur articu-lates with the pelvic girdle at the acetabulum; this region is often called the *hip joint*.

The knee is the point of articulation of the femur and the bones of the leg. It is covered with a piece of cartilage called the *patella* (kneecap). The leg runs

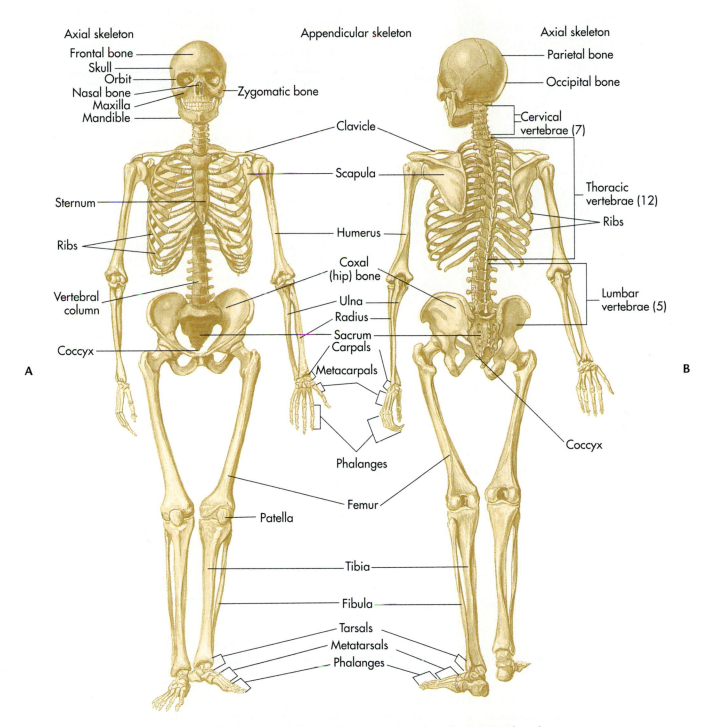

Axial skeleton

Frontal bone
Skull
Orbit
Nasal bone
Maxilla
Mandible

Zygomatic bone

Sternum

Ribs

Vertebral
column

Coccyx

A

Appendicular skeleton

Clavicle

Scapula

Humerus

Coxal
(hip) bone
Ulna
Radius
Sacrum
Carpals

Metacarpals

Phalanges

Femur

Patella

Tibia

Fibula

Tarsals
Metatarsals
Phalanges

Axial skeleton

Parietal bone

Occipital bone

Cervical
vertebrae (7)

Thoracic
vertebrae (12)

Ribs

Lumbar
vertebrae (5)

Coccyx

B

Fig. 7-8 The human skeleton. A, An anterior view. B, A posterior view.

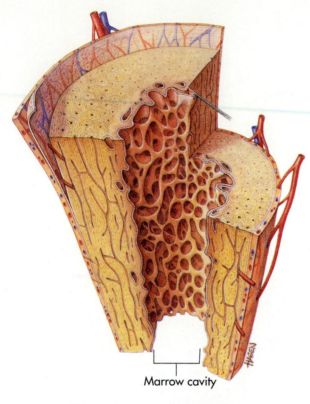

Fig. 7-9 Bone marrow cavity.

from the knee to the ankle and contains two bones: the tibia and the fibula. The tibia is longer and thicker than the fibula. The anterior portion of the tibia, covered only by skin, is commonly called the *shin*. A number of irregular bones, the tarsals, comprise the ankle. Beyond the ankle are the metatarsals, which make up the foot. The toe bones, like the finger bones of the hand, are called *phalanges* (Fig. 7-17).

The muscular system

 Describe the structure and function of the muscular system and identify three types of muscle.

 MUSCULAR SYSTEM: The body system composed of contractile tissue that allows for movement.

The **muscular system** is composed of contractile tissues (muscle) responsible for movement. Muscle is categorized into three distinct types: skeletal, smooth, and cardiac (Fig. 7-18). Skeletal muscle is voluntary and is under conscious control. There are more than 350 skeletal muscles in the body.

Smooth muscle is involuntary and is not under conscious control. Examples of smooth muscle include the muscle that dilates the pupils of the eyes and the muscle of the intestinal wall. Smooth muscle works automatically; humans cannot consciously influence the contraction of involuntary muscles.

Cardiac (heart) muscle is a special type of involuntary muscle. This type of muscle has the ability to generate its own stimulus to contract if necessary. This property, called *intrinsic automaticity,* allows the heart to continue to pump in extreme circumstances, such as when its external nerve supply is damaged.

The circulatory system

 Describe the structure and function of the circulatory system.

 CIRCULATORY SYSTEM: The body system composed of the heart, blood, and blood vessels that is responsible for the circulation of blood.

The **circulatory system,** sometimes referred to as the cardiovascular system, consists of the heart, blood, and blood vessels.

The heart is a muscular, cone-shaped organ, and its function is to pump blood throughout the body. It is located behind the sternum (breastbone) and is about the size of a closed fist—approximately 5 inches long, 3 inches wide, and 2.5 inches thick. It weighs 10 to 12 ounces in men and 8 to 10 ounces in women. Roughly two thirds of the heart lies in the left side of the chest cavity (Fig. 7-19).

Functionally, the heart is divided into right and left sides, which are separated by a thick wall called the interventricular septum. The heart muscle is referred to as the myocardium (Fig 7-20). Surrounding the heart is a thick set of two membranes, the pericardium. Together, these membranes form the pericardial sac around the heart. Normally, the pericardial sac contains only a small amount of lubricating fluid that allows the heart to contract and expand smoothly within the chest cavity.

> **HELPFUL HINT**
> If the pericardial sac rapidly fills with fluid, such as blood, the heart is no longer able to adequately fill and the signs and symptoms of shock result. This condition is known as **cardiac tamponade** and is a common result of penetrating chest trauma.

The normal human heart consists of two upper chambers, the atria, and two lower chambers, the ventricles. The atria receive blood returned to the heart from other parts of the body, whereas the ventricles pump blood out of the heart. The atria and ventricles are separated by valves that prevent backward flow of blood. Other valves are located between the ventricles and the arteries into which they pump blood (Fig. 7-21).

Blood and its components

Blood is the fluid tissue that is pumped by the heart through the arteries, veins, and capillaries. Blood

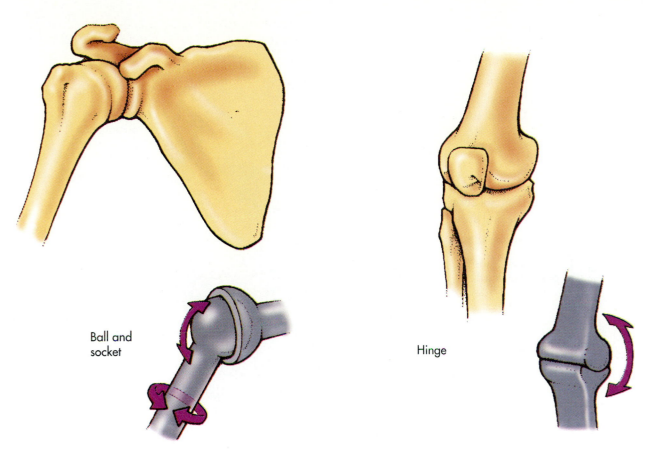

Ball and
socket

Hinge

Fig. 7-10   Examples of joints in the human body.

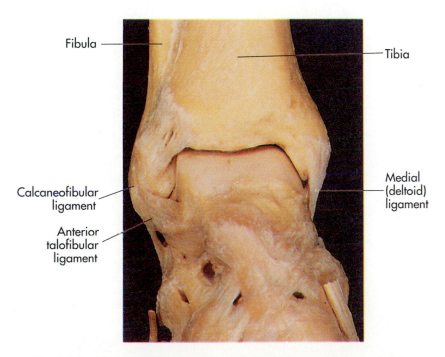

Fibula

Tibia

Calcaneofibular
ligament

Medial
(deltoid)
ligament

Anterior
talofibular
ligament

Fig. 7-11   Ligaments bind bones and cartilage together at a joint.

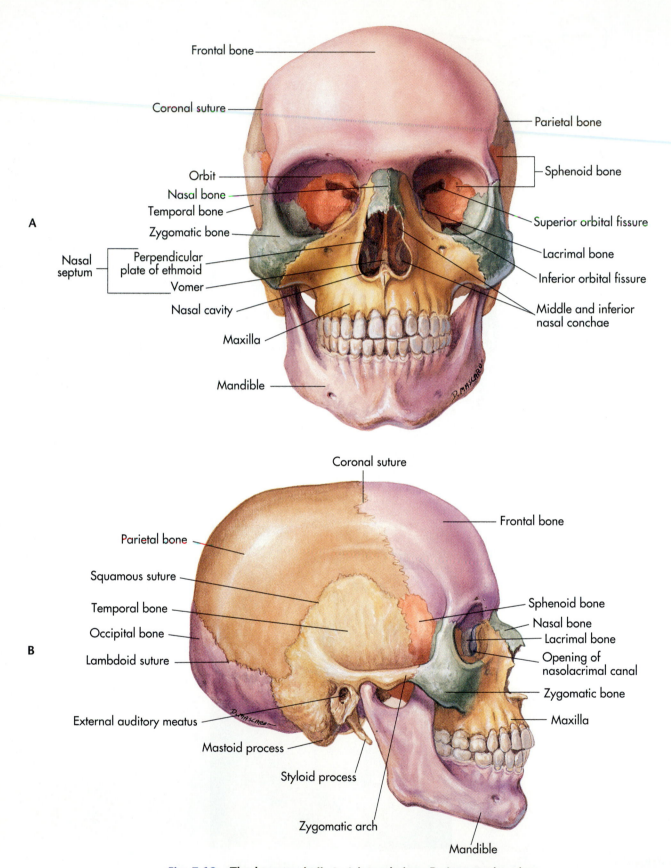

A

Frontal bone

Coronal suture

Parietal bone

Orbit

Nasal bone

Temporal bone

Zygomatic bone

Nasal septum

Perpendicular plate of ethmoid

Vomer

Nasal cavity

Maxilla

Mandible

Sphenoid bone

Superior orbital fissure

Lacrimal bone

Inferior orbital fissure

Middle and inferior nasal conchae

B

Coronal suture

Frontal bone

Parietal bone

Squamous suture

Temporal bone

Occipital bone

Lambdoid suture

External auditory meatus

Mastoid process

Styloid process

Zygomatic arch

Mandible

Sphenoid bone

Nasal bone

Lacrimal bone

Opening of nasolacrimal canal

Zygomatic bone

Maxilla

Fig. 7-12   The human skull. A, A lateral view. B, An anterior view.

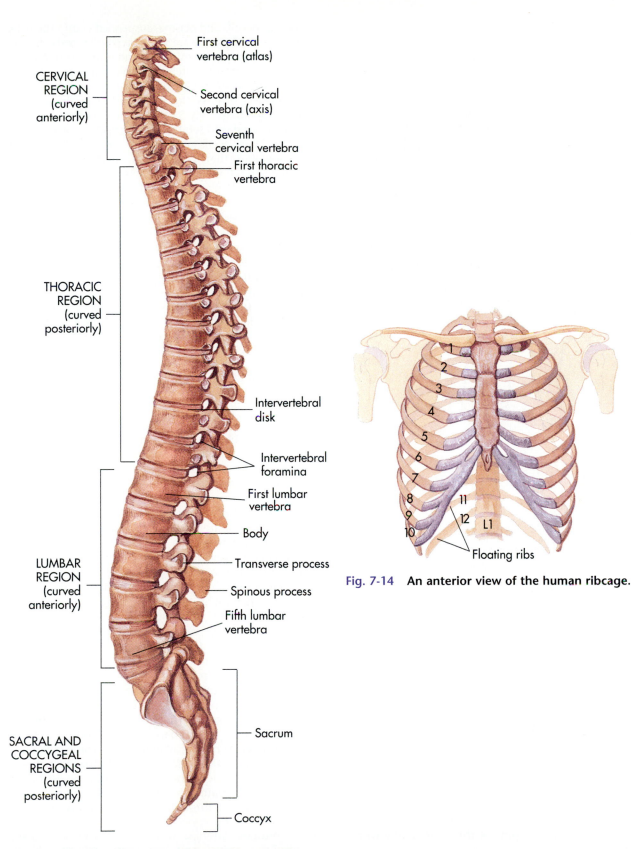

CERVICAL
REGION
(curved
anteriorly)

First cervical
vertebra (atlas)

Second cervical
vertebra (axis)

Seventh
cervical vertebra

First thoracic
vertebra

THORACIC
REGION
(curved
posteriorly)

Intervertebral
disk

Intervertebral
foramina

First lumbar
vertebra

LUMBAR
REGION
(curved
anteriorly)

Body

Transverse process

Spinous process

Fifth lumbar
vertebra

SACRAL AND
COCCYGEAL
REGIONS
(curved
posteriorly)

Sacrum

Coccyx

Floating ribs

Fig. 7-14   **An anterior view of the human ribcage.**

Fig. 7-13   **The sections and bones in the vertebral column (spine).**

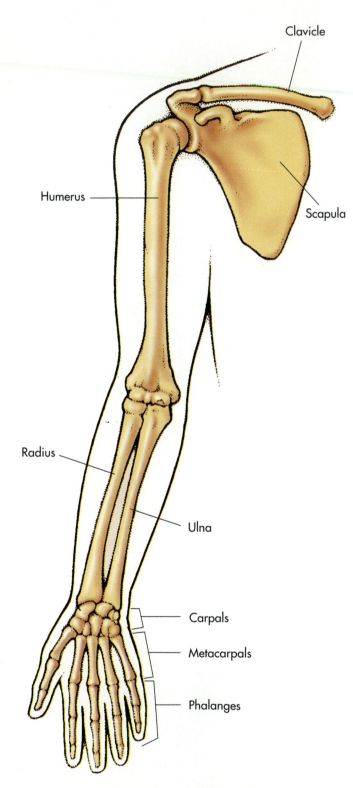

Fig. 7-15 **The anatomy of the upper and lower arm and hand.**

Clavicle

Humerus

Scapula

Radius

Ulna

Carpals

Metacarpals

Phalanges

consists of cells and plasma. Suspended within the pale, straw-colored plasma are several types of blood cells and dissolved chemicals, minerals, and nutrients (Fig 7-22). Men have approximately 70 cubic centimeters (cc) of blood per kg of body weight, whereas women have slightly less, 65 cc per kg. In an adult man, this amount equals approximately 5 or 6 liters (L) of blood.

Red blood cells (erythrocytes) are disc-shaped blood cells. These cells contain a protein known as hemoglobin that gives them their reddish color. Hemoglobin binds oxygen that is absorbed in the lungs and transports it to the tissues where it is needed.

White blood cells (leukocytes) fight infection and help eliminate foreign materials from the body. There are five types of leukocytes, each of which has a role. Neutrophils fight bacterial infections, whereas lymphocytes and monocytes help eliminate viruses and fungal infections. Eosinophils and basophils are important in allergic reactions.

Platelets are small cells in the blood that are essential for clot formation. Blood clots as a result of a series of chemical reactions. During this process, platelets aggregate together in a clump and form much of the foundation of the blood clot. The remainder of the clot consists of blood proteins, made primarily by the liver.

Blood flow

Arteries are blood vessels that carry blood away from the heart to the body. Veins transport blood from the body back to the heart (Fig. 7-23). Arteries decrease in size as they move away from the heart, branching into many small arterioles. Arterioles then divide many times until they form capillaries.

Capillaries are microscopic thin-walled vessels through which oxygen, carbon dioxide, and other nutrients and waste products are exchanged (Fig. 7-24). To return deoxygenated ("used") blood to the heart, groups of capillaries gradually enlarge to form venules. Venules then merge together forming larger and larger veins. Eventually, the veins merge together into the immense superior vena cava and inferior vena cava, which empty into the right atrium.

Blood passes from the right atrium into the right ventricle and is pumped to the lungs via the pulmonary artery. In the lungs, the blood is oxygenated and waste products are removed.

Freshly oxygenated blood is returned to the left atrium via the pulmonary veins. Blood then flows into the left ventricle, which pumps the oxygenated blood through the aorta, and then to the entire body. The left ventricle is the strongest and largest of the four cardiac chambers, because it is responsible for pumping blood through literally thousands of miles of arterial blood vessels.

Coronary arteries, which arise from the aorta, supply oxygen and nutrients to the heart. Deoxygenated venous blood from the heart drains into five different coronary veins that empty into the right atrium via the coronary sinus (Fig. 7-25).

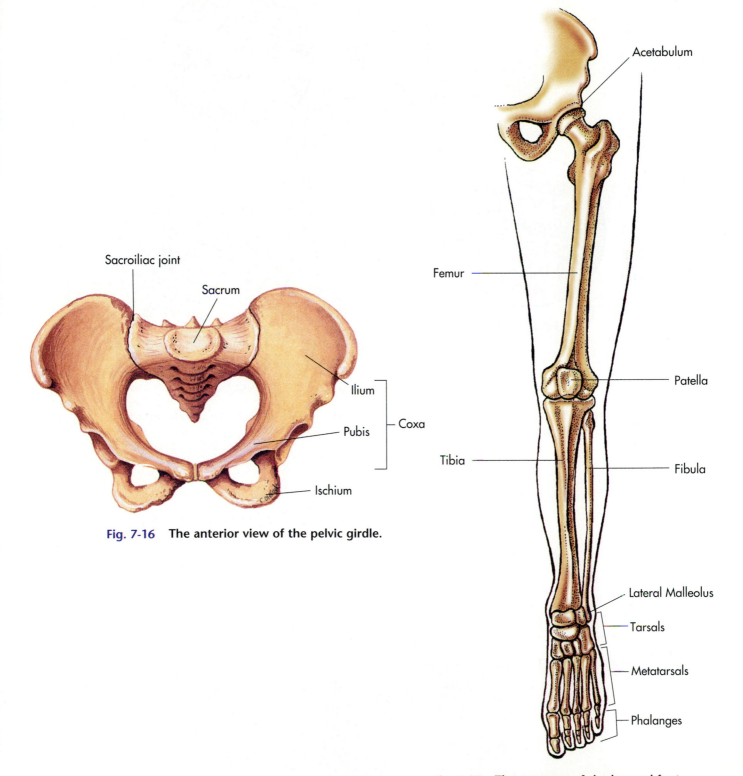

Sacroiliac joint

Sacrum

Ilium

Pubis

Ischium

Coxa

Fig. 7-16   **The anterior view of the pelvic girdle.**

Acetabulum

Femur

Patella

Tibia

Fibula

Lateral Malleolus

Tarsals

Metatarsals

Phalanges

Fig. 7-17   **The anatomy of the leg and foot.**

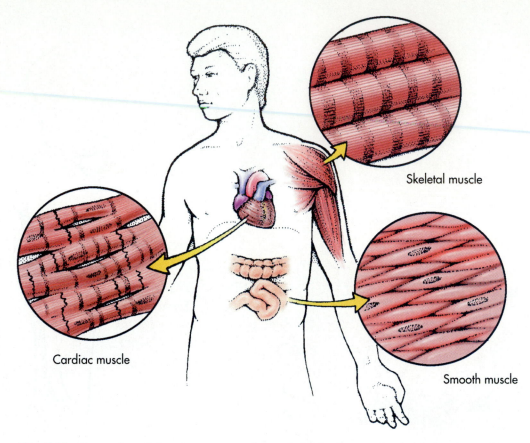

Fig. 7-18 Examples of the three types of muscle in the human body: skeletal muscle, smooth muscle, and cardiac muscle.

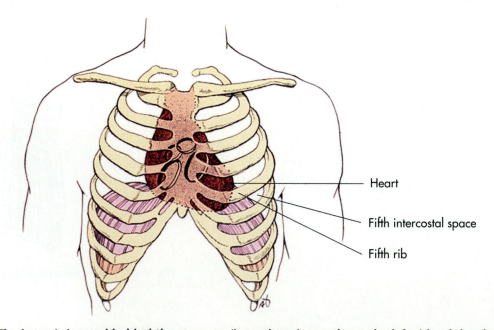

Fig. 7-19 The heart is located behind the sternum (breastbone), mostly on the left side of the chest cavity.

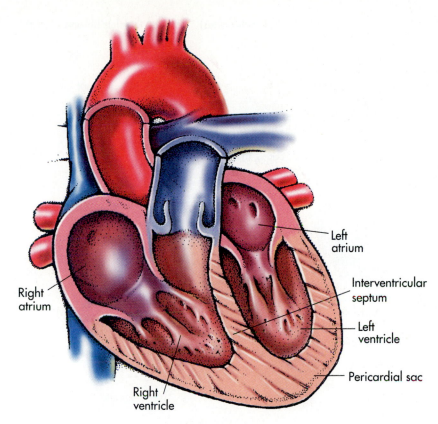

Left
atrium

Interventricular
septum

Left
ventricle

Right
atrium

Pericardial sac

Right
ventricle

Fig. 7-20   The external anatomy of the human heart.

Normal blood flow

Aorta

Superior
vena cava

Left pulmonary
arteries

Aortic
semilunar
valve

Pulmonary trunk

Pulmonary veins

Pulmonary
semilunar
valve

Right
atrium

Left atrium

Tricuspid valve

Bicuspid valve

Papillary muscles

Inferior
vena cava

Right
ventricle

Left ventricle

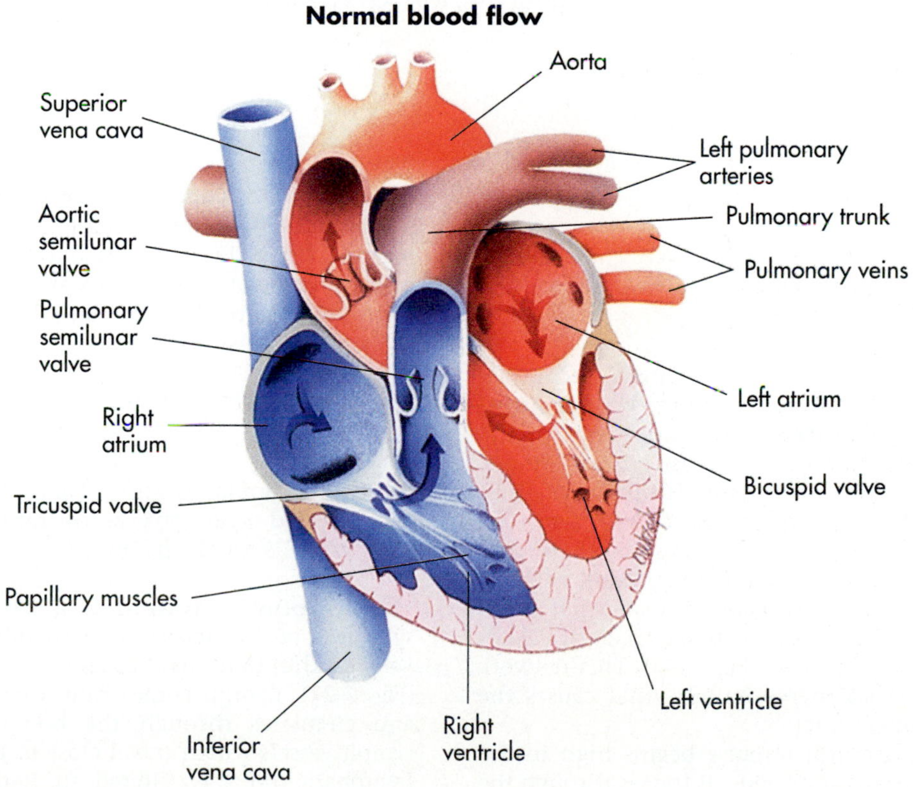

Fig. 7-21   The internal anatomy of the human heart.

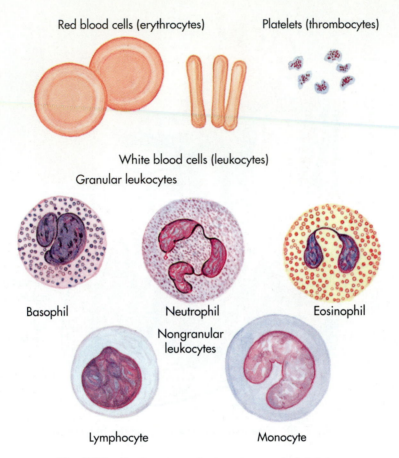

Red blood cells (erythrocytes)   Platelets (thrombocytes)

White blood cells (leukocytes)
Granular leukocytes

Basophil   Neutrophil   Eosinophil

Nongranular
leukocytes

Lymphocyte   Monocyte

Fig. 7-22   Erythrocytes, leukocytes, and platelets.

Control of the heart

🔑 **CARDIAC CONDUCTION SYSTEM:** The pathway through which electrical impulses travel in the heart.

Control of the heart's rate and strength of contraction comes partially from the brain, via the **autonomic nervous system,** from hormones of the endocrine system, and from the heart tissue. Contraction of myocardial tissue is initiated within the heart itself in a group of electrical tissues called the *sinus node.* The electrical impulse then goes through the **cardiac conduction system,** which is a complex grouping of specialized tissues that forms a network of connections, much like an electrical circuit, throughout the heart (Fig. 7-26). This network carries the electrical nerve impulse that causes the heart muscle to contract.

The initial electrical impulse begins high in the right atrium, in the sinus node. It travels through the atria via intraatrial pathways to the atrioventricular (AV) node. The stimulus then passes into the bundle of His where the conduction system divides into two portions: the right bundle branch and the left bundle branch. These fibers spread out to their respective sides of the heart. Finally, very small Purkinje's fibers take the current from the bundle branches to the individual myocardial cells.

The lymphatic system

🔑 **LYMPHATIC SYSTEM:** The body system comprised of capillaries, thin vessels, valves, ducts, nodes, and organs that allows for the transport of lymph through the body.

The **lymphatic system** is a passive circulatory system that transports a plasmalike liquid called *lymph,* a thin fluid that bathes the tissues of the body (Fig. 7-27). Lymph comes from excess cellular fluid and circulates through the body in thin-walled lymph vessels which travel close to the major veins. Lymphatic fluid is filtered in lymph nodes and returns to the main circulatory system via the thoracic duct, which empties into the superior vena

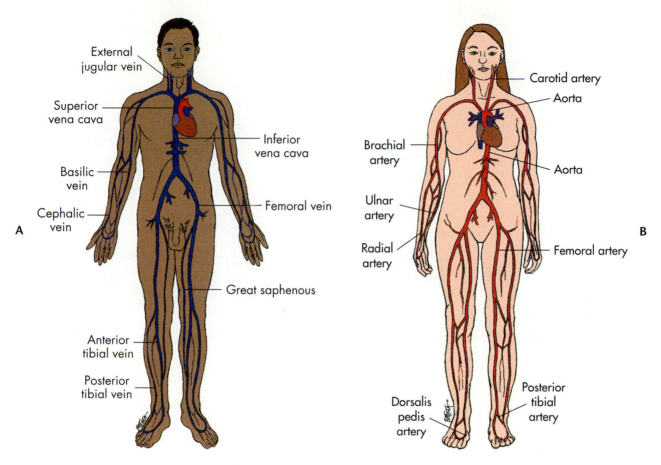

Fig. 7-23   A, Major veins of the body. B, Major arteries of the body.

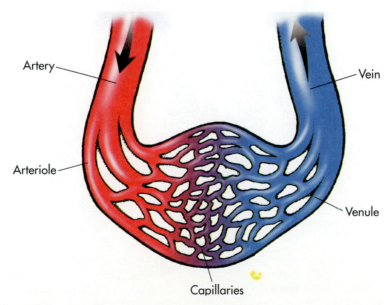

Fig. 7-24   Oxygen, carbon dioxide, and other nutrients and waste products are exchanged through capillares.

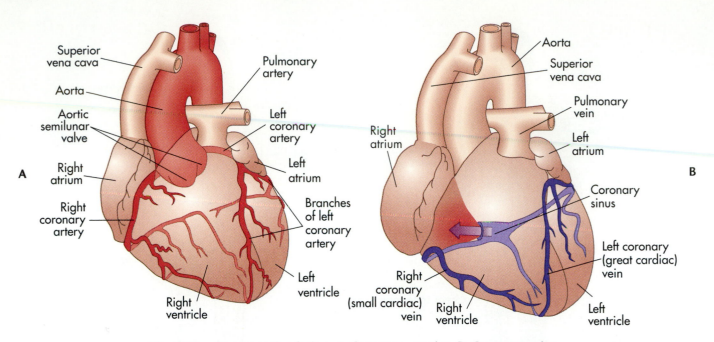

Fig. 7-25   Coronary circulation. A, Coronary arteries. B, Coronary veins.

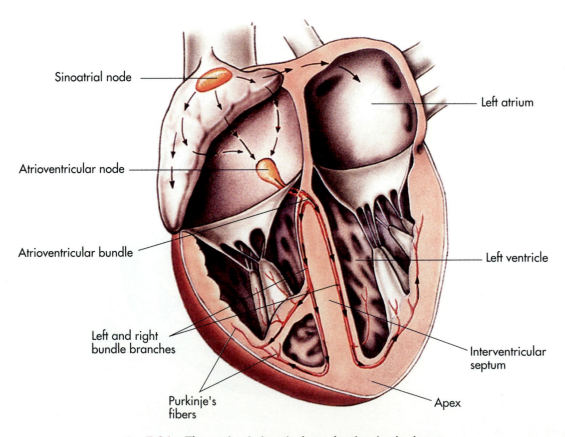

Fig. 7-26   The path of electrical conduction in the heart.

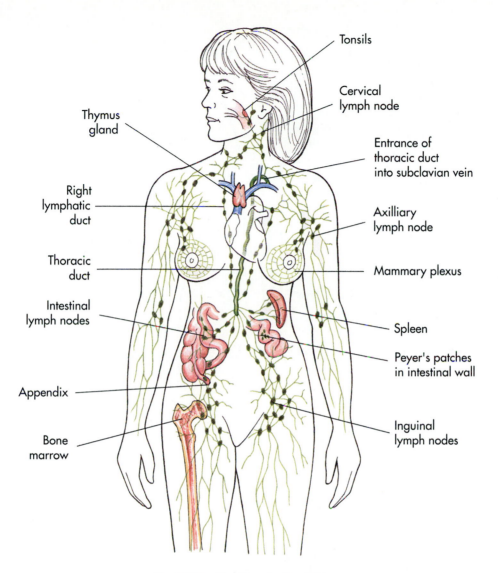

Tonsils

Cervical
lymph node

Entrance of
thoracic duct
into subclavian vein

Axilliary
lymph node

Mammary plexus

Spleen

Peyer's patches
in intestinal wall

Inguinal
lymph nodes

Thymus
gland

Right
lymphatic
duct

Thoracic
duct

Intestinal
lymph nodes

Appendix

Bone
marrow

Fig. 7-27   The lymphatic system.

cava. The lymphatic system functions primarily to absorb fat from the intestines and to trap infection-causing organisms (such as viruses and bacteria).

 CLINICAL NOTES
The lymph nodes are the site where bacteria or viruses are trapped. They are held here until they can be destroyed by cells of the immune system. As a result, the lymph nodes or "glands" may become swollen during an infection. This swelling is an indication that the lymphatic system is properly performing its function.

The respiratory system

 Describe the structure and function of the respiratory system.

RESPIRATORY SYSTEM: The body system that allows for the exchange of oxygen and carbon dioxide in blood.

The **respiratory system** consists of the organs and structures associated with breathing and gas exchange in the body. The respiratory system is divided into two parts: the upper respiratory system

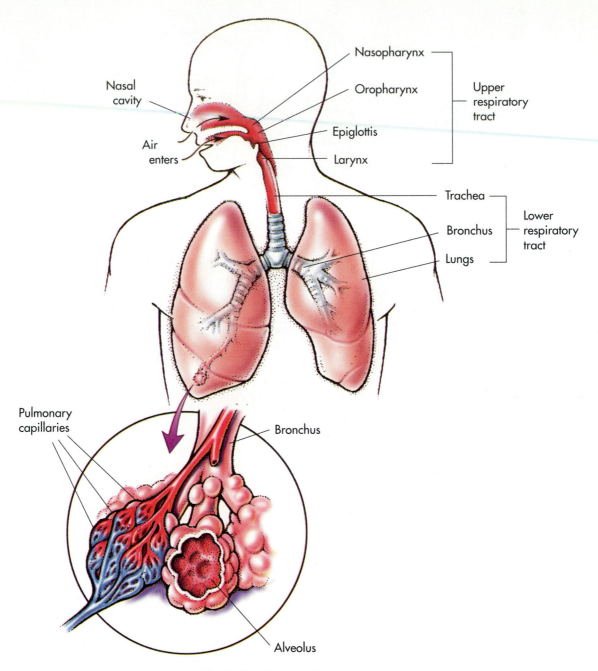

Nasal cavity

Air enters

Nasopharynx

Oropharynx

Epiglottis

Larynx

Upper respiratory tract

Trachea

Bronchus

Lungs

Lower respiratory tract

Pulmonary capillaries

Bronchus

Alveolus

Fig. 7-28   The respiratory system.

(mouth, nasal cavity, oral cavity, larynx, and vocal cords) and the lower respiratory system (trachea, bronchi, bronchioles, and alveoli) (Fig. 7-28).

Inspired air flows into the body through either the nose or the mouth. The nasal cavity is referred to as the nasopharynx, and the oral cavity, the oropharynx. These two cavities connect together posteriorly to form a common cavity, the pharynx. Air then travels downward through the larynx, which contains the vocal cords, and into the trachea.

The lower respiratory system begins with the trachea, which is a tube of cartilage and other connective tissue that extends from the larynx to the bronchi. Its purpose is to convey air to the lungs. In most adults, the trachea is approximately 4 inches long (Fig. 7-29).

The trachea divides into the right and left mainstem bronchi; this region is known as the carina. At this point, the air enters the lungs through the mainstem bronchi. The mainstem bronchi divide into secondary bronchi, each going to a separate lobe of the lung. The bronchi divide into progressively smaller branches called *bronchioles,* ending as alveoli.

Alveoli are tiny sacs of lung tissue where gas exchange takes place (Fig. 7-30). The lung contains

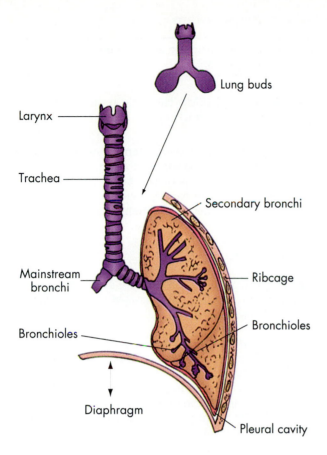

Fig. 7-29   The upper airway.

Labels: Lung buds, Larynx, Trachea, Secondary bronchi, Mainstream bronchi, Ribcage, Bronchioles, Bronchioles, Diaphragm, Pleural cavity

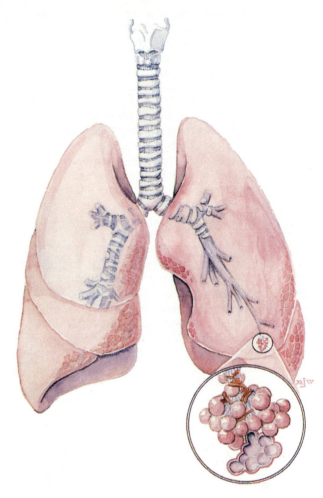

Fig. 7-30   Gas exchange takes place in the alveoli.

300 million alveoli, each about one-third mm in diameter. Alveoli are surrounded by capillaries. The membrane between the alveolus and the capillary is very thin, consisting of only one cell layer. Respiratory exchange between the lung and blood vessels occurs in the alveoli.

There are two lungs, the right lung and the left lung. The right lung has three lobes (upper, middle, and lower), whereas the left lung has only two (upper and lower). The lungs are covered with two connective tissue membranes known as the pleura. These membranes envelop each lung and line the inner borders of the rib cage, or pleural cavity.

CLINICAL NOTES

The membrane closest to the lung is referred to as the visceral pleura. The other membrane forms the parietal pleura. There is a potential space between the visceral and parietal pleura, known as the pleural space. Normally, the two membranes are close together and a space does not exist, other than enough to contain a small amount of lubricating fluid. Under certain disease conditions, or following trauma, fluid and/or air may accumulate in the pleural space, leading to respiratory problems. An abnormal collection of air in the pleural cavity is called a pneumothorax and an abnormal collection of fluid is called a pleural effusion.

Respiratory physiology

Oxygen is essential for the function of body processes. Inspired air contains approximately 21% oxygen. The primary waste product of the human body is carbon dioxide. Carbon dioxide is carried in the blood to the lungs. Expired air contains carbon dioxide and approximately 16% oxygen.

The primary function of the respiratory system is to provide for the exchange of gases at the alveolar-capillary membrane, the point where a single alveolus lies against a single capillary. At the alveolar-capillary exchange surface, the alveolus and the red blood cell come very close together. Oxygen and carbon dioxide diffuse across the membrane. Oxygen moves from the alveolus to the hemoglobin molecule of the red blood cells. Carbon dioxide flows from the blood into the alveolus. When the individual exhales, carbon dioxide is breathed into the atmosphere and eliminated from the body.

CLINICAL NOTES

The large number of alveoli allow an extremely large surface area for respiratory exchange in the relatively limited space of the thoracic cavity. By wrapping the small capillaries around an enormous number of alveoli, a total surface area of more than 85 square meters occurs. If each lung consisted of only a single sphere, like a large balloon, the surface area would be only 0.01 square meters (1 meter = 39.37 inches).

The brain controls respiration. The respiratory center of the brain responds to the levels of carbon dioxide in the blood. Excess levels of carbon dioxide cause the brain to stimulate ventilation, whereas decreased levels of carbon dioxide force the brain to decrease ventilation. The brain also responds to levels of oxygen in the blood; however, the brain's response to oxygen is less predictable than its response to carbon dioxide.

CLINICAL NOTES

The lungs are important in maintaining the degree of acid and base in the blood. When a person hyperventilates, an excess of carbon dioxide is exhaled or "blown off." This deficit of carbon dioxide causes the blood to turn more basic. This condition is known as a **respiratory alkalosis.** Certain conditions, such as severe chronic obstructive pulmonary disorder (COPD) and respiratory failure may block the lungs' ability to blow off carbon dioxide. The gas is then retained in the blood, causing a build-up of acid. This state is known as a **respiratory acidosis.**

CLINICAL NOTES

Technically, **ventilation** refers to the movement of carbon dioxide in and out of the lungs. **Oxygenation** is a separate, but somewhat related, process. For example, a person may hyperventilate, causing a decrease in the carbon dioxide level in the blood (respiratory alkalosis) but no change in the level of oxygen.

When a person inhales, the diaphragm contracts, creating a negative pressure in the chest cavity. This negative pressure "sucks" in air, expanding the lungs. Air is expired when the lung tissue collapses due to its natural elasticity—much like a balloon that has had the air suddenly released. Exhalation is a passive progress, and normally requires no muscular effort.

The nervous system

> Describe the structure and function of the nervous system.

 NERVOUS SYSTEM: The body system that controls the body's functions.

The **nervous system** is an extensive network of cells that conducts information that controls and coordinates all the functions of the body. Nerve cells are called *neurons.* The nervous system is divided into two parts: the central nervous system, and the peripheral nervous system.

The central nervous system

CENTRAL NERVOUS SYSTEM: The portion of the nervous system comprised of the brain and spinal cord.

The **central nervous system** consists of the brain and spinal cord (Fig. 7-31). The brain, which lies in the cranial cavity, is divided into three major parts: the cerebrum, the cerebellum, and the medulla. The cerebrum is the top portion of the brain and consists of the left and right hemispheres. The cerebrum is further subdivided into four lobes. Thinking, sensation, and voluntary movement are controlled by the cerebrum.

The cerebellum is located behind and below the cerebrum. Its primary function is to control the body's coordination. The medulla, also known as the brainstem, is the most inferior portion of the brain. This portion of the brain contains important centers that control involuntary respiration, heart, and blood vessel function (Fig. 7-32).

The spinal cord

The spinal cord is a cylindrical cord of nervous tissue extending from the brain. It runs the length of the vertebral canal from the foramen magnum, a large opening at the base of the skull, to the level of the second lumbar vertebra. Below this level, the cord divides into individual nerves known as cauda equina.

The spinal cord receives motor nerve impulses from the brain and transmits these to the body, causing muscles to contract and movement to occur. Sensory nerve impulses from the organs of special sensation are transmitted to the spinal cord, then to the brain. Both motor and sensory impulses are carried by spinal nerves from the spinal cord.

The brain and spinal cord are covered by three layers of membranes known as meninges. The outer layer is the dura mater and is the thickest. The middle layer is the arachnoid membrane, and the inner layer, which is closely adherent to the brain tissue, is the pia mater (Fig. 7-33). Cerebrospinal fluid (CSF), a clear substance produced in the brain (Fig. 7-34),

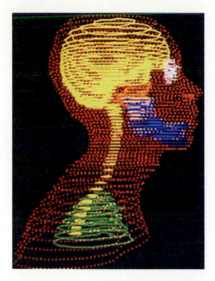

Fig. 7-31 A computer-generated image of the brain and spinal cord.

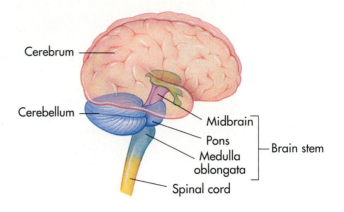

Fig. 7-32 **The anatomy of the brain.**

circulates between the pia mater and the arachnoid in the subarachnoid space. This space is continuous from the cranial cavity to the sacrum. It fills and protects the cranial and spinal cavities, cushioning the brain and spinal cord. In the adult there is normally approximately 140 mL of CSF.

The peripheral nervous system

PERIPHERAL NERVOUS SYSTEM: The portion of the nervous system comprised of cranial nerves, the spinal nerves, and the autonomic nervous system.

The **peripheral nervous system** includes the cranial nerves, the spinal nerves, and the autonomic nervous system.

There are three types of peripheral nerves: 1) Sensory nerves transmit impulses from the organs to the spinal cord. 2) Motor nerves transmit impulses that stimulate muscle contraction and movement from the spinal cord to the muscles. 3) Mixed nerves carry both sensory and motor messages.

Twelve pairs of cranial nerves extend directly from the brain. Thirty-one pairs of spinal nerves leave the spinal cord—each pair leaves at a separate level of the vertebral column. The nerves pass from the spine via the intervertebral foramina. These nerves are numbered according to the regions of the vertebral column with which they are associated: eight cervical, twelve thoracic, five lumbar, five sacral, and one coccygeal. The spinal nerves subdivide into numerous peripheral nerves that extend to the entire body.

The autonomic nervous system

AUTONOMIC NERVOUS SYSTEM: The division of the nervous system that controls involuntary functions such as heart rate.

The autonomic nervous system, a specialized subdivision of the peripheral nervous system, regulates involuntary functions of the body (Fig. 7-35). Examples of autonomic nervous system responsibilities include activity of the heart and smooth muscle. There are two divisions of the autonomic nervous system: the sympathetic and the parasympathetic nervous systems.

SYMPATHETIC NERVOUS SYSTEM: Division of the autonomic nervous system that is responsible for constriction of blood vessels, elevation of blood pressure and heart rate, and a feeling of nervousness in a stressful situation.
PARASYMPATHETIC NERVOUS SYSTEM: Division of the autonomic nervous system responsible for slowing the heart rate, intestinal activity, respiratory rate, and pupillary responses.

The **sympathetic nervous system** generates what we typically think of as the "fight or flight" response—constriction of blood vessels, elevation of the blood pressure and heart rate, and a feeling of nervousness. The **para-sympathetic nervous system** works the opposite way causing slowing of the heart rate. The parasympathetic nervous system controls intestinal activity, respiratory rate, and

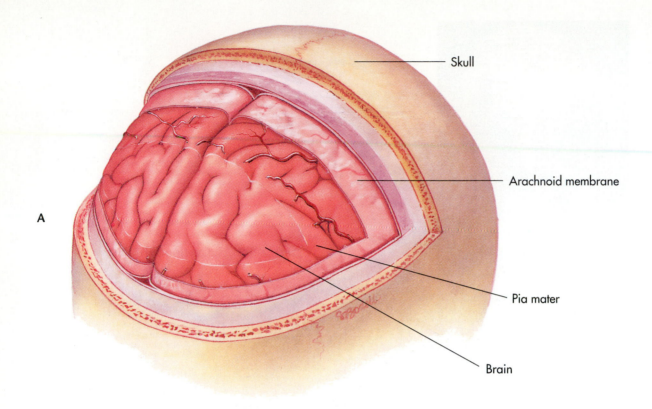

A

- Skull
- Arachnoid membrane
- Pia mater
- Brain

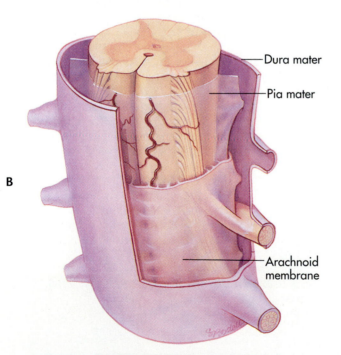

B

- Dura mater
- Pia mater
- Arachnoid membrane

Fig. 7-33 Meningeal covering of: A, The brain. B, The spinal cord.

pupillary responses. In extreme instances, excess stimulation of the parasympathetic nervous system can lead to cardiac arrest.

> **HELPFUL HINT**
> Typical sympathetic responses include tachycardia, elevated blood pressure, and a feeling of nervousness. Typical parasympathetic responses are nausea, vomiting, fainting (due to slow heart rate), and abdominal distress.

The gastrointestinal system

> **GASTROINTESTINAL SYSTEM:** The body system responsible for digestion.

The **gastrointestinal system** is composed of structures and organs involved in the consumption, digestion, and elimination of food. Digestion begins in the mouth where food is chewed by the teeth and mixed with saliva from the salivary glands. The partially digested food is then swallowed and travels via the esophagus to the stomach.

The abdomen is divided into imaginary quadrants. Due to the large number of organs in the abdomen, these quadrant enable emergency providers to distinguish the location of problems. The umbilicus (navel) serves as the central reference point. The diaphragm is the top of the abdominal cavity, and the pelvic bones, the bottom. The

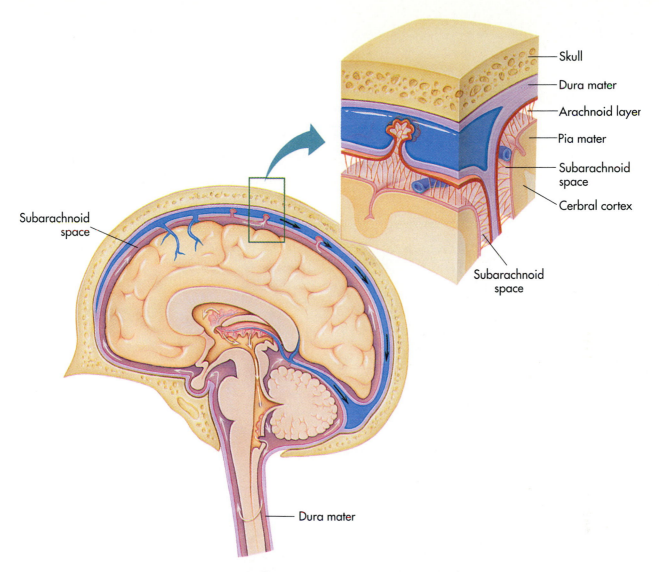

Fig. 7-34 Circulation of cerebrospinal fluid in the subaradnoid space.

quadrants are divided by a set of imaginary perpendicular lines intersecting at the umbilicus (Fig. 7-36).

 Identify the four quadrants of the abdomen.

The abdominal organs are identified by their location within these quadrants. Some of the organs are located in more than one quadrant. There is anatomic overlap between organs of the gastrointestinal, urinary, and reproductive systems. The major organs in each quadrant are:

- Right upper quadrant (RUQ)—liver, gallbladder, part of the large intestine, right kidney
- Left upper quadrant (LUQ)—stomach, spleen, pancreas, part of the large intestine, left kidney
- Right lower quadrant (RLQ)—appendix, part of the large intestine, right ovary, right ureter, uterus, urinary bladder

- Left lower quadrant (LLQ)—part of the large intestine, left ovary, left ureter, uterus, urinary bladder

The kidneys and pancreas are not located in the abdominal cavity *per se*, but in an area behind the peritoneal membranes called the *retroperitoneal space*. However, injuries and illness affecting these organs often cause abdominal symptoms that are best classified by location. For this reason, these organs are included as being located within these quadrants.

The hollow abdominal organs

Abdominal organs are classified as hollow or solid. Hollow organs generally comprise the digestive system, through which foodstuffs move (Fig. 7-37).

The esophagus, or swallowing tube, carries food and liquid from the pharynx to the stomach, an expandable organ located below the diaphragm in the left upper quadrant. Here, the food is churned

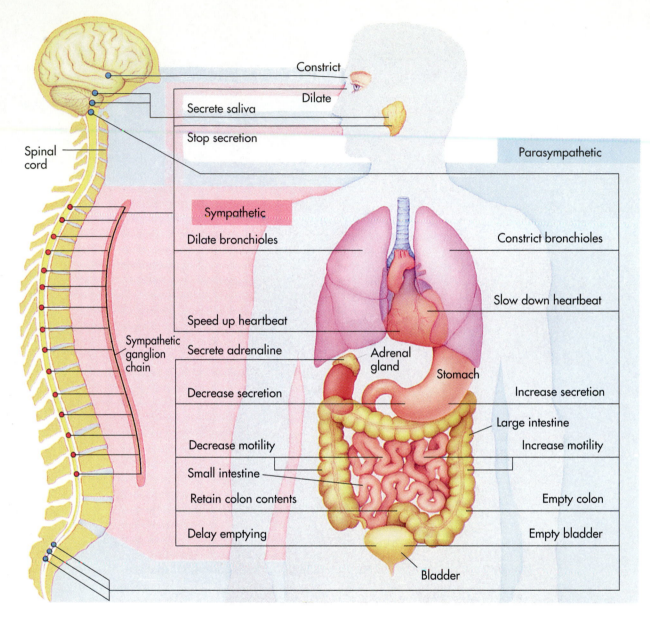

Fig. 7-35 Organ regulation by the autonomic nervous system. The sympathetic nervous system is highlighted in red, the parasympathetic in blue.

and mixed with digestive juices, forming a semiliquid mass called *chyme*.

Food moves through the pyloric valve into the small intestine, which is the longest part of the digestive tract and the major site of food digestion and absorption of nutrients. There are three parts of the small intestine: the duodenum, the jejunum, and the ileum. Together, the entire small intestine is often 20 feet in length.

The ileum empties into the large intestine. Here, the collection and removal of the wastes from digestion, including water, occurs. Stool is formed in the longest portion of the large intestine, the colon. It is stored in the rectum and excreted through the anus.

The appendix is a fingerlike attachment to the first part of the large intestine in the right lower quadrant. It has no known function, and may become inflamed, causing appendicitis.

The gallbladder is a pear-shaped organ located on the lower surface of the liver. It acts as a reservoir for bile, an important digestive enzyme. When a person eats fatty foods, the gallbladder contracts, releasing bile into the small intestine.

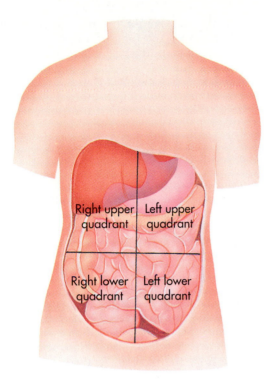

Fig. 7-36   Organs of the abdomen.

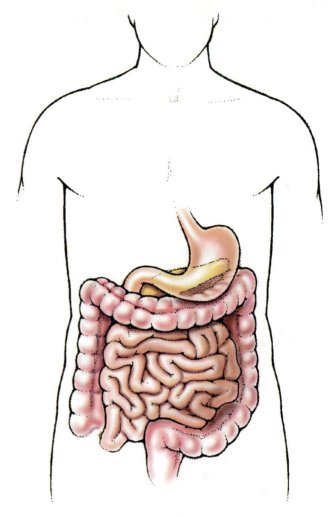

Fig. 7-37   Hollow abdominal organs.

 CLINICAL NOTES
Injury to a hollow organ may cause it to be punctured or to rupture. In either case, the internal contents are dumped into the abdominal cavity, which may lead to infection or irritation.

The solid abdominal organs

The liver is a large solid organ in the right upper quadrant. It has many functions, including storage of glucose, protein synthesis, and filtering the blood of body wastes. Many drugs and chemicals also are broken down (detoxified) here.

The spleen is a highly vascular organ located in the left upper quadrant behind the stomach. It aids in the removal of old blood cells from the circulation as well as in fighting infection.

The pancreas is an elongated gland located in the left upper quadrant behind the stomach. It has several functions, including the manufacture of digestive juices as well as the hormones insulin and glucagon.

 HELPFUL HINT
Injury to a solid organ may result in significant bleeding into the abdominal cavity. This injury is very serious because the patient can be in severe shock and may even bleed to death, without any signs of external bleeding.

The urinary system

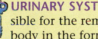 **Describe the structure and function of the urinary system.**

URINARY SYSTEM: The body system responsible for the removal of waste products from the body in the form of urine.

The **urinary system** removes waste products from the blood by a complex filtration process. It also is involved in maintaining a proper balance between water and salts in the blood.

The major structures of the urinary tract are anatomically intertwined with those of the digestive system. The kidneys are located behind the abdominal cavity, in the retroperitoneal space. These solid, bean-shaped organs filter blood and excrete body wastes in the form of urine. The kidneys also are important in the regulation of the body's fluid balance and blood pressure. The ureters are a pair of thick-walled hollow tubes that carry urine from the kidneys to the urinary bladder.

The urinary bladder is a hollow, muscular sac in the midline of the lower abdominal area that stores urine until it is excreted. The urethra is a hollow, tubular structure that drains urine from the bladder, passing it to the outside.

The reproductive system

 Describe the structure and function of the male and female reproductive systems.

REPRODUCTIVE SYSTEM: The body system responsible for sexual reproduction.

The **reproductive system** includes all of the male and female structures responsible for sexual reproduction.

Female reproductive organs
The uterus is a hollow, pear-shaped organ located in the midline of the lower quadrants. It is the site of implantation, growth, and nourishment of the fetus during pregnancy. The cervix is the part of the uterus that extends into the vagina. During childbirth, the baby passes through the dilated cervix into the vaginal birth canal. The vagina is the muscular tube that forms the lower part of the female reproductive tract.

The fallopian tubes are two hollow tubes that extend from the uterus to the region of the ovary.

These serve as a passage for the movement of the ovum from the ovary and for sperm from the uterus upward. The fallopian tube is where fertilization usually occurs.

The ovaries are the female sex glands, and there is usually one on each side of the lower quadrants. These glands produce hormones that regulate female reproductive function and secondary sexual characteristics (breast and pubic hair development), as well as serve as the source of the ovum, or egg (Fig. 7-38).

Male reproductive organs
The testicles, or testes, are the male gonads. The testes are held in a pouch of skin known as the scrotum. The testes produce sperm and secrete male hormones such as testosterone, which are responsible for secondary sexual characteristics.

The prostate gland is a chestnut-shaped structure located at the base of the urethra. Together with an associated set of glands, the seminal vesicles, the prostate produces secretions that become part of semen.

The urethra is a hollow, tubular structure that drains urine from the bladder. It also provides the pathway by which sperm and semen are released from the penis, the external male reproductive organ, during sexual intercourse. (Fig. 7-39).

The immune system

 Describe the structure and function of the immune system.

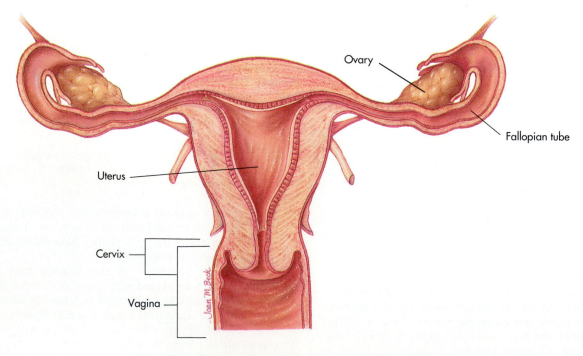

Fig. 7-38   The anatomy of female reproductive system.

IMMUNE SYSTEM: The body system that protects the body from foreign materials.

The **immune system** defends the body against bacteria, viruses, and other foreign matter. The body has two types of immunity, which is the ability to resist damage from foreign substances or harmful chemicals: nonspecific immunity and specific immunity. Nonspecific immunity occurs via three mechanisms. Mechanical barriers, such as the skin, prevent the entry of many bacteria. In addition, tears, saliva, and mucous in the respiratory tract continuously wash foreign matter away. Secondly, chemicals such as histamine promote inflammation in response to foreign invaders to the body. Finally, white blood cells (leukocytes) ingest and destroy bacterial invaders and foreign matter.

Two types of specific immunity exist. Foreign substances, known as antigens, lead to the formation of antibodies by the immune system. These antibodies form the basis of antibody-mediated immunity. When the body is exposed to a foreign antigen, the antibody attacks it and initiates a series of reactions designed to eliminate the antigen from the body. Cell-mediated immunity is achieved by the actions of lymphocytes. These cells seek out and destroy foreign materials, such as viruses, fungi, bacteria, and particles.

The endocrine system

 Describe the structure and function of the endocrine system.

ENDOCRINE SYSTEM: The body system comprised of ductless glands that are responsible for hormone production.

The **endocrine system** consists of several glands located throughout the body (Fig. 7-40). These glands secrete proteins called *hormones,* which regulate many body functions, such as growth, reproduction, temperature, metabolism, and blood pressure.

- The pituitary gland, sometimes known as the "master gland," is located at the base of the brain in the cranial cavity. It manufactures hormones that regulate the function of the other endocrine glands in the body.

- The thyroid gland is a large gland situated at the base of the neck. It manufactures and secretes hormones that influence growth, development, metabolism, and levels of calcium in the body.

- The parathyroid glands are embedded in the posterior portion of the thyroid. They produce

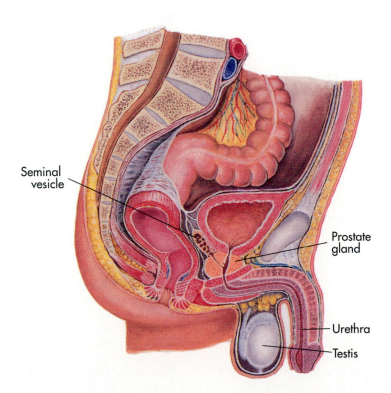

Seminal vesicle

Prostate gland

Urethra

Testis

Fig. 7-39   The anatomy of male reproductive system.

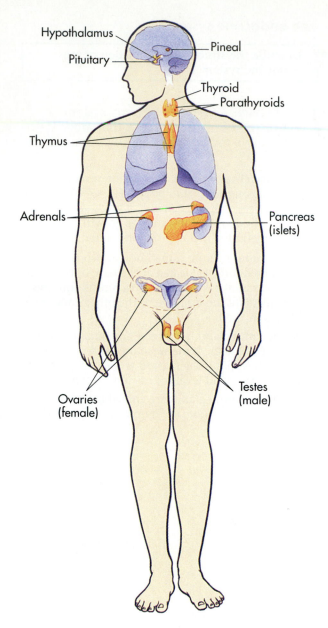

Hypothalamus
Pituitary
Pineal
Thyroid
Parathyroids
Thymus
Adrenals
Pancreas (islets)
Ovaries (female)
Testes (male)

Fig. 7-40 Endocrine glands in the human body.

hormones that maintain normal levels of calcium in the blood.

- The pancreas is considered an organ of both the digestive and the endocrine systems. In addition to producing digestive enzymes, it manufactures the hormones insulin and glucagon. Both of these hormones are vital in control of the body's metabolism and blood sugar level. Lack of insulin leads to diabetes mellitus.

- The adrenal glands are located on top of each kidney. They manufacture and secrete certain sex hormones as well as other hormones vital in maintaining the body's water and salt balance.

During stress, the adrenal gland produces epinephrine and norepinephrine, which mediate the "flight or fight" response of the sympathetic nervous system mentioned previously.

- The reproductive glands, or gonads, are the ovaries in the woman and the testes in the man. These glands produce hormones responsible for development of secondary sex characteristics (such as a deep voice and facial hair in men and breast development in women), as well as for reproduction.

The integumentary system

INTEGUMENTARY SYSTEM: The body system comprised of the skin and its appendixes.

The **integumentary system** refers to the body's external surface and includes the skin, nails, hair, sweat, and oil glands. The major functions of the integumentary system are temperature regulation, defense against disease-causing organisms, and maintenance of fluid balance.

There are two major layers of the **skin**. The outermost layer is the epidermis. It contains no blood vessels but is rich in hair (in many locations), openings from sweat and oil glands, and nerves. Below the epidermis is the dermis, a thick layer that contains connective tissue, hair follicles, glands (which extend upward into the epidermis), and nerve endings for temperature, touch, pain, and pressure.

Below the skin (epidermis and dermis) is the hypodermis, sometimes called *subcutaneous tissue*. It attaches the skin to the underlying bone or muscle and contains much of the body's fat stores. Most nerves and blood vessels run through the dermis, extending only small branches into the epidermis (Fig. 7-41).

The special sensory system

SPECIAL SENSORY SYSTEM: The system of the body responsible for the five senses.

The **special sensory system** of the body consists of special nerve receptors that perceive light, sound, taste, odors, and sensations from the skin or areas outside of the body.

The eyes—vision
The eyes lie within the bony orbits of the skull (Fig. 7-42). They are held in place by loose connective tissue and several muscles. The muscles also control eye movements. The optic nerve enters the globe, or eyeball, posteriorly, through an opening in the orbit called the *optic foramen*.

The white part of the eye is called the *sclera*. The colored part of the eye is the iris. The iris surrounds the pupil, a circular opening through which light

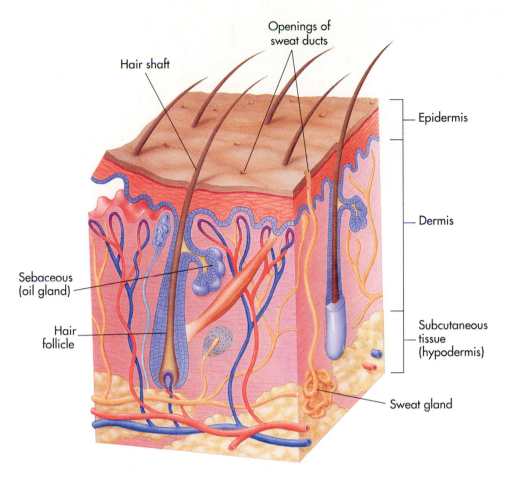

Openings of
sweat ducts

Hair shaft

Epidermis

Dermis

Sebaceous
(oil gland)

Hair
follicle

Subcutaneous
tissue
(hypodermis)

Sweat gland

Fig. 7-41   **The integumantary system in the human body.**

passes to the lens. The cornea is the transparent ante-rior portion of the eye that overlies the iris and pupil. The anterior chamber is the portion of the globe between the lens and the cornea. The anterior chamber is filled with a clear, watery fluid known as *aqueous humor.*

The conjunctiva is a thin, transparent membrane that covers the sclera and internal surfaces of the eye-lids and stops at the iris. Tears come from the lacrimal sacs and pass through the lacrimal ducts, located on the nasal border of the eyelids. Tears are drained by ducts that lead to the nose.

The interior of the eye contains a jellylike material known as *vitreous humor.* At the rear of the interior of the globe lies the retina. The retina is a delicate 10-layered structure of nervous tissue continuous with the optic nerve. The function of the retina is to receive light, which generates nerve signals that are conducted to the brain by the optic nerve and inter-preted as vision.

The mouth and tongue—taste
The mouth and tongue contain various nerves, called *taste receptors* or *taste buds* that sense salt and sweet sensations separately. These nerves then transmit

impulses back to the taste center of the brain, where they are converted into sensations we perceive as taste (Fig. 7-43).

The ears—hearing
Sound waves enter the ear through the large outside portion, the auricle, or pinnae. They travel down the ear canal to the eardrum, or tympanic membrane. Vibration of sound waves against the tympanic mem-brane sets up vibrations in three small bones on the other side, called *ossicles.* Vibrations of the ossicles are converted into nerve impulses, which are trans-mitted to the brain via the auditory nerve. The brain then converts these impulses into what we experi-ence as sound. The inner portion of the ear helps in maintaining balance.

The nose—smell
Special receptors, known as *olfactory nerves,* line the nasal cavity. These receptors detect various odors and transmit the message to a large nerve at the base of the brain, the olfactory bulb. Sensations of smell from the olfactory bulb are then transmitted to the brain and translated into sensations of smell (Fig. 7-44).

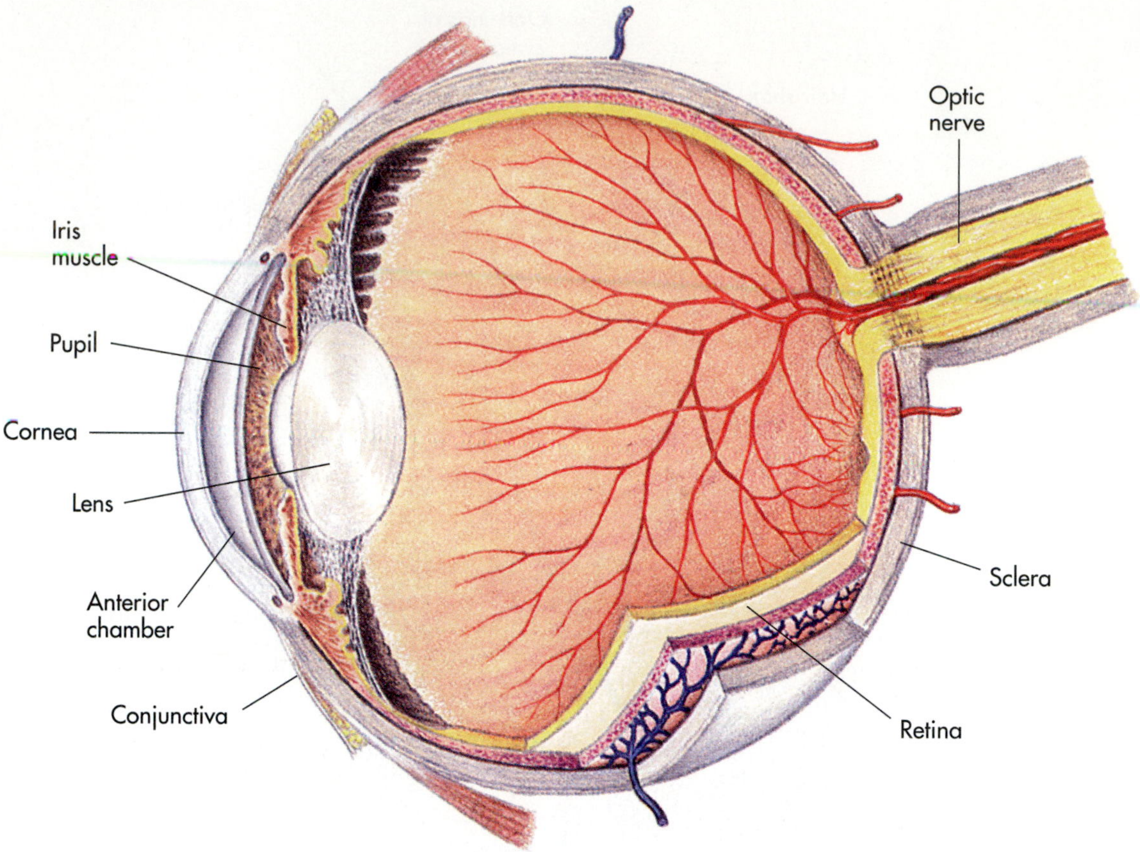

Iris
muscle

Pupil

Cornea

Lens

Anterior
chamber

Conjunctiva

Optic
nerve

Sclera

Retina

Fig. 7-42   A horizontal section of the human eye, as viewed from above.

The skin—touch

The special sense of touch is interrelated with the function of the peripheral nervous system. Various touch receptors on the skin detect when and what we touch. Similar receptors also detect heat, cold, and pain. These impulses are transmitted to the spinal cord and then to the brain, where they are brought into conscious reality.

CASE HISTORY FOLLOW-UP

EMT–I Jackson and her crew arrive at the trauma center in approximately 7 minutes. The trauma team meets them at the door and takes the patient immediately to the OR.

When EMT–I Jackson returns to the station, she asks the EMT-I student to explain the significance of the anatomic locations of the stab wounds.

"Well," he says, "nothing like putting me right on the spot. So, here goes. . .

"First, the wound at the right anterior axillary line at T4. T4 is the "nipple line," and an anterior axillary entry for a knife wound could cause an injury to the right lung, resulting in a pneumothorax, hemothorax, or both, as well as an abdominal injury, including liver, gallbladder, pancreatic, or intestinal injury, or major vessel injury in the mediastinum,

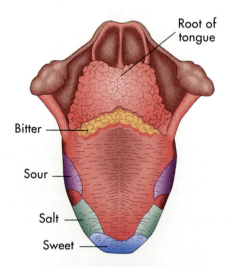

Root of
tongue

Bitter

Sour

Salt

Sweet

Fig. 7-43   **The surface of the tongue and the various regions sensitive to taste.**

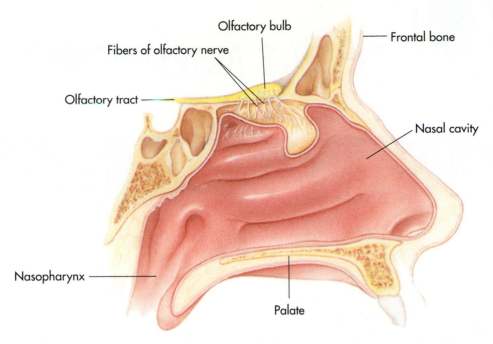

Olfactory bulb

Fibers of olfactory nerve

Frontal bone

Olfactory tract

Nasal cavity

Nasopharynx

Palate

Fig. 7-44   Sensations of smell are transmitted from the nasal cavity to the olfactory bulb in the brain.

including inferior or superior vena cava. Any of these thoracic injuries could rapidly become fatal, whereas the abdominal injuries would pose a great risk for death from hemorrhage and infection.

"Second, the wound at the left midaxillary line at T6. This wound not only poses a serious risk for lung injuries, but also poses an even greater risk for cardiac injury. Abdominal penetration would likely involve gastric injury, and should a major vessel have been injured in the mediastinum, it would probably have involved the descending thoracic or abdominal aorta. The patient would most likely have been dead in seconds.

"Third, the left epigastric region wound. If the knife were thrust upward, toward the head, it could have caused diaphragmatic trauma, as well as cardiac injury—and don't men often stab upward? If the knife went in perpendicular to the skin, it may have penetrated the spleen, stomach, pancreas, small intestine, or even a kidney. The patient would definitely have a hemoperitoneum. Depending on the path of the knife, the organs on the right side of the upper left abdomen could have been injured as well, including the liver or gallbladder.

"Fourth, the left midbuttock wound. This one may have injured his ischiadic or sciatic nerve, which may account for the lack of a pain response in his left leg.

"And last, the right anterior midthigh wound. This one typically wouldn't be life-threatening unless it struck a major vessel and the patient was losing a significant amount of blood. However, with the 5-cm larger circumference in the right thigh, that may just be the case.

"Well, what do you think?"
EMT–I Jackson responds, "I have to admit, I'm impressed. I'll bet you pass your anatomy test."

SUMMARY

Anatomy is the study of body structures. Physiology is the study of the function of these structures. The various organ systems of the body provide support (skeletal system), movement (muscular system), and overall control of body functions (nervous system). The respiratory system facilitates intake and absorption of oxygen into the blood, which is then delivered to the tissues by the circulatory system.

Food and water are absorbed by the digestive and lymphatic systems, whereas the endocrine system produces hormones that aid in the metabolism of food, as well as in other chemical processes. Body wastes are excreted by combined actions of the urinary (urine), gastrointestinal (stool), and respiratory (carbon dioxide) systems.

The immune system defends the body against invasion by organisms and foreign substances. An important component of immunity is the integumentary system consisting of the skin, nails, hair, and sweat and oil glands. This system provides the body's external covering and provides for temperature regulation and protection. Special sensory systems allow for the senses of vision, taste, hearing, smell, and touch.

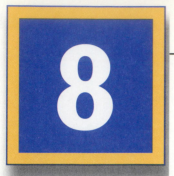

8 PATIENT ASSESSMENT

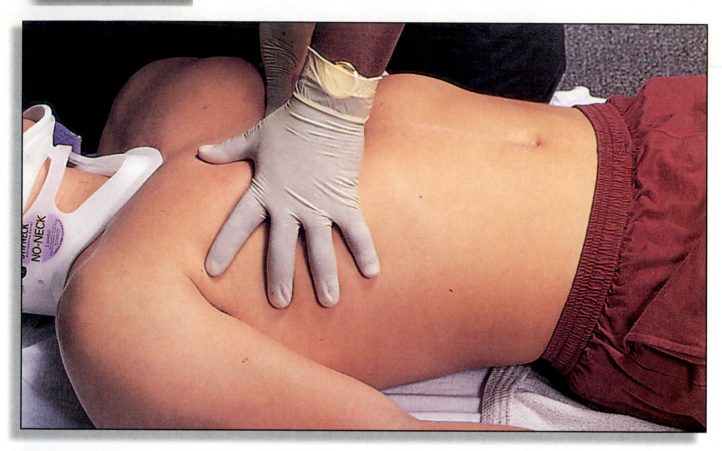

CASE HISTORY

It's early afternoon on a rainy, winter day. EMT–Intermediates Smith and Jones are eating lunch at the base when the alarm sounds: "Unit 3...Respond as backup to a motor vehicle accident with injuries...Intersection of Highway K and Mexico Road...Time out 1230." En route, the EMT–Is are advised that three cars are involved and there are multiple patients. Police are on the scene, and fire/rescue personnel have been dispatched. The air/medical crew has been placed on standby. ETA is 5 minutes.

As the EMT–Is approach the crash site, they see warning lights and police blocking access to the intersection. There are cars and people everywhere, and the scene looks very busy. Two of the cars are still on the roadway, and the third car is on its side as a result of the impact. The EMT–Is don their protective gear and report to the command post established by the fire department.

Case History, continued

The EMT–Is are directed to the first ambulance that arrived on the scene. In the patient compartment they find a woman holding a child in her lap, talking to a police officer. They hear her say that she and her 3-year-old child were front-seat passengers in one of the cars at the intersection, and they were able to exit the car after impact. The patients are visibly shaken but have no apparent injuries. EMT–I Smith performs a brief initial assessment on the woman and obtains an initial set of vital signs. The child is whimpering and clinging to his mother. He will not cooperate for an examination, so EMT–I Smith attempts to palpate major body regions through his winter clothing. His mother states that she thinks he's OK and is just scared from the accident. She wants him to be "checked out" at the emergency department. The police officer offers to stay with them so that EMT–I Smith can care for other patients at the scene. EMT–I Smith returns to the command post and assists EMT–I Jones and the other crews.

There were a total of seven patients, two of whom had serious injuries and were flown out to the trauma center. EMT–Is Smith and Jones transported the mother and her child and one other patient with minor injuries to a local hospital. The other crew transported the remaining patients. En route back to base, EMT–I Smith is advised by Dispatch to contact his medical direction physician. She wants to talk to him about one of the patients he transported.

LEARNING OBJECTIVES

Upon completion of this chapter, the EMT-Intermediate should be able to:

- DESCRIBE the six phases of patient assessment.
- IDENTIFY potential scene hazards that may endanger the EMT–I or the patient.
- DESCRIBE the self-protection measures required for body substance isolation precautions.
- DESCRIBE the problems an EMT–I might encounter in a hostile situation and suggest mechanisms of management.
- DESCRIBE the initial assessment and what areas are critical to evaluate.
- DESCRIBE the need for and methods of cervical spine immobilization throughout the phases of patient assessment.
- DESCRIBE techniques for evaluating the effectiveness of ventilation.
- DESCRIBE the mechanism of evaluating the effectiveness of perfusion including pulse and skin color.
- DEFINE a "priority" patient and discuss several illnesses or suspected injuries that would lead you to classify a patient in this fashion.
- DESCRIBE the components of the focused assessment for both the medical and the trauma patient.
- DESCRIBE the components of the detailed assessment and discuss various conditions that determine whether or not the EMT–I must perform this phase of patient assessment.
- DESCRIBE the need for on-going assessment; list the components and discuss the frequency of this part of the patient evaluation.
- DISCUSS factors that must be considered when determining to which hospital a patient should be transported.
- DESCRIBE the need for communication with either medical direction or the receiving facility when transporting a patient.
- DISCUSS the benefits of accurate documentation.

ANISOCORIA	NECK VEIN DISTENSION
APNEA	NORMOTENSION
AVPU	OPQRST
BATTLE'S SIGN	ORTHOSTATIC HYPOTENSION
BODY SUBSTANCE ISOLATION PRECAUTIONS	PARESTHESIAS
CARDIAC DYSRHYTHMIA	PULSE OXIMETER
CEREBROSPINAL FLUID	PULSE PRESSURE
CHEYNE-STOKES	PUPILLARY REACTIVITY
COSTOVERTEBRAL ANGLE	RALES
DETAILED ASSESSMENT	RAPID TRAUMA ASSESSMENT
DIASTOLE	RHONCHI
EUPNEA	RIGIDITY
FOCUSED HISTORY AND PHYSICAL EXAMINATION	SAMPLE HISTORY
GLASGOW COMA SCALE	SCENE SIZE-UP
HEMIPLEGIA	SCLERA
HYPERTENSION	SUBCUTANEOUS EMPHYSEMA
HYPOTENSION	SYSTOLE
INITIAL ASSESSMENT	VISUAL ACUITY EXAMINATION
KUSSMAUL	WHEEZES

INTRODUCTION

 Describe the six phases of patient assessment.

Patient assessment is a structured method of evaluating a patient's physical condition. An organized, well-developed patient assessment is a valuable tool for providing patient care. The patient assessment is the process of looking for, asking about, and recognizing the symptoms and signs of an abnormal condition.

A symptom is a subjective indication of a disease or condition as perceived by the patient. For example, the patient may complain of the symptom chest pain. A sign is an objective finding such as a rash or a deformed arm.

Patient assessment is a process that continues throughout the time spent with a patient, because a patient's condition can change quickly. Continual assessment allows the EMT-I to recognize critical situations early and to positively influence patient outcome.

Patient assessment is a team process. While an EMT–I is assessing a patient, other team members are initiating life-saving care, gathering additional information, and ensuring that equipment is ready for use. Typically, one individual acts as team leader. This person may be assigned as part of the shift schedule or determined by the members of the crew. Designating a team leader in advance will minimize confusion at the scene.

Patient assessment skills are best mastered by practice and experience. This chapter will provide direction and guidance for properly developing patient assessment skills. It is up to the individual EMT–I to put this information into daily practice and to develop proficiency.

The patient assessment and care process will be discussed in six phases: scene size-up (scene assessment), initial assessment (primary survey), resuscitation, focused history and physical examination, detailed assessment (secondary survey), and ongoing assessment (which includes definitive field management and transportation) (Fig. 8-1).

Prior to 1994, the Department of Transportation (DOT) curriculum for basic-level prehospital care providers divided patient assessment into four phases:

- Scene assessment
- Primary survey
- Resuscitation
- Secondary survey

The revised curriculum now teaches six phases of patient assessment:

- Scene size-up
- Initial assessment
- Resuscitation
- Focused history and physical examination
- Detailed assessment
- On-going field management

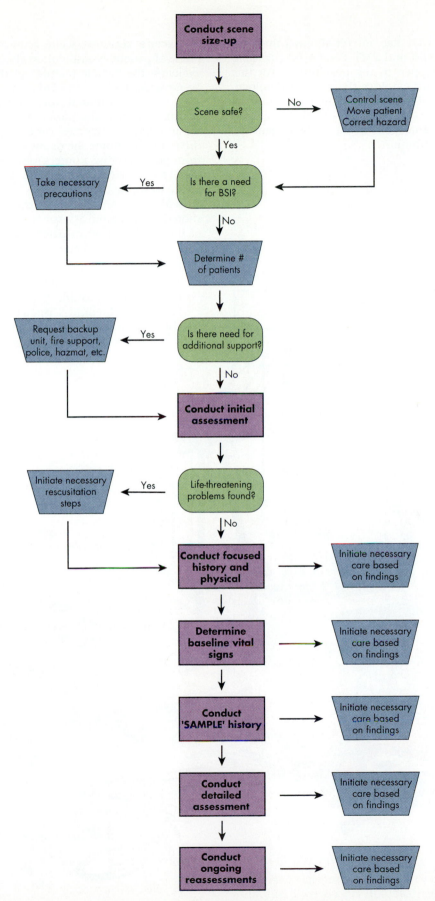

Fig. 8-1 Algorithm demonstrating the necessary steps in patient care and assessment.

Although the DOT has not yet adopted these six phases to the EMT–I and EMT–Paramedic curricula, this will likely happen in the near future. For this reason, this chapter employs the new terminology. Parenthetic references are made, where necessary, to the older terms. For example, the "initial assessment" in this chapter is analogous to the "primary survey" in the older curriculum.

SCENE SIZE-UP

 SCENE SIZE-UP: The immediate evaluation of an emergency scene for safety of the crew, patient, and bystanders.

🍎 **Identify potential scene hazards that may endanger the EMT–I or the patient.**

The **scene size-up** (scene assessment) is the first phase of patient assessment. At this point, the EMT–I evaluates the "whole picture" of the call (Fig. 8-2). Scene size-up allows the EMT–I to ensure a reasonably safe environment for rescuers and patients, anticipate potentially hazardous situations, and call for appropriate resources. For example, as the EMT–I drives up to a home, he or she notices a man on the front porch waving a butcher knife. From the immediate scene size-up the EMT–I knows to wait for police to secure the scene.

Before any care is given to the patient, the EMT–I should begin a rapid assessment of the circumstances of the call based on dispatch information, previous knowledge, and on-scene observations.

1. Dispatch information—In many area dispatchers are trained to gather more information than just location and possible problems (Fig. 8-3). The Emergency Medical Dispatcher (EMD) may be able to provide information on:

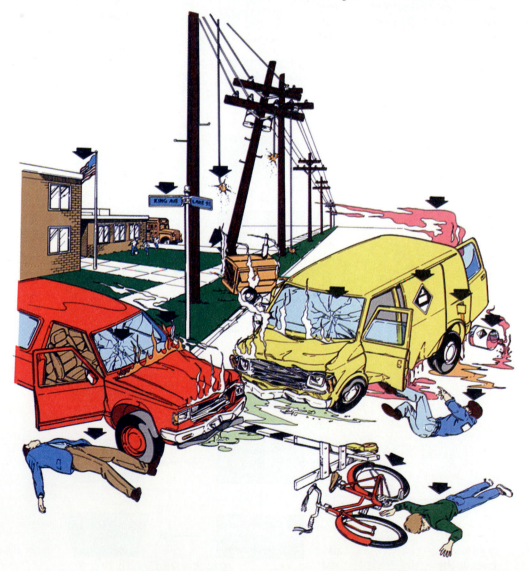

Fig. 8-2 Many different hazards can be present at an emergency scene.

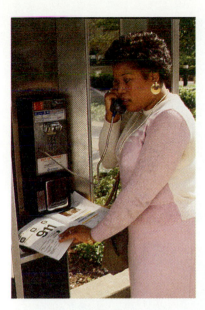

Fig. 8-3 Bystanders can often provide detailed information about an emergency scene including scene conditions, number of patients, and their conditions and patient histories.

- Scene conditions
- Number of patients
- Patient conditions
- Medical history

 HELPFUL HINT
Not all dispatchers are trained as EMDs. To qualify as an EMD, a person must undergo specific training, including the use of pre-arrival instructions and call-prioritizing.

2. Previous knowledge—if the EMT–I is aware of a situation potentially requiring special assistance, he or she may need to direct the EMD to dispatch police or other emergency agencies immediately. Potentially hazardous situations include calls to high-risk parts of a response area (high crime or drug use areas), known unsafe situations (gang fights, shootings, stabbings), and sometimes just a "gut feeling" based on the EMD's information.

3. On-scene observations—there are five considerations regarding on-scene observations:

- Is the scene safe? Is it safe for responders, the patient, and the bystanders? If the scene is unsafe, the EMT–I should attempt to make it safe, if possible. Otherwise, the EMT–I should NOT enter the scene.
- Should body substance isolation precautions be taken? In general, the answer to this question should always be YES.

- Is this a medical or a trauma patient? If medical, what is the nature of the illness? If trauma, what is the mechanism of injury?
- How many patients are involved?
- Is additional help required? The EMT–I should recognize and request backup immediately on arrival (or en route). It is better to cancel a request for additional help during the response than to have not requested necessary assistance in the first place.

Body substance isolation precautions

 Describe the self-protection measures required for body substance isolation precautions.

The EMT–I can be exposed to numerous contagious diseases during normal patient contact. Some of these diseases, such as AIDS, hepatitis, and meningitis can be deadly. Other diseases, such as chickenpox, influenza, and common colds are not deadly but may cause an EMT–I to miss work or spread disease to family members and colleagues.

BODY SUBSTANCE ISOLATION PRECAUTIONS: The use of protective equipment to minimize the chances of the EMT–I being exposed to contagious diseases.

Body substance isolation precautions (formerly called universal precautions) are a set of guidelines for healthcare providers that minimize exposure to contagious diseases. The Centers for Disease Control and Prevention recommends that healthcare providers use the following set of body substance isolation precautions during all patient encounters:

- *Wear latex or vinyl gloves when in contact with blood or other body fluids, mucous membranes, or nonintact skin of any patient or when handling items soiled with blood or body fluids.* For those incidents in which large amounts of blood or body fluids are present, the EMT–I should wear thicker gloves or use two pairs of gloves. Although medical gloves provide a good barrier, they may not provide protection from sharp objects such as wood, metal, or glass. Work-type gloves, with latex or vinyl gloves underneath, are appropriate until the hazard has been removed (Fig. 8-4 A).
- *Wear protective eyewear or masks whenever blood or body fluids may splash or spray near the eyes, nose, or mouth.* EMT–Is are often victims of splash exposure. Blood and other body fluids splashed into the eyes can transmit certain diseases. When the potential for splash exposure is high, EMT–Is should wear eye protection such as safety glasses. These glasses resemble regular glasses with the sides near the eyes also covered. Some healthcare professionals recom-

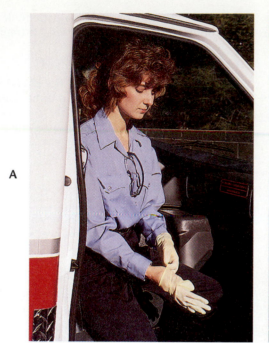 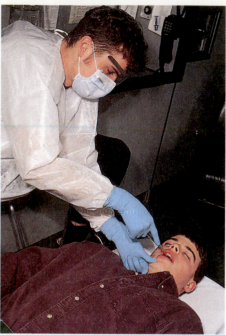

Fig. 8-4 Body substance isolation precautions **A,** Latex or vinyl gloves must be worn whenever there is a potential for contact with blood or other body fluids of any patient. **B,** Protective eyewear, a facial mask, and a gown should be worn whenever there is a potential for splash exposure to blood or other body fluids of any patient.

mend that basic eye protection be worn during any incident.

- A mask provides protection against splash exposure to the mouth and nose, as well as against airborne pathogens. Because different manufacturing standards are used for masks that protect against body fluid exposure and those that protect against airborne disease, the EMT–I should check the package labeling to be certain the right mask is being used. The mask works best when worn by the EMT–I, not by the patient. An anti-infection mask placed over the patient's mouth and nose may interfere with the EMT–I's ability to assess the patient's airway. However, an alert, cooperative patient with a productive cough may be asked to wear a mask (particularly if an infectious airborne disease is suspected). EMT–Is should follow their local protocols (Fig. 8-4 B).

- *Hands should be washed thoroughly if they are contaminated with blood or body fluids. The EMT–I also should wash his or her hands before and after treating each patient, even if gloves have been worn* (Fig. 8-5).

- *Avoid recapping needles—always dispose of sharp objects in medical waste containers.*

Many items used by EMT–Is for patient care are now disposable, such as sheets, pillowcases, airway masks, and splints. Disposable items are usually designed for

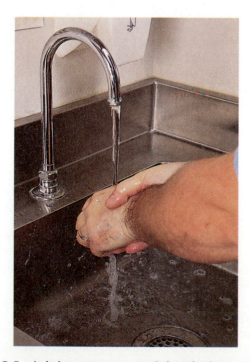

Fig. 8-5 It is important to wash hands thoroughly before and after dealing with each patient. Hands should also be washed if they come in contact with a patient's blood or body fluid.

single use only. Single-use items are the best way to prevent transmission of diseases, but it is not practical to make all equipment disposable. Nondisposable items must be properly decontaminated after potential infectious disease exposure. Equipment manufacturers may provide helpful guidelines.

The EMT–I must dispose of medical waste properly. Single-use items should be placed in plastic bags and disposed of in the proper containers. Each EMT–I must become familiar with the waste disposal policy of his or her EMS system.

These guidelines are not simply good protection for the EMT–I and the patients, they are the law. EMS systems and hospitals are required to ensure that protective equipment and proper medical waste disposal areas are available. The United States Occupational Safety and Health Administration (OSHA) and state agencies may levy significant civil penalties against EMS systems that fail to comply with these procedures.

Scene safety

The main purpose behind scene safety is to prevent illness or injury to EMT–Is or bystanders and to prevent further illness or injury to the patient(s). EMT–Is should look for potential hazards such as collapsed structures, chemical spills, fire, weapons, and violent people. If the scene is unsafe, the EMT–I should NOT enter. No matter how critically ill or injured the patient is, a dead or injured EMT–I will not be of help. Dispatch should be instructed to notify the appropriate agencies for emergency assistance.

To assess scene safety, the EMT–I should consider the environment whether or not a hostile situation exists, or if any special equipment or personnel (*eg*, fire department, hazardous materials teams) will be required:

- *Consider the environment.* What is the location of the emergency? Will the patient have to be moved, and if so, are there numerous flights of steps, narrow corridors, or nonfunctioning elevators? Is there a fire (or risk of fire)? Is the patient in the wilderness or at a great height? What is the weather like? If the patient is inside, and it is snowing outside, he or she will need protection against the environment. Is there a possibility of air or fluid chemical contamination? ALL of these factors must be considered when determining whether or not a scene is safe.

- *Preserve patient modesty* as much as possible during all phases of patient contact. Sometimes, it is difficult to hide the patient from the view of onlookers. In most cases, however, the best solution is to assess the patient in back of the ambulance, if available, or in another private location.

- *Is the situation hostile?* If a crime has occurred, have the perpetrators been captured? Is their location known? The EMT–I should not assume that there is only one perpetrator. Also, the EMT–I

should note the bystanders' mood—are they hostile or supportive? If any doubts exist, the EMT–I should not enter (or remain on) the scene unless law enforcement assistance is present.

- *Is special equipment required?* At this time, the EMT–I must decide whether self-contained breathing apparatus or protective clothing is required. This decision should be made BEFORE entering the scene. The EMT–I should NOT attempt water rescue or entry into a fire or hazardous materials incident without proper training and equipment.

It can be very stressful and difficult to decide not to enter an unsafe scene. This is a decision, however, that must occasionally be made. The EMT–I must remember that an injured or otherwise incapacitated EMT–I is of no benefit to a patient. The EMT–I should not increase the number of victims that must be cared for by the remaining rescue personnel. Self-protection MUST be the EMT–I's primary concern.

Personal protection

 Describe the problems an EMT–I might encounter in a hostile situation and suggest mechanisms of management.

In some cases, a patient or bystander may pose a threat to an EMT–I. It is important to recognize potential danger signs and follow a few key rules to reduce the chance of death or injury:

- Potentially violent situations may not be obvious. If outright signs or even "gut feelings" reveal possible danger, do not enter until police have secured the area.

- If a patient becomes violent during the incident, move to a safe area and await police arrival.

- Take a position to avoid being cornered or injured by doors, objects, or vehicles.

- Realize that persons of both sexes and of any race, age, and economic status have the potential to injure an EMT–I. Do not let size or an initially calm disposition catch you off guard.

- Avoid being judgmental. Some patients become violent because of medical problems, medication, or simple emotional stress. Do not attribute all violent behavior to alcohol or illicit drug abuse.

- After the scene and patient are secured, provide care as needed.

- Documentation is important, especially when the care given differs from that set by protocols. If physical restraints are needed, carefully document this fact in the run report. EMS systems should have well-established protocols regulating the use of force to facilitate patient care (*see* Chapter 3, "Medical/Legal Considerations").

- In some systems body armor (bulletproof vests) is worn. The carrying of weapons is discouraged except by EMS personnel who function in law enforcement capacities. Persons untrained and unfamiliar with proper weapon use can be injured or killed with their own weapons.

INITIAL ASSESSMENT (PRIMARY SURVEY)

 Describe the initial assessment and what areas are critical to evaluate.

INITIAL ASSESSMENT: A quick evaluation of the patient to determine immediate life-threatening emergencies.

The next step in patient assessment is the **initial assessment** (formerly called the *primary survey*) (Fig. 8-6). The initial assessment is a rapid, organized, and systematic evaluation during which the following should be completed:

- Form a general impression of the patient.
- Quickly determine the nature of the illness or the mechanism of injury.
- Provide spinal stabilization if indicated.
- Are any life-threatening conditions present? If so, manage these conditions immediately.
- Evaluate the patient's level of responsiveness.
- Assess the airway. Is it patent? Is the patient responsive or unresponsive?
- Assess breathing. Is it present? Is it adequate?
- Assess circulation. Determine the pulse rate. At the same time, check for bleeding and evaluate the skin for color, temperature, and moisture. In children under 6 years of age, determine adequacy of capillary refill.
- Identify priority (unstable) patients. At this point, a decision should be made whether to begin transport or wait for paramedic backup. Local protocols should be followed. Throughout the assessment process, the EMT–Is should speak to the patient and state their names, explain their level of training, and make it clear that they are there to help.

General impression of the patient
The EMT–I's immediate sensory assessment of the situation, combined with the patient's chief complaint, forms the general impression (Fig. 8-7). Everything seen, heard, or smelled when approaching the patient should be noted. Is the patient comfortable, or is he or she writhing in pain? Does the patient look healthy, or does he or she look

barely alive? What is the patient's chief complaint? Is there a medical problem (such as chest pain), or has trauma occurred (such as a shooting)?

Mechanism of injury/nature of illness
As part of the general impression, the EMT–I must decide whether the patient has been the victim of trauma or if a medical problem exists (Fig. 8-8). Sometimes, the decision is obvious—a person struck by a moving car, or a man collapsed with shortness of breath and no known trauma. Other times, the picture may not be quite so clear, such as the person who suffers a heart attack while driving a car, causing a crash. The EMT–I should make the best decision possible based on the information available at the time.

If trauma is involved, the EMT–I should try to determine what happened. Did the patient fall, was the patient stabbed, was there a motor vehicle accident? What was the size of the knife blade? What was the caliber of the gun? How much damage was done to the car?

The EMT–I should attempt to obtain information from the patient, family members, or from bystanders (including other emergency care professionals) regarding the trauma (Fig. 8-9). While assessing the mechanism of injury, the EMT–I should determine how many patients are present and decide whether or not additional help will be required. The need for spinal immobilization also should be considered. If multiple patients are involved, the triage procedure should be started at this point.

In the medical patient, the EMT–I should try to identify the nature of the illness. Is the patient short of breath, does the patient have chest pain, is the patient dizzy? The patient, family, or bystanders may provide invaluable information. While determining the nature of the medical illness, the EMT–I should determine how many patients are present and decide whether or not additional help will be required. As in a trauma scene, if multiple patients are involved, the triage procedure should begin at this point (Fig. 8-10).

If trauma and potential injury to the cervical spine are suspected, the patient's spine should be stabilized.

Life-threatening problems or injuries
Note: The information in this chapter is NOT designed to replace formal American Heart Association or American Red Cross courses on cardiopulmonary resuscitation. The authors assume that the reader has already successfully completed a basic life support (CPR) course.

The EMT–I should look for life-threatening problems or injuries (such as marked difficulty breathing or severe bleeding) and treat these immediately. A general impression of the patient's condition forms the basis for the rest of patient care. If the patient does not look well, the patient should be considered unstable (priority) and treated according to the local protocols. However, not all sick patients "look

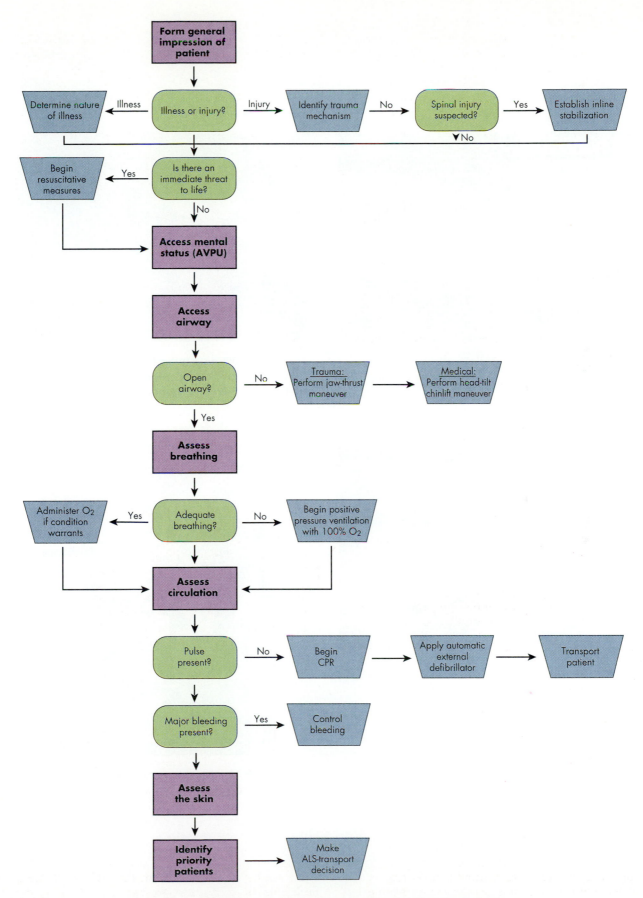

Fig. 8-6   Algorithm showing steps for initial patient assessment.

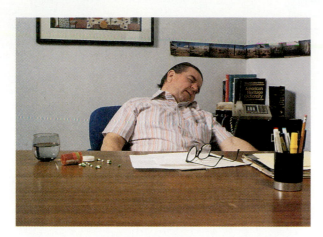

Fig. 8-7 Form a general impression of the scene using all of your senses to take in information.

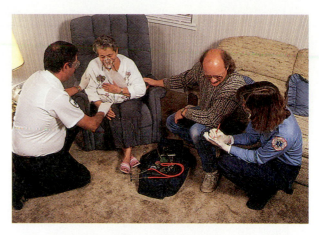

Fig. 8-9 Talking with family members or bystanders can be an excellent way to gather information about an emergency scene.

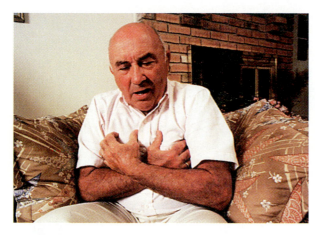

Fig. 8-8 Emergencies can be either medical or trauma in nature.

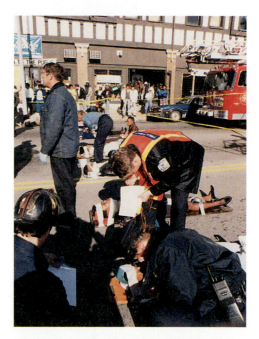

Fig. 8-10 Many emergency scenes involve a number of patients.

bad." Appearance is only one criterion by which patients are assessed.

Level of responsiveness

Determine the patient's level of responsiveness using the **AVPU** mnemonic:

A = Patient is <u>A</u>wake and <u>A</u>lert.

V = Patient responds to <u>V</u>erbal stimulus.

P = Patient responds to <u>P</u>ainful stimulus.

U = Patient is <u>U</u>nresponsive.

A patient who is unresponsive, especially if he or she has no gag or cough, should be considered priority. Even a patient who responds verbally but does not follow commands appropriately should be treated as a priority case.

Airway assessment
Initial approach

The EMT–I should approach the patient face-to-face, if possible. This approach allows for the development of rapport with the patient. This approach also saves the patient from having to turn his or her head to see who is coming. The EMT–I should make eye contact with the patient and introduce himself or herself: "I am EMT–Intermediate Smith, and we are here to help you." If spinal injuries are suspected, tell the patient not to move.

Techniques of airway management

The patient who is responsive and can speak clearly has an open airway. For these patients, the initial survey can continue. For patients who are unresponsive, the EMT–I must open the airway.

Describe the need for and methods of cervical spine immobilization throughout the phases of patient assessment.

For semiresponsive or unresponsive medical patients, the head-tilt/chin-lift should be performed.

If the airway is not clear, the EMT–I should clear it. For trauma patients or those patients with an unknown nature of illness, the cervical spine should be stabilized and the jaw thrust maneuver performed (Fig. 8-11). While one EMT–I provides airway and spine protection, the other EMT–I continues the initial survey. If a second EMT–I is not available, the first EMT–I must maintain the airway and protect the spine. Once the jaw thrust is performed, the EMT–I stabilizes the neck until it is properly immobilized (Figs. 8-12 to 8-15).

There are numerous forms of mechanical airway adjuncts that the EMT–I may find helpful. These adjuncts are discussed in detail in Chapter 9, "Airway Management."

Breathing assessment

The EMT–I should immediately assist ventilation or ventilate patients with inadequate breathing. These patients include:

- Patients who are not breathing (respiratory arrest).

- Patients whose respiratory rate (number of breaths per minute) is less than 10 per minute or greater than 30 per minute.

- Patients who have decreased levels of responsiveness.

Look, listen, and feel

The EMT–I should quickly determine whether the patient is breathing by looking, listening, and feeling for air exchange.

- *Look* for rise and fall of the chest.

- *Listen* for air moving in and out of the patient's nose or mouth.

- *Feel* exhaled air against your chin, face, or palm of your hand with the rise and fall of the chest (Fig. 8-16).

All three of these sensations must be present to conclude that the patient is breathing adequately. If any of these signals is absent, the patient may not be breathing enough to oxygenate the body tissues and remove carbon dioxide. Also, a patient whose rate of respiration is greater than 20 or less than 12 breaths per minute often will be unable to maintain sufficient air exchange and will become hypoxic and hypercarbic. At a minimum, these patients should receive a high concentration of supplemental oxygen. If hypoventilation is suspected, the EMT–I should assist the patient's breathing with a ventilatory adjunct.

Ventilation maneuvers
In general

The patient should be ventilated by either mouth to mask or by adjunct devices whenever inadequate air exchange is suspected. In all cases, supplemental oxygen should be used. Two initial ventila-

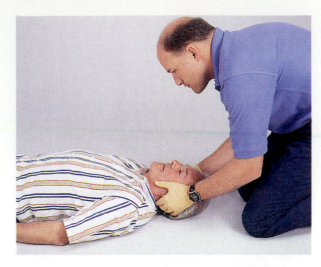

Fig. 8-11 For patients with suspected trauma injuries, perform the jaw thrust maneuver.

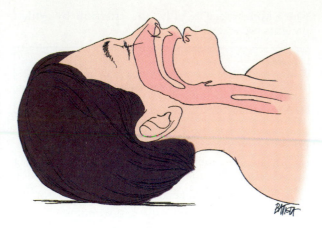

Fig. 8-12 A normal airway—the patient is breathing adequately.

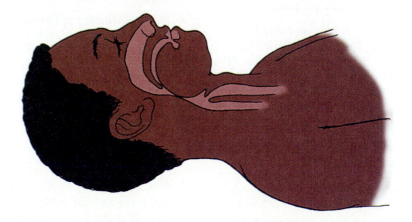

Fig. 8-13 If the patient becomes unconscious, the tongue may slide back in the mouth, obstructing the airway.

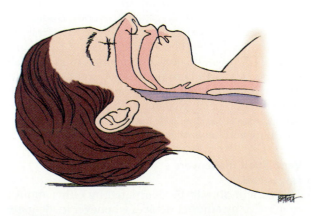

Fig. 8-14 Fluid in the airway may obstruct a patient's respiration.

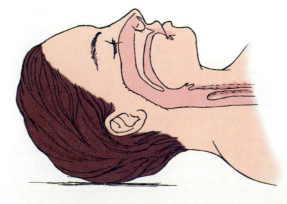

Fig. 8-15 The airway can also become constricted, blocking the patient's ability to breathe adequately.

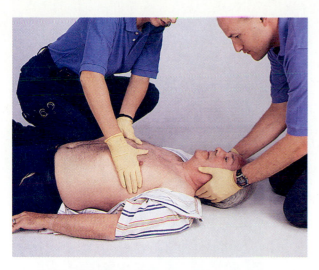

Fig. 8-16   Feel the patient's chest to check for adequate ventilations.

tions of 1.5 to 2.0 seconds each should be given, followed by one breath every 5 seconds. Some EMS physicians recommend ventilating the apneic or unresponsive patient every 3 to 5 seconds. Any patient with difficulty breathing should be treated as a priority case.

 Describe techniques for evaluating the effectiveness of ventilation.

Assessment of effective ventilation
There are several ways to determine whether or not the patient is receiving effective ventilatory assistance. A combination of the following indicators is usually most helpful:

- Rise in chest wall—the chest wall should rise with inhalation and fall with exhalation.
- Auscultation of the lungs—good movement of air in all the lung fields during inspiration should be heard.
- Skin color—as the patient becomes better oxygenated, his or her color should improve; ie, the patient should "pink up."
- Heart rate—typically, persons develop tachycardia and then bradycardia with respiratory compromise. A change toward normal in the heart rate with proper ventilation should be seen.
- Pulse oximetry—if a person is not being effectively ventilated, the pulse oximetry reading may be low.

Even if breathing is present and the patient is responsive, high-concentration oxygen (15 L/min nonrebreather mask) still may be required. All patients with a serious illness or injury should

receive high-concentration oxygen. An unresponsive patient with adequate respirations should receive high-concentration oxygen.

Circulation assessment
Rapid pulse check

 Describe the mechanism of evaluating the effectiveness of perfusion including pulse and skin color.

If the patient is responsive, the EMT–I should quickly check for a radial pulse (Fig. 8-17). In a child less than 1 year of age, the brachial pulse should be palpated. If no radial pulse is present, the carotid pulse should be palpated. If the patient is unresponsive, the EMT–I should feel for the carotid pulse first (Fig. 8-18).

If the patient is pulseless:

- Medical patient greater than 12 years of age—start CPR and apply the automated external defibrillator (AED) or standard defibrillator.
- Medical patient less than 12 years of age—start CPR.
- Trauma patient—start CPR.

Even if carotid and radial pulses are present, a pulse rate less than 60 beats per minute or greater than 100 beats per minute should be considered potentially life-threatening if combined with other pertinent findings, such as hypotension, chest pain, or severe dizziness.

The presence of certain pulses often indicates that various minimum systolic blood pressure levels are present. These numbers are only estimates, however. For example, if a radial pulse is present, the patient's systolic blood pressure is approximately 80 mm Hg. Knowing these limits will help with a more rapid estimation of the patient's blood pressure:

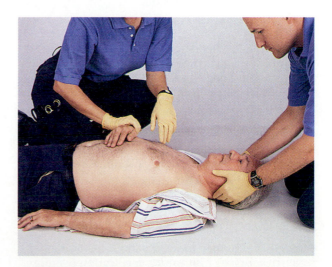

Fig. 8-17   An EMT-I assessing a patient's skin.

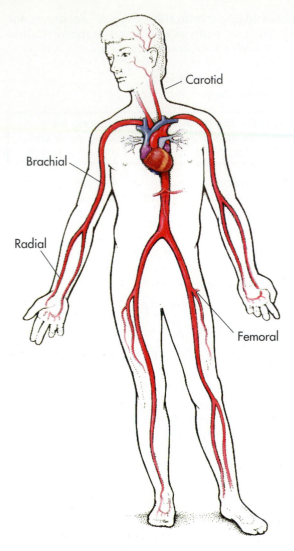

Fig. 8-18   Major pulse points on the human body.

Carotid—60 mm Hg systolic

Femoral—70 mm Hg systolic

Radial—80 mm Hg systolic

Check for major bleeding
If major bleeding is present, it should be controlled using standard measures. These measures include direct pressure, elevation, pressure points, bandages, and tourniquets.

Assess the skin
The color, temperature, and moisture of the patient's skin can be recognizable signs of abnormal situations:

• Warm, pink, dry skin usually indicates adequate circulation. This is the normal skin condition.

• Pale, cool, and clammy skin indicates shock.

• Hot, dry skin may indicate serious medical emergencies such as heat injury, medication overdose, or infection.

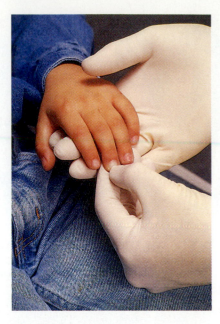

Fig. 8-19   Capillary refill may be assessed in children under the age of six.

The patient's face, lips, nailbeds, mouth, earlobes, and eyelids are all places where color may be assessed. In dark-skinned patients, look for color changes in the nailbeds, under the tongue, and in the conjunctiva.

Some abnormal skin colors and conditions leading to them are:

• Red—alcohol or cocaine ingestion, anaphylactic (allergy) shock, hyperthermia, stroke, heart attack

• Pale—shock, stress, heart attack, anemia, hypothermia

• Yellow (jaundice)—liver disease, gallbladder disease, kidney disease

• Mottled red, pale, or blue—poor perfusion; often seen in cardiac arrest

Another sign assessed at the time of evaluating skin color and temperature is capillary refill. Capillary refill is assessed by pressing on the patient's nailbed or palmar surface of the hands or feet. Normally a pink color returns within 2 seconds when the pressure is released. If refill is slow or absent, the patient's circulation may be inadequate.

This test has been the subject of much controversy in recent medical literature. Some experts state that the test is questionable in adults. For example, some women and elderly patients of both sexes may have refill times of up to 10 seconds and still have adequate circulation. The new 1994 DOT EMT–Basic curriculum recommends that this test be used only in children under 6 years of age (Fig. 8-19). Even in young children, the test is unreliable if the patient is in a cold environment or has just come out of the cold. EMT–Is should follow their local protocols and medical direction instructions.

To better assess and care for the patient it may be necessary to remove some or all clothing. The nature of the incident will dictate to what extent this must be done. It is important to protect the patient from embarrassment as much as possible without compromising patient care.

> **HELPFUL HINT**
> Other points to remember when removing a patient's clothing to facilitate examination and care are:
> - Use caution in extremely cold environments, especially when transferring the patient to metal backboards or scoop stretchers.
> - Prevent further exposure to toxic substances that may burn or irritate the skin.
> - In hot weather, remember that skin contact with certain surfaces (such as metal parts of a stretcher) can cause burns.

Identify priority (unstable) patients

 Define a "priority" patient and discuss several illnesses or suspected injuries that would lead you to classify a patient in this fashion.

Priority patients are unstable patients who require more advanced level care as soon as possible. Depending on the EMT–I's location and protocols, identification of a patient as "priority" may simply mean rapid transportation to the nearest medical facility. In certain cases, paramedic backup may be requested at the scene or en route. In some EMS systems, an aeromedical helicopter service may be activated. EMT–Is should follow their local protocols when making these decisions.

Availability of care also may play a role in the EMT–I's decision-making. For instance, if paramedic care is 20 minutes away and the appropriate hospital is 5 minutes away, it would be more prudent to transport the patient to the hospital. In other situations, initiating transportation and meeting the paramedic unit at a point en route may be appropriate. "Priority" does not necessarily mean a high-speed ambulance ride with lights and siren. The important factor is starting transportation or providing advanced care rapidly. EMT–Is should always follow their local EMS protocols and the recommendations of medical direction.

It is impossible to list all conditions or situations that would make a patient a priority. In general, it is best to err on the side of caution. Some general guidelines for the identification of priority patients include:

- Poor general impression
- Unresponsive patients, especially if there is no gag reflex
- Responsive patients who are unable to follow simple commands
- Difficulty breathing

- Shock (hypoperfusion)
- Complicated childbirth
- Chest pain with blood pressure less than 100 systolic
- Hypoxia that fails to rapidly correct (within 1 to 2 minutes of field intervention)
- Multiple trauma (including severe burns)
- Severe hypertension
- Uncontrolled bleeding
- Severe pain anywhere

Resuscitation

In the resuscitation phase, life-saving procedures should be performed as needed. These procedures include techniques such as relief of airway obstruction, control of hemorrhage, artificial respiration, CPR, defibrillation of cardiac arrest victims, initiation of shock management (*eg*, administration of epinephrine in anaphylactic shock and administering glucose (sugar) in severe hypoglycemia). The resuscitation phase is performed concurrently with the initial survey. Thus, if an obstructed airway is noted during the initial survey, steps should be taken immediately to relieve the obstruction.

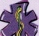

> **STREET WISE**
> Perform the resuscitation phase concurrently with the initial survey, "treating as you go." If an obstructed airway is detected during the initial survey, stop and take care of the problem before continuing the survey.

FOCUSED HISTORY AND PHYSICAL EXAMINATION

 Describe the components of the focused assessment for both the medical and the trauma patient.

 FOCUSED HISTORY AND PHYSICAL EXAMINATION: An in-depth examination to determine the severity and cause of the patient's condition. It includes both a hand's-on examination and a gathering of the patient's history.

During the **focused history and physical examination** (Fig. 8-20), the patient should be evaluated on the suspected condition only. The information that is sought during this phase is limited and is specifically related to the acute problem for which care is being provided. The focused history and physical examination will differ for medical and trauma patients.

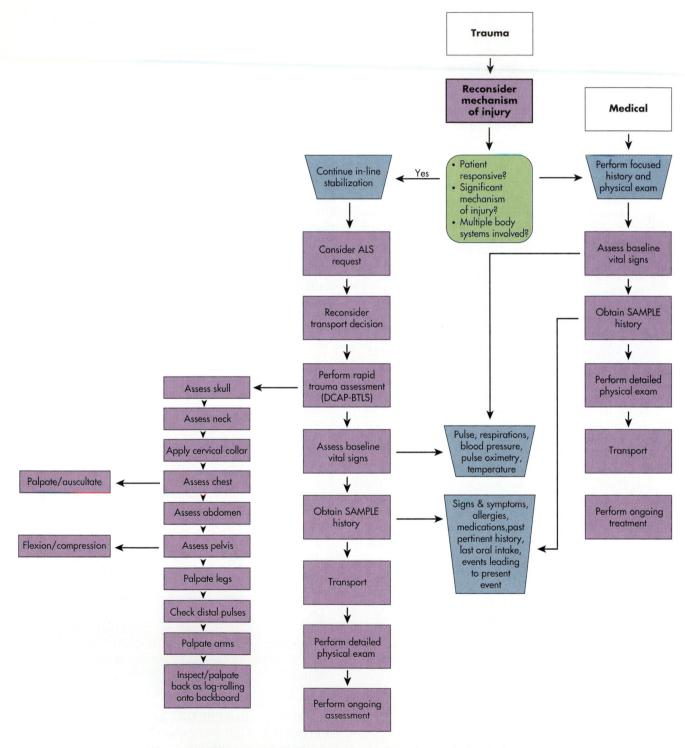

Fig. 8-20 Algorithm showing the procedures for a focused physical assessment.

Trauma patients
Reconsider mechanism of injury and transport decision

The EMT–I should reconsider the patient's mechanism of injury prior to proceeding with the history and physical examination. Also, the EMT–I should review the decision about whether to transport the patient and/or call for paramedic assistance. Did the patient fall from a significant height? Is the patient very young (infant or child) or elderly? These factors may worsen the potential significance of seemingly minor injuries.

Perform rapid trauma assessment

> **RAPID TRAUMA ASSESSMENT:** A quick and thorough hands-on examination of the trauma patient to evaluate his or her condition.

The next step in patient assessment is to perform the **rapid trauma assessment.** The EMT–I should reassess the patient's mental status and continue spinal stabilization. The acronym for the rapid head-to-toe examination in a trauma patient is DCAP-BTLS. The EMT–I should look and feel for the following signs of injury:

D = Deformity
C = Contusions
A = Abrasions
P = Punctures/Penetrations
B = Burns
T = Tenderness
L = Lacerations
S = Swelling

The patient should be carefully evaluated for each of these signs of injury. The patient should be rolled, using spinal precautions, to inspect the posterior body. This inspection can be done while the patient is being placed onto a backboard.

The head and neck should be assessed first (Figs. 8-21 and 8-22). The EMT–I should quickly inspect and palpate the neck for:

- Obvious blunt trauma (Fig. 8-23)
- Neck vein distention (suggestive of chest injury) (Fig. 8-24)
- Deviation of the trachea away from the midline
- Tenderness over the posterior cervical spine bones (Fig. 8-25).

If a cervical spine injury is present or suspected, the EMT–I should apply a cervical spine immobilization device (Fig. 8-26). A second EMT–I should continue to stabilize the head until the patient is secured to a long backboard.

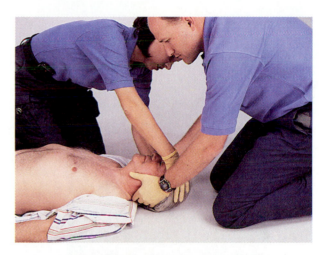

Fig. 8-21   An EMT-I assesses a patient's head, checking for signs of trauma, deformity, or bleeding.

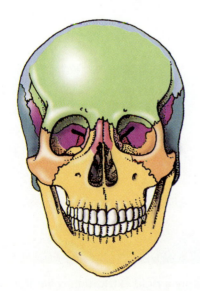
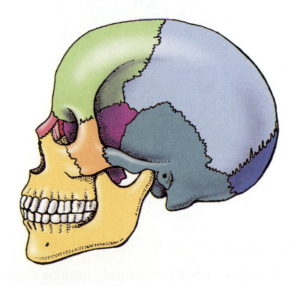

Fig. 8-22   A normal skull, with no trauma or injury.

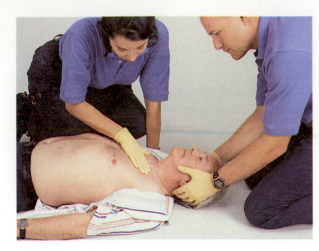

Fig. 8-23 An EMT-I assesses a patient's neck for signs of trauma.

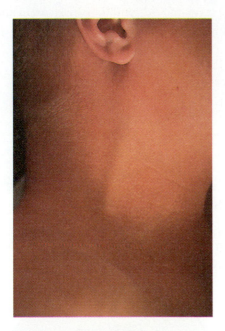

Fig. 8-24 Distended neck veins may suggest chest injury.

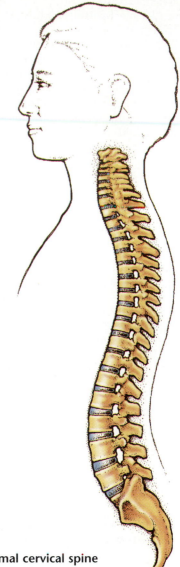

Fig. 8-25 A normal cervical spine without trauma or injury.

A second EMT–I or an extrication collar may not always be immediately available. In this case, the EMT–I should continue with the initial assessment, stabilizing the patient's head between his or her knees until additional assistance is obtained.

Next, the EMT–I should quickly inspect and palpate the patient's chest for the following (Figs. 8-27 and 8-28):

• Paradoxic respirations—unequal expansion of the chest due to a defect in the chest wall (flail chest) (Fig. 8-29).

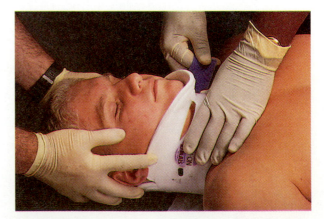

Fig. 8-26 Apply a rigid extrication collar if a cervical spine injury is suspected.

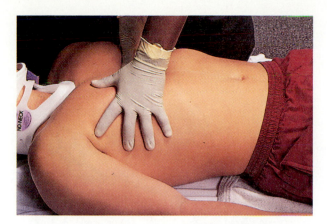

Fig. 8-27   **An EMT-I assesses a patient's chest, looking for paradoxical breathing or major injuries.**

- Obvious major injuries—such as open chest wounds (quickly seal the wound with a gloved hand), burns, deformities, bruises, lacerations, or crepitation, indicating subcutaneous emphysema (Fig. 8-30).

Chest inspection is followed by auscultation of the lungs, listening to air movement into and out of the patient's chest with a stethoscope (Fig. 8-31). Each lung is auscultated at a point approximately 2 to 3 inches below the axilla (armpit) in the midline. This location is referred to as the midaxillary point. Another location for auscultating lung sounds is immediately inferior to each clavicle in the mid-clavicular line. The earpieces of the stethoscope should fit snugly into the ears. The chest piece is placed tightly over the midaxillary point, and the EMT–I listens for 5 to 10 seconds on each side (Fig. 8-32).

During this part of the survey, it is necessary for the EMT–I to determine only that breath sounds are present and equal in intensity on both sides of the chest. Unequal breath sounds may indicate potentially life-threatening conditions such as pneumothorax, tension pneumothorax, or hemothorax.

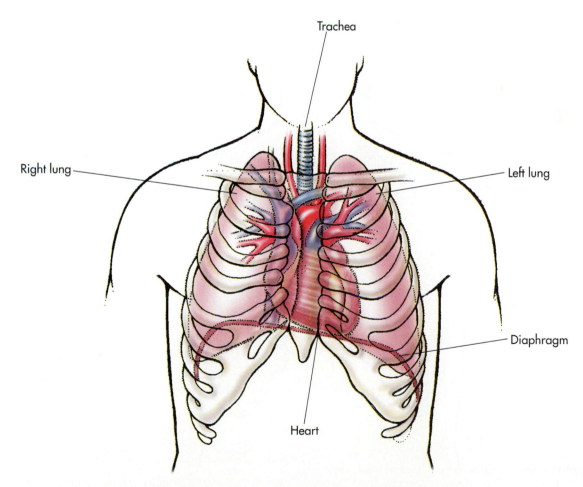

Fig. 8-28   Normal chest structures, without trauma or injury.

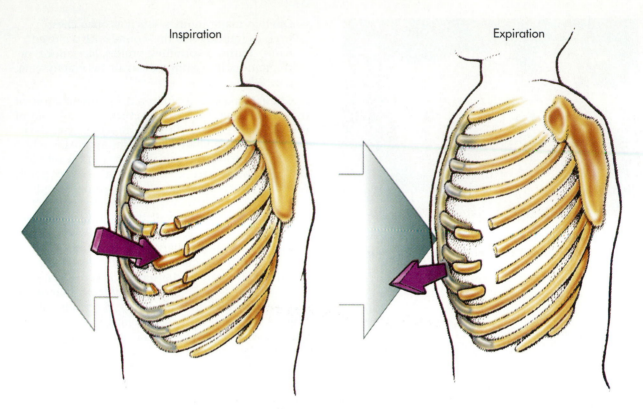

Inspiration   Expiration

Fig. 8-29   Paradoxic respirations result from damage to the ribs.

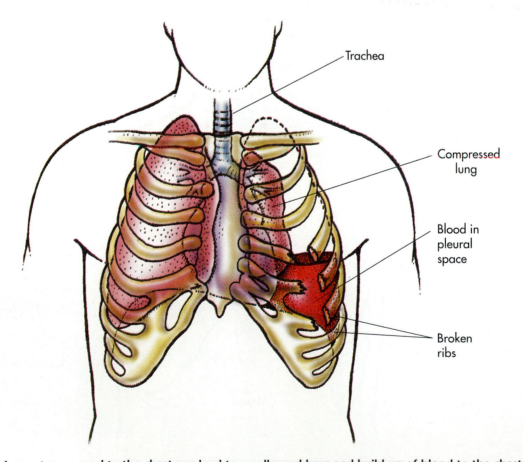

Trachea

Compressed lung

Blood in pleural space

Broken ribs

Fig. 8-30   A puncture wound to the chest can lead to a collapsed lung and build-up of blood to the chest cavity.

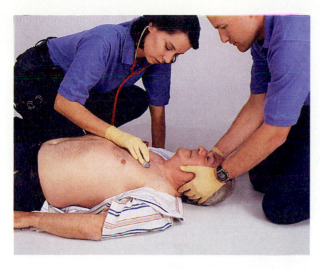

Fig. 8-31   An EMT-I auscultating a patient's lungs, listening to the flow of air in and out of the chest.

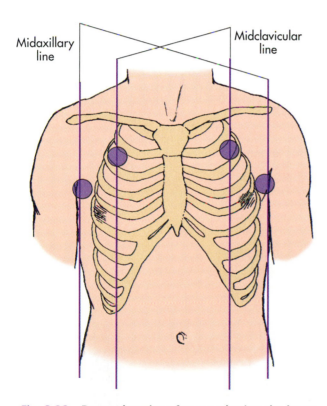

Midaxillary line

Midclavicular line

Fig. 8-32   Proper locations for auscultating the lungs

Next, the EMT–I should palpate the ab-domen (Figs. 8-33 and 8-34). The abdomen may be firm, soft, or distended. The pelvis is gently compressed at the iliac crests with bilateral pressure to determine tenderness or instability (Figs. 8-35 and 8-36). All four extremities are assessed for distal pulse, motor function, and sensation (Figs. 8-37 to 8-42).

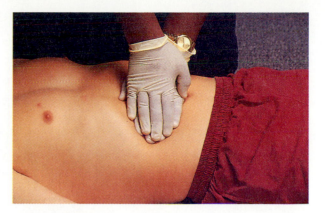

Fig. 8-33   An EMT-I palpating a patient's abdomen, checking to see if it is soft, firm, or distended.

Obtain baseline vital signs

Next, baseline vital signs are obtained. These signs should include pulse, respirations, blood pressure, pulse oximetry, and temperature. Vital signs will provide an objective guideline by which to evaluate the function of the body's vital systems.

Remember three important points concerning vital signs:

1. Vital signs are evaluated as a "set." No one vital sign will provide adequate information concerning a patient's condition.

2. "Normal" is not a constant. Just as people come in all shapes and sizes, "normal" vital signs can vary within fairly large ranges. Vital signs also vary considerably by age.

3. Vital signs require continual monitoring. After initial readings, monitor trends in vital signs constantly to determine if the patient is getting better, worse, or staying the same. Protocols vary from system to system, but a good "rule of thumb" is to recheck vital signs every 5 to 10 minutes. Reassess vital signs more frequently if the patient's condition changes.

Pulse

When assessing vital signs the most commonly used pulse points are the radial, carotid, brachial, and femoral arteries. In the responsive patient, the radial pulse is used most often (Fig. 8-43). In patients with signs or symptoms of shock or poor circulation, the radial pulse either may be absent or difficult to assess. In these patients, the carotid or femoral pulse should be used.

When palpating the pulse, three characteristics are important: rate, regularity, and character.

The pulse rate (sometimes called *heart rate*) is measured in terms of beats per minute (BPM). The normal adult pulse rate is 60 to 100 BPM. A heart rate that is greater than 100 BPM is called *tachycardia*, whereas a heart rate less than 60 BPM is referred to as *bradycardia*. Athletes and patients on certain blood pressure or cardiac medications may have a resting

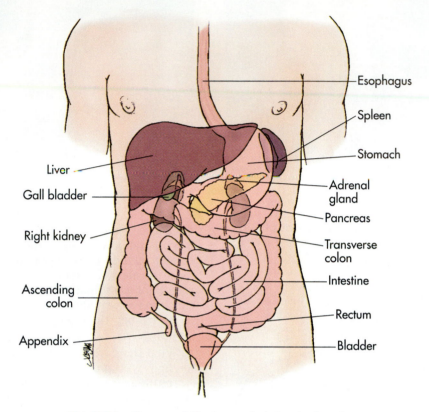

Fig. 8-34 **Organs of the normal abdominal cavity.**

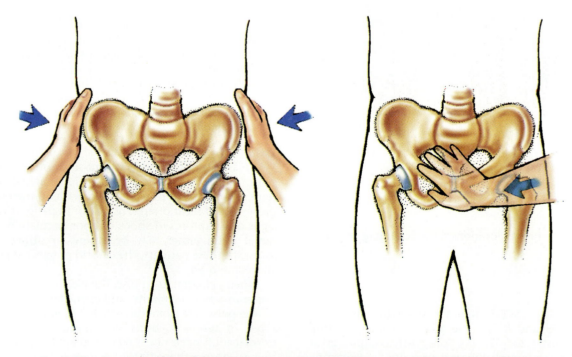

Fig. 8-35 **To assess the pelvis, gently compress at the iliac crests with bilateral pressure.**

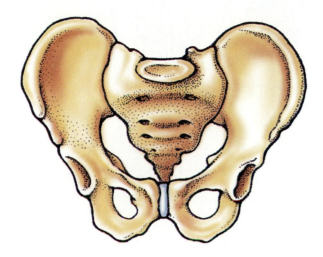

Fig. 8-36   A normal pelvis.

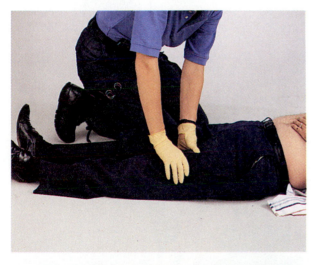

Fig. 8-37   An EMT-I palpating a patient's upper leg, checking for pulse, motor function, and sensation.

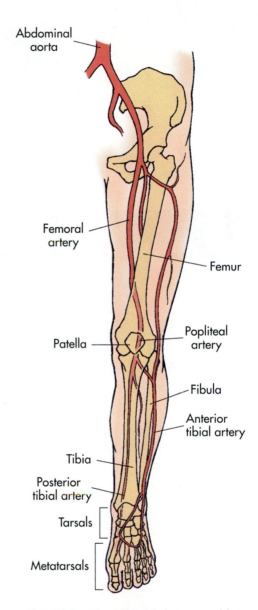

Fig. 8-38   Structure of the normal leg.

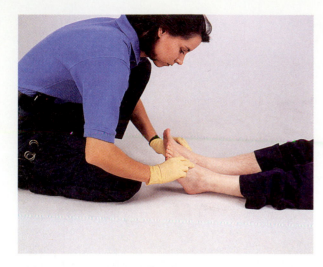

Fig. 8-39 An EMT-I palpating a patient's lower leg, checking for pulse, motor function, and sensation.

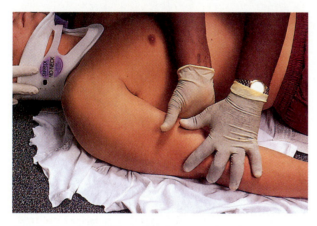

Fig. 8-40 An EMT-I palpating a patient's arm, checking for pulse, motor function, and sensation.

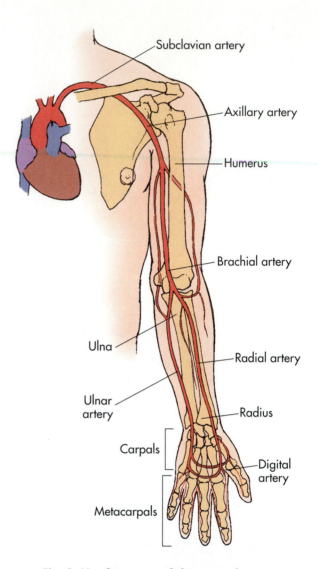

Subclavian artery

Axillary artery

Humerus

Brachial artery

Ulna

Radial artery

Ulnar artery

Radius

Carpals

Digital artery

Metacarpals

Fig. 8-41 Structure of the normal arm.

pulse rate as low as 40 BPM. This rate may be considered normal for these patients, as long as they are not dizzy or showing other signs or symptoms of hypoperfusion.

Normal pulse ranges for various age groups are as follows:

- Newborn to 3 years of age: 100 to 160 BPM
- Child (3 to 8 years of age): 70 to 150 BPM
- Older child (8 to 12 years of age): 55 to 110 BPM
- Adolescent (older than 12 years of age): 60 to 110 BPM
- Adults: 60 to 100 BPM

CARDIAC DYSRHYTHMIA: A disorder of cardiac rhythm.

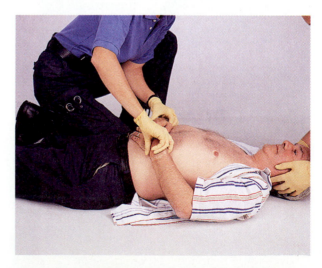

Fig. 8-42 An EMT-I checking the distal pulses of the arm.

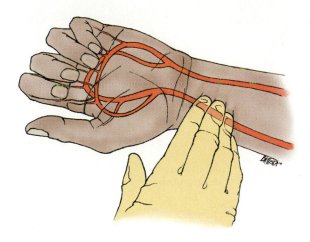

Fig. 8-43 The radial pulse point is used most often to assess an adult patient's pulse.

The regularity of the patient's pulse also should be assessed. Under normal circumstances, the pulse has very regular intervals between beats. Certain conditions such as heart disease or drugs can cause the pulse to be irregular. An irregular pulse may indicate a rhythm disturbance of the heart called a **cardiac dysrhythmia.** Some patients will complain that they feel dizzy, or notice "skipped" or "extra" heart beats. If the patient has an irregular pulse, it is helpful to count the rate for a full minute. The EMT–I should determine the frequency and nature, if possible, of the irregularities. For example, the pulse may skip every four beats, or pause every third beat, and this information may be helpful in determining the cause of the problem.

If an irregular pulse is detected after repeated checks, cardiac abnormalities should be suspected. The combination of a rapid and irregular pulse may be dangerous because the heart's chambers do not have enough time to refill with blood between contractions. The amount of blood that the heart pumps out during each contraction decreases significantly, resulting in a reduction in perfusion.

Character is another important component of the pulse. Pulse character is usually described as:

- *Strong*—easily palpated
- *Weak*—difficult to palpate
- *Bounding*—visible through the skin
- *Thready*—weak, unsteady, and usually rapid

Weak and thready pulses are associated with the signs and symptoms of shock. A bounding pulse may be caused by exercise, heat injury, stroke, or high blood pressure.

Respirations
Under normal circumstances an adult breathes about 12 to 20 times per minute. Children and infants breathe at a faster rate than adults. An adult

patient whose respiratory rate is less than 10 or above 30 is often experiencing some type of compromise that requires appropriate care. The normal respiratory rates are:

- Newborn: 40 breaths per minute
- Infant (less than 1 year of age): 20 to 30 breaths per minute
- Child: 18 to 26 breaths per minute
- Adult: 12 to 20 breaths per minute

Bradypnea is a respiratory rate that is too slow, and tachypnea is a respiratory rate that is too fast.

Along with rate, assess the depth and quality of respirations. Depth of respiration is assessed by watching the rise and fall of the patient's chest while assessing respirations. Some patients are abdominal breathers whose abdomens may move more than the chest during respiration. Quality of respirations includes the adequacy of air exchange and ease of respirations. Hearing and feeling air exchange is important. Chest movement is not proof of adequate breathing.

> **STREET WISE**
> Some patients may try to consciously control their respiratory rates when they know the EMT–I is monitoring them. Some tips on gaining a more accurate rate are:
> - After assessing the pulse, keep your hands in place but count respirations instead.
> - When counting a radial pulse, place the patient's arm across his or her chest; when you finish taking the pulse, count the respirations instead.

Ease of respirations also is an important component to assess. Signs of respiratory distress include:

- *Nasal flaring*—Widening of the nostrils during inspiration. This finding is more common in infants and children.

- *Paradoxic or asymmetric chest movements*—A portion of the chest wall moves in a direction opposite to the rest of the chest. The most common reason for this is damage to a portion of the chest wall. With the loss of the normal mechanical function, the injured section is unable to move in synchrony with the normal sections.

- *Use of accessory muscles*—The neck and intercostal muscles (the muscles between the ribs) only participate in breathing when respiratory difficulty is present. Their contractions can be seen as indentations between the patient's ribs and above the clavicles during inhalation. These are sometimes called *intercostal or supraclavicular retractions* (Fig. 8-44).

- *Lip pursing*—Exhaling through puckered-out lips, indicating strained breathing. Patients subconsciously breathe this way in an attempt to increase the pressure in the lungs. Increased pressure causes more alveoli to remain open for

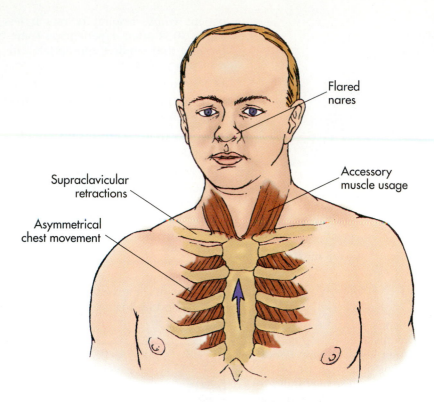

Flared nares

Accessory muscle usage

Supraclavicular retractions

Asymmetrical chest movement

Fig. 8-44   Signs of respiratory distress: nasal flaring, asymmetric chest movements, and the use of accessory muscles to breathe.

a longer period of time, increasing the amount of oxygen delivered to the patient (Fig. 8-45).

- *Noisy breathing*—Stridor is a high-pitched sound usually heard on inspiration, and indicates obstruction in the airway. Grunting is abnormal, short and loud breaks during exhalation, which may indicate pain or severe respiratory distress, particularly in an infant or child. Gurgling is a bubbling sound from fluid in the airways, such as from heart failure, excessive oral secretions, or pneumonia.

- *Obvious difficulty in inhalation or exhalation*

- *Cyanosis*—bluish discoloration of the skin and lips; a late sign of respiratory difficulty (Fig. 8-46).

Some common breathing patterns are (Fig. 8-47):

- **Eupnea**—normal inhalation and exhalation
- **Apnea**—absence of breathing
- Bradypnea—slow respirations
- Tachypnea—rapid and usually shallow respirations
- **Kussmaul**—rapid and deep respirations usually found in patients with diabetes or others with imbalances of the acid content in their bodies
- **Cheyne-Stokes** (pronounced "chain"-stokes)— series of rapid then slow respirations followed by periods of apnea.

Blood pressure

Note: The authors assume that the reader is familiar with the process of taking a patient's blood pressure using auscultation (stethoscope), palpation, or an automated device.

The blood pressure is a measurement of the force within the arteries created by the flow of blood. Blood pressure is measured with a sphygmomanometer, also referred to as a blood pressure (BP) cuff. Blood pressure is measured in millimeters of mercury (mm Hg). A measurement of 120 mm Hg means that there is enough pressure within the blood vessel to support a column of mercury 120 mm tall. Although most sphygmomanometers use mercury, air and electronic devices are becoming increasingly common.

SYSTOLE: The contraction of the heart.
DIASTOLE: The relaxation of the heart.

Each contraction of the heart, or **systole,** generates a wave of pressure in the arterial tree. The peak level of this wave is known as the systolic pressure. The diastolic pressure is the low point of the wave and reflects the force maintained between beats, or **diastole,** when the heart is at rest.

Blood pressure readings are recorded as a figure that looks like a fraction, *eg,* 120/80 mm Hg. The first

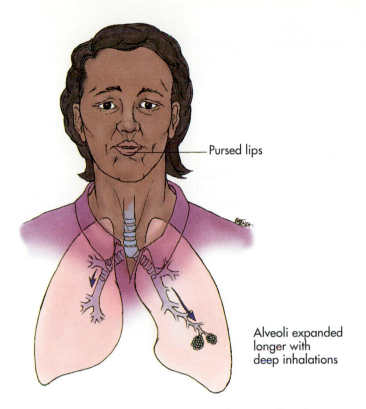

Pursed lips

Alveoli expanded
longer with
deep inhalations

Fig. 8-45 **Pursed lips may indicate that a patient is
having trouble breathing.**

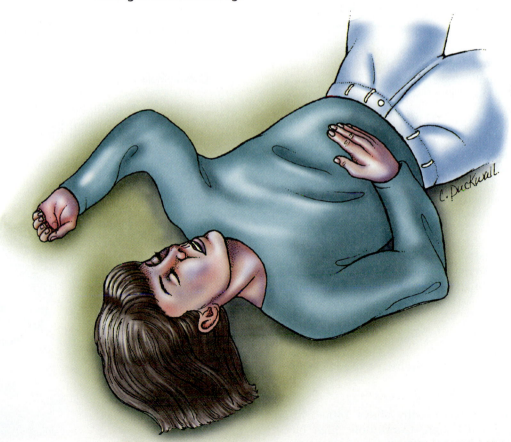

Fig. 8-46 **Cyanosis is a late sign of respiratory difficulty.**

or upper number is the systolic pressure. The second or bottom number is the diastolic pressure. Because most gauges have a scale in increments of 2 mm Hg, blood pressure is read as an even number. In contrast, digital units may show odd numbers (Fig. 8-48).

NORMOTENSION: The condition of having normal blood pressure.

As with other vital signs, there is no single blood pressure that is normal for everyone. The normal systolic blood pressure range (**normotension**) for an adult at rest is 90 to 140 mm Hg. Diastolic pressure ranges from 60 to 90 mm Hg. Blood pressure ranges may be affected by:

- *Age*—Blood pressure usually increases in the elderly.
- *Sex*—Women tend to have lower blood pressure.
- *Body size*—Smaller patients may normally have a lower blood pressure.

Normotensive ranges for various age groups are as follows:

- Newborn (average): 70/40 mm Hg
- Up to 1 year of age: 86/60 mm Hg
- Over 2 years of age: see formula below
- Adult (average): 90-140/60-90 mm Hg

CLINICAL NOTE

The lower limit of normal for systolic BP in a child over 2 years of age may be estimated by the following formula:

Systolic lower limit = 70 + (2 × (times) age in years)

Levels below this number in a child should be considered abnormal under the appropriate circumstances (*eg,* a sick patient or evidence of injury). Other signs of shock are usually present in a child before his or her blood pressure drops. A decrease in blood pressure in a child is a LATE sign of shock and should indicate a need for priority care.

HELPFUL HINT

It is difficult to measure blood pressure in infants or newborns in the field. It is important for EMT–Is to follow their local protocols in these situations.

HYPERTENSION: The condition of having high blood pressure.
HYPOTENSION: The condition of having low blood pressure.

Blood pressure consistently above 140/90 in an adult is considered high. Continuous high blood pressure is called **hypertension.** Blood pressure that is below 90/60 in an adult is considered low. Continuous low blood pressure is known as **hypotension.**

In certain circumstances, such as in a noisy moving ambulance or an aircraft, it may be easier and more accurate to use the palpation method to determine a patient's systolic blood pressure.

ORTHOSTATIC HYPOTENSION: A condition in which a patient's blood pressure suddenly drops upon standing up.

In some individuals, the blood pressure drops suddenly when the person stands up. This condition is known as **orthostatic hypotension.** Orthostatic hypotension is more common in smaller women or girls, the elderly, and patients who are dehydrated or bleeding internally. There are numerous causes of orthostasis, including volume

Normal (Eupnea)	
Bradypnea	
Tachypnea	
Hyperventilation (hyperpnea)	
Cheyne-Stokes	
Kussmaul	

Fig. 8-47   Common breathing patterns.

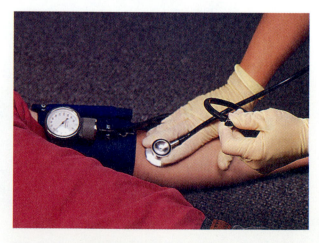

Fig. 8-48   A patient's blood pressure is measured with a sphygmomanometer.

loss for any reason such as bleeding or diarrhea. Remember that orthostatic changes are somewhat subjective, and normals vary from patient to patient. In general, "positive" orthostatic changes include:

- An increase in the pulse rate of 10 to 20 beats per minute or greater.
- A decrease in the systolic blood pressure of 10 to 20 mm Hg or greater.
- Symptoms in the patient. These symptoms may include weakness, dizziness, or light headedness. Even if the pulse and BP do not change, many experts consider a patient who develops symptoms with positional changes to have a positive test.

When checking for changes, the EMT–I should take the BP and pulse with the patient lying down. The patient should be placed in a seated position for 2 minutes and the procedure repeated. If the test is positive (blood pressure decreases, pulse increases, or patient is symptomatic), the patient is orthostatic. If the test is negative, the EMT–I should recheck pulse and BP after allowing the patient to stand for 2 minutes. The most helpful sign of orthostasis is if the patient develops symptoms—regardless of whether or not the pulse or blood pressure changes.

> **HELPFUL HINT**
> In many cases, there is no need to determine orthostatic vital signs, especially if the patient is obviously unstable in the initial position found. Perform this part of the assessment only if you feel it will contribute to patient care.

PULSE PRESSURE: Obtained by subtracting the diastolic pressure from the systolic pressure.

The difference between systolic blood pressure and diastolic blood pressure is the **pulse pressure.** The normal value is 40 mm Hg. During early shock, cardiac tamponade, or tension pneumothorax, the resistance to flow in the blood vessels goes up, which is reflected as an increase in diastolic blood pressure and a narrowing of the gap between systolic and diastolic BP (a decrease in the pulse pressure). As shock progresses and the body's compensatory mechanisms fail, this finding is no longer reliable.

Certain cardiovascular conditions may cause the blood pressure to be different in each of the upper extremities. If time permits, measure the blood pressure in each arm.

Electronic blood pressure monitors are excellent for continuous monitoring of blood pressure. In emergencies they are not appropriate for initial measurements because:

- The initial readings tend to be inaccurate.
- They take more time to put into use than manual methods.
- As with any electronic device, they are subject to operator and equipment failure.

Maintain proficiency in traditional BP monitoring, and use a manual sphygmomanometer for the initial assessment.

Errors can occur in the measurement of blood pressure. Generally, most are avoidable:

1. If the cuff size is too small, it will act as a tourniquet and the reading will be falsely high.
2. If the cuff size is too large, the reading will be falsely low.
3. Sounds may be heard incorrectly.
4. The cuff may be put on too loosely. The recorded BP will not be correct, but it is impossible to reliably predict whether it will be falsely high or falsely low.

Pulse oximetry

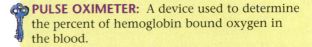

PULSE OXIMETER: A device used to determine the percent of hemoglobin bound oxygen in the blood.

The **pulse oximeter** (Fig. 8-49) is a device that monitors the arterial oxygen saturation, the amount of oxygen in the tissues, by way of a probe connected to the patient's finger, toe, or ear lobe. The pulse oximeter is very sensitive and usually will report changes in the arterial oxygen saturation level before the patient develops any signs or symptoms of respiratory problems. Generally, a pulse oximetry reading of 95% (90% to 92% in areas of higher elevation) or better is considered within normal limits.

The pulse oximeter sends an infrared beam of light through the finger, toe, or earlobe. There is a direct relationship between the amount of oxygen in the blood and the ability of the blood to absorb this light. The device compares the amount of light sent into the measurement area to the amount of light exiting the other side of the finger. Using a mathematical formula, the pulse oximeter converts this difference into oxygen saturation.

Pulse oximetry is unreliable if a patient is hypothermic or hypotensive. Patients with carbon monoxide poisoning, severe vascular disease, anemia, and abnormal hemoglobins (thalassemia) also may demonstrate unreliable readings. Thus, the use of oximetry is significantly limited in unstable patients and persons with cardiac arrest.

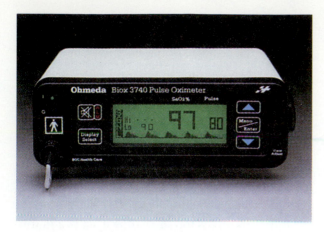

Fig. 8-49 A pulse oximeter measures the amount of oxygen in a patient's blood using an infrared beam of light.

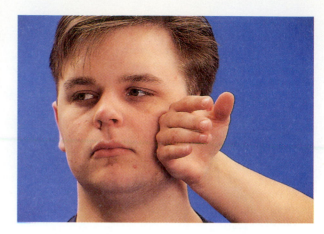

Fig. 8-50 A patient's skin temperature is an important vital sign during assessment.

Temperature

Body temperature is another important vital sign. The temperature is assessed by touching the patient's skin with the back of the hand (Fig. 8-50). The forehead is the most commonly used location. The EMT–I should avoid using the patient's hands or feet to assess body temperature, especially if the patient is found in a cold environment. The lower back, the cheek, and abdomen also are helpful sites to assess the skin temperature. Cool skin may indicate shock or exposure to the cold. Warm skin may indicate fever or heat injury.

In some EMS systems, temperature is measured with a thermometer. In the responsive adult patient, oral or tympanic membrane measurement is most appropriate. In the nonalert or very young patient, axillary or rectal temperature may be better. The advent of electronic thermometers has made temperature monitoring quicker and more accurate. If a patient has a very low body temperature (less than 90° F), a special thermometer is required, because most thermometers start at 94° or 95° F.

Several newer thermometers are now available that use a beam of infrared light to measure the temperature of the eardrum (tympanic membrane). This infrared light provides a rapid and reasonably accurate measurement of the patient's temperature and correlates with both oral and rectal temperature determinations.

> **HELPFUL HINT**
> Taking a patient's temperature in the field is a controversial practice. EMT–Is should follow local protocols.

Signs for concern

Vital signs consist of pulse, respiration (including pulse oximetry), blood pressure, and temperature (Table 8-1). These signs are collective indicators of the patient's condition. Persons who have any vital sign in the range listed in Table 8-1 are potential "Priority" patients.

Take a SAMPLE history

After obtaining vital signs, the EMT–I should take a **SAMPLE history,** using these letters as an acronym to record the following:

S = Signs and Symptoms

A = Allergies

M = Medications (prescription or over-the-counter)

P = Past pertinent medical history

L = Last oral intake, fluid or solid

E = Events leading to present event

Medical patient
Initial steps

In the unresponsive medical patient, the EMT–I should perform rapid airway assessment and protect the airway as necessary. The EMT–I also should attempt to obtain whatever information possible from relatives and bystanders. A complete SAMPLE history as previously outlined will provide the best information about the patient. The EMT–I must remember to look for MedicAlert tags on the patient's wrist or chest. The EMT–I then assesses baseline vital signs and provides care based on signs and symptoms.

Assess the complaint, signs, and symptoms

In the responsive medical patient, the complaint, signs, and symptoms are assessed using the **OPQRST** acronym:

- **O** = Onset—when did the problem begin?
- **P** = Provocation—what makes the problem worse?

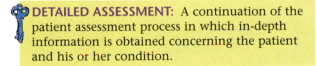

AGE	SYSTOLIC BP	PULSE	RESPIRATIONS
TABLE 8-1	**Vital Signs for Potential "Priority" Patients**		
Newborn to 2 years of age	< 60	< 80, >180	< 15 or > 40
2 to 5 years of age	< 70	< 60, >160	< 10 or > 30
Older than 5 years of age	< 90	< 50, >120	< 10 or > 25

- **Q** = Quality—what is the problem (usually pain) like; is it sharp, crushing, viselike?
- **R** = Radiation—does the pain go (move) anywhere?
- **S** = Severity—on a scale of 0 to 10 (0 = no pain, 10 = the worst pain imaginable), how bad is the pain?
- **T** = Time—does the symptom come and go, or is it always there?

Detailed assessment

 Describe the components of the detailed assessment and discuss various conditions that determine whether or not the EMT–I must perform this phase of patient assessment.

Introduction

DETAILED ASSESSMENT: A continuation of the patient assessment process in which in-depth information is obtained concerning the patient and his or her condition.

The **detailed assessment** (Fig. 8-51) (sometimes called the *secondary survey*) is an organized subjective and objective examination of the patient. This examination is patient- and injury-specific; it gathers more detailed patient information than that provided in the initial and the focused assessments. The patient's injury or illness will indicate whether or not the EMT–I should perform this part of the patient assessment. A simple cut finger, for example, would not require a detailed assessment. However, a victim of multiple trauma would. Identifying illness or injuries also allows the EMT–I to begin patient care, which may prevent further injury and decrease pain.

The detailed assessment is divided into three parts:

- The chief complaint
- The patient history
- The head-to-toe survey

For "priority" patients, the detailed assessment (if indicated) should be performed en route to the hospital (Fig. 8-52). In some cases, the time required to care for life-threatening conditions will not allow for completion of the detailed assessment.

 STREET WISE
For "priority" patients, perform the detailed assessment en route to the hospital.

The chief complaint
The chief complaint is the reason that EMS assistance was summoned. The chief complaint will indicate why EMS was requested and which areas should be explored in the detailed assessment.

The chief complaint is best elicited from the responsive patient by asking a direct but open-ended question, such as "Why did you call 9-1-1 today, sir?" or "How can we assist you today?" The EMT–I should then listen because most patients will tell the EMT–I what is wrong with them. The most common chief complaint deals with pain, followed by loss of function and abnormal states.

For the unresponsive patient the chief complaint may be provided by a bystander or family member. If the chief complaint is not readily obvious, the EMT–I should ask, "Did anyone see what happened?" or "Can you tell me what happened?" In these situations it is especially important to note the information discovered during the scene survey.

The patient history
Introduction
The history consists of information about the patient including events leading to the EMS call. This information may be obtained from the patient, a family member, or bystanders.

Communication principles
To obtain a patient history, the EMT–I must ask questions appropriately and listen carefully to the patient's answers. Patients will usually communicate what is wrong. When a patient describes a problem in his or her own words, regardless of medical accuracy, remember that it is the patient's perception of the problem.

Communication is essential in any professional interaction. The following suggestions will help make communication with patients more effective:

- Make an introduction, and give the purpose for responding to the scene: "Hello, I am Joe Smith. I am an EMT–I with the Fire Department, and I'm here to help you."

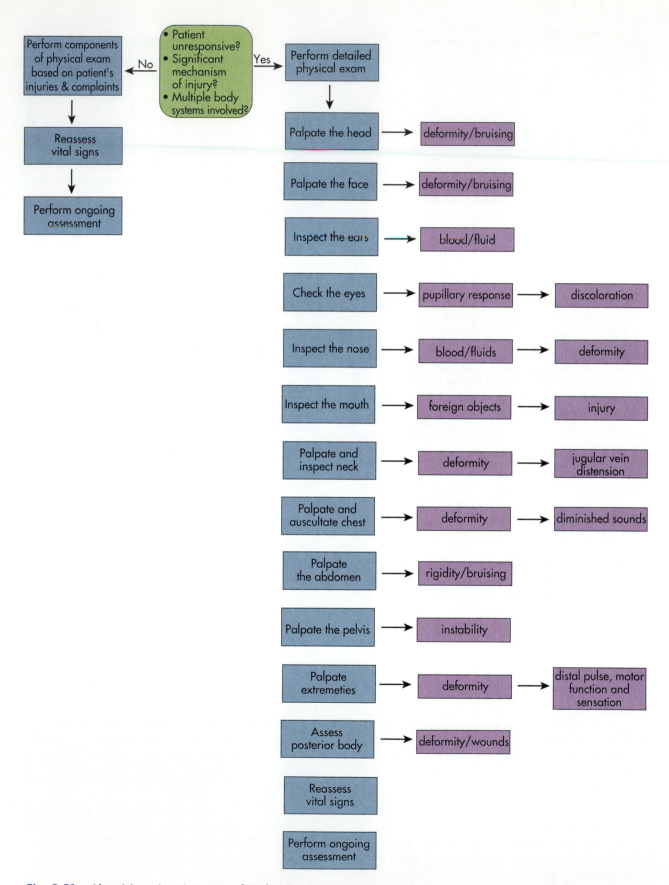

Fig. 8-51 **Algorithm showing steps for the detailed patient assessment (sometimes referred to as the secondary survey).**

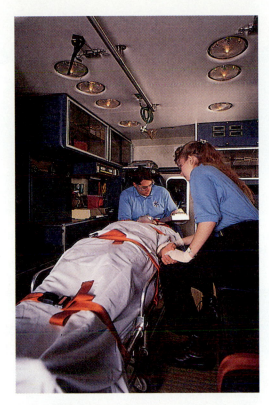

Fig. 8-52 It may be necessary to perform the detailed assessment while en route to the receiving facility if the patient is a "priority."

- Look the patient in the eye when speaking to him or her.
- Ask the patient's name and use it. First names are inappropriate unless requested by the patient or unless the patient is a child. Never use terms such as "buddy," "honey," or "sweetheart," which may offend some people.
- Explain, in simple terms, what actions are being taken: "I'm going to be holding your head so that it won't move. This is to protect you in case the accident hurt your neck. The other EMT–Is are going to put some material around your neck to hold it steady."
- Allow the patient to speak freely and ask questions.
- Periodically repeat to the patient what you understand him or her to be saying, paraphrasing his or her words: "So, I understand that you've been having this heaviness under your breastbone for the last couple of hours. You're a little short of breath and sick at your stomach, but you haven't vomited. Is that right?"
- Answer the patient's questions in lay terms that can be easily understood. Someone who is sick or injured will have more difficulty understanding than a healthy person would.

- Do not patronize the patient or make his or her concerns sound trivial. People seek EMS assistance because to them, the problem is truly an emergency.
- Maintain a calm, self-assured, and caring attitude.
- Listen carefully to family members and witnesses as well as to the patient. If the patient is a child, talk to both parents and child.
- Assume that all patients, even if they are unable to speak, are able to hear and understand what you and your colleagues say.

Some tips for interviewing the geriatric patient follow:

1. Use the patient's formal name (*eg*, Mrs. Jones) unless asked by the patient to do otherwise.
2. Avoid slang terms such as dear, honey, sweetheart, or buddy.
3. Make sure you have the patient's attention.
4. Don't assume the patient is hard of hearing just because he or she is older. Start to talk in a normal tone of voice, then determine if you need to "turn up the volume."
5. Move slowly, and avoid sudden movements.
6. Ask only one question at a time; use simple, clear language.
7. Provide enough time for the patient to respond to your questions.

Specific questions to ask

The EMT–I should ask open-ended questions that require the patient to answer with more than a "yes" or "no." "Yes/no" questions tend to lead to inaccurate conclusions. Patients tire from a series of rapid-fire questions and may begin saying what they think EMS personnel want to hear, instead of the truth.

It is impossible to list all of the questions to ask a patient when obtaining a patient history. Some of the basic questions about the patient's chief complaint include:

- What is the problem?
- Where is the problem?
- When did it start?

Elicit specific features of the patient's complaint such as:

- Quality—describe the symptoms.
- Intensity—how strong is the symptom? If the patient has pain, ask him or her to rate it on a scale of "0 to 10," with "0" being pain-free and "10" indicating the very worst pain possible.
- Frequency—how often do you have the symptom?
- Aggravating factors—what makes the symptom worse?
- Relieving factors—what makes the symptom better?

Although these questions are often asked for complaints of pain, they are helpful in evaluating any type of symptom. The EMT–I should be sure to determine if more than one complaint is present.

Other patient information

Basic patient identification information should be recorded for all patients, such as name, address, telephone number, insurance information, and name of regular physician. The exact information needed depends on the EMS system. The patient's caregivers (such as visiting nurse or relative) and bystanders also should be questioned.

The head-to-toe examination
Introduction

The head-to-toe examination (secondary survey) is a thorough examination of the body to identify wounds, fractures, and other injuries or signs of illness. Perform the secondary survey for "priority" patients while en route to the hospital.

Some tips for performing a detailed assessment on a geriatric patient include:

1. Elderly patients have decreased temperature–regulating mechanisms; they are more sensitive to cold and to changes in the temperature.

2. Preserve the patient's modesty as much as possible.

3. Remember that the geriatric patient may have slowed physical and verbal response times.

4. The skin normally loses its elasticity with aging, and skin turgor is routinely diminished even in well-hydrated patients.

5. Observe the patient's surroundings carefully for clues as to the problem, or abuse or neglect.

6. Depression, suicide attempts, and overdoses (deliberate and accidental) are more common with geriatric patients.

7. New onset wheezing or shortness of breath is likely to be cardiac in cause.

Head

Look for obvious signs of injury, such as discolorations, lacerations, or deformities (Fig. 8-53). Gently palpate for deformities and areas of tenderness. Hair matted with blood usually indicates a scalp injury. Gently palpate the neck (unless already inaccessible due to extrication collar placement) for swelling, pain, and bruises. Suspect cervical spine injury in patients with head injuries.

Eyes

Inspect the eyes for obvious trauma (8-54). Dark circles or bruises around the eyes may be *raccoon eyes,* which may indicate a skull fracture. Examine the pupils with a penlight, and note and compare their size and reactivity. Pupil size is classified as normal, dilated, constricted, or unequal. Unequal pupils in any patient with an altered level of responsiveness may be a sign of head injury or brain dysfunction.

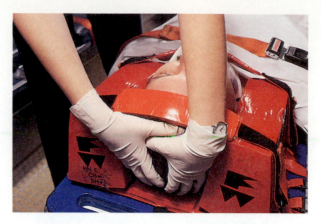

Fig. 8-53 **Palpate the head, feeling for deformities or tender spots.**

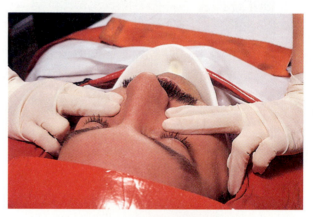

A

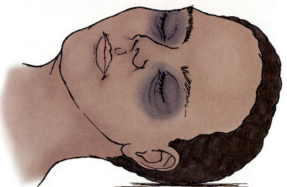

B

Fig. 8-54 **A, Inspect the patient's eyes, checking for deformities, pain or bruises. B, Raccoon eyes may indicate a skull fracture.**

PUPILLARY REACTIVITY: The reactivity of a patient's pupils to light.

Pupillary reactivity is the speed at which the patient's pupils constrict when exposed to bright light. The response is classified as reactive, slow, or nonreactive. The best way for the EMT–I to acquire a

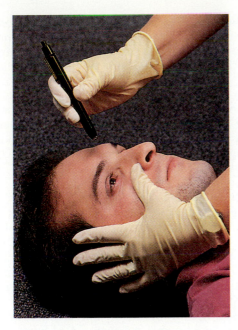

Fig. 8-55 An EMT-I checking a patient's pupils for size and reactivity.

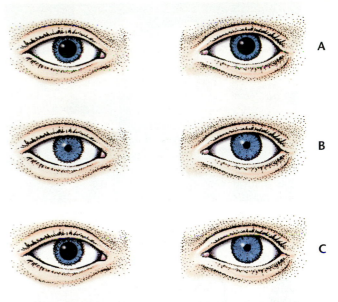

Fig. 8-56 A, Dilated pupils may indicate fear, shock, or cardiac arrest. B, Constricted pupils may indicate shock, head injury or poisoning. C, Unequal pupils may indicate a head or eye trauma in a patient.

sense for the normal response is to practice on friends and colleagues.

To check for pupillary size and reactivity, do the following (Fig. 8-55):

1) Briefly direct your light at one eye.
2) Observe for pupil constriction.
3) Remove the light and observe for dilation.
4) Repeat for the other eye and compare the responses.

 HELPFUL HINT
In a brightly lighted area, the pupils normally will be constricted; it may be difficult to see much change when checking for reactivity. In this case, shade the eyes with the other hand.

The commonly used abbreviation PERRL stands for Pupils are Equal, Round, and React to Light. Abnormal pupillary responses and their causes include (Fig. 8-56):

- Dilated pupils—fear, shock, cardiac arrest, brain injury, drug use, blindness
- Constricted pupils—head injury, bleeding in the brain, stroke, drug use, poisoning
- Unequal pupils—head injury, bleeding in the brain, direct trauma to the eye, cataract surgery

HELPFUL HINT
Two percent to four percent of people have unequal pupils normally. This condition is known as **anisocoria.**

- Unresponsive pupils—coma, death, artificial eye, drug use

SCLERA: The whites of a patient's eyes.
VISUAL ACUITY EXAMINATION: A brief exam to determine how accurately the patient is seeing.

Observe the **sclera** (white part of the eye). Reddened or bloodshot sclera may indicate alcohol consumption, drug use, or injury. Retract the lower eyelids and look at the color of the mucous membrane. Pale color may indicate poor perfusion. Palpate the orbits for fractures. Perform a brief **visual acuity examination** by asking the patient to count fingers. Visual acuity is a measure of the accuracy of a patient's vision. Note any blurring, double vision, or blindness.

Ears

CEREBROSPINAL FLUID: Clear fluid surrounding the brain and spinal cord that acts as a cushion.

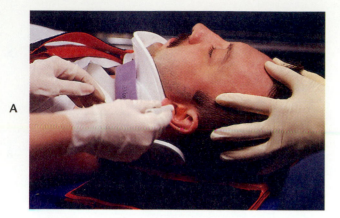

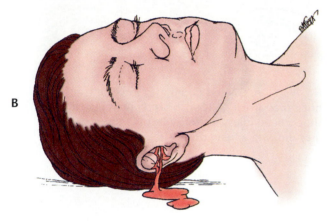

Fig. 8-57 A, Inspect the patient's ears for blood or fluid. B, Always suspect cervical spine injury or skull fracture in a patient with blood or other fluid in the ear.

Examine the outer ear for lacerations, bleeding, or other evidence of soft-tissue trauma (Fig. 8-57). Visually inspect the ear canals. Blood or clear, watery fluid, **cerebrospinal fluid** (CSF), in the ear may indicate basilar skull fracture. CSF may be mixed with blood.

A drop of blood that is mixed with CSF will form a brown ring when placed onto a gauze. This test is known as the "halo test," or "Bull's eye sign." For years, this test was standard in determining whether or not fluid contained CSF. However, the efficacy of this test recently has been questioned in the medical literature. Current trends suggest that a chemical dipstick for glucose, such as those used in blood glucose monitoring, should be used instead. EMT–Is should follow their local protocols and medical direction recommendations.

BATTLE'S SIGN: A discoloration of the area behind the ear; indication of the possibility of skull fracture, but considered a late sign.

Check the area behind the ears for discoloration. Bruising of this area is called **Battle's sign** and may indicate a basilar skull fracture. This sign usually takes time to develop and may not be visible at the scene.

Nose
Observe for deformities indicating a fracture or dislocated nasal cartilage. Note lacerations or other soft-tissue injuries. A skull fracture may cause blood or CSF fluid to drain into the nasopharynx, which may compromise the patient's airway.

Mouth and throat
In the unresponsive patient, gently separate the lips and inspect the mouth for foreign material, broken teeth, or dentures (remove dentures only if loose). Note soft-tissue injuries within the mouth. Lacerations on the floor of the mouth, the inner surface of the cheek, and the base of the tongue are often overlooked (Fig. 8-58).

Bleeding into the mouth can obstruct the upper airway. Suction may be required to keep the airway open and to get a clear view. If the patient's airway is compromised, clear the airway and reclassify the patient as a priority patient. If spinal injury is not suspected, position the patient to allow for blood drainage.

While assessing the mouth, note the patient's breath odor. Alcohol ingestion usually gives off a distinct odor. A fruity odor may indicate diabetes mellitus.

Face
Observe the face for obvious deformities, swelling, or discoloration. Gently palpate the maxilla and mandible for possible fractures.

Neck
Observe the neck for ecchymosis, neck vein distention, and open injuries (Fig. 8-59). Gently palpate the anterior neck for tracheal positioning and ask if the patient feels pain. Never palpate both sides of the neck at the same time because blood flow to the brain could be disrupted. *Do not remove the extrication collar if already in place.*

NECK VEIN DISTENSION: A bulging outward of the veins in the neck.

Ecchymosis in the neck region may signify trauma and impending airway obstruction. Normally, the neck veins are barely visible. If these veins appear to be bulging outward, they should be considered distended. **Neck vein distention** may be seen in conditions such as congestive heart failure and cardiac tamponade.

SUBCUTANEOUS EMPHYSEMA: A condition in which air enters the subcutaneous tissue through a hole in the trachea.

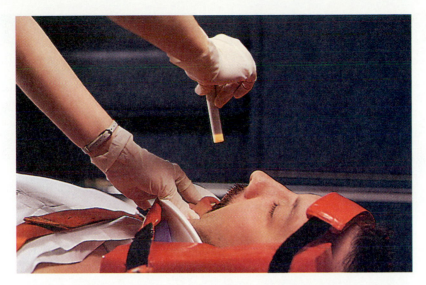

Fig. 8-58   An EMT-I inspecting a patient's mouth for foreign objects and soft tissue injuries.

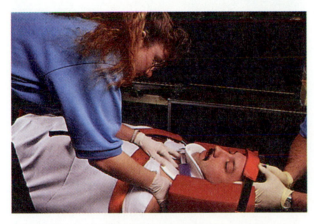

Fig. 8-59   An EMT-I carefully palpating a patient's cervical spine.

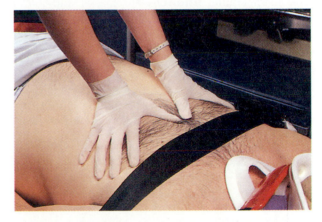

Fig. 8-60   An EMT-I observing a patient's chest for expansion or injury.

An open wound to the anterior neck, even if it appears relatively minor, is an emergency. If swelling develops, pressure on the trachea may obstruct the airway. If the trachea is injured, air may leak into the subcutaneous tissue, a condition known as **subcutaneous emphysema**. A patient may describe this condition as feeling like a crunching or crackling below the skin.

Chest
If not already done, expose the chest and observe for symmetric breathing, equal expansion, obvious injuries, or open wounds. Palpate the chest by beginning with the clavicles then palpating the rib cage (Fig. 8-60). Note pain, tenderness, possible fractures, or subcutaneous emphysema.

After palpation, auscultate the chest to verify breath sounds (Fig. 8-61). The chest should be aus-cultated in at least six different areas. Ascertain that breath sounds are equal on each side. If cervical spine injury is not suspected, perform both anterior and posterior auscultation. It also is possible to check the posterior breath sounds while moving the patient onto a backboard. Depending on the EMS system, the EMT–I may be asked to classify breath sounds as well as to determine whether or not they are present.

WHEEZES: A high-pitched squeal in the lungs during the process of breathing.
RHONCHI: A coarse gurgling sound in the lungs during the process of breathing.
RALES: A crackling or bubbling sound in the lungs.

Breath sounds are classified as one of three types. **Wheezes** are squeaking, high-pitched sounds that

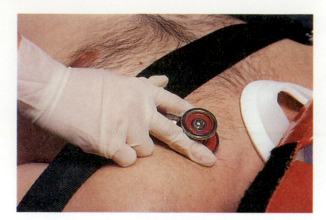

Fig. 8-61 An EMT-I auscultating a patient's lungs during the head-to-toe examination.

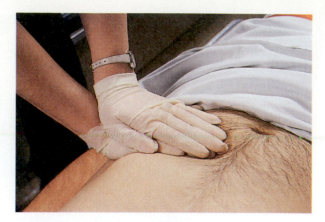

Fig. 8-62 Palpate all four quadrants of the abdomen for injury or tenderness.

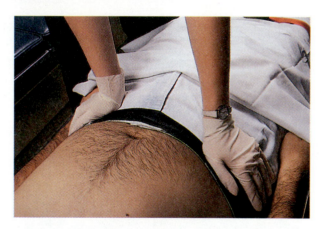

Fig. 8-63 Palpate the patient's pelvis by applying bilateral pressure at the iliac crests.

may occur on either inspiration, expiration, or both. They represent spasm in the airways and are present in asthma, chronic obstructive pulmonary disease, and heart failure. **Rhonchi** are coarser and sound like gurgling. They are often present over the larger airways only and may be present on both inspiration and expiration. Rhonchi indicate mucus or some other type of material in the larynx, trachea, or bronchi. They often are present in upper respiratory infections such as bronchitis. **Rales** (sometimes called crackles) are crackling or bubbling sounds that represent fluid in the alveoli and are present in heart failure and pneumonia.

Abdomen

> **RIGIDITY:** A condition characterized by hardness and stiffness.
> **COSTOVERTEBRAL ANGLE:** Angle formed where the lowest rib meets the spinal column.

Inspect the abdomen for signs of obvious injury, ecchymosis, or swelling. Palpate each quadrant of the abdomen lightly first, then deeper (Fig. 8-62). Observe the patient's face for any painful response or grimace. Also note if abdominal **rigidity,** hardness or stiffness of the abdominal wall, is present. Palpate posteriorly at the **costovertebral angle** (CVA) at the junction of the twelfth rib and the twelfth thoracic vertebra. CVA tenderness may indicate a kidney disorder.

Findings of discoloration, rigidity, exposed intestines (evisceration), or severe pain indicate a serious problem. Classify these patients as "priority."

Pelvis

Examine the pelvis by gentle palpation at the iliac crests (Fig. 8-63). Place your hands on the patient's iliac crests and gently push in and downward. If the pelvis is injured, the responsive patient will feel extreme pain. Trauma to the pelvic structures usually causes critical injuries. If pelvic injury is suspected, proceed under the "priority" criteria.

Genitourinary

It usually is not necessary to inspect the genitourinary area when no abnormalities or injuries are suspected. When examination is necessary, only assess the external genitalia; internal examinations of the female genitals are not appropriate in the prehospital setting unless conditions related to labor and delivery are present. Observe for blood on the groin area of the clothing. If found, visualize the external genitalia. Also inspect the perineum, which is the area between the anus and the genitals.

In the male patient also examine for priapism, which is spontaneous prolonged erection sometimes seen in spinal injury, kidney disease, or sickle cell anemia. Also observe for avulsion of the penis.

For the female patient observe for soft-tissue injuries and obvious bleeding. If the patient is actively bleeding from the vagina, suspect uterine bleeding until proven otherwise.

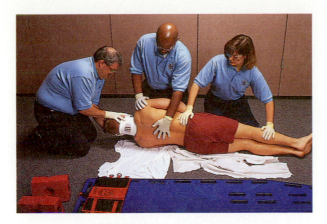

Fig. 8-64   Carefully palpate the patient's back as he or she is being log rolled to a long board.

Extremities

When examining the arms and legs, start with the lower extremities because injuries to the legs are potentially more serious than those of the arms.

Inspect the lower extremities for obvious deformities, discoloration, and soft-tissue injuries. Palpate the legs, including the calf, to find injuries and pain. Palpate a distal pulse and recheck capillary refill in each extremity.

Back

Initially examine the back of a supine patient by placing your hands under the voids on each side. Further assessment of the back and buttocks can be accomplished as the patient is moved to a long backboard (Fig. 8-64).

Inspect for obvious soft-tissue and skeletal injuries. Gently palpate the back for deformities and pain. Minimize patient movement because back injuries can be easily aggravated.

Neurologic assessment

An important part of the neurologic assessment is the evaluation of patient's level of responsiveness—the patient's degree of awareness of his or her surroundings. The level of responsiveness is the best indicator of the condition of the central nervous system. Any changes should be noted. Deterioration indicates the need for urgent medical attention and reclassification as a "priority" patient.

Glasgow coma scale

GLASGOW COMA SCALE: A numerical scale used for neurologic assessment in a critical patient.

In addition to the AVPU scale, another helpful neurologic assessment is the **Glasgow coma scale.** Although this scale has become somewhat controversial in recent medical literature, it is still widely used. The three main areas assessed are eye opening, verbal response, and motor response.

The maximum score possible is 15 and the minimum is 3. Adults scoring below 9 have a poor neurologic prognosis. A separate scale has been devised for children.

Evaluate motor response on the patient's best response to either a verbal command or a painful stimulus. Six points is the maximum possible score in this category. The motor response is scored as follows:

- 6 = patient obeys a simple command such as "lift your right hand up"
- 5 = patient moves a limb in an attempt to locate a painful stimulus and remove it
- 4 = patient attempts to withdraw from a painful stimulus
- 3 = patient flexes the arms and wrists in response to painful stimuli (decorticate posturing)
- 2 = patient extends the arms at the elbows in response to painful stimuli (decerebrate posturing)
- 1 = no motor response to pain on any limb

Evaluate verbal response on the best answer to questions of time, place, and person: "what day is this," "what place is this," "what is your name?" There are a maximum of five possible points in this category, which is scored as follows:

- 5 = patient is oriented to time, place, and person
- 4 = patient is able to converse but is not oriented to time, place, or person
- 3 = patient speaks in only short phrases or uses words that make no sense
- 2 = patient responds with incomprehensible sounds such as moans and groans
- 1 = patient has no verbal response

Evaluate eye opening on the basis of what stimuli, if any, are required for the patient to open his or her eyes without assistance. The maximum points possible in this category are four. Eye opening is scored as follows:

- 4 = patient opens eyes spontaneously
- 3 = patient opens eyes in response to your speech (spoken or shouted)
- 2 = patient opens eyes only in response to pain
- 1 = patient exhibits no response

CLINICAL NOTES
The AVPU scale evaluates what stimulus it takes to get a response. The Glasgow coma scale evaluates what response results from the stimulus given. Both scales are valuable tools for the EMT–I during patient assessment.

Sensory and neurologic function in the lower extremities are assessed as follows:

- Sensory—Provide a mild pain stimulus, such as a pinch, and note the patient's response. Avoid sticking a pin or needle into the foot to assess sensation. While pinching distally with one hand, stabilize the proximal tibia/fibula with the other hand. This may prevent further damage should the stimulus cause excessive movement.

- Motor—Ask the patient to move his or her toes, then to press his or her feet against your hands. Note any inability to move. If spine or back injury is suspected, do not have the patient move his or her feet.

Examine the upper extremities in the same way as the lower extremities. Observe for needle tracks and rashes. When palpating a distal pulse, the radial pulse is most convenient. When assessing neurologic function, ask the patient to perform the following:

- Sensory—Provide a mild stimulus, such as a pinch, to the wrist. Stabilize the proximal forearm to avoid excessive motion.

> **HELPFUL HINT**
> To assess equality of sensation, stroke the outside of one extremity, then the outside of the other extremity. Ask the patient if it feels the same on both sides.

- Motor—Ask the patient to move his or her fingers, then to squeeze your hands. Note any loss or deficit of grip strength. If spine or back injury is suspected, do not have the patient move his or her arms.

PARALYSIS: The loss of movement, the loss of sensation, or both. Paralysis of both arms and both legs is quadriplegia. Paralysis of the arm and leg on one side of the body is hemiplegia. Paraplegia is the paralysis of both legs.
PARESTHESIA: A condition in which the patient complains of tingling or numbness in the arms or legs.

When assessing the responsive patient, the EMT–I should ask about any numbness or tingling sensation in the arms or legs. These sensations, known as **paresthesias,** could indicate possible spinal cord damage or local circulatory problems. Any patient who complains of numbness or tingling in the extremities or inequality of sensation, particularly following an injury, should be cared for as though a spinal injury exists.

Other information to evaluate on a continuing basis includes:

- Changing levels of responsiveness
- Orientation to person, place, and time

- Speech quality
- Pupillary reaction to light

The most important thing for the EMT–I to remember in assessing neurologic function and level of responsiveness is to look for changes. Deterioration in these parameters is very important to note. If a patient's level of responsiveness or neurologic function worsens, handle as a "priority" patient.

Should the patient become unstable at any time during the detailed assessment, repeat the initial survey and initiate "priority" procedures.

ON-GOING ASSESSMENT, FIELD MANAGEMENT, AND TRANSPORTATION

On-going assessment

> Describe the need for on-going assessment; list the components and discuss the frequency of this part of the patient evaluation.

Patient assessment is an on-going process that must be continued while the EMT–I is providing definitive field management and transportation. In a stable patient, the assessment should be repeated every 15 minutes. In an unstable patient, the assessment should be repeated every 5 minutes.

On-going assessment includes the following parameters:

- Reassess mental status
- Monitor the airway
- Monitor breathing—rate and quality
- Reassess pulse—rate and quality
- Monitor skin color, temperature, and condition
- Realign patient priorities as needed
- Reassess vital signs
- Repeat focused examination regarding complaint or injuries
- Check efficacy of interventions

Definitive field management
Definitive field management includes life-saving modalities described previously, as well as treatment of less-threatening problems to the extent possible in the field. This process includes airway maintenance and ventilation, as well as the use of intravenous (IV) fluids and pneumatic antishock garment for shock. In many patients, cardiac monitoring is appropriate. If a patient has trauma, fracture stabilization, bandaging, and immobilization to the stretcher will improve comfort and ensure a safer transport to the hospital.

If an IV line is started, it is helpful to draw blood for the hospital to analyze. The EMT–I's local protocols also may include use of the fingerstick blood glucose test in the field.

Transportation

 Discuss factors that must be considered when determining to which hospital a patient should be transported.

The facility to which the patient is transported depends on factors such as patient condition, available facilities, and available transport modes. It is generally accepted that patients should be directly transported to the most appropriate facility for their condition. If possible, and if allowed by local protocols, the EMT–I also should consider the patient's wishes to be taken to a certain hospital.

Many EMS system now include specialty centers for:

- Multiple system trauma
- Acute myocardial infarction (chest pain emergency departments)
- Burns
- Spinal cord injuries
- Pediatric trauma
- Eye injuries
- Extremity reimplantation
- Neonatal emergencies
- Hyperbaric medicine
- Behavioral and psychiatric emergencies

In many EMS systems, the EMT–Is determine which patients are referred to a specialty center based on written protocols. Other systems require transport authorization from medical direction. Depending on the level of care available, transport time, and patient condition, some patients are directed to the closest emergency department for initial evaluation and life-saving treatment. In most cases, however, direct transportation to the appropriate specialty center is best for the patient.

Different modes of transportation are available—conditions, local protocols, and medical direction will dictate which mode is used. Aeromedical transportation, especially EMS helicopter transport, has become a common vehicle for transporting critically ill and injured patients to the appropriate specialty center. General guidelines for when helicopter transport is *not* appropriate include:

- During lightning or high wind conditions
- During heavy cloud periods (unless the helicopter can fly on instruments)
- Combative patients
- Patients contaminated by hazardous materials
- Patients whose size prohibits proper securing inside the aircraft

- When ground transport is faster, including waiting time for the helicopter to reach the scene

In summary, the EMT–I should follow the "3 Rs" rule of medical transportation: Get the "right person" to the "right place" in the "right amount of time."

Some tips for transporting the geriatric patient include:

1. A geriatric patient may think he or she is being brought to the hospital to die, and many will resist transport.

2. Explain clearly everything that is being done to the patient.

3. Give these patients choices whenever possible.

4. Ensure that someone will take care of the patient's possessions.

5. Use family members whenever possible to help reassure the patient.

Communication—contacting medical direction

 Describe the need for communication with either medical direction or the receiving facility when transporting a patient.

Once transport is begun, it is imperative to contact the receiving facility, either directly or through the medical direction facility. Some EMS systems require that units also call in during the resuscitation phase of the incident. At this point, the EMT–I should take the time to provide only "need to know" information such as:

- Nature of the incident
- Number of patients to be transported
- Life-threatening problems
- Care being rendered
- Results of that care
- Estimated time of arrival (ETA) at the facility

If additional information is necessary, a follow-up call can be made en route to update information about the patient's condition. Some EMS systems require medical direction contact to be made at specific times. If a certain skill requires permission from medical direction, more information (such as vital signs or specific injuries) may be needed before making contact with medical direction.

 Discuss the benefits of accurate documentation.

The EMT–I should be certain to fill out the appropriate run reports in a clear and readable form. A well-documented report is essential for proper transfer of care to the receiving facility, as well as for defense if patient care ever needs justification in a hearing or negligence suit.

CASE HISTORY FOLLOW-UP

EMT–I Smith is back at base and feeling a little nervous as he places the call to the hospital. A million things are running through his mind. Did he miss a major injury to one of the patients? Did he leave out some important patient information? Was his radio report inaccurate? Was his paperwork not complete? He hates emergency responses like this car crash. The scenes are always busy, and there are so many things that need to be done at one time. It's so easy to overlook something important.

The medical direction physician comes to the phone. Her voice is friendly, yet she sounds concerned. She asks EMT–I Smith about his assessment of the 3-year-old child. EMT–I Smith feels sick to his stomach and before answering the physician's question, he asks if the child is okay. The physician tells him that the boy will be fine but that he had a right midshaft femur fracture and had lost quite a bit of blood by the time he got to the emergency department. According to the mother, the child was sitting on her lap when the crash occurred and was thrown to the floorboard of the car.

EMT–I Smith mentally reviews his physical examination of the child. He remembers that the child had a lot of winter clothing on and did not want to be touched. He recalls feeling the boy's chest, abdomen, arms, and legs and thinking that his right thigh felt a little larger than the left as he palpated through the boy's clothes. If only the boy had grimaced or shown some reaction, EMT–I Smith would have removed his clothing and performed a more thorough examination.

EMT–I Smith apologizes to the physician and refrains from making excuses. She tells him not to be too hard on himself and that "we all need to learn from our mistakes." But, EMT–I Smith knows the bottom line is that he did not do a good patient assessment. He was distracted by the scene and by the number of patients. He knows that he is ultimately responsible for this error. He vows never to let this kind of thing happen again.

SUMMARY

Patient assessment is a structured method of evaluating a patient's physical condition. The process involves six phases: scene size-up (scene assessment), initial assessment (primary survey), resuscitation, focused history and physical examination, detailed assessment (secondary survey), and on-going assessment (which includes definitive field management and transportation).

During the scene size-up, the EMT–I must evaluate the "whole picture" of the call. The purpose of this phase is to provide a safe environment for EMS personnel and the patient. On arrival, five critical decisions must be made:

- Is the scene safe?
- How many patients are involved?
- Is additional help needed?
- Is this a medical or a trauma patient?
- Is there a need for body substance isolation precautions?

The initial assessment is an organized approach to the patient in which the following tasks are performed:

- Form a general impression of the patient.
- Determine if any life-threatening conditions are present. If so, treat these immediately.
- Evaluate the patient's level of responsiveness.
- Assess the airway. If the patient is responsive and can speak clearly, the airway is open. Otherwise, it must be opened.
- Assess breathing. Immediately ventilate patients with inadequate breathing.
- Assess circulation by checking the pulses. Look for and treat bleeding and assess the skin.
- Identify priority (unstable) patients who require more advanced level care as soon as possible.

During the resuscitation phase, the EMT–I should perform life-saving procedures as needed, if not already done.

The focused history and physical examination evaluates the patient based on the suspected condition. In trauma patients, the EMT–I must first reconsider the mechanism of injury and the transport decision and then perform the rapid trauma assessment. The acronym for this examination is DCAP-BTLS:

D = Deformity

C = Contusions

A = Abrasions

P = Punctures/penetrations

B = Burns

T = Tenderness

L = Lacerations

S = Swelling

The EMT–I should follow the rapid trauma assessment and obtain baseline vital signs. These vital signs should include pulse, respirations, blood pressure, pulse oximetry, and temperature (as per local protocol). Finally, a SAMPLE history is taken:

S = Signs and symptoms

A = Allergies

M = Medications

P = Past pertinent medical history

L = Last oral intake—fluid or solid

E = Events leading to present event

The detailed assessment is a more detailed examination, which is patient- and injury-specific. The patient's illness or injury should indicate whether or not this part of the patient assessment needs to be performed. There are three parts to the detailed assessment. The chief complaint is the main problem for which EMS was called. During the patient history, details of the chief complaint and related problems are explored in detail. Finally, a head-to-toe survey is performed as indicated by the patient's conditions.

Patient assessment is an on-going process (on-going assessment) that is continued while the EMT–I provides definitive field management and transportation to the hospital. During this process, the EMT–I reassesses mental status, airway, breathing, pulse, the skin, and the vital signs. Treatment priorities are modified as needed, and the focused examination repeated as necessary. The effects of any treatment provided to the patient should be continuously monitored.

Many conditions cannot be completely managed in the field. The job of the EMT–I is to provide life-saving care when necessary, stabilize the patient, and appropriately "package" the patient for transportation to more definitive care, usually at a hospital. Local protocols will most often determine to which medical facility the patient is taken. Medical direction and/or the receiving facility should be contacted as per the EMT–I's local protocols. The EMT–I should be sure to document all care given on the appropriate run report in a clear and legible fashion.

9

AIRWAY MANAGEMENT

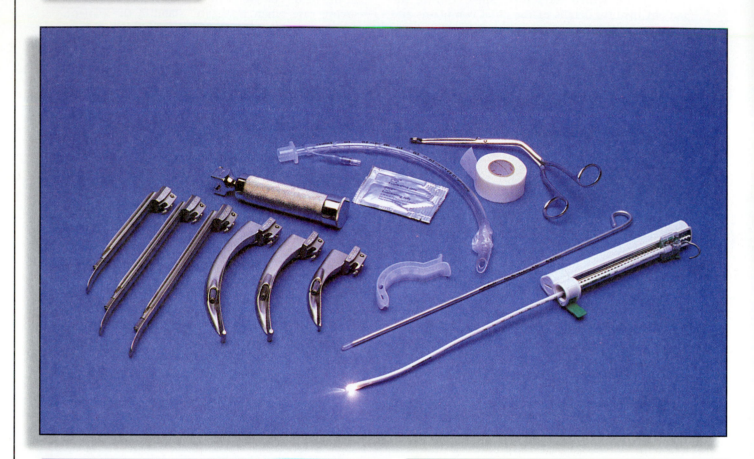

CASE HISTORY

It is early Sunday morning, 2:30 AM, when the dispatch comes in for a multiple vehicle collision on Country Meadows Road. EMT–Intermediates Simms and Brown arrive to find a car that had crashed into a pole at high speed.

EMT–I Simms gains access to the patient, a man approximately 20 years of age, through the driver's side rear window. EMT–I Simms maintains cervical spine immobilization with her gloved hands as she says, "Hi, I'm an EMT–Intermediate. Don't move. Can you hear me?" The patient doesn't answer. "Can you speak? Say something," EMT–I Simms says in a loud, firm voice. Again, no answer.

EMT–I Simms holds the patient's head immobile and upright in straight anatomic alignment while she leans over his mouth to hear and feel if he is breathing. She can hear gurgling and stridorous respirations. They are slow and shallow. "We've got to intubate right away!" EMT–I Simms

Case History, continued

calls out to her crew. She feels the patient's carotid pulse while she holds his head immobile and notes that it is 140 and thready.

Her partner, EMT–I Brown, places a nonrebreather mask on the patient with oxygen at 12 L/min and prepares to ventilate and suction. The crew extricates the patient rapidly while EMT–I Simms maintains his head alignment with her hands. A cervical spine immobilization device is applied, and the patient is secured to the backboard with padding. EMT–I Simms asks EMT–I Brown to hyperventilate and suction the patient while she prepares to place the tube.

EMT–I Simms inserts an endotracheal tube and inflates the balloon with 10 cc of air. She then confirms placement by auscultation for equal bilateral breath sounds and double-checks placement by auscultating the epigastrium to ensure there are no sounds of air movement in the stomach.

LEARNING OBJECTIVES

Upon completion of this chapter, the EMT–Intermediate should be able to:

- DESCRIBE the anatomy of the upper airway including the mouth, nose, pharynx, epiglottis, and larynx.
- IDENTIFY the three regions of the pharynx.
- RECALL the anatomic relationship of the larynx to the:
  - tongue
  - pharynx
  - epiglottis
  - vocal cords
  - esophagus
- RELATE the difference between the true and false vocal cords.
- RECALL and demonstrate the essential elements of assessing airway patency, breathing effectiveness, and oxygenation in the ill or injured patient.
- IDENTIFY the common mechanisms of upper airway compromise and describe the procedures for resolving each.
- DESCRIBE and demonstrate the procedures used to manually open the airway.
- DISCUSS indications, contraindications, and methods for insertion and use of the following:
  - oropharyngeal airway
  - nasopharyngeal airway
  - esophageal obturator airway
  - esophageal gastric tube airway
  - pharyngotracheal lumen airway
- DISCUSS the indications, contraindications, and methods of performing suctioning.
- IDENTIFY the common mechanisms of ventilatory failure and describe the procedures for resolving each.
- DISCUSS indications, contraindications, and methods for use of the following:
  - pocket mask
  - bag-valve-mask device
  - demand valve resuscitator
- IDENTIFY the common mechanisms of hypoxia and describe its treatment.
- LIST the indications and oxygen delivery concentrations of the following:
  - nasal cannula
  - simple face mask
  - nonrebreather mask
  - Venturi mask
- RECALL the indications, contraindications, and alternatives of endotracheal intubation.
- ASSEMBLE and check the equipment used to perform endotracheal intubation.
- LIST and demonstrate the steps for performing endotracheal intubation.
- DEMONSTRATE the methods used to ensure correct placement of the endotracheal tube.

KEY TERMS

ADULT RESPIRATORY DISTRESS SYNDROME
AMBIENT AIR
ANOXIA
APNEA
ASPIRATED
BREATH SOUNDS
CARINA
CRICOTHYROID MEMBRANE
CYANOSIS
DIAPHRAGM
DIFFUSION
DIGITALLY
DYSRHYTHMIA
ENDOTRACHEAL INTUBATION
EPIGLOTTIS
FIBROSIS
FIO$_2$
GAG REFLEX
GLOTTIS
HYPERCARBIA
HYPOVENTILATION
HYPOXEMIA
HYPOXIA
INTRAPULMONARY SHUNTING

KYPHOSCOLIOSIS
LATERAL
MANDIBLE
MAXILLA
MINUTE VOLUME
MUCOUS MEMBRANE
NASAL SEPTUM
OCCIPUT
OROTRACHEAL
PATENT AIRWAY
PARTIAL PRESSURE OF CARBON DIOXIDE (PCO$_2$)
PHONATION
PARTIAL PRESSURE OF OXYGEN (PO$_2$)
RED BLOOD CELLS
REGURGITATION
RETRACTION
SEROUS MEMBRANE
SNORING BREATHING
STRIDOR
STYLET
SUBCUTANEOUS EMPHYSEMA
TRACHEAL LUMEN
TRACHEAL TUGGING
VENTILATION

INTRODUCTION

In the prehospital setting, the EMT–I must be prepared to treat patients who are experiencing obstructed airway, aspiration, inadequate ventilation, or hypoxia. Each is a life-threatening condition that requires immediate intervention if the patient is to survive. This chapter presents information related to the adult patient. Oxygenation, ventilation, and airway management for infants and children are discussed in Chapter 17, "Pediatric Emergencies."

PATENT AIRWAY: An open, unblocked airway.

Some of the procedures employed by the EMT–I are done manually whereas others require adjunctive equipment or advanced techniques. In contrast to the hospital environment, where care is provided in a controlled setting, managing patients in the field is often done with too few hands, little lighting, and an anxious crowd who expects the patient to be saved no matter how severe his or her condition. All these factors make the EMT–I's job challenging. Of all the components of the EMT–I training program, learning how to maintain a **patent airway** and provide ventilatory assistance and oxygenation are among the most important. To learn these skills, it is important for the EMT–I to understand the normal anatomy and physiology of the respiratory system.

ANATOMY OF THE RESPIRATORY SYSTEM

The job of the respiratory system is to move air in and out of the lungs, bringing oxygen into the body and removing carbon dioxide. Oxygen is required for the conversion of essential nutrients into energy. Carbon dioxide is a waste product of metabolism and must be removed. For normal breathing to occur a person must have a patent airway, intact ventilatory musculoskeletal system, unobstructed respiratory passageways, adequate pulmonary blood flow, and appropriate neurologic stimulation.

MUCOUS MEMBRANE: A thin layer of connective tissue lining many of the body cavities through which air passes; usually contains small, mucus-secreting glands. Mucus is a thick, slippery secretion that functions as a lubricant and protects various surfaces.

CLINICAL NOTES
Inflammations of the various membranes of the body are assigned names by adding the suffix *-itis* to their anatomic name.

All of the respiratory structures leading to the microscopic alveoli (where the actual exchange of gases takes place) are lined with a highly vascular **mucous membrane.** This membrane filters the air. When inspired air finally reaches the distal passageways it is the same temperature as the body, 100% humidified, and essentially sterile. The respiratory passageway can be thought of as being divided into the upper and lower airways.

Upper airway

 Describe the anatomy of the upper airway including the mouth, nose, pharynx, epiglottis, and larynx.

Structures of the upper airway include the nose, mouth, pharynx, and larynx (Fig. 9-1). The nose and mouth provide passageways into the respiratory system.

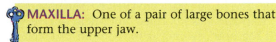 **MAXILLA:** One of a pair of large bones that form the upper jaw.

Nose
The nose is the uppermost aspect of the airway. Its external portion, the part that protrudes from the face, is made up of a bony and cartilaginous framework covered by skin. It is surrounded by the **maxilla** along the sides and below at its base. On the front surface of the nose are two openings to the outside of the body. These openings are referred to as *nostrils* or *nares*.

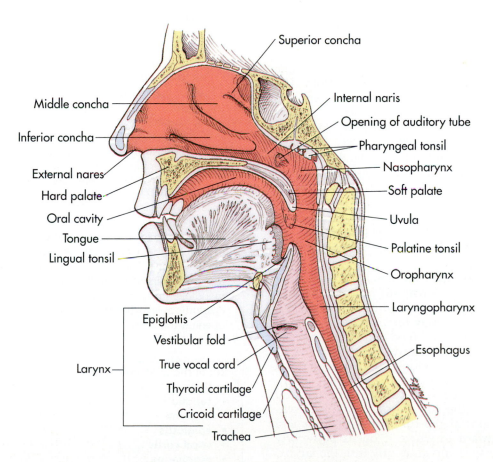

Fig. 9-1 **Anatomy of the upper airway.**

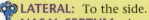

LATERAL: To the side.
NASAL SEPTUM: An anatomic wall dividing the nostrils. It is made up of bone and cartilage covered by mucous membrane.

The internal portion of the nose is separated into the right and left cavity by the **nasal septum.** Each cavity has three bones: the superior, middle, and inferior turbinates (also referred to as *conchae*) located on their **lateral** walls. The turbinates can be compared to shelves. The purpose of the turbinates is to cause turbulent air flow through the nose, forcing it to rebound in several directions during its passage. This action traps finer particles, which the cilia of the mucous membrane then propel back to the pharynx to be swallowed. On the back surface of the internal nose are two nares that serve as a passageway into the nasopharynx. Because its walls have a rich blood supply, serious bleeding can occur if the nasal passages are injured.

MANDIBLE: The large bone forming the lower jaw.

Mouth

The mouth, also referred to as the *oral cavity,* is formed by the cheeks, hard and soft palates, and tongue. The lips are the fleshy folds that surround the opening, and the gums and teeth are located inside the mouth. The top of the mouth is covered by the hard and soft palates, whereas the tongue, a large mass of muscle, can be found on the bottom. The tongue attaches to the **mandible** as well as to the hyoid bone through a series of muscles and ligaments. It assists with speech and the swallowing of food. The hyoid bone, shaped like a "U," is located just under the chin. It is unique in that it is the only bone of the axial skeleton that does not articulate with any other bone. Rather, it is suspended from the temporal bone by ligaments.

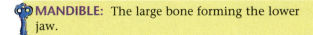 **Identify the three regions of the pharynx.**

Pharynx

The pharynx, also called the *throat,* is a muscular conduit that extends downward from the back of the soft palate to the upper end of the esophagus. It serves as the passageway for air into the respiratory tract (anteriorly) and food and liquid into the digestive system (posteriorly). The pharynx is divided into three regions: the nasopharynx (located immediately behind the nasal cavity), oropharynx (located behind the mouth), and laryngopharynx (the lower portion). The laryngopharynx begins at the tip of the epiglottis and extends downward to where it opens posteriorly into the esophagus and anteriorly into the larynx. It is also called the *hypopharynx.*

GAG REFLEX: Retching or striving to vomit; it is a normal reflex triggered by touching of the soft palate or the throat.

Because the mouth and pharynx serve a dual purpose of conveying air and food and/or liquid, they are lined with sensitive nerves that activate the cough, **gag reflex,** and swallowing mechanisms to prevent the airway from being accidentally blocked or foreign matter being drawn into the lungs.

CLINICAL NOTES
A cough is a forceful exhalation of a large volume of air. To initiate a cough, approximately 2.5 L of air is drawn into the respiratory passageways. Next, the glottic opening closes tightly shut to trap the air within the lungs. The abdominal and thoracic muscles then contract, pushing against the diaphragm and increasing the pressure within the tracheobronchial tree. The vocal cords suddenly open in a cough, forcing air and foreign particles out of the lungs.

Located in the front of the pharynx, just below the base of the tongue, are the epiglottis, laryngeal inlet, and mucous membrane-covered arytenoid and cricoid cartilages of the larynx. Just behind the hypopharynx are the fourth and fifth cervical vertebrae.

The epiglottis is a leaf-shaped, flexible cartilage that hangs over the larynx. It is connected to the hyoid bone and mandible by a series of ligaments and muscles. Its most important function is to prevent food or liquid from entering the respiratory tree during swallowing. Just above the epiglottis is the vallecula, the depression between the epiglottis and base of the tongue. To the sides are indentations called *pyriform fossa.*

HELPFUL HINT
Because of their attachment to the mandible (directly and indirectly), both the tongue and epiglottis can fall back against the posterior wall of the pharynx, closing off the airway when the jaw goes slack. This problem can be corrected by using the chin-lift or jaw-thrust, which moves the mandible forward, lifting the tongue and epiglottis away from the posterior pharynx and opening the airway.

Recall the anatomic relationship of the larynx to the:
• **tongue**
• **pharynx**
• **epiglottis**
• **vocal cords**
• **esophagus**

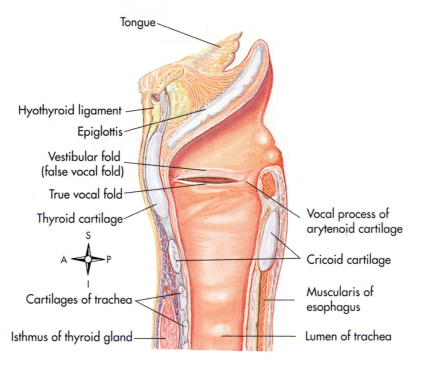

Figure 9-2   **Sagittal view of the larynx.**

Labels (clockwise from top):
- Tongue
- Hyothyroid ligament
- Epiglottis
- Vestibular fold (false vocal fold)
- True vocal fold
- Thyroid cartilage
- Cartilages of trachea
- Isthmus of thyroid gland
- Vocal process of arytenoid cartilage
- Cricoid cartilage
- Muscularis of esophagus
- Lumen of trachea

Larynx

The larynx is the triangular-shaped structure that connects the pharynx with the trachea. Positioned midline in the neck, below the hyoid bone and in front of the esophagus, the larynx is made up of the thyroid cartilage, cricoid cartilage, vocal cords, and arytenoid folds. It performs several functions including protecting the lower airway and producing voice (Fig. 9-2).

The walls of the larynx consist of cartilages that prevent it from collapsing during inspiration. The main laryngeal cartilage is the thyroid cartilage. It is also referred to as the *Adam's apple* and is more prominent in men than women. The thyroid cartilage consists of two large shield-shaped pieces that form the anterior wall of the larynx and give it its V-shaped appearance. The posterior wall is open and consists of muscle.

 CRICOTHYROID MEMBRANE: Membrane situated between the cricoid and thyroid cartilages of the larynx.

Below the thyroid cartilage is the cricoid cartilage. It is attached to the first ring of tracheal cartilage. Unlike the thyroid and tracheal cartilages, which are open on their posterior surfaces, the cricoid cartilage is the only complete ring. It is shaped like a signet ring with the bulky portion located posteriorly. In children, the narrowest part of the laryngeal airway is the cricoid cartilage. Connecting the bottom border of the thyroid cartilage with the top aspect of the cricoid cartilage is the **cricothyroid membrane.** Just behind the cricoid cartilage is the esophagus.

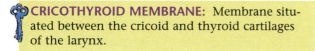 **CLINICAL NOTES**
Above and behind the cricoid cartilage are the two pyramid-shaped arytenoid cartilages. They attach to the vocal folds and pharyngeal wall and, by their action, open and close the vocal cords.

 GLOTTIS: The slitlike opening between the vocal cords.

🍎 **Relate the difference between the true and false vocal cords.**

The cavity of the larynx extends from its triangular-shaped inlet at the epiglottis to the circular outlet at the lower border of the cricoid cartilage where it is continuous with the lumen of the trachea. At the upper end of the laryngeal cavity, extending from the anterior surface of the arytenoid cartilages to the posterior surface of the thyroid cartilage, lie the true and false vocal cords. The superior pair form the false vocal cords (also called *vestibular folds)* and consist of elastic connective tissue covered by folds of mucous membrane. When these cords come together, they stop air from leaving the lungs (when a person holds his or her breath) and prevent foreign

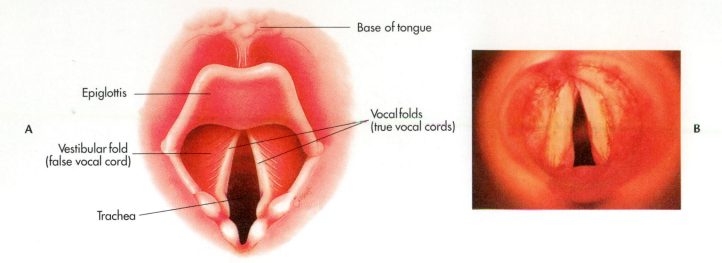

Base of tongue

Epiglottis

A

Vocal folds
(true vocal cords)

B

Vestibular fold
(false vocal cord)

Trachea

Fig. 9-3 A, B   Vocal cords viewed from above.

materials such as food or liquids from entering the airway. Below the false cords are the true vocal cords. They are cordlike structures that can vibrate to produce sound as expired air passes over them. The space between the true vocal cords is referred to as the glottic opening or **glottis.** In the adult, the glottic opening is the narrowest portion of the upper airway (Fig. 9-3).

> ### STREET WISE
> The passage of an endotracheal tube between the vocal cords interferes with the creation of sound used for voice production and coughing. If the patient is able to make sounds (*eg,* speak, moan, and so forth) it means the endotracheal tube is not in the correct location.

> ### CLINICAL NOTES
> The most common ailment of the larynx is inflammation, or laryngitis, often accompanying colds and followed by a temporary diminishing or complete loss of voice. Other diseases commonly attacking the larynx include croup, diphtheria, and cancer. Laryngeal cancer has been shown to be caused by cigarette smoking and by the intake of large amounts of alcohol. Persons who smoke and drink excessively run an especially high risk of developing cancer of the larynx.

Most of the larynx is richly lined with nerve endings from the vagus nerve. Due to the degree of vagal innervation, stimulation of the pharyngeal and laryngeal mucous membrane (by a laryngoscope or endotracheal tube) can cause bradycardia, hypotension, and a decreased respiratory rate.

Lower airway
The lower airway consists of the trachea, right and left mainstem bronchi, secondary bronchi, bronchioles, and alveoli.

Trachea
The trachea is the cylindrical tube, approximately 10 to 15 cm long, which extends from the lower rim of the larynx to the bronchi at the level of the fifth or sixth thoracic vertebra. It is situated in front of the esophagus and supported by C-shaped cartilaginous rings that extend throughout its length. These cartilages keep the tracheal walls from collapsing. The purpose of the trachea is to conduct air between the larynx and the lungs (Fig. 9-4).

> **CARINA:** Point at which the trachea divides (bifurcates, or separates into two sections) into the right and left mainstem bronchi.

Bronchial tree
At the **carina,** the trachea branches into right and left mainstem bronchi. There is one bronchus for each lung. The right bronchus is a more direct passageway from the trachea, because it is wider, shorter, and more vertical than the left. For this reason, aspirated foreign bodies—or mispositioned endotracheal tubes—are more likely to enter the right mainstem bronchus than the left. Like the trachea, the bronchi are lined with a ciliated mucus layer and reinforced with cartilaginous rings. On entering the lung each bronchus branches into secondary bronchi, one for each lobe of the lungs (three on the right and two on the left). This subdivision continues again and again, forming progressively smaller divisions. As the branches get smaller, the cartilaginous rings begin to

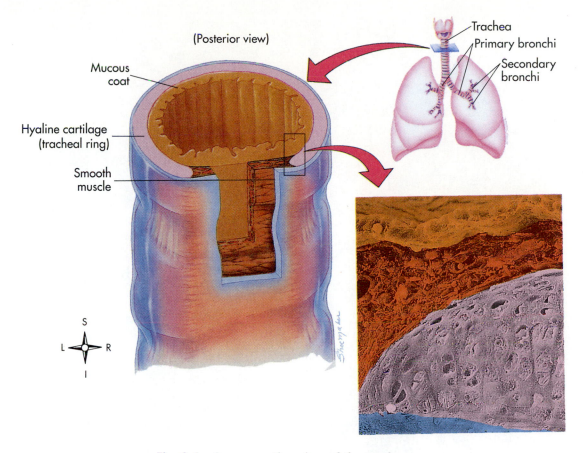

Fig. 9-4   A cross-section view of the trachea.

disappear and the structures are mostly smooth muscle. The more distal portions are referred to as *bronchioles*. Bronchioles, in turn, branch into even smaller tubes called *terminal* and *respiratory bronchioles,* which eventually divide into microscopic branches called *alveolar ducts*. These ducts then terminate in clusters of air sacs, called *alveoli*. The continuous branching of the trachea into primary bronchi, secondary bronchi, bronchioles, and terminal bronchioles resembles a tree trunk (with its branches) and is commonly referred to as the *bronchial tree* (Fig. 9-5).

Alveoli

The alveoli are hollow, grapelike structures only one or two cell layers thick (Fig. 9-6). They are the most important functional units of the respiratory system, because they serve as the primary site for oxygen and carbon dioxide exchange. Each alveoli lies in contact with a blood capillary, and there are millions of alveoli in each lung. The surface of the respiratory membrane inside the alveoli is covered with surfactant. This important substance keeps the alveoli from collapsing as air moves in and out during respiration.

Each microscopic alveolus is in contact with a rich capillary network arising from the pulmonary artery

(Fig. 9-7). The blood at the arteriole end of the pulmonary capillary is high in carbon dioxide and low in oxygen. As the blood passes through the capillaries most of the carbon dioxide in the blood diffuses into the alveoli, and oxygen from the alveoli diffuses into the capillary blood. Diffusion is the process whereby particles move from an area of greater concentration to an area of lesser concentration until the distribution of particles is equal. Therefore, the exchange of gases depends on differences in the concentration of gases on each side of the pulmonary membrane, which is referred to as the *diffusion gradient*.

SEROUS MEMBRANE: A two-layer epithelial membrane that lines body cavities and covers the surfaces of organs.

Lungs

The lungs are cone-shaped, light, spongy, elastic organs; one lung is located on each side of the heart in the thoracic cavity. The right lung has three lobes, whereas the left has two. Each lung is enclosed in a **serous membrane** called the *pleura*. This membrane is in the form of a sack and includes two layers: the visceral pleura and the parietal

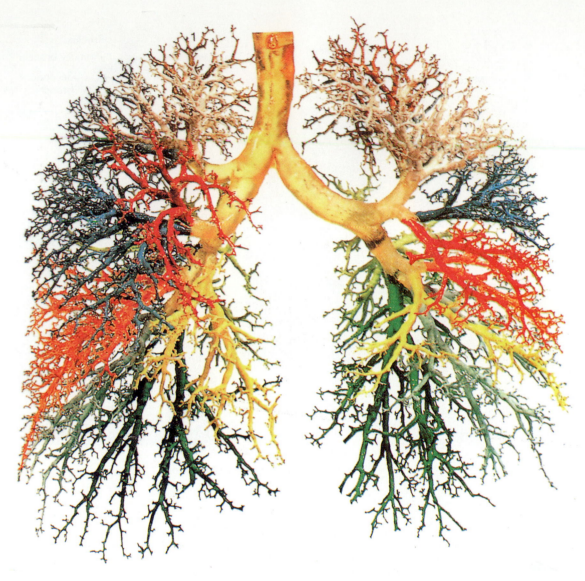

Fig. 9-5   A plaster cast of the bronchial tree.

pleura. The visceral layer of this membrane closely covers the lungs. The parietal layer of the pleura lines the inner surface of the chest wall, diaphragm, and mediastinum. The visceral pleura is separated from the parietal pleura by a potential space, the pleural space, that contains just a few drops of pleural fluid. The fluid acts to prevent friction as the lung tissue expands and contracts in the chest cavity (Fig. 9-8).

The tissues of the lungs are perfused via the bronchial arteries with oxygenated blood containing nutrients. After the bronchial arterial blood has passed through the capillaries and collected carbon dioxide from the lung tissues, it empties into the pulmonary veins and left atrium.

PHYSIOLOGY OF THE RESPIRATORY SYSTEM

In the preceding anatomy of the respiratory system section, the structures responsible for moving air in and out of the body were reviewed. This section reviews the mechanism or process of breathing and gas exchange.

Respiration

Respiration is the exchange of gases between the body cells and the atmosphere. There are three parts of respiration:

- External respiration—Involves the exchange of gases between the circulating blood and air and

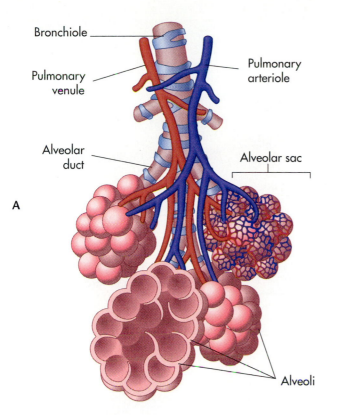

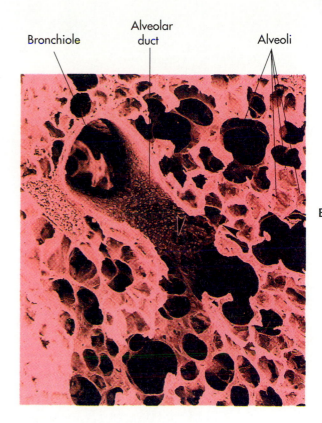

Fig. 9-6   **Anatomy of the alveoli. A, Terminal bronchioles branch into alveolar ducts, which terminate in alveoli. B, Electron micrograph scan of bronchiole, alveolar duct and alveoli. Arrowhead indicates opening of aveoli into the alveolar duct.**

is carried on by the expansion and contraction of the lungs.

- Internal respiration—Involves the exchange of dissolved gases between the circulating blood and interstitial fluids in the peripheral tissues.
- Cellular respiration—Actual use of oxygen by cells in the process of metabolism.

Respiration requires close interaction between the respiratory, central nervous, musculoskeletal, and circulatory systems. The process and rate at which respiration proceeds are controlled by a nervous center in the brain. The regulation of respiration is largely involuntary, and is controlled through chemical, physical and nervous reflexes that monitor the body's changing carbon dioxide levels and oxygen needs.

DIAPHRAGM: A wide muscular partition separating the thoracic, or chest, cavity, from the abdominal cavity. It is attached to the lumbar vertebrae, the lower ribs, and the sternum, or breastbone. It slants upward, higher in front than in the rear, and is dome-shaped when relaxed. Three major openings in the diaphragm allow passage of the esophagus, aorta, veins, nerves, and lymphatic and thoracic ducts.

Ventilation
The process of moving air in and out of the lungs is referred to as *ventilation*. It includes inspiration (breathing in) and expiration (breathing out).

Changes in the size and gross capacity of the chest are controlled by contractions of the **diaphragm** and of the muscles between the ribs (Fig. 9-9 A). Inspiration is initiated by the respiratory center in the medulla of the brain signaling the muscles of respiration to increase the size of the chest cavity (Fig. 9-9 B). The diaphragm and the intercostal muscles are stimulated to contract. The diaphragm, the major inspiratory muscle (accounting for 70% of the air flow in and out of the lungs), flattens downward against the abdominal structures. This action increases the vertical dimensions of the thoracic cavity in which the lungs are suspended, causing them to expand. Normal quiet breathing is accomplished almost entirely by this muscle. At the same time, the intercostal muscles lift the rib cage upward and outward, thus increasing the horizontal and transverse dimensions of the thoracic cavity. These actions create a potential vacuum that draws air into the enlarged lungs, filling them. Airway resistance must be overcome to generate flow through the airways. Changes in airway diameter affect airway resistance.

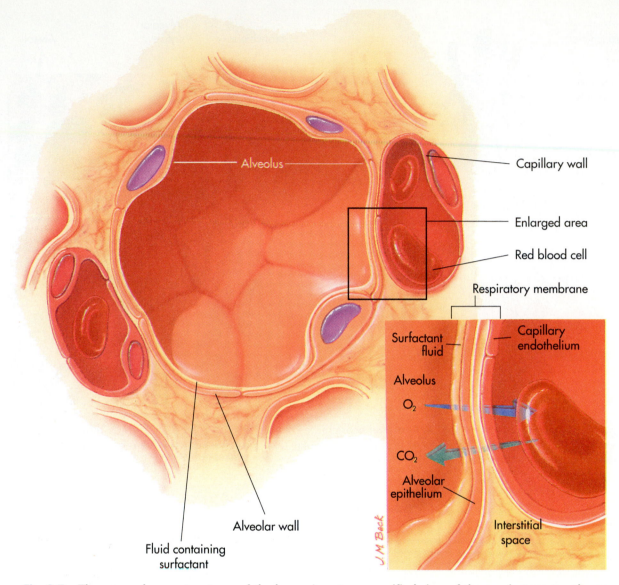

Fig. 9-7 The gas exchange structures of the lungs. Insert, a magnified view of the respiratory membrane.

Expiration occurs when the diaphragm and respiratory muscles relax and the chest cavity decreases in size (Fig. 9-9 C). The decreasing thoracic volume increases the intrathoracic pressure, and air is forced out of the lungs. This act is passive (unless forced), and the driving force stems from lung recoil.

MINUTE VOLUME: The volume of air exchanged in one minute.

Respiratory volume

Under normal circumstances people exchange sufficient volumes of air to accommodate normal as well as extraordinary physiologic requirements. On average, adults inhale and exhale between 500 to 800 cc of air, 12 to 20 times every minute. The air inhaled and exhaled in a single respiratory cycle is referred to as the *tidal volume*. Of the 500 to 800 cc of air inhaled and exhaled, dead air space, or the amount of air remaining in the air passageways (unavailable for gas exchange), equals approximately 150 cc. The alveolar air (that which reaches the alveoli for gas exchange) equals approximately 350 cc. The air exchanged over the course of a minute is referred to as the **minute volume.** The average minute volume ranges between 6000 and 16,000 cc. These volumes of air are necessary to remove carbon dioxide and to bring in sufficient supplies of oxygen.

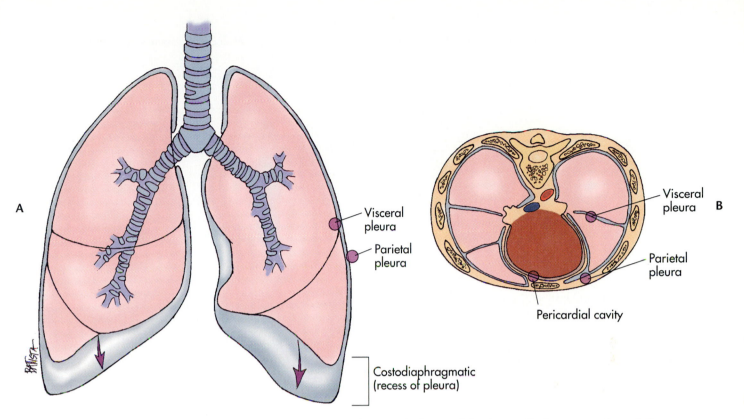

Fig. 9-8 A, An anterior view of the visceral pleura and parietal pleura of the lungs. B, A cross-section of the visceral pleura and parietal pleura of the lungs.

Exchange and transport of oxygen and carbon dioxide

DIFFUSION: A passive process of molecules moving from an area of higher concentration to an area of lesser concentration.
RED BLOOD CELLS: Round disks, concave on two sides, and approximately 7.5 thousandths of a millimeter in diameter.

CLINICAL NOTES
The mature red blood cell contains no nucleus. Hemoglobin, a protein in red blood cells, is the most prevalent of the special blood pigments that transport oxygen from the lungs to the body cells, where it picks up carbon dioxide for transport back to the lungs to be expired. The red blood cells are formed in the bone marrow. After an average life of 120 days, during which they incur substantial damage, they are broken down and removed by the spleen.

PO$_2$: Abbreviation for partial pressure of oxygen.
PCO$_2$: Abbreviation for partial pressure of carbon dioxide.

CLINICAL NOTES
To understand how oxygen and carbon dioxide are carried in the blood, it is helpful to understand about partial pressures of gases. Usually, gases are found as mixtures of several gases together, like the air we breathe. Dalton's law of partial pressures states that the pressure exerted by a mixture of gases is equal to the sum of the partial pressures of each (Fig. 9-10), and each gas acts as if it were present alone. The symbol used to designate partial pressure is the capital P preceding the chemical symbol for the gas. Some references still use the older symbol, a capital P and small *a* (Pa) to denote partial pressure. In air, the pressure of 760 mm Hg is the sum of the partial pressures of oxygen, nitrogen, carbon dioxide, water vapor, and trace gases. The partial pressure of each gas is directly related to its concentration in the total mixture. Atmospheric air contains 21% oxygen, 0.03% carbon dioxide, 78% nitrogen, and 0.97% other gases. The partial pressure of each is determined by multiplying its percentage by the sum (760 mm Hg).
Atmospheric PO2 = 21% × 760 = 159.6 mm Hg (rounded off to 160 mm Hg).

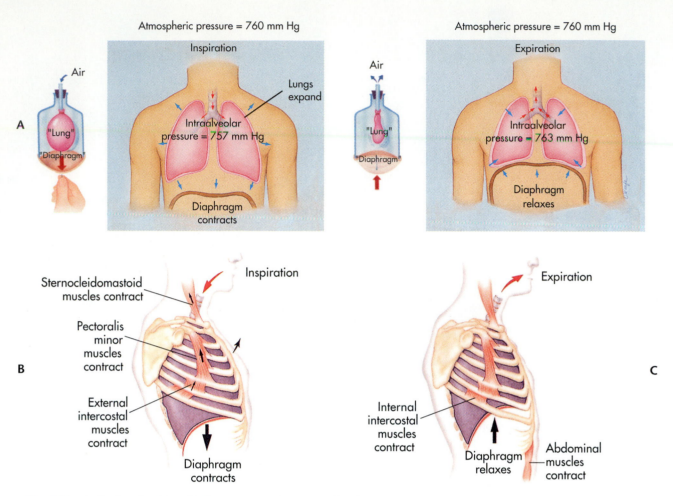

Fig. 9-9 **A, On inspiration, the lungs expand as a result of decreased pressure in the thoracic cavity. On expiration, the diaphragm relaxes and the lungs recoil as a result of increased pressure in the thoracic cavity. B, Mechanisms of inspiration. C, Mechanisms of expiration.**

Oxygenation

During inspiration, atmospheric air containing 21% oxygen is drawn into the respiratory passageways. At this concentration, oxygen has a partial pressure of 160 mm Hg. By the time inspired air reaches the alveoli, a number of factors combine to reduce the **partial pressure of oxygen (PO$_2$)** to 104 mm Hg. The warming and humidification of the atmospheric air in the upper respiratory tract results in an increase in the partial pressure of water vapor from 5.7 mm Hg to 47 mm Hg with partial pressures of other gases declining (because the total pressure must remain at 760 mm Hg). Also, in the respiratory passageways, inspired air mixes with gas that was not exhaled on the previous exhalation (150 mL of dead space). Because dead space air contains more carbon dioxide and less oxygen than inspired air, the PO$_2$ is reduced

further. Air that finally reaches the alveoli for diffusion across the respiratory membrane registers even more partial pressure changes but still remains high in oxygen (104 mm Hg) and low in carbon dioxide. In the alveoli this air is met by capillary venous blood oxygen that has a PO$_2$ of just 40 mm Hg. In a physiologic process called **diffusion**, oxygen moves across the alveolar/capillary membrane into the bloodstream until gas pressures are equal on both sides (Fig. 9-11).

Oxygen is transported in arterial blood in two ways: physically, dissolved in plasma; and chemically, attached to hemoglobin. While the blood is in the alveolar capillary, it absorbs enough oxygen to raise its PO$_2$ to 104 mm Hg. Because fluids can hold little gas in solution, just a small portion (3%) of oxygen is carried in plasma. Hemoglobin carries the majority (97%) of oxygen (Fig. 9-12). When

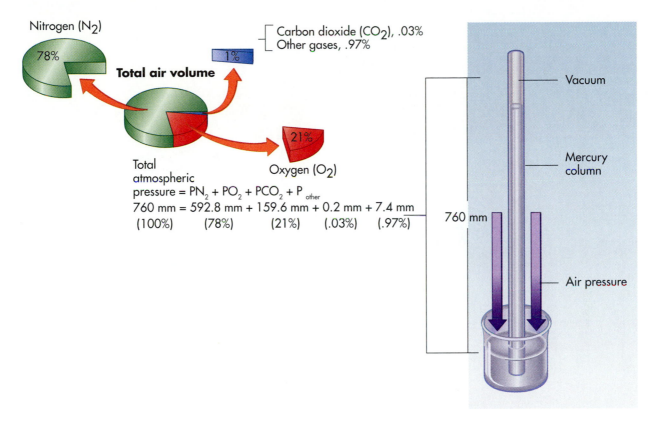

Nitrogen (N2)

78%

Total air volume

1%

Carbon dioxide (CO2), .03%
Other gases, .97%

21%

Total atmospheric pressure = $PN_2 + PO_2 + PCO_2 + P_{other}$

Oxygen (O2)

760 mm = 592.8 mm + 159.6 mm + 0.2 mm + 7.4 mm
(100%)   (78%)   (21%)   (.03%)   (.97%)

Vacuum

Mercury column

760 mm

Air pressure

Fig. 9-10   Partial pressures of various gases in atmospheric air.

hemoglobin is in the presence of high PO_2, (*eg*, in the pulmonary capillaries), oxygen binds to hemoglobin's iron molecules to form oxyhemoglobin. Hemoglobin bound to oxygen to its fullest extent (each gram of saturated hemoglobin carrying 1.34 mL of oxygen) is considered 100% saturated. Hemoglobin is close to being fully saturated at a PO_2 of 80 to 100 mm Hg. In this state the blood is bright red or scarlet.

Oxygenated blood leaving the pulmonary capillaries has a PO_2 of 104 mm Hg. This blood then mixes with shunted (deoxygenated) blood. This lowers the PO_2 of the blood leaving the lungs through the pulmonary arteries to 95 mm Hg. This oxygen-enriched blood is then transported back to the heart via the pulmonary bloodstream where it is then pumped to the systemic capillaries. There it comes into contact with tissues having a PO_2 of close to 40 mm Hg. Just like what occurred in the pulmonary capillaries, oxygen diffuses from an area of greater concentration (the bloodstream) to the area of lesser concentration (into the tissues). Oxygen then moves through the tissues to the cells where it plays an essential role in the Kreb's cycle (described further in Chapter 10, "Shock"), assisting with the production of energy. Because oxygen is constantly

being used by the cells, a low PO_2 in the tissues continually exists. This condition makes for easy diffusion of oxygen from the bloodstream into the tissues.

The pressure of oxygen in the blood after it has passed through the capillaries and reached the veins is lowered to 40 mm Hg. This decrease in oxygen concentration results in the blood turning bluish-red. The blood then is returned to the right side of the heart through the venous circulation. The heart then pumps this blood through the pulmonary arteries to the lungs where the cycle begins again (Fig. 9-13).

Carbon dioxide

While oxygen is moving into the tissues, carbon dioxide, a waste product of metabolism, is diffusing from the tissues (where the **partial pressure of carbon dioxide [PCO2]** is 50 mm Hg) into the blood (where the PCO_2 is 40 mm Hg). The venous blood returning to the lungs has a PCO_2 of 46 mm Hg. In the lungs, the carbon dioxide is removed.

Once in the blood, carbon dioxide is carried to the lungs in three ways (Fig. 9-14):

- Dissolved in plasma (produces the PCO_2 of the blood)

- Coupled with hemoglobin

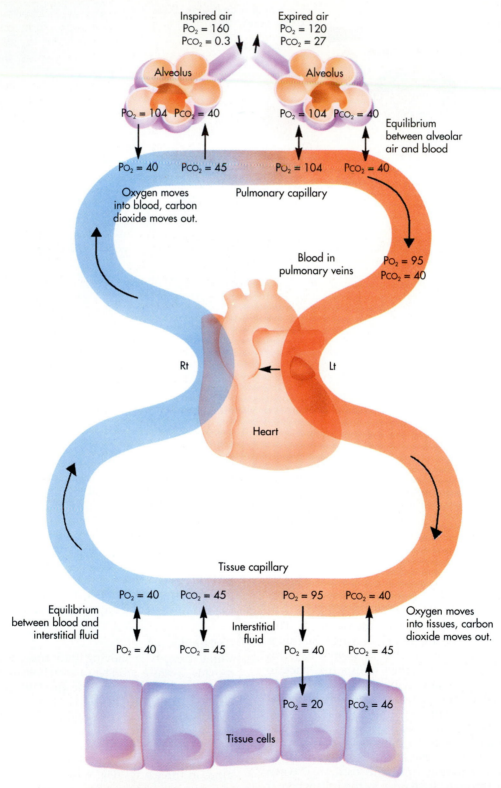

Fig. 9-11 Oxygen and carbon dioxide diffuse across the alveolar capillaries as a result of differences in partial pressure.

- Combined with water as carbonic acid and its components

Only 10% of the carbon dioxide is carried in blood plasma. Some of this 10% has a partial pressure; the rest reacts very slowly with water to form carbonic acid (H_2CO_3), which may break down further into hydrogen ions (H^+) and bicarbonate ions (HCO_3^-). Both processes are reversible.

Approximately 20% of the carbon dioxide reacts somewhat faster with hemoglobin in the **red blood cells** (RBCs) to form the compound carbaminohemoglobin.

Approximately 70% of the carbon dioxide converts to carbonic acid in the RBCs. This process occurs in a split second due to the presence of carbonic anhydrase, a catalyzing enzyme. Just as fast, the carbonic acid breaks down into hydrogen ions and bicarbonate ions; the hydrogen ions remain cell-bound and are neutralized by the hemoglobin, while the bicarbonate ions trade places with chloride ions in the surrounding plasma. RBCs expel excess bicarbonate yet remain electrically neutral in this process, called the *chloride shift*.

When venous blood enters the lung for gas exchange, all reversible chemical processes reverse, and CO_2 is once again formed. The gas diffuses into the alveoli and is expired. The exhaled air is high in carbon dioxide and low in oxygen. The amount of carbon dioxide in the body is dependent on ventilatory effectiveness. Under normal conditions, if ventilations are increased, the carbon dioxide will decrease. If ventilations are decreased, the carbon

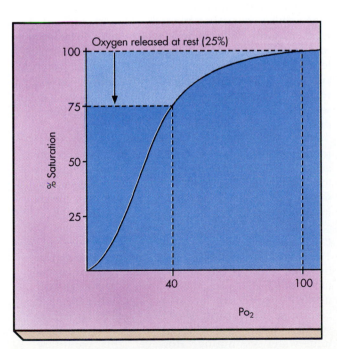

Fig. 9-12 Hemoglobin allows blood to transport up to 20ml of dissolved O_2 per 100 ml of blood.

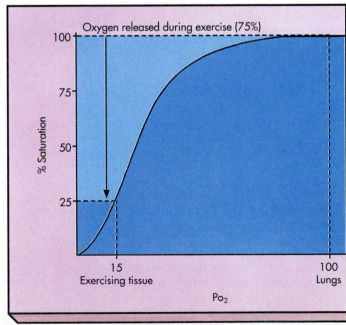

Fig. 9-13 Oxygen-hemoglobin dissociation curve. The graphs indicate the percentage of the hemoglobin saturated with oxygen as the PO_2 increases.

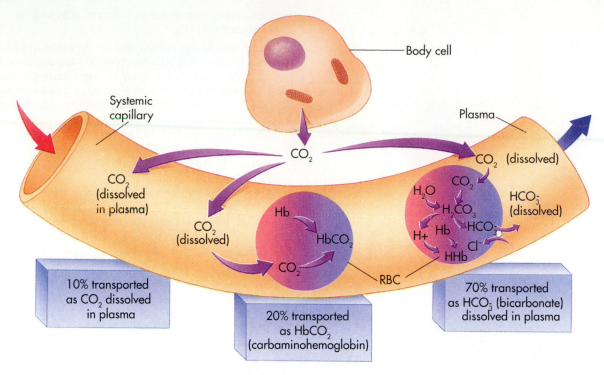

Fig. 9-14 Carbon dioxide is transported from the body's tissues back to the lungs. Ten percent of the CO_2 is carried in blood plasma; twenty percent is transported in carbaminohemoglobin; seventy percent converts to bicarbonate and is transported in blood plasma.

dioxide will increase. In other words, carbon dioxide levels vary inversely with ventilations (Fig. 9-15).

Nitrogen
Atmospheric air also contains 79% nitrogen. Although nitrogen has no metabolic function, it is necessary for maintaining inflation of body cavities that are gas filled.

Stimulus to breathe
Medulla and pons
Unlike heart muscle, which contracts rhythmically even when separated from the nervous system, the respiratory muscles do not possess inherent rhythmicity. Stimuli from the brain are needed to produce the pattern of sequential inspiration-expiration. The main nervous centers for controlling the rate and depth of breathing are located in the medulla oblongata and the pons of the brainstem. Called *respiratory centers,* they are really scattered neurons that act as a unit to control respirations (Fig. 9-16). Under resting conditions, nervous activity in the medulla produces a normal rate and depth of respirations (12 to 20 breaths per minute). The receptors of the medulla also sense the need for changing the rate and depth of respirations to maintain homeostasis. Central chemoreceptors, located in the medulla, are sensitive to slight changes in the concentration of carbon dioxide in the blood plasma. It is

not a direct effect, because the carbon dioxide must first diffuse across the blood-brain barrier into the cerebral spinal fluid that bathes the chemosensitive area of the medulla. There, the carbon dioxide combines with water to form carbonic acid, which then dissociates into bicarbonate and hydrogen ions. The increased level of hydrogen ions stimulates the chemosensitive area, which then stimulates the respiratory center, resulting in a greater rate and depth of breathing. Consequently, carbon dioxide levels decrease as carbon dioxide is eliminated from the body.

When excess carbon dioxide is present, the respiratory center stimulates the respiratory muscles to greater activity. When the carbon dioxide concentration is low, breathing is depressed. The control centers in the medulla are in turn regulated by a number of inputs from receptors located in various areas of the body.

Cerebral cortex
The cerebral cortex can influence respiration by modifying the rate at which the neurons in the medulla fire. This response allows a person to voluntarily speed up or slow down his or her breathing rate during activities such as speaking, singing, eating, or holding his or her breath during underwater swimming. However, this voluntary control has limits. Other factors such as blood carbon dioxide levels are much more powerful in

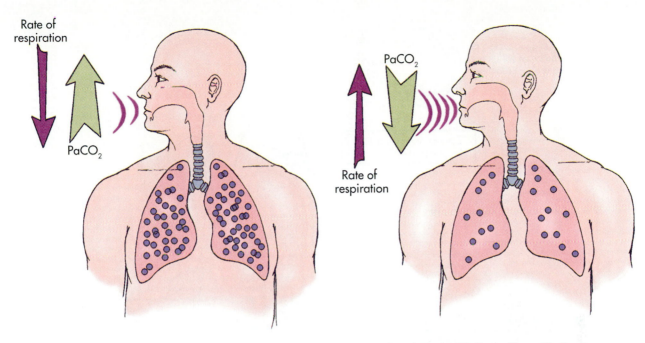

Fig. 9-15 Carbon dioxide levels in the body are inversely proportional to ventilations. If ventilations are high, carbon dioxide levels are low. If ventilations are low, carbon dioxide levels are high.

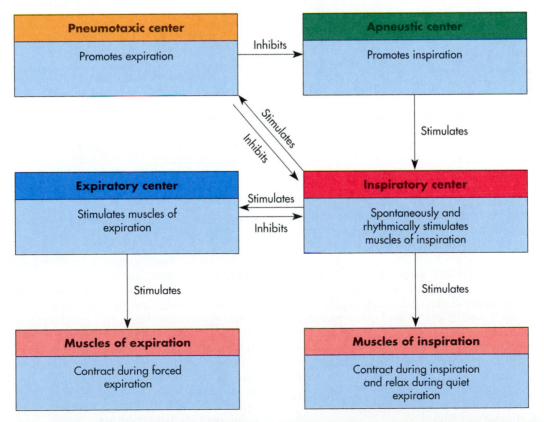

Fig. 9-16 A, Respiratory centers act as a unit to control respiration. Active neurons in the respiratory center stimulate inspiration; inactive neurons cause the muscles of inspiration to relax.

(Continued)

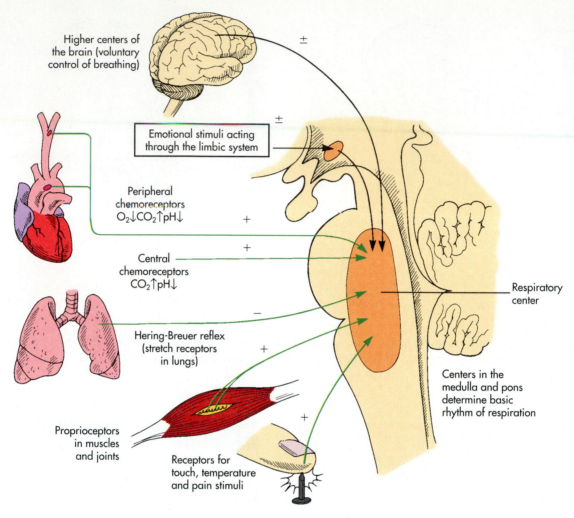

Higher centers of the brain (voluntary control of breathing)

Emotional stimuli acting through the limbic system

Peripheral chemoreceptors $O_2\downarrow CO_2\uparrow pH\downarrow$

Central chemoreceptors $CO_2\uparrow pH\downarrow$

Hering-Breuer reflex (stretch receptors in lungs)

Proprioceptors in muscles and joints

Receptors for touch, temperature and pain stimuli

Respiratory center

Centers in the medulla and pons determine basic rhythm of respiration

Fig. 9-16 cont'd. B, The regulatory mechanisms that affect the depth and rate of ventilation.

controlling respirations than voluntary control. Regardless of the intent, a person will resume breathing when the body senses the need for more oxygen or if carbon dioxide levels increase to certain levels.

Emotions, *(eg,* sobs and gasps of crying), acting through the limbic system of the brain, also can affect the respiratory center. Additionally, the activation of touch and thermal and pain receptors also can stimulate the respiratory center, as can body movements that occur during exercise. These movements stimulate proprioceptors in the joints of the limb, which in turn pass along afferent nerve fibers to the spinal cord and brain.

Peripheral chemoreceptors
Located peripherally in the aorta arch and carotid bodies are specialized receptors called *chemoreceptors.* These receptors are sensitive to

- Increased carbon dioxide levels
- Increased blood acid levels
- Decreased blood oxygen levels

The carotid body receptors are found at the point where the common carotid arteries divide, and the aortic bodies are small clusters of chemosensitive cells located adjacent to the aortic arch near the heart. When stimulated, these receptors send nerve impulses to the respiratory control centers in the medulla that in turn modify the respiratory rate. The peripheral chemoreceptors are sensitive to large increases in carbon dioxide and significant decreases in oxygen.

Pulmonary stretch receptors
Specialized stretch receptors (also referred to as the *Hering-Breuer reflex),* located throughout the pulmonary airways and in the alveoli of the lungs, influ-

ence the normal pattern of breathing and act to protect the respiratory system from excessive stretching caused by harmful overinflation. When the tidal volume of air has been inspired, the lungs are expanded enough to stimulate microscopic stretch receptors. Inhibitory impulses follow afferent pathways to the medulla where the inspiratory act is curtailed. Relaxation of inspiratory muscles occurs, and expiration follows (Fig. 9-16).

CLINICAL NOTES
Individuals with chronic respiratory disease have a decreased ability to remove carbon dioxide. This condition results in a progressive increase in the carbon dioxide concentrations of the body. Over time, the respiratory centers adjust to tolerate high carbon dioxide levels. The medullary respiratory centers become dulled to these changes. The body then relies on peripheral chemoreceptors to control respirations. Respiration in these individuals is controlled by oxygen level: the rate and depth of respiration increases in response to PO_2 levels below 60 mm Hg. Because the peripheral chemoreceptors respond to low PO_2, any treatment involving high concentrations of oxygen can act to suppress the hypoxic drive, thus suppressing respirations. For this reason, oxygen therapy should be administered carefully in patients who have a history of chronic respiratory disease. In those situations in which a high oxygen concentration is required (eg, acute myocardial infarction, shock) the EMT–I should be prepared to assist the patient's breathing if respiratory depression or apnea occurs.

ASSESSMENT OF THE PATIENT

> Recall and demonstrate the essential elements of assessing airway patency, breathing effectiveness, and oxygenation in the ill or injured patient.

The EMT–I must be skilled in assessing and managing patients who present with upper airway obstruction. Intervention in these cases may require the EMT–I to employ several skills at the same time. The first step is to determine if an open airway is present. When the possibility of spinal injury exists, airway patency must be assessed and ensured in conjunction with in-line cervical spine stabilization. If airway compromise is identified, it must be resolved. Once a patent airway is ensured, respiratory effectiveness must be assessed. If the patient is not breathing adequately, the EMT–I must provide assisted breathing. Following that, circulatory effectiveness must be evaluated and measures taken to resolve any life-threatening deficiencies.

Body substance isolation precautions must be employed during assessment and management of patients. At a minimum, protective rubber gloves and goggles should be worn whenever airway management is performed. If there is a chance that body fluids may be splashed, the EMT–I also should wear a mask and protective gown or overalls.

A good assessment becomes a window to the patient's condition and can make the difference between the patient surviving or not surviving. Indications of airway obstruction, hypoxia, and hypoventilation are usually evident to the EMT–I during those first critical minutes. Intervention can resolve many life-threatening conditions.

Initial impression
A great deal of information is available during the approach to the patient. Is the patient responsive? Is the patient breathing? Does the patient appear to have adequate air exchange? These questions often are answered by the time the EMT–I reaches the patient. The absence of an open airway and/or the lack of effective breathing efforts requires the EMT–I to take immediate steps to correct the problem.

Once the EMT–I is at the patient's side, and then throughout the provision of care, the EMT–I should continue the assessment in a logical and systematic manner. The EMT–I must assess and ensure an open airway, check respiratory function and evaluate circulation. The patient's level of responsiveness also should be evaluated, because restlessness, agitation, disorientation, coma, and so forth indicate decreased cerebral oxygenation. Once the initial examination is complete and the necessary intervention taken, a more thorough, focused examination can be done. However, even when the airway is initially patent, continuous reassessment is warranted, because airway patency may change at any time.

Indicators of respiratory function include airway patency, appearance of the neck, breathing efforts, color of the skin, breath sounds, outward signs (flaring of the nares, retraction, noisy breathing), air movement at the nose and mouth, compliance (felt with ventilatory assistance provided with a bag-valve-mask device), and the pulse rate. Devices such as the pulse oximetry unit can be used to determine the oxygen saturation. Another sign of respiratory function is silence, which indicates a complete absence of air movement.

Airway patency
Air movement and sounds typically indicate airway patency. Sounds such as gurgling, snoring, and so forth suggest obstruction of the upper airway (Table 9-1). If an obstruction is identified, immediate steps must be taken to correct the problem.

Neck
After assessing and ensuring a patent airway, the neck should be quickly inspected for distended

TABLE 9-1	The Sounds and Causes of Some Common Airway Obstructions
SOUND	**COMMON TYPES OF AIRWAY OBSTRUCTION**
Snoring respirations	The tongue
Gurgling sounds	Accumulation of blood, vomitus, or other secretions
Stridor (a harsh, high-pitched sound heard on inhalation)	Laryngeal edema or constriction

jugular veins, tracheal shift, or tugging. The presence of any of these indicates a likely respiratory problem.

Breathing efforts

The adequacy of air exchange should be assessed by observing the patient's breathing efforts. The EMT–I should feel for air movement at the patient's nose and mouth. When an endotracheal tube is in place, the proximal end can be checked for air movement. Normally, the chest rises and falls with each respiratory cycle. In the adult patient, the respiratory rate ranges between 12 to 20 breaths per minute. Breathing should be spontaneous and regular. Slow, fast, or irregular breathing indicates a significant problem and requires the EMT–I to intervene with assisted breathing (bag-valve-mask, demand valve, automatic ventilator).

When assisting a patient's breathing with a ventilatory device or after placing an airway adjunct (nasopharyngeal airway, esophageal obturator airway, endotracheal tube) the EMT–I should observe the rise and fall of the patient's chest to determine correct use and placement. When assisting a patient's breathing with the bag-valve-mask device, the EMT–I can gauge the effectiveness of air flow into the lungs by noting the compliance and how quickly the bag empties. *Compliance* is defined as the stiffness or flexibility of the lung tissue. It is noted by how easily air flows into the lungs. When compliance is good, air flow occurs with a minimum amount of resistance. When compliance is poor, ventilation is harder to achieve. Compliance is poor in diseased states of the lungs, chest wall injuries, or with tension pneumothorax. Compliance also decreases when the upper airway is obstructed by the tongue. If poor compliance occurs during assisted breathing the EMT–I should look for potential causes. Is the airway open? Is the head properly extended or jaw-thrust properly employed? Is the patient developing a tension pneumothorax? Is the endotracheal tube occluded? Has the endotracheal tube been inadvertently pushed into the right or left mainstem bronchus? A bag that empties too quickly or "collapses" also should be regarded as ominous. It may indicate incorrect placement of the endotracheal tube into the esophagus or a defect in the bag-valve-mask device. An end-tidal carbon dioxide ($ETCO_2$) detector also can be used to monitor the effectiveness of ventilations.

Pulse oximetry

Pulse oximetry is a simple, noninvasive procedure used to determine the effectiveness of patient oxygenation. It allows for continuous monitoring, detecting trends in patient's oxygenation status within 6 seconds. Pulse oximetry can:

- Reaffirm perceived hypoxia
- Reveal hidden hypoxia
- Assist in determining what oxygen adjunct should be applied and liter flow to be administered
- Aid in monitoring clinical improvement or deterioration in acutely dyspneic patients
- Identify when to intubate
- Identify changes during intubation or other airway manipulations

Pulse oximetry should be taken on all patients and recorded as part of their vital signs, because normal evaluation of oxygenation is notoriously unreliable. Also, saturation readings should be taken before and after oxygen is administered to any patient.

It is important to keep a patient's oxygen saturation in a normal range, because declines in saturation result in a reduction in oxygen content.

- With **90%** saturation, PO_2 drops to 60 mm Hg.
- With **75%** saturation, PO_2 drops to 40 mm Hg.
- With **50%** saturation, PO_2 drops to 27 mm Hg (Fig. 9-17).

In addition to oxygen saturation (SaO_2), a visual pulse rate is displayed (and is audible). However, this unit should not be used in place of the cardiac monitor when the situation dictates the use of one.

Prior to use, the EMT–I should test the unit on himself or herself to confirm that it is in good operating condition. To do this, the EMT–I should turn on the unit and follow all operating recommendations set forth by the manufacturer. After it is found that the unit is in good operating condition, the

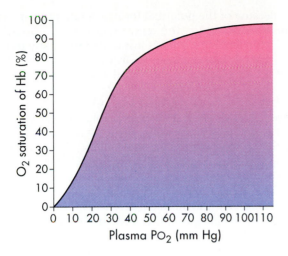

**Fig. 9-17   Oxygen-hemoglobin dissociation curve.
At lower levels of O$_2$ saturation the levels of plasma
PO$_2$ decrease.**

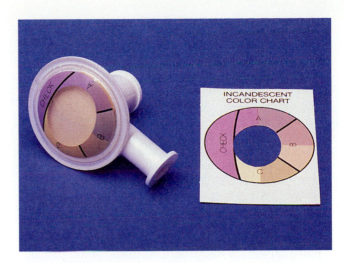

Fig. 9-18   A colormetric end-tidal CO$_2$ detector.

EMT–I should place the finger clip on the patient's index finger with the outline of the finger facing up. All dirt and nail polish or any obstructive covering should be removed to prevent the unit from giving a false reading. When these steps are completed, the unit will show a red number on the left, which is the SaO$_2$, and a red light on the right showing the patient's heart rate.

The EMT–I should consider pulse oximetry as only another tool to assist in patient monitoring. A variety of circumstances produce false readings, including:

- Carbon monoxide
- Excessive ambient light on the sensor probe
- Patient movement
- Hypotension (low flow states)
- Hypothermia
- Use of vasoconstrictive drugs by the patient
- Nail polish
- Jaundice

Also, pulse oximetry cannot give information about alveolar ventilation. For this reason the EMT–I should be careful not to accept adequate SaO$_2$ values while neglecting gross hypoventilation. Another consideration is that patients with chronic obstructive pulmonary disease may have a normally low SaO$_2$, so adequate histories must be obtained.

HYPOXEMIA: Insufficient oxygenation of the blood.

Oxygen therapy is used to treat **hypoxemia.** SaO$_2$ readings can help determine which oxygen adjunct should be placed on the patient and the liter flow to be administered. A SaO$_2$ in the 95% to 99% range is ideal, and no supplemental oxygen is needed unless the patient's chief complaint or injury mechanism warrants. An SaO$_2$ of 91% to 94% represents mild hypoxemia and indicates that the airway should be checked and oxygen therapy started at 4 to 6 L via nasal cannula. An SaO$_2$ of 85% to 90% represents moderate hypoxemia. The airway must be checked and aggressive oxygen therapy started at 15 L/min via nonrebreather mask. An SaO$_2$ reading of less than 85% indicates severe hypoxemia. In these cases, the EMT–I should prepare to intubate or assist ventilations with a bag-valve-mask and 100% oxygen.

End-tidal carbon dioxide detectors

End-tidal carbon dioxide detectors are an effective way of verifying correct endotracheal tube placement. These devices detect the presence of carbon dioxide in the intubated patient's expired air (Fig. 9-18). End-tidal air, which closely correlates with the percentages of gases found in mixed venous blood, contains approximately 6% carbon dioxide. A lack of carbon dioxide in the end-tidal air strongly suggests the tube has been misplaced into the esophagus.

The two types of end-tidal carbon dioxide detectors available to date are the disposable colormetric device and the electronic monitor. Both are attached in-line between the endotracheal tube and the ventilatory device after intubation.

The least expensive of the two devices, the disposable colormetric device, is designed for single patient use and contains a nontoxic chemical indicator that reacts instantly to expired tracheal carbon dioxide by changing color. The reversibility of this color change allows the EMT–I to determine esophageal or tracheal intubation (after the required six breaths). The presence of a yellow color on expiration indicates correct placement in the trachea, whereas a purple color indicates improper placement in the esophagus. The color varies from expiration to inspiration as carbon dioxide levels rise and fall in a phasic manner.

The electronic device is a more expensive portable or hand-held end-tidal carbon dioxide detector, which uses an infrared analyzer to measure the percentage of carbon dioxide gas at each phase of respiration. This information is displayed on a digital readout or printout. This device can provide verification of correct endotracheal intubation or provide continuous carbon dioxide monitoring with a cannula during transport. Newer models combine pulse oximetry, pulse rate, and respiratory rate in one unit.

The end-tidal carbon dioxide detector has two potential weaknesses. First, sometimes carbon dioxide inadvertently enters the stomach. It has been shown that six breaths can quickly wash out any retained carbon dioxide. The second weakness is that adequate circulation and pulmonary perfusion are required to obtain diffusion of carbon dioxide from the pulmonary capillary bed. Thus, initial end-tidal carbon dioxide levels may be considerably lower during cardiac arrest. However, with adequate cardiopulmonary resuscitation (CPR), these levels should rise enough to allow the end-tidal carbon dioxide detector to verify proper intubation.

Because of the potential for inaccurate readings in some conditions, the end-tidal carbon dioxide detector should be used as just one of the many tools the EMT–I has available to assess correct endotracheal tube placement and ventilatory status.

Esophageal intubation detectors

Two relatively new devices available for use by the EMT–I to verify correct placement of an endotracheal tube are the esophageal intubation detector and esophageal intubation detector bulb (Fig. 9-19). Neither of these devices is a carbon dioxide detector. Rather, these simple and easy-to-use devices take advantage of the anatomic differences between the trachea and esophagus. Other benefits of these devices include that they are inexpensive; provide fast, immediate results; require no calibration; reduce the risk of ventilating the stomach; are durable; have unlimited shelf life; and are usable in low-light conditions.

The esophageal intubator device resembles a large syringe with a 15-mm adapter at its distal end. After the endotracheal tube is placed and before any ventilation attempts, the device is attached (with the compression plunger fully inserted into the syringe barrel) to the endotracheal tube. The compression plunger is then withdrawn. If the tube is in the esophagus, its soft, unsupported walls will collapse around the end of the endotracheal tube, preventing

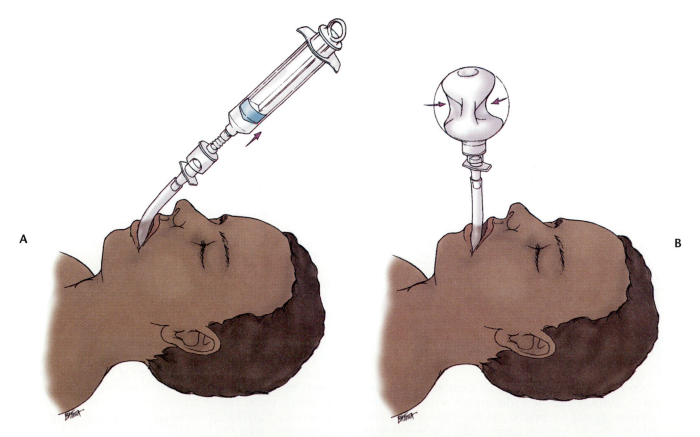

A

B

Fig. 9-19   **Esophageal intubation detector. A, Syringe. B, Bulb.**

air from being drawn out of the device. If the endotracheal tube is in the trachea, the rigid trachea remains patent, allowing the plunger to be easily withdrawn from the device.

The esophageal intubation detector bulb works in a similar way. It is a disposable device that is compressed before it is attached to the endotracheal tube. As compression on the bulb is released, a vacuum is created. If the tube is in the esophagus, the bulb will not reinflate. However, if the endotracheal tube is properly placed, the bulb will reinflate.

Appearance of the chest

The EMT–I should note the presence of intercostal retraction or accessory muscle usage. Manifestations of respiratory compromise include the presence of nasal flaring (nostrils wide open during inspiration), tracheal tugging, retraction of the intercostal muscles, and use of the diaphragm and neck muscles to assist with inspiration.

> **BREATH SOUNDS:** Sound of air passing in and out of the respiratory passageways as heard with a stethoscope.

Breath sounds

Auscultation of the chest provides information about airflow into and out of the lungs. The sites usually auscultated include: 1) just beneath the right and left clavicles (apexes of the lungs) and 2) the right and left lateral sides of the chest in the midaxillary line (at the level of the eighth or ninth intercostal spaces). At each site, the EMT–I should listen to first one side of the chest and then the other. **Breath sounds** should be equal. There also are six locations on the posterior chest that can be auscultated. However, given that the patient is usually in a supine position during airway management, the anterior and lateral positions are most accessible. The presence of airflow with auscultation over the sternal notch reveals the correct placement of an endotracheal tube in the trachea.

In some cases air movement into the stomach may mimic lung sounds. Obese or barrel-chested patients are most likely to present this problem, because their breath sounds may seem distant or muffled. For this reason it is important to ensure the presence of clear, equal, bilateral lung sounds.

Epigastric sounds

Auscultation of the chest is only one means of assessing air movement with assisted breathing or correct placement of an airway adjunct. Auscultation of the epigastrium should immediately follow assessment of breath sounds. It should be silent, with no sounds audible during ventilation.

Gastric distention

Whenever providing ventilatory support, the EMT–I should watch for signs of gastric distention.

Gastric distention is suggestive of inadequate hyperextension of the head, too much pressure being generated by the ventilatory device, or improperly placed airway adjuncts.

Skin

The color and texture of the skin provide information regarding oxygenation. Early in respiratory compromise the sympathetic nervous system is stimulated in an effort to offset the lack of oxygen. This stimulation makes the skin appear pale and diaphoretic. Cyanosis is another sign of respiratory distress. When oxygen binds with hemoglobin the blood appears bright red. Unoxygenated hemoglobin is blue and imparts a bluish color to the skin. However, this sign is not truly reliable, because severe tissue hypoxia is possible without cyanosis. In fact, cyanosis is considered a late sign of respiratory compromise. When it does appear, cyanosis is usually seen at the lips, fingernails, and/or the skin.

> **ANOXIA:** Deficiency of oxygen.

Circulatory status

The pulse rate also can tell of respiratory compromise. Tachycardia usually accompanies hypoxemia whereas bradycardia suggests **anoxia** with imminent cardiac arrest.

History

The history of the patient with airway obstruction or compromise may be evident, as in the case of upper airway obstruction in the responsive patient. Other causes usually are not so easily defined. When time and the patient's condition permit, appropriate questions should be asked to establish the past medical history, history of present complication, and/or the mechanism of injury.

UPPER AIRWAY PROBLEMS

 Identify the common mechanisms of upper airway compromise and describe the procedures for resolving each.

Upper airway obstruction is defined as the interference of air flow through the upper airway and can represent an immediate threat to life. It may be caused by a number of factors, including:

- The tongue
- Foreign bodies
- Vomitus
- Blood, teeth
- Swelling due to allergic reaction, smoke inhalation
- Epiglottitis

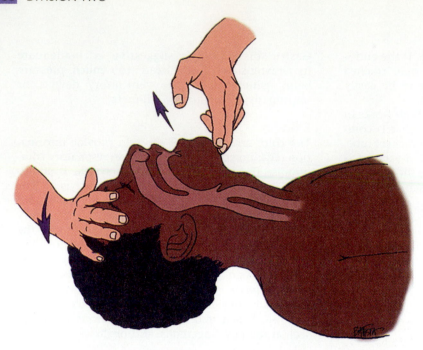

Fig. 9-20 Unconscious patients lose muscle control, allowing the tongue to fall back against the back of the throat, causing airway obstruction.

Blockage of the airway must be corrected promptly if the patient is to survive.

The tongue
Pathophysiology
The tongue is the most common cause of upper airway obstruction in the unresponsive patient (Fig. 9-20). It occurs when muscle tone is depressed or absent in the supine patient. This condition allows the tongue to fall back against the soft palate and posterior pharyngeal wall infringing on the airway. To further aggravate the problem, the epiglottis can occlude the airway at the level of the larynx. With the tongue and epiglottis in obstructing positions, airflow into the respiratory system is reduced or absent. Additionally, inspiratory efforts may draw the tongue and epiglottis into more of an obstructing position. Airway obstruction by the tongue depends on the position of the head and jaw and can occur regardless of whether the patient is in a lateral, supine, or prone position.

In some cases, after a person has collapsed, the EMT–I will arrive to find that bystanders or family members have placed a pillow under the patient's head in an attempt to make him or her more comfortable. This movement can obstruct the airway even more. Public education efforts should tell citizens what to do *and* what not to do in these types of emergencies.

SNORING BREATHING: Noisy, raspy breathing, usually with the mouth open.
APNEA: Absence of breathing.

In the breathing patient, **snoring breathing** is a characteristic sign of airway obstruction caused by the tongue. **In apnea,** the initial clue to this type of obstruction is that it is difficult to ventilate the patient. After repositioning the patient's head and neck, assisted breathing should be easier to deliver.

Basic treatment

 Describe and demonstrate the procedures used to manually open the airway.

Manual manipulations
Treatment of this problem is directed at moving the tongue out of the way. The EMT–I must lift the mandible forward, displacing the hyoid anteriorly. This movement pulls the tongue forward and keeps the epiglottis elevated away from the back of the throat and glottic opening.

Any of the following procedures can be used to lift the mandible forward:

- Head-tilt/chin-lift maneuver
- Jaw-thrust maneuver
- Jaw-lift maneuver

In some cases, such as in the spontaneously breathing patient, opening the airway with manual maneuvers may be all that is required to ensure a patent airway.

Caution must be used whenever trauma is suspected. Those cases require use of the chin-lift without head-tilt maneuver or modified jaw-thrust maneuver to open the airway.

Head-tilt/Chin-lift
The preferred procedure for opening the airway is the head-tilt/chin-lift (Fig. 9-21). This technique is considered superior to the other procedures because direct manipulation of the jaw lifts the tongue and epiglottis out of their obstructing positions. To perform this procedure, the EMT–I should:

1. Employ body substance isolation precautions.
2. With the patient in a supine position, move next to his or her side by the upper arm.

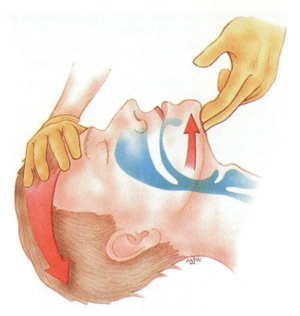

Fig. 9-21   **Head-tilt/chin-lift maneuver**

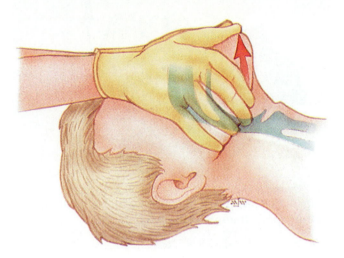

Fig. 9-22   **Jaw-thrust maneuver.**

3. Place the uppermost hand on the patient's fore-head and apply firm downward pressure with the palm to tilt the patient's head back.

4. Grasp the patient's chin with the other hand by placing the thumb on the front of the jaw and positioning the index finger under the jaw. This step should be done without putting undue pressure on the jaw.

 STREET WISE
The EMT–I should be careful not to compress the soft tissues underneath the patient's chin, because that can obstruct the airway. Rather, the EMT–I should keep his or her fingers on the bony part of the chin.

5. Lift the jaw anteriorly to open the airway.

Jaw-thrust

The jaw-thrust is another useful technique for opening the airway (Fig. 9-22). When employed with the head-tilt and retraction of the lower lip, it is referred to as the *triple airway maneuver*. To perform the jaw-thrust, the EMT–I should:

1. Employ body substance isolation precautions.

2. With the patient in a supine position, move to the top of the patient's head.

3. Rest both elbows on the same surface as the patient is lying.

4. Place fingertips on each side of the patient's lower jaw, at the angles.

5. Firmly push the jaw forward while gently tilting the patient's head back.

6. Retract the patient's lower lip with both thumbs.

Jaw-lift

The jaw-lift also may be used to open the airway, although it must be employed carefully because the EMT–I is required to put his or her fingers into the patient's mouth. To perform the jaw-lift, the EMT–I should:

1. Employ body substance isolation precautions.

2. With the patient in a supine position, move to the top of his or her head.

3. Use one hand to grasp the mandible by placing the thumb deep into the mouth, pressing downward on the tongue and positioning the index finger under the mandible.

4. Pull the jaw anteriorly to open the airway.

Because these procedures cause manipulation of the head and neck, they should not be used in patients with suspected spine injury. Rather, the chin-lift or jaw-thrust without head-tilt maneuver should be used.

Chin-lift or jaw-thrust without head-tilt

In trauma patients with suspected spine injury, initial attempts at opening the airway should be done with the head kept in a neutral position. The chin-lift or jaw-thrust often can be successfully employed without the head-tilt. If the airway remains obstructed, then the head-tilt should be slowly and gently added until the airway is open (Fig. 9-23).

Airway adjuncts

Discuss indications, contraindications, and methods for insertion and use of the following:
- oropharyngeal airway
- nasopharyngeal airway
- esophageal obturator airway
- esophageal gastric tube airway
- pharyngotracheal lumen airway

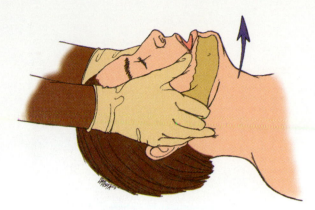

Fig. 9-23 Jaw-thrust maneuver without head-tilt when spinal trauma is suspected.

Two basic adjuncts that can be used to supplement the manual procedures previously described are the oropharyngeal airway and the nasopharyngeal airway.

However, placement of airway adjuncts should follow manual maneuvers. Potential side effects of airway devices, such as activation of the gag, cough, and/or swallowing mechanisms, can cause significant cardiovascular stimulation as well as an increase in intracranial pressure.

Both the oropharyngeal and nasopharyngeal airways are designed to lift the base of the tongue forward, away from the poste-rior oropharynx. As their names imply, the oropharyngeal airway is inserted into the mouth, and the nasopharyngeal airway is placed into the nostril.

> **HELPFUL HINTS**
> Proper head position must be maintained even when an oropharyngeal or nasopharyngeal airway is in place, because these adjuncts only assist in maintaining an open airway.

Oropharyngeal airway
The oropharyngeal airway is a plastic J-shaped device that conforms to the curvature of the palate (Fig. 9-24 A). Once in place, it holds the base of the tongue forward, away from the posterior oropharynx, allowing air to pass around and through the tube (Fig. 9-24 B). Oropharyngeal airways come in several sizes, ranging from #0 (infant) to #6 (large adult). The proper size must be used because an airway that is too long can press the epiglottis against the laryngeal entrance, thereby obstructing the airway. An airway that is too short fails to hold the tongue forward and may actually push it back against the posterior oropharynx.
Indications
Primary uses of the oropharyngeal airway are:

- To maintain an open airway in an unresponsive, breathing patient who has no gag reflex or a

patient being ventilated with a bag-valve-mask or other positive pressure device.

- As a bite block to prevent patients from biting down on and occluding an endotracheal tube.

Advantages and disadvantages of the oropharyngeal airway include:
Advantages
- It can be inserted quickly.
- It acts to counter obstruction by the teeth and lips.
- It facilitates suctioning of the pharynx because a large suction tube can pass on either side.
Disadvantages
- It does not isolate the trachea.
- It cannot be inserted when the patient's teeth are clenched shut.
- It can obstruct the airway if not inserted properly.
- It can easily be dislodged.
Contraindications
Oropharyngeal airways should not be used in patients who have a gag reflex because they can stimulate vomiting (by putting pressure on the posterior gag reflexes) or laryngospasm. Its use also should be avoided in patients who have severe maxillofacial injuries (trauma to the mandible or maxilla or significant soft-tissue damage to the tongue or pharynx).
Procedure
To insert the oropharyngeal airway, the EMT–I should:

1. Employ body substance isolation precautions.
2. Use the head-tilt/chin-lift or jaw-thrust to open the airway.
3. Ensure or maintain effective breathing, hyperventilate the patient with 100% oxygen if indicated.
4. Measure the airway to determine the appropriate size by holding it next to the patient's cheek. The proper size airway extends from the corner of patient's mouth to the tip of the ear lobe on the same side of the face, or to the angle of the lower jaw (Fig. 9-25 A).
5. If the patient's mouth is closed, the crossfinger technique can be used to open it. This technique is performed by crossing the thumb and forefinger of one hand and placing them on the upper and lower teeth at the corner of the patient's mouth, then spreading the fingers apart to open the patient's jaws.
6. Move the tongue out of the way by grasping the jaw and tongue between the thumb and index finger of the left hand, lifting it anteriorly.
7. With the other hand, hold the airway at its flange end and insert it into the mouth with the curve reversed and the tip pointing toward the roof of the patient's mouth (Fig. 9-25 B).

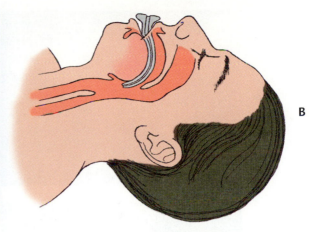

Fig. 9-24   A, Oropharyngeal airways. B, Oropharyngeal airway in proper use.

8. Slide in the airway along the roof of the mouth. Use caution to avoid pushing the tongue posteriorly (Fig. 9-25 C).

9. Once the tip is past the uvula, approaching the back of the throat near the base of the tongue, rotate the airway 180° until it comes to rest over the tongue (Fig. 9-25 D). The flange of the airway should rest on the patient's lips (Fig. 9-25 E).

10. Hyperventilate the patient with a bag-valve-mask device supplied with 100% oxygen or demand valve resuscitator if indicated (Fig. 9-25 F).

11. Check for proper placement of the airway by looking for chest rise. Then auscultate both sides of the chest and over the stomach with a stethoscope.

Precautions
Care must be taken to ensure that the airway is correctly positioned because improper placement can push the tongue back against the posterior oropharynx, thus obstructing the airway (Fig. 9-26).

If the airway is too short or too long, it must be removed and replaced with the correct size. An indicator of improper placement is when the airway advances out of the mouth during ventilatory efforts.

An alternative method for inserting the oropharyngeal airway is to use a tongue blade to depress the tongue while pushing the airway past it.

Because its presence can stimulate vomiting or regurgitation, the airway must be immediately removed and the EMT–I must be prepared to suction if the patient gags and/or becomes responsive.

Nasopharyngeal airway
The nasopharyngeal airway is an uncuffed soft plastic tube. One end is funnel-shaped, preventing it from slipping inside the nose, whereas the other end is bevel-shaped to facilitate its passage into the nostril. It is designed to follow the natural curvature of the nasopharynx, extending from the nostril to the posterior pharynx just below the base of the tongue (Fig. 9-27).

The proper size airway is slightly smaller in diameter than the opening of the patient's nostril (about the diameter of the patient's little finger) and extends from the tip of the nose to the tip of his or her earlobe. Selecting the appropriate size is important because a tube that is too short will not extend past the tongue. Conversely, a tube that is too long may pass into the esophagus resulting in hypoventilation and gastric distention when artificial ventilation is delivered.

Indications
The nasopharyngeal airway is used to relieve soft-tissue upper airway obstruction when an oropharyngeal airway is contraindicated.

Advantages and disadvantages of the nasopharyngeal airway are listed below:

Advantages
- It can be inserted quickly.
- It bypasses the tongue.
- It may be used when a gag reflex is present.
- It can be used in the presence of injuries to the oral cavity (trauma to the mandible, maxilla, or significant soft-tissue damage to the tongue or pharynx).
- It can be used when the patient's teeth are clenched shut.

Disadvantages
- It is smaller than the oropharyngeal airway.
- It does not isolate the trachea.
- It is difficult to suction through.
- It can cause severe nosebleed if inserted too forcefully.
- It may cause pressure necrosis of the nasal mucosa.
- It may kink and clog, obstructing the airway.

Contraindications
Use of the nasopharyngeal airway should be avoided in patients who have nasal obstructions or who are

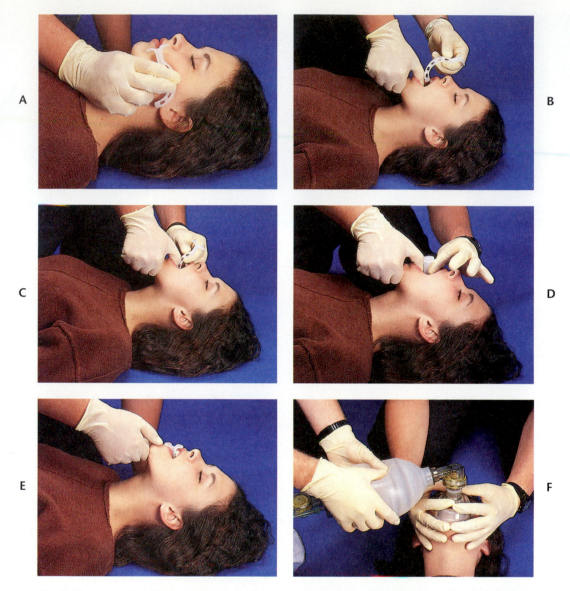

Fig. 9-25 Inserting the oral airway (adult patient only). **A,** Measure the airway to determine the appropriate size. **B,** Open the patient's mouth and begin to insert the airway with the tip pointing toward the roof of the mouth. **C,** Slide the airway along the roof of the mouth. **D,** Rotate the airway 180 degrees. **E,** The flange of the airway should rest on the patient's lips. **F,** Ventilate the patient with 100% oxygen through a BVM.

prone to nosebleeds or when there are indications of nasal injury. Also, its use should be avoided when basilar skull fracture is likely because the airway can be inadvertently passed into the brain.

Procedure

To insert the nasopharyngeal airway, the EMT–I should:

1. Employ body substance isolation precautions.

2. Open the airway manually using the head-tilt/chin-lift or jaw-thrust.

3. Ensure or maintain effective ventilatory function. If indicated, hyperventilate the patient with 100% oxygen.

4. Measure to determine the appropriate size airway for patient (Fig. 9-28 A).

5. Lubricate the exterior of the tube with a water-soluble gel to ease its insertion (Fig. 9-28 B). If possible a lidocainegel should be used in the responsive or semi-responsive patient because its anesthetic properties make insertion more comfortable.

6. Gently push the tip of the nose upward.

7. Pass the tube into the patient's right nostril (Fig. 9-28 C). The curve of the airway should be upward, toward the patient's forehead, the bevel of airway toward the nasal septum.

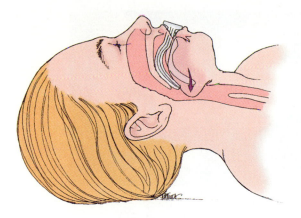

Fig. 9-26 Improper placement of an oropharyngeal airway can lead to an airway obstruction.

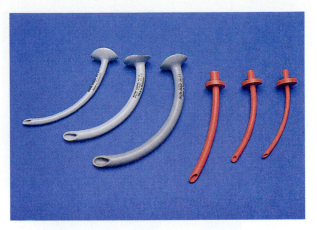

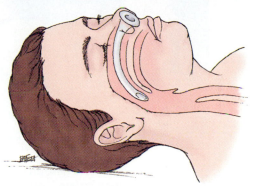

Fig. 9-27 A, Nasopharyngeal airways. B, Nasopharyngeal airway in use.

8. Pass the airway along the floor of the nasal cavity until the flange rests firmly against the patient's nostril (Fig. 9-28 D). Avoid pushing against any resistance because it can cause tissue trauma and airway kinking. In some cases the septum may be deviated, and insertion into the right nostril cannot be accomplished, thus the left nostril must be used.

9. Verify appropriate position of the airway. Clear breath sounds, chest rise, and air flow at the proximal end of the device on expiration indicate correct placement.

10. Hyperventilate the patient with 100% oxygen (if indicated).

If resistance is met while inserting a nasopharyngeal airway, the EMT–I should not force it into the nose. Rather, he or she should pull the tube out and try the other nostril. If resistance is such that the tube cannot be easily inserted, the EMT–I should try a smaller size tube. If the patient gags as the last 1/2 inch (or so) is inserted, the airway may be too long and should be withdrawn slightly until it is tolerated.

Precautions
Although the nasopharyngeal airway is better tolerated in semiresponsive patients than the oropharyngeal airway, its use may precipitate vomiting and laryngospasm. It also may injure the nasal mucosa causing bleeding and aspiration of clots into the trachea. Suctioning may be required to remove the secretions or blood. For these reasons, appropriate body substance isolation precautions must be used.

Foreign bodies
Pathophysiology
A foreign body that becomes lodged in the laryngopharynx is another cause of upper airway obstruction. In the adult, the source is usually food (particularly meat). Common factors associated with choking on food include large, poorly chewed pieces of meat; alcohol consumption; laughing, talking, or

exercising while eating; or dentures. This emergency often occurs in restaurants and is mistaken for a heart attack, giving rise to the name, "cafe coronary." In children, the obstruction typically is due to food or other objects such as bubble gum, balloons, marbles, beads, coins, or small toy parts.

STRIDOR: A high-pitched noise heard on inspiration.
CYANOSIS: Bluish color to the skin, seen with hypoxia.

Assessment
Airway obstruction may be partial or complete. With partial airway obstruction, air exchange may be good or poor. Good air exchange exists when the patient is able to generate an effective cough. Poor air exchange is present when the patient is unable to generate an effective cough, when stridor is heard during inhalation, and when there is increased breathing difficulty and cyanosis.

TRACHEAL TUGGING: Condition in which the Adam's apple appears to be pulled upward on inspiration. It occurs in the presence of airway obstruction.

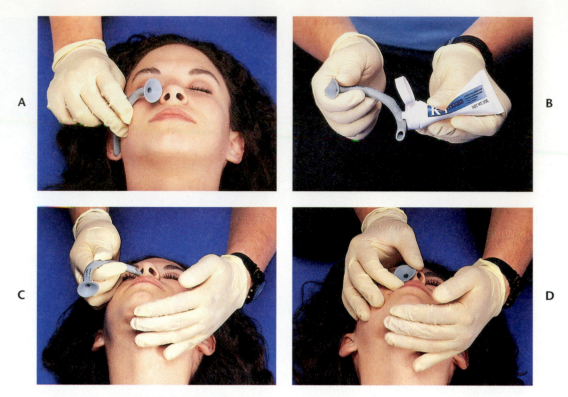

Fig. 9-28 Inserting the nasopharyngeal airway (all ages). **A,** Measure the airway to determine the appropriate size. **B,** Lubricate the airway with a water-soluble lubricant. **C,** Insert the airway into the nostril with the bevel facing the septum. **D,** Advance the airway until the flange rests against the patient's nostril.

> **RETRACTIONS:** The inward movement of the soft tissues of the chest, commonly the suprasternal notch and the intercostal spaces. Usually associated with respiratory compromise or airway obstruction.

Airway obstruction is complete when the patient is unable to speak, breathe, or cough; air flow is not felt or heard from the nose and mouth; and spontaneous breathing efforts result in **retraction** of the supraclavicular and intercostal areas. **Tracheal tugging** as well as an absence of chest expansion also occur. The classic sign of complete upper airway obstruction is the patient clutching his or her neck between the thumb and fingers. This gesture is referred to as the "universal distress signal" (Fig. 9-29).

In complete airway obstruction, the patient becomes unresponsive quickly and death occurs if the obstruction is unrelieved. When spontaneous breathing is absent, complete airway obstruction can be recognized by persistent difficulty encountered when attempting to deliver assisted breathing to the patient.

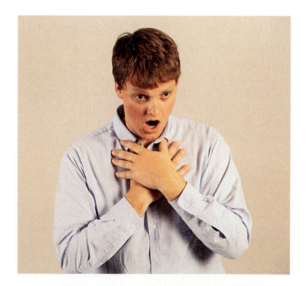

Fig. 9-29 The typical sign that a patient is experiencing an upper airway obstruction.

Basic treatment

With adequate air exchange, treatment is directed toward supporting and encouraging the patient to cough. Supplemental oxygen should be provided if the patient is becoming hypoxic. In poor air exchange or with complete obstruction, treatment is aimed at relieving the obstruction. This relief is accomplished by using abdominal thrusts (also referred to as the *Heimlich maneuver*).

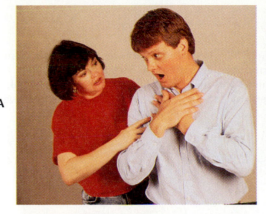

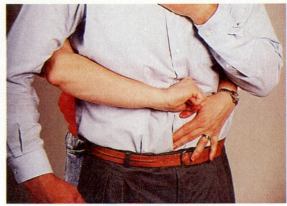

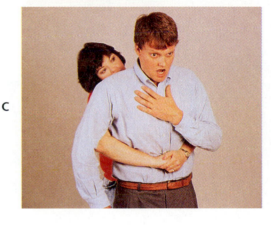

Fig. 9-30 Relieving airway obstruction in conscious patients. A, Ask the victim, "Are you choking?" B, Make a fist and place the thumb side against the patient's abdomen just above the navel. C, Grasp the fist with the other hand and press into the victim's abdomen in an upward motion.

Procedure

To relieve airway obstruction in the responsive patient, the EMT–I should:

1. Ask the victim, "Are you choking?" (Fig. 9-30 A)
2. Determine if complete airway obstruction is present (as previously described).
3. Deliver abdominal thrusts.
   - Stand behind the patient and wrap the arms around the patient's abdomen.
   - Make a fist and place the thumb side against the patient's abdomen in the midline slightly above the navel but well below the xiphoid process (Fig. 9-30 B).
   - Grasp the fist with the other hand and press into the victim's abdomen with quick upward thrusts (Fig. 9-30 C).
4. Continue these procedures until the obstruction is dislodged or the patient becomes unresponsive.

Procedure

To relieve airway obstruction in the unresponsive patient, the EMT–I should:

1. Check for responsiveness (if in a bystander role, [eg, off duty], activate the EMS system).
2. Open the airway using the head-tilt/chin-lift.
3. Check for breathing.

4. Attempt to deliver two slow breaths.
5. Reposition the head and try to give rescue breaths again.
6. Straddle the victim's thighs and give up to five subdiaphragmatic abdominal thrusts (Fig. 9-31 A).
7. Perform tongue-jaw lift and finger sweep (Figs. 9-31 B, C).
8. Repeat steps until the obstruction is resolved.

Aspiration

REGURGITATION: A passive, backward flow of gastric contents from the stomach into the oropharynx.
ASPIRATE: The taking of foreign material into the lungs during inhalation.

Pathophysiology

Other objects including dentures, teeth, blood, fluids, and vomitus also can obstruct the upper airway.

HYPERCARBIA: Excessive partial pressure of carbon dioxide in the blood.

Vomitus, typically **regurgitated** from the stomach into the oropharynx during states of decreased responsiveness, contains partially dissolved food, protein dissolving enzymes, and hydrochloric

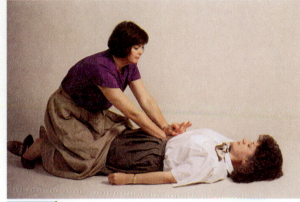

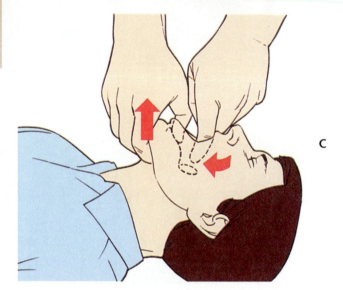

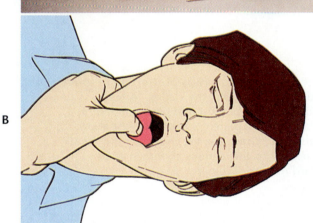

Fig. 9-31   Relieving an airway obstruction in an unresponsive patient. A, Straddle the victim's thighs and give up to five abdominal thrusts. B, Perform tongue-jaw lift. C, Perform a finger sweep.

acid. If allowed to be **aspirated** into the lungs, this combination can lead to increased interstitial fluid, pulmonary edema, and destruction of the alveoli. This condition seriously impairs gas exchange and leads to hypoxemia and **hypercarbia.** Furthermore, food particles can obstruct the bronchiolar airways, thus compromising air flow. Saliva, like vomitus, contains certain digestive enzymes. It, too, can fill the alveoli, causing similar problems.

Assessment
Gurgling sounds heard on inspiration and/or expiration indicate the accumulation of fluids or vomitus in the upper airway.

Basic treatment
Prompt intervention with cricoid pressure, suctioning, and positioning of the patient usually can prevent aspiration.

Cricoid Pressure
Cricoid pressure (also referred to as the *Sellick maneuver*) is a quick, effective way of preventing gastric distention and/or regurgitation. It is performed by applying firm pressure (about the same amount as is necessary to stop bleeding) over the cricoid cartilage and directing it posteriorly against the esophagus (Fig. 9-32). This pressure closes the esophagus off to pressures as high as 100 cm H_2O. The cricoid cartilage can be located by palpating the depression just below the thyroid cartilage. This depression is the cricothyroid membrane. The projection just below this membrane is the cricoid cartilage. Pressure is applied with the

thumb and index finger of one hand to the front of the cartilage just to the sides of the midline. More pressure is required to prevent regurgitation than gastric distention. This technique is invaluable when assisting a patient's breathing (*eg,* with a bag-valve-mask device, demand valve resuscitator) and during attempts at endotracheal intubation.

Suctioning

 Discuss the indications, contraindications, and methods of performing suctioning.

Suctioning is used to remove vomitus, blood, fluids, and secretions from the airway. A variety of devices are available for the prehospital setting, including portable and stationary units (Fig. 9-33 A-C). Each device is capable of generating vacuum levels of at least 300 mm Hg when the distal end is occluded and allows a free air flow rate of at least 30 L/min when the tube is open.

Portable units allow suctioning to be done immediately rather than waiting until the patient is in the ambulance. Some are hand-, foot-, or oxygen-powered, whereas others are battery-powered. Many of today's hand-held units are capable of generating excellent suctioning pressures, and, because of their small size (often weighing only 1 pound or so), can be easily stored in an airway kit.

The two most common types of suction catheters are the tonsil tip and whistle tip. The tonsil tip (also

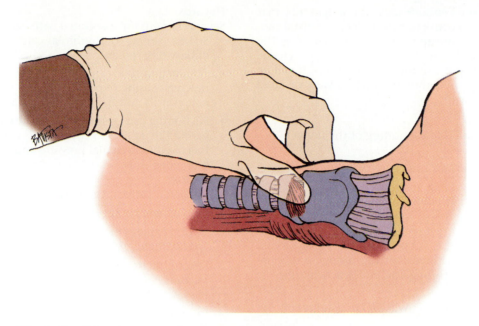

Fig. 9-32   Cricoid pressure, known as the Sellick maneuver, prevents gastric distention and regurgitation in patients receiving artificial ventilations.

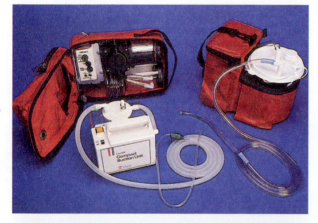

A

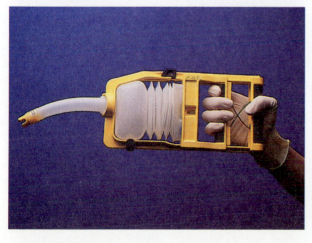

B

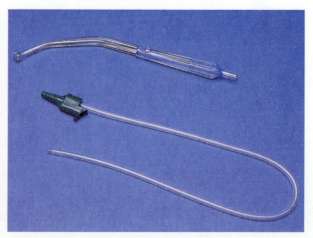

C

Fig. 9-33   Types of suction units. A, Portable suction unit. B, Hand-held portable suction unit. C, Rigid (top) and soft (bottom) suction catheters.

referred to as the *Yankauer suction)* is a rigid tube that has a ball-like tip with multiple holes at its distal end. Some catheters are supplied with an open tip. The tonsil-tip suction catheter is designed to remove larger particles and voluminous secretions. It can be inserted along an oropharyngeal airway or used during laryngoscopy.

Disadvantages

- Its use is limited to suctioning of the upper airway.
- Vigorous insertion can cause lacerations or other injuries.

The whistle-tip suction catheter is a small, easy-to-use, flexible tube that is long enough to extend into the lower respiratory tract. It can be inserted through the nares, into the oropharynx or nasopharynx, through a nasopharyngeal airway, along an oropharyngeal airway, or through an endotracheal tube.

Disadvantages

- It is ineffective in removing large volumes of secretions rapidly.
- Is often unable to retrieve even smaller food particles.

Precautions

Each suctioning attempt should be restricted to 15 seconds or less. The reason is that during suctioning, breathing assistance is interrupted and the air the patient receives is depleted of oxygen. If possible, the patient should be hyperventilated with 100% oxygen both before and after each suctioning attempt. However, when fluids are present in the upper airway and assisted breathing may lead to aspiration, the airway should be cleared before suctioning is begun.

STREET WISE
Suction should not be activated during insertion of the catheter because it depletes the air of oxygen.

Once the catheter is properly positioned, suction should be applied and the catheter withdrawn. Most suction catheters have a control opening at the proximal end that allows suction through the catheter to be started or stopped. If the suction catheter is not equipped with a control opening, the EMT–I can create one by making a small slit in the catheter or suction tubing. Alternatively, suction can be controlled by turning the suction unit on and off as needed.

When fluids in the upper airway are so voluminous or thick that the tonsil-tip or whistle-tip suction catheters cannot provide adequate suctioning, the EMT–I should remove the catheter and use the thick-walled, wide-bore suction tubing alone. Water should be suctioned through the tubing between suctioning attempts to dilute the secretions and facilitate flow through the tubing. Any blockage of the tubing, even partial, can cut down on suction pressure and make the device less effective. It is important to keep the tubing as clean as possible.

Hazards

Several hazards are associated with suctioning:

- Serious cardiac dysrhythmias can occur secondary to hypoxia.
- The suction tube can stimulate the airway mucosa causing hypertension and tachycardia or bradycardia and hypotension (vagal stimulation).
- Suctioning can stimulate the airway mucosa, triggering the patient to cough. This can result in increased intracranial pressure and reduced cerebral blood flow.

Procedure

To suction a patient, the EMT–I should:

1. Employ body substance isolation precautions.
2. Hyperventilate the patient (if possible) for approximately 30 seconds.
3. Determine the depth for catheter insertion by measuring from the patient's lips to the earlobe (Fig. 9-34 A).
4. Insert the suction catheter to the proper depth (Fig. 9-34 B).
5. Turn the suction unit on or place the thumb over suction control opening, limiting suction to 15 seconds.
6. Withdraw the catheter. When using a whistle-tip catheter, rotate it between the fingertips to keep it from adhering to the pharyngeal wall (Fig. 9-34 C).
7. Flush out the suction catheter and tubing with saline and evaluate the need for additional suctioning.
8. Hyperventilate the patient with a bag-valve-mask device supplied with 100% oxygen or a demand valve resuscitator.

Alternative Procedures

It also may be necessary for the EMT–I to place the patient on his or her side and use the fingers to clear substances from the patient's mouth.

Trauma
Pathophysiology

Trauma to the head, face, or neck can lead to airway obstruction by cluttering the airway with broken teeth, facial bones, tissue, and blood. When blood is aspirated into the lungs it can clog the bronchi and alveoli with clots that obstruct air flow. A fractured mandible when displaced backward can push the tongue backward with it and obstruct the airway. Also, direct injury to the larynx and trachea from a blunt instrument, bullet, or knife can result in airway obstruction due to the rapid accumulation of blood in the tissues surrounding the wound or by fracturing or displacing the larynx, allowing the vocal cords to collapse into the tracheal opening.

Assessment

As with aspiration, gurgling sounds heard on inspiration and expiration indicate the accumulation of

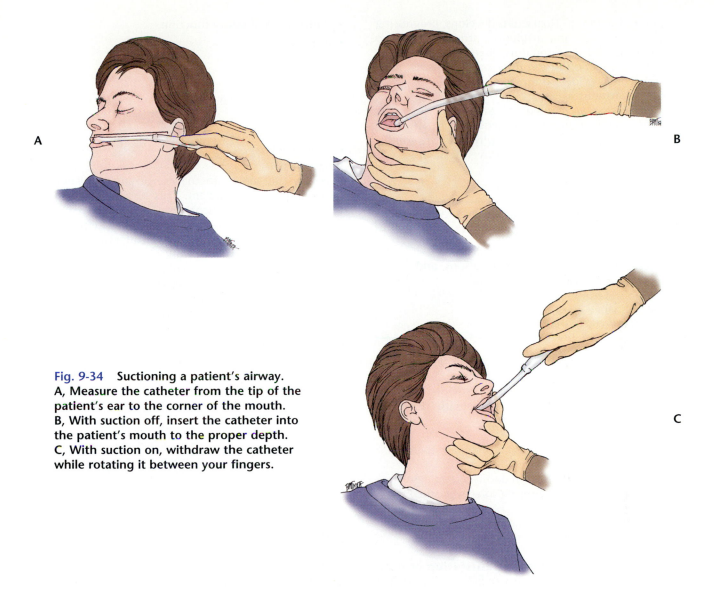

Fig. 9-34 Suctioning a patient's airway.
A, Measure the catheter from the tip of the patient's ear to the corner of the mouth.
B, With suction off, insert the catheter into the patient's mouth to the proper depth.
C, With suction on, withdraw the catheter while rotating it between your fingers.

fluids or blood in the upper airway. Stridor is indicative of upper airway obstruction due to swelling.

Basic treatment

Steps used to manage the trauma patient depend on the location and extent of the injuries. Suctioning is used to remove blood and small particles from the upper airway. In extreme cases, the patient's whole body should be rolled to the side while maintaining in-line support of the head to allow drainage of blood from the patient's mouth. If the trauma is limited to the mandible, insertion of a nasopharyngeal airway may be useful. Placement of an endotracheal tube can be used to seal off the trachea, preventing aspiration.

Laryngeal edema/spasm
Pathophysiology

Laryngeal edema and spasm also can lead to upper airway obstruction. As discussed earlier, the glottis is the narrowest part of the adult's upper airway.

Edema or spasm of the vocal cords is a potentially lethal condition, because even moderate swelling can severely obstruct air flow through the glottis, resulting in asphyxia.

In adults, laryngeal edema can result from anaphylaxis, epiglottitis, and inhalation of super-heated air, smoke, or toxic substances. In children, upper airway obstruction related to laryngeal edema typically is caused by epiglottitis or croup. Epiglottitis can develop rapidly, causing the epiglottis to swell. In extreme cases it can enlarge to the point where it obstructs the glottis and causes suffocation. With croup, there is edema of the loose tissues just below the larynx. In the smaller-diameter tracheas of children, this partial airway obstruction can cause complete airway obstruction.

Assessment

The patient with allergies may report an itching sensation in the palate followed by the sensation of a lump in the throat. Hoarseness develops, progressing rapidly to cough and inspiratory stridor. Hives also may be present. As respiratory distress becomes more marked, retraction of the intercostal and neck muscles becomes evident on inspirations.

Basic treatment
Emergency management is aimed at reversing swelling and improving oxygenation. In the presence of allergic reaction or anaphylaxis, the administration of epinephrine can prove life-saving.

Ventilatory problems

> Identify the common mechanisms of ventilatory failure and describe the procedures for resolving each.
>
> Discuss indications, contraindications, and methods for use of the following:
> • pocket mask
> • bag-valve-mask device
> • demand valve resuscitation

Once a patent airway is ensured, the EMT–I then must determine if there is a need for ventilatory support. Assisted breathing must be provided to those patients who are apneic or experiencing depressed respiratory function.

VENTILATION: Breathing, moving air in and out of the lungs.
HYPOVENTILATION: A reduced rate or depth of breathing, often resulting in an abnormal rise of carbon dioxide.
HYPOXIA: Reduced oxygen supply to the cells.

Pathophysiology
As discussed earlier, adequate **ventilation** or respiratory minute volumes are needed for a sufficient intake of oxygen and removal of carbon dioxide. A decrease in either the respiratory rate or volume will lead to a reduction in the respiratory minute volume. This condition is referred to as **hypoventilation.** Hypoventilation leads to the accumulation of carbon dioxide (also referred to as *hypercarbia*), development of **hypoxia,** and a lowered pH. Hypoventilation also can occur when the respiratory rate is so fast that the depth of breathing is reduced, or when breathing is deep, but the rate is excessively slow. In both situations, too little air exchange takes place due to an overall reduction in respiratory minute volumes. Ultimately, if left uncorrected, respiratory and/or cardiac arrest can occur.

A number of mechanisms can bring about hypoventilation including:

• Depressed respiratory function
• Drug overdose
• Spinal injury
• Head injury

• Impaired ventilatory function
• Fractured ribs
• Flail chest
• Pneumothorax
• Chronic obstructive pulmonary disease (COPD), asthma
• Muscular paralysis
• Poliomyelitis

Assessment
A critical component to the use of any ventilatory device is proper assessment. This assessment begins with looking at each patient during those first seconds of exposure and continuously thereafter to determine if there is sufficient air exchange. Observant evaluation of the level of responsiveness, work of breathing, respiratory rate, mucous membrane color, and pulse oximetry readings all provide the EMT–I with critical information. For those EMT–Is who are permitted, the use of the electrocardiogram monitor also can provide invaluable information. If respiratory failure is imminent or present, supportive measures must be instituted. Even patients who are spontaneously breathing may require ventilatory support, because respiratory efforts that are too slow or too shallow result in hypoxia and hypercarbia and eventually lead to death. In some cases, hypoventilation will not be obvious. Thus, patients who have a respiratory rate outside the normal parameter, less than 12 or greater than 20 breaths per minute, may require ventilatory assistance. These patients must be closely watched and provided with ventilatory assistance as needed. Certainly, patients with respiratory rates of less than 10 or greater than 30 breaths per minute should receive ventilatory assistance.

Basic treatment
When illness or injury adversely affects a person's ability to breathe, it may be necessary to intervene and provide ventilatory support. In the prehospital setting, several procedures and devices are available for providing ventilatory assistance in the hypoventilating or apneic patient.

Assisting breathing
To effectively assist a patient's breathing, the EMT–I must deliver adequate volumes of air (at least 800 mL each breath) at a fast enough rate (12 to 20 breaths per minute). This is true regardless of the procedure or equipment used. Three factors challenge the EMT–I's ability to do this:

• The difficulty associated with maintaining an open airway
• Resistance to airflow
• The need to maintain a closed ventilatory system

Difficulty associated with maintaining an open airway
During the act of assisting a patient's breathing, rescuers often push down on the patient's chin or face in an attempt to maintain a seal. This action forces the jaw and the tongue backward into an obstructing

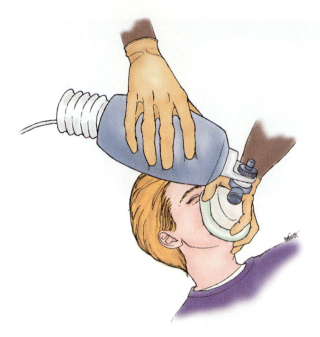

Fig. 9-35   For effective ventilatory assistance, the EMT-I must make certain that a good seal is created and maintained, and that the lower jaw is forced forward to keep the airway open.

position, closing off the airway. When assisting a patient's breathing, the EMT–I must employ a technique that ensures both an adequate seal and a forward disposition of the lower jaw (Fig. 9-35).

Resistance to airflow

In a nonbreathing patient there is frictional resistance in the respiratory passageways as well as elastic resistance of the lungs and chest wall. To expand the lungs, this resistance must be overcome. It can be like blowing up a balloon—initially it is hard to inflate the balloon, but after it begins to expand, inflation becomes much easier. The EMT–I must be careful because the high pressure required to expand the lungs can force air into the esophagus.

Need to maintain a closed ventilatory system

A closed ventilatory system must be maintained to deliver adequate volumes of air to the patient's lungs. The reason is very simple: air travels the path of least resistance. If the EMT–I does not maintain a tight seal between the patient's face and the mask, air will leak out. Ventilating with a bag-valve-mask device equipped with pop-off valve can lead to the same problem when there is a great deal of airway resistance. Air tends to blow off through the valve rather than be pushed through the air passageways.

Pop-off valves should be deactivated or devices equipped with them should not be used.

The EMT–I must not forget that the patient must be allowed to passively exhale between delivered breaths in order to remove carbon dioxide.

Procedures and devices used to provide assisted breathing include:

- Mouth-to-mouth/nose breathing
- Mouth-to-mask breathing
- Bag-valve-mask device
- Demand-valve resuscitator
- Automatic ventilator

Mouth-to-mouth/nose

Mouth-to-mouth or mouth-to-nose breathing is a quick, effective means of assisting a patient's breathing, and, when applied properly, good ventilatory volumes can be delivered because an effective seal over the patient's mouth (or nose) is easily maintained. Although this procedure requires no adjunctive equipment, the EMT–I should employ the use of a protective barrier. The most significant limitation of mouth-to-mouth breathing is that it provides little oxygen (because expired air from the EMT–I only contains 17% oxygen). Additionally, the patient may have copious secretions, bleeding, or gastric regurgitation or may be suffering from a transmittable disease.

Pocket mask

The pocket mask is a clear plastic device that covers the patient's mouth and nose, preventing contact between the EMT–I and patient and reducing the risk of contamination during resuscitation. Mouth-to-mask breathing has been shown to be more effective at delivering adequate tidal volumes than a bag-valve-mask. This is because the EMT–I's lungs are of greater capacity than the bag-valve-mask device, and, because the pocket mask is easier to employ than a bag-valve-mask device, both hands can be used to hold the mask to the patient's face.

A variety of pocket masks are available; some are reusable, whereas others are disposed of after a single use. Most are small and compact, allowing the EMT–I to always have one device available, whether at work or off-duty. Pocket masks often are supplied with a one-way valve that keeps the EMT–I from coming into contact with the patient's expired air. This valve reduces the risk of infection.

Oxygen delivery

Many pocket masks are supplied with an inlet for delivery of supplemental oxygen to the patient. Mouth-to-mask breathing, combined with an oxygen flow rate of 10 L/min can deliver an inspired oxygen concentration of approximately 50%.

Procedure

To use the pocket mask, the EMT–I should:

1. Employ body substance isolation precautions.

2. Connect the oxygen tubing to the oxygen inlet of the mask.

3. Adjust the oxygen flow rate to 10 L/min or greater.

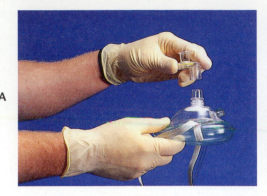
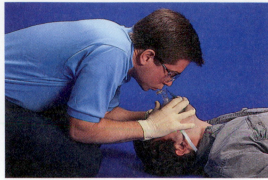

Fig. 9-36 Mouth-to-mask ventilation with supplemental O$_2$. A, Connect a one-way valve to the mask. B, After creating an appropriate seal, ventilate the patient through the one-way valve on top of the mask.

4. Attach a one-way valve to the ventilatory inlet/outlet port of the mask (Fig. 9-36A).

5. Kneel at the top of the patient's head and open the airway using the head-tilt procedure (provided there is no likelihood of a cervical spine injury).

6. If needed, insert an oropharyngeal airway.

7. Place the mask on the patient's face with the:
   • Narrow end (apex) over the bridge of the nose
   • Wide end (base) in the groove between the lower lip and chin.

8. Position both hands over the mask with the thumbs on the dome and index and middle fingers extended across the base. Press downward on the mask with the thumbs and fingers to maintain an effective seal between the patient's face and the mask.

9. Hook the ring and little fingers under the patient's jaw. Use the fingers to keep the patient's head tilted back (in nontrauma related cases) and the jaw displaced forward.

10. Take a deep breath and ventilate the patient through the one-way valve on top of the mask (Fig. 9-36 B). Each breath should be delivered in a slow and steady manner (minimum inspiratory time of 2 seconds). This method helps prevent gastric distention and reduces the possibility of regurgitation and aspiration.

11. Check for ventilatory effectiveness by observing chest rise and feeling for lung resistance.

12. Remove your mouth and allow the patient to passively exhale. Listen for air flow from the mask's inlet port during passive exhalation and watch the patient's chest fall.

13. Ventilate the patient with no less than 800 mL volume with each breath at a rate of at least 12 times a minute.

14. Continue the procedure until effective spontaneous breathing is restored or resuscitation efforts are ordered terminated.

Bag-valve-mask device

Another tool used to provide ventilatory support is the bag-valve-mask device. It consists of a self-inflating silicone or rubber bag and two valves, the nonrebreathing valve and inlet valve. Typically, the bag-valve-mask is available in three sizes: adult (capable of storing between 1000 to 1600 mL of air), child (capable of storing 500 to 700 mL of air), and infant (capable of storing 150 to 240 mL of air). The bag-valve-mask may be used with a mask, endotracheal tube, esophageal obturator airway, or other airway devices. At a minimum, the bag-valve-mask should:

1. Consist of a self-inflating bag that is easy to grip and compress.

2. Be easy to clean and sterilize. With the concern over the potential transmission of infectious disease, there are a number of disposable units available for use in the prehospital care setting.

3. Include a nonjam valve system (even in the presence of large particles of vomitus).

4. Have a standard 15 mm/22 mm fitting, which allows for attachment of the device to a standard mask, esophageal obturator, pharyngotracheal lumen airway, or endotracheal tube.

5. Provide satisfactory performance under extremes of environmental temperatures.

6. Include a system for delivery of 85% to 100% oxygen with an oxygen reservoir and supplemental oxygen source.

7. Contain only a few parts and be easy to assemble in an emergency.

As mentioned earlier, bag-valve-mask devices used in the field setting should not be equipped with a pop-off valve. Pressures required to ventilate the patient during delivery of CPR in cardiac arrest may exceed the pop-off limit. Additionally, in patients who have poorly compliant (stiff) lungs, the tidal volume delivered may be insufficient.

The mask used with a bag-valve-mask should be transparent, so that the EMT–I can see any vomitus or secretions around the patient's mouth. Also, it should have an air cushion or inflatable cuff. Selecting the proper size mask is important; one that is too small or too large will make it difficult to get a good seal. The mask should just cover the area between the bridge of the nose and the indentation beneath the lower lip. Ideally, the mask should only be applied for a short period of time, being quickly replaced by the insertion of an endotracheal tube. Endotracheal intubation eliminates the need for a tight seal between the patient's face and a mask (the most common cause of ineffective ventilation) and protects the patient's airway from collapse.

Advantages and disadvantages of the bag-valve-mask device include the following:

Advantages

- It provides an immediate means of ventilatory support.
- It conveys a sense of compliance of patient's lungs to the EMT–I.
- It can be used with spontaneously breathing patients.
- It can deliver an oxygen-enriched mixture to patient.

Disadvantages

- It is hard to maintain adequate seal while delivering required volume of air.
- It is sometimes difficult to deliver the required tidal volume (squeeze the bag adequately).

Oxygen delivery

When used without a supplemental oxygen source, the bag-valve-mask will only deliver 21% oxygen. When supplied with an oxygen source set at a flow rate of 15 L/min, approximately 40% to 60% oxygen will be delivered. This result typically is accomplished by attaching oxygen tubing from an oxygen regulator to the oxygen inlet nipple located on the bottom or top end (depending on the manufacturer) of the bag-valve-mask. To deliver 85% to 100% oxygen, the bag-valve-mask must be equipped with a reservoir. The reservoir may consist of a bag-type unit or tubing. The purpose of the reservoir is to collect a volume of 100% oxygen equal to the capacity of the bag. When the bag reexpands after having been squeezed, the 100% oxygen is drawn from the reservoir into the bag. Another device capable of delivering 85% to 100% oxygen through a bag-valve-mask is a demand valve. It delivers 85% to 100% oxygen (depending on the capability of the device) when negative pressure from within the bag (after the bag has been squeezed and is reexpanding) triggers the demand valve to release high-flow oxygen in a sufficient volume to refill the bag. When the demand valve is attached to the reservoir port of the bag-valve-mask, the oxygen inlet nipple must be occluded to prevent inadvertent leaking of ambient air into the bag (Fig. 9-37).

> **INTRAPULMONARY SHUNTING:** The circulation of blood to nonventilated alveoli, which results in the blood having the same oxygen content as systemic venous blood.

In life-threatening conditions such as shock, drug overdose, and cardiac arrest, severe hypoxemia may be caused by **intrapulmonary shunting,** alveolar collapse, and decreased perfusion. For this reason the highest concentration of oxygen (as close to 100% as possible) should always be used in conjunction with providing ventilatory assistance to a patient.

Precautions

Although its use has gained widespread acceptance in the prehospital care setting, the bag-valve-mask also has been characterized as cumbersome and difficult to use. The most frequent problem encountered is the inability to provide adequate ventilatory volumes to patients who are not endotracheally intubated. This situation occurs because of the difficulty providing a leakproof seal to the face while maintaining an open airway. Mask leak is a serious problem, decreasing the volume delivered to the oropharynx by as much as 40% or more. While providing ventilatory support to the patient, the EMT–I should continually listen for air leaks from around the mask. Air leak indicates that a better seal needs to be established and maintained.

Poor ventilation also occurs when the bag is not squeezed completely enough to force adequate amounts of air into the patient's lungs. At least 800 to 1200 mL of air per breath is needed. With four fingers on top and the thumb underneath, the bag is compressed with the right hand as completely as possible. Unfortunately, EMT–Is with smaller hands may not be able to empty the bag enough to achieve the needed ventilatory volumes.

However, the problems of not maintaining an adequate seal, keeping an open airway, and compressing the bag sufficiently can be overcome with adequate skill practice and modifications in procedure.

When delivering assisted breathing, the resistance in the bag must be continually noted. Increased resistance (indicated by a bag that is hard to squeeze) suggests airway obstruction. A tongue that falls back against the posterior oropharynx is the most likely culprit. Unless trauma is suspected, further hyperextension of the patient's head corrects this problem. If an oropharyngeal airway has not been placed yet, it should be inserted at this point. Other possible causes include foreign body obstruction, tension pneumothorax, or severe bronchospasm. Conversely, a bag that compresses too easily indicates a leak somewhere in the system. The best indicator of effective ventilations is the rise and fall of the patient's chest.

To effectively use the bag-valve-mask with the mask attached, the EMT–I must assume a position at the top of the patient's head. Otherwise, is it

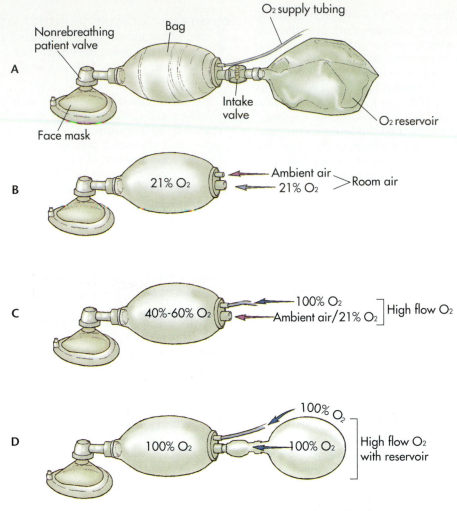

Fig. 9-37 A, Components of the bag-valve-mask device. B, A bag-valve-mask device without a supplemental oxygen supply delivers 21% O_2 to the patient. C, A bag-valve-mask device with an oxygen source delivers 40% to 60% O_2 to the patient. D, A bag-valve-mask device equipped with a reservoir delivers nearly 100% O_2 to the patient.

nearly impossible to maintain an effective seal between the mask and the patient's face while keeping the airway open.

Procedure

To use the bag-valve-mask, the EMT–I should (Fig. 9-38):

1. Employ body substance isolation precautions.

2. Unless the likelihood of trauma is present, tilt the patient's head back and mandible anteriorly using an appropriate airway maneuver.

3. If the patient is unresponsive, insert an oropharyngeal airway. If a gag reflex is present, a nasopharyngeal airway may be used.

4. Select the appropriate size mask.

5. Place mask on patient's face with narrow end (apex) over bridge of nose and wide end (base) in groove between the lower lip and chin.

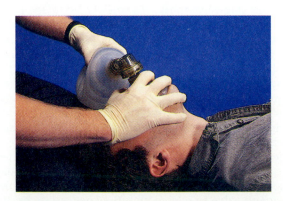

Fig. 9-38 BVM ventilation procedure with one rescuer.

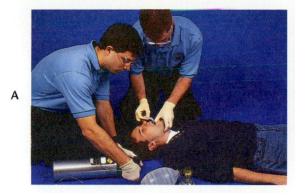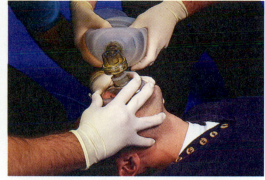

Fig. 9-39   BVM ventilation procedure with two rescuers. A, One EMT-I opens the airway while a second EMT-I sets up the BVM. B, One EMT-I holds the mask in place while a second EMT-I ventilates.

6. Obtain a tight seal by applying firm downward pressure over the mask with the thumb on the dome and index and middle fingers on the base.

7. Hook the last two or three fingers under the jaw, then pull the chin backward to maintain the head-tilt.

8. Squeeze the bag with one hand or between one hand and the arm, chest, or thigh (if kneeling). Compression of the bag should be as complete as possible using a smooth, steady action. Between each compression, the bag should be allowed to refill completely.

9. Watch for the patient's chest to rise during ventilation and fall during passive exhalation.

10. Auscultate the chest to make sure that appropriate ventilation is occurring.

11. Connect reservoir and oxygen tubing to the oxygen inlet of the bag-valve-mask and deliver oxygen at 12 to 15 L/min.

12. Hyperventilate patient (12 to 20 times per minute or once every 2 to 5 seconds with at least 800 mL of air with each breath). Allow for adequate exhalation after each delivered breath.

13. Auscultate the chest to be sure adequate ventilation is being delivered.

Because of the problems inherent to this device it only should be used by trained and experienced personnel. Additionally, because of the potential for skill degradation after only a short while, ventilating with a bag-valve-mask device should be practiced on a CPR manikin with appropriate frequency.

Ventilation with a bag-valve-mask device may be more effectively delivered using two EMT–Is: one holding the mask in place and maintaining an open airway, the other squeezing the bag with two hands (Fig. 9-39).

Demand valve

The demand valve resuscitator is a manually triggered, oxygen-powered (delivering 100% oxygen at

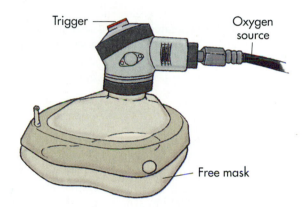

Fig. 9-40   The demand valve allows a steady stream of O_2 to be delivered to the patient while the button is depressed.

40 to 60 L/min) ventilatory device. Connected to an oxygen supply through high-pressure tubing, it is small, easy to use, rugged, and has an easily accessible manual control button (Fig. 9-40). When the demand valve is opened or activated, a steady stream of oxygen flows to the patient. On the delivery end, it can be attached to a face mask, esophageal obturator, endotracheal tube, or tracheostomy tube.

Most of these devices contain an inspiratory release valve that also allows the demand valve to be used to provide 100% oxygen to spontaneously breathing patients. The slight negative pressure created by the inspiratory effort of the patient triggers the valve from a nonflow state to a flowing state. The greater the inspiratory effort, the higher the flow. When the inspiratory effort ceases, oxygen stops flowing.

Advantages

- It is easy to use.
- It provides high oxygen concentrations.

Disadvantages

- The device fails to provide a sense of chest compliance during ventilation; thus care must be taken not to overinflate the lungs.

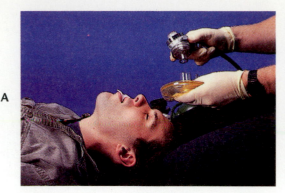 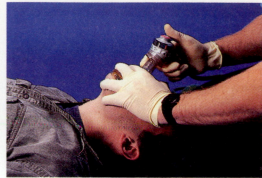

Fig. 9-41 Ventilating a patient. A, Select the appropriate sized mask and attach it to the oxygen supply. B, Firmly hold the mask to the patient's face and deliver ventilations.

- High pressures generated by the device may cause barotrauma to lungs, resulting in pneumothorax and subcutaneous emphysema.
- It may open the esophagus causing gastric distention.
- The high oxygen flow rate quickly expends portable oxygen cylinders.

Precautions
Because the device is dependent on an oxygen source for power, another means of ventilatory support is needed if the oxygen cylinder requires changing during patient ventilation. Due to the sudden high pressure that the demand valve resuscitator provides, it should not be used in pediatric patients (under 16 years of age). It should be used with extreme caution in patients who are endotracheally intubated.

Procedures
To ventilate a patient with a demand valve resuscitator, the EMT–I should:

1. Employ body substance isolation precautions.
2. Assume a position at the top of the patient's head.
3. Unless the likelihood of trauma is present, tilt the patient's head back and mandible anteriorly using an appropriate airway maneuver.
4. If the patient is unresponsive, insert an oropharyngeal airway. If a gag reflex is present, a nasopharyngeal airway may be used.
5. Open the regulator valve to the oxygen supply.
6. Select the proper size mask for the patient (Fig. 9-41 A).
7. Place the mask on the patient's face with the narrow end (apex) over bridge of the nose and the wide end (base) in the groove between the lower lip and chin.
8. With both hands, firmly hold the mask to the patient's face to make a seal while maintaining an appropriate head and neck hyperextension.

9. Deliver a ventilation by pushing the button of the device (Fig. 9-41 B).
10. Watch for chest rise and auscultate the lung sounds to ensure proper ventilation.
11. As soon as the chest rises, release the pressure on the button to allow passive expiration. The flow of oxygen then ceases, and the expired air is vented out a one-way valve to the atmosphere.

Automatic ventilators
Automatic ventilators employed in the prehospital setting are:

- Time-cycled, constant-flow, gas-powered devices.
- Lightweight, compact, and easy to use.
- Designed to operate in temperature extremes from -30° to 125° F, making them dependable in emergency situations.

Like the devices described earlier, automatic ventilators are equipped with a standard 15-mm inside diameter/22-mm outside diameter adapter that allows them to be attached to various airway devices and masks (Fig. 9-42).

Automatic ventilators are often equipped with two controls: one that regulates the ventilatory rate and one regulating tidal volume. Some devices deliver controlled ventilation only, whereas others function as intermittent mandatory ventilators, reverting to controlled mechanical ventilation in nonbreathing patients. The inspired oxygen concentration is usually fixed at 100%, but it may be adjustable depending on the device.

ADULT RESPIRATORY DISTRESS SYNDROME (ARDS): Pulmonary insufficiency that occurs due to a number of bodily insults. Pathologic findings include alveolar and interstitial edema due to leaking capillaries.

Automatic ventilators are typically supplied with a pop-off feature that works to prevent barotrauma. The

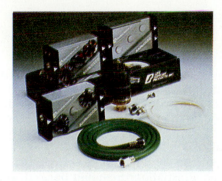

Fig. 9-42   *Automatic ventilators: Autovent 1000, 2000, and 3000.*

pop-off valve vents a portion of the tidal volume to the atmosphere when the preset level of airway pressure is exceeded. Unfortunately, pop-off valves can be detrimental in the presence of cardiogenic pulmonary edema, **adult respiratory distress syndrome** (ARDS), pulmonary contusion, bronchospasm, or other disorders in which high airway pressures must be exerted. To ensure proper working order, these devices must be checked regularly.

When providing ventilatory support to patients who are endotracheally intubated, use of the automatic ventilator allows the EMT–I to perform other vital tasks. When it is used in conjunction with a face mask the EMT–I must continue to maintain proper positioning of the patient's head as well as an effective seal between the mask and the patient's face.

Gastric distention

If the airway is obstructed by inadequate positioning or when high pressures are used during ventilation, air can enter the stomach instead of the lungs. This occurrence can lead to gastric distention and severe complications including regurgitation of the stomach contents with possible aspiration, decreased vital capacity due to elevation of the diaphragm, and gastric rupture due to overdistention. When gastric distention occurs in the field setting and is interfering with ventilations, measures must be taken to relieve it. After turning the patient onto his or her side, the EMT–I should place one hand over the epigastrium, between the umbilicus and the rib cage, and exert moderate pressure. A suction unit should be available to clear the upper airway in case of regurgitation. **Relieving gastric distention is performed using extreme caution and only when absolutely necessary.**

HYPOXIA

 Identify the common mechanisms of hypoxia and describe its treatment.

Oxygen therapy is an essential treatment of seriously ill or injured patients. The EMT–I must be knowledge-able and skilled in the application of all supplemental oxygen delivery devices and the rationale for their use.

Pathophysiology

Oxygen plays a vital role in the body's production of energy. Without it, normal metabolism cannot occur. The movement and utilization of oxygen in the body is dependent on having:

- An adequate concentration of inspired oxygen
- Appropriate movement of oxygen across the alveolar/capillary membrane into the arterial bloodstream
- An adequate number of red blood cells to carry the oxygen
- Proper tissue perfusion
- Efficient off-loading of oxygen at the tissue level

These elements are collectively known as the *Fick Principle*.

DYSRHYTHMIA: A disturbance in the normal rhythm of the heart.

Hypoxia is defined as a decreased or inadequate supply of oxygen. It has several adverse effects on the body. At the cellular level, it leads to anaerobic metabolism, a physiologic process that can result in metabolic acidosis, cellular depression, and, eventually, cellular death. In the brain, it brings about swelling that results in reduced blood flow to the cerebral tissues and a worsening of the hypoxia. In the heart, it can cause cardiac **dysrhythmias** and decreased cardiac output. Hypoxia also increases myocardial and respiratory workloads, because these systems are used by the body to offset the hypoxia. Causes of hypoxia include:

- Insufficient oxygen in inspired air due to:
  - Smoke
  - Toxic gases
  - High altitude
- Failure of the ventilatory mechanism due to:
  - Pneumothorax
  - Fractured ribs
  - Muscular paralysis
  - **Kyphoscoliosis**
- Upper airway compromise caused by:
  - Foreign body obstruction
  - Epiglottitis
  - Croup
  - Edema of vocal cords
- Lower airway compromise caused by:
  - Chronic bronchitis
  - Acute asthma attack
  - Tumors

- Pneumonia
- Pulmonary edema
- Emphysema
- **Fibrosis**
- Circulatory deficiency due to:
  - Pump failure
  - Congestive heart failure
  - Congenital defects
  - Blood loss (hemorrhage)
  - Shock
  - Anemia
  - Carbon monoxide poisoning
- Cellular deficiency as a result of:
  - Cyanide poisoning
  - Toxic shock syndrome

KYPHOSCOLIOSIS: Lateral curvature of the spine; can interfere with normal breathing.
FIBROSIS: Abnormal formation of scar tissue in the connective tissue framework of the lungs following inflammation or pneumonia and in pulmonary tuberculosis.

Assessment

Signs of hypoxia may include changes in the patient's mental status, tachycardia, and/or a pulse oximetry saturation reading of less than 95% and so forth. Dyspnea and cyanosis are late signs.

 List the indications and oxygen delivery concentrations of the following:
- **nasal cannula**
- **simple face mask**
- **nonrebreather mask**
- **Venturi mask**

Treatment

Treatment of hypoxia is directed at increasing the patient's oxygen level through supplemental oxygen administration. Indications include chest pain due to myocardial ischemia, cardiorespiratory arrest, and suspected hypoxia of any cause, including major blood loss, major trauma, congestive heart failure, lung disease or injury, airway obstruction, stroke, shock, head injury, and carbon monoxide poisoning.

Supplemental oxygen raises the oxygen level by increasing the:

- Percentage of oxygen provided to the patient (increased **FIO$_2$** of inspired air)
- Oxygen concentration at the alveolar level
- Arterial oxygen levels
- Amount of oxygen delivered to the cells

 FIO$_2$: Percentage of oxygen in inspired air.

Through these actions, supplemental oxygen decreases hypoxia and reduces the intensity of the breathing efforts and myocardial work that the body must keep up to maintain a given oxygen level.

Precautions

Although there are no absolute contraindications to oxygen administration, it should be used with caution in patients prone to carbon dioxide retention and in premature infants. Recommended flow rates with the patient with COPD are 1 to 3 L delivered via nasal cannula or 24% to 28% via Venturi mask. If a patient develops respiratory depression, his or her breathing must be supported with a bag-valve-mask supplied with 15 L of oxygen (85% to 100%) or other ventilatory device.

> **STREET WISE**
> Never withhold oxygen from a patient who is hypoxic.

AMBIENT AIR: Environmental or room air.

Supplemental oxygen is administered through high-flow and low-flow systems. High-flow systems are equipped with a Venturi adapter that draws in large amounts of room air for each liter of oxygen delivered from the oxygen regulator. This action ensures delivery of precise oxygen concentrations regardless of how well the patient is breathing. In low-flow systems, oxygen travels directly from the regulator to the patient, allowing **ambient air** to be drawn into the respiratory passageways with each breath. This process dilutes the oxygen concentration from 100% (being delivered through the oxygen tubing) to a mixture of the two (100% oxygen and ambient air). The concentration delivered to the patient depends on the flow rate and type of oxygen-delivery device used. With some oxygen-delivery devices, the oxygen concentration varies in concert with changes in the respiratory minute volume. A patient who is breathing faster and/or deeper receives less oxygen, because he or she is taking in more ambient air, thus greatly diluting the oxygen flow of the low-flow system. Conversely, a patient whose breathing is slow and/or shallow dilutes the delivered oxygen flow with less ambient air and receives a higher concentration of oxygen. Devices that allow greater variation in the percentage of oxygen delivered to the patient are the nasal cannula and simple face mask.

Supplemental oxygen should be provided at a liter flow that delivers an appropriate concentration

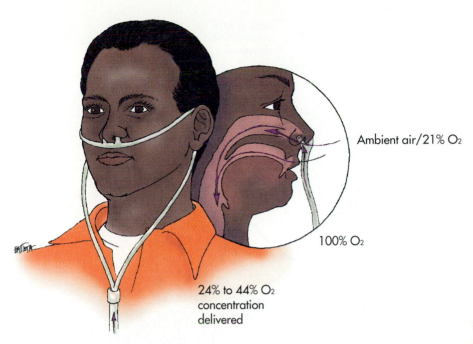

Ambient air/21% O₂

100% O₂

24% to 44% O₂
concentration
delivered

Fig. 9-43   A nasal cannula and the oxygen concentration delivered.

based on the patient's condition and medical history and local protocols. A variety of devices are used to deliver supplemental oxygen in spontaneously breathing patients:

- Nasal cannula
- Simple face mask
- Partial rebreather mask
- Nonrebreather mask
- Venturi mask

Patients needing assisted breathing usually receive high concentrations of oxygen through the device used to provide ventilatory assistance. The pocket mask, bag-valve-mask, demand valve, and automatic ventilator each can provide high concentrations of oxygen.

Nasal cannula

The nasal cannula is a comfortable and easily tolerated device capable of delivering an oxygen concentration of 24% to 44% when supplied with flow rates of between 1 and 6 L/min. (Fig. 9-43).

The flow rate should be limited to 6 L/min. Anything greater does little to increase the inspired oxygen concentration, because the anatomic reserve (nasal cavity) is already filled. Additionally, higher flow rates dry the mucous membranes and can cause headaches.

Use of the nasal cannula is recommended for patients who are:

- Experiencing minor to moderate hypoxia
- Predisposed to carbon dioxide retention
- Frightened or feel suffocated with other delivery devices
- Feeling nauseous or vomiting

A benefit of the nasal cannula is that it does not interfere with assessment because the patient's response to questions can be easily heard. Additionally, there is no rebreathing of expired air. The presence of nasal obstruction is the only contraindication for use of the nasal cannula.

Applying the nasal cannula

To use the nasal cannula, the EMT–I should:

1. Explain to the patient the need for oxygen and apply the cannula.
2. Attach the nasal cannula to the oxygen.
3. Adjust the flow meter to deliver 6 L/min or less.
4. Place the two prongs of the cannula into the patient's nostrils with the tab facing up (prongs should curve upright).
5. Hook the tubing behind each ear and under the patient's chin.
6. Gently secure the cannula by sliding the adjuster upward under the patient's chin. The type that has an elastic strap fits over the ears and around the back of the head and it is tightened by adjusting the strap on both sides simultaneously until the cannula is secure, yet comfortable.
7. Continuously monitor the oxygen level in the tank.

Simple face mask

Components of the simple face mask include oxygen tubing and a cone-shaped face mask that has two inlet/outlet ports (one on each side). It fits over the patient's nose, mouth, and chin. The inlet/outlet ports allow ambient air to be drawn in with each breath and carbon dioxide-filled air to escape on expiration. Oxygen is delivered to the mask through an inlet port located at its base.

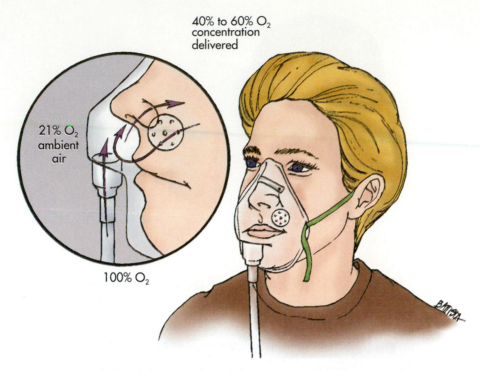

40% to 60% O₂
concentration
delivered

21% O₂
ambient
air

100% O₂

Fig. 9-44   **A simple face mask and the oxygen concentration delivered.**

Oxygen concentration delivered

In the patient who is breathing normally, the simple face mask can deliver a concentration of 40% to 60% oxygen (Fig. 9-44). Recommended flow rates used with the simple face mask range between 8 and 12 L/min. No less than 8/L should be administered through the device, because expired carbon dioxide can accumulate in the mask, resulting in hypercarbia. Flow rates of at least 8 L are needed to wash out the carbon dioxide exhaled by the patient. The simple face mask is used to provide oxygen to patients who are suffering from moderate hypoxia.

Disadvantages

- It may feel restrictive to the patient, particularly those patients experiencing severe dyspnea.
- It is hot and confining, and may irritate the skin.
- It is difficult to hear the patient speaking when the device is in place.
- It requires a tight face seal to prevent oxygen leakage.

Precautions

Because the mask covers the patient's face it should be used with caution in the presence of nausea and vomiting. In the pediatric patient, flow rates of 6 to 8 L/min are generally used.

Nonrebreather mask

The nonrebreather mask looks similar to the simple face mask. The difference is that, in addition to the oxygen tubing and face mask, there is a reservoir bag attached to the mask base and a rubber flap covering each of the air inlet/outlet ports (Fig. 9-45). The reservoir collects 100% oxygen delivered through the oxygen tubing. As the patient breathes in, the 100% oxygen (contained in the reservoir) is drawn into the mask and the patient's respiratory passageways. Ambient air is kept from entering the mask during inspiration by the rubber flaps that close over the inlet/outlet ports. During expiration the flapper valves are forced open, allowing the expired air to pass to the outside. A one-way valve, positioned between the mask and the reservoir, keeps expired air from diluting the oxygen contained in the reservoir bag.

Oxygen concentration delivered

When supplied with 10 to 15 L/min the nonrebreather mask is capable of delivering a 60% to 100% concentration of oxygen.

Precautions

Because it is a closed system that prevents breathing in of ambient air, the reservoir bag should not be allowed to totally deflate, which can cause the patient to suffocate. The EMT–I should observe the reservoir bag as the patient breathes. If it collapses more than slightly during inspiration, the flow rate should be increased until only a slight deflation is seen. The reservoir bag should be kept from twisting or kinking and should be positioned outside the sheets or blankets so it is completely free to expand. To move sufficient oxygen into the reservoir bag and remove

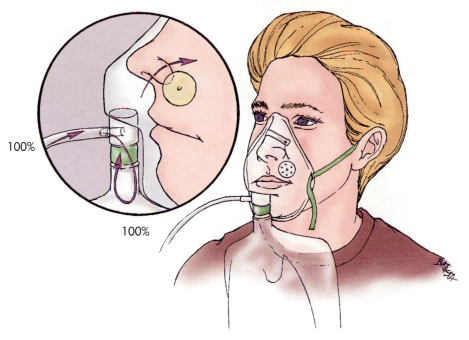

60% to 100% O₂
concentration
delivered

100%

100%

Fig. 9-45 **A nonrebreather mask and the O₂ concentration delivered.**

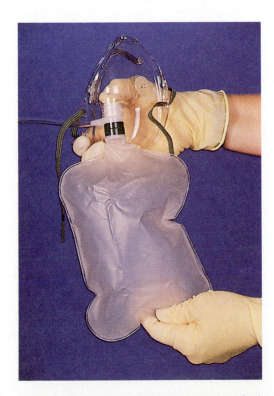

Fig. 9-46 **Inflate the reservoir bag with O₂ before placing it on the patient.**

exhaled carbon dioxide, at least 10 L of oxygen is needed. Also, the nonrebreather mask requires the use of a tight seal. With some patients, this tight seal may be difficult to obtain or may feel confining. Lastly, the nonrebreather mask should be employed with caution in patients who report nausea.

Use of the nonrebreather mask is recommended for the treatment of severely hypoxic patients, such as respiratory compromise, shock, acute myocardial infarction, trauma, carbon monoxide poisoning, and so forth.

Procedure

To use the nonrebreather mask, the EMT–I should:

1. Attach the nonrebreather mask to the oxygen flow meter nipple.
2. Prefill the reservoir by using a finger to cover the exhaust portal (the connection between the mask and reservoir) (Fig. 9-46).
3. Adjust the flow meter to deliver 10 to 15 L/min.
4. Apply the mask by placing it over the patient's nose, mouth, and chin.
5. Press the flexible metal nosepiece so that it fits the bridge of the patient's nose.
6. Tighten the mask by adjusting the elastic strap on both sides simultaneously until the mask is secure.
7. Make sure the one-way flaps are secure and functioning.

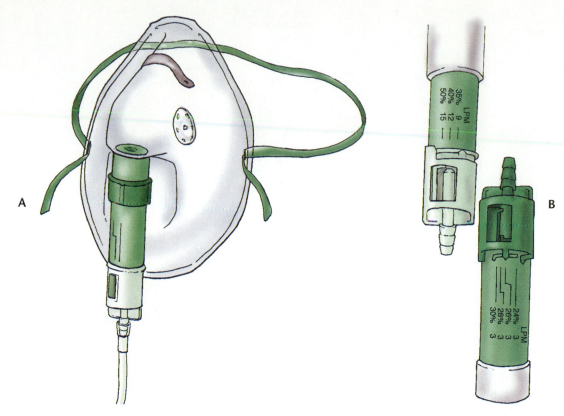

Fig. 9-47 A, A Venturi mask. B, Some Venturi masks are equipped with a control that regulates the amount of ambient air that can enter.

8. Observe the reservoir bag as the patient breathes (if it collapses more than slightly during inspiration, increase the flow rate).

9. Keep the reservoir from kinking or twisting.

10. Continuously monitor the oxygen level in the tank.

Venturi mask

The Venturi mask is a high-flow device that includes oxygen tubing, a face mask, and a Venturi system. As oxygen passes through the jet orifice in the mask, it draws in ambient air. The resulting mixture is delivered to the patient through the face mask. The same amount of ambient air is always entrained regardless of the rate or depth of respirations, thus, fixed concentrations of oxygen (within 1%) can be provided. This mask is particularly useful with patients with COPD, with whom careful control of the inspired oxygen concentration is needed. Some Venturi masks are supplied with a dial that controls the amount of ambient air entrained, whereas others come with interchangeable caps.

Oxygen concentration delivered

Typically, the device delivers oxygen concentrations of 24%, 28%, 35%, or 40%. The liter flow needed depends on the oxygen concentration desired (Fig. 9-47).

As mentioned earlier, oxygen also can be delivered to the patient via a partial rebreather mask, bag-valve-mask unit, or demand valve resuscitator.

ADVANCED AIRWAY MANAGEMENT

In most cases, manual airway control, ventilation, and oxygenation should precede the use of advanced airway adjuncts. This guideline is particularly important when the patient has been apneic or in cardiac arrest for several minutes prior to help arriving. Use of ventilatory support procedures allows the EMT–I to correct profound hypoxia and hypercarbia. However, due to the high pharyngeal pressures (leading to gastric insufflation) created by most ventilatory support procedures, an advanced airway adjunct should be placed as soon as possible to prevent aspiration. The next four adjuncts to be discussed are advanced-level procedures.

- Esophageal obturator airway and esophageal gastric tube airway
- Pharyngotracheal lumen airway
- Esophageal tracheal combitube
- Endotracheal tube

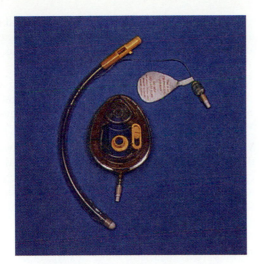

Fig. 9-48 Components of the esophageal obturator airway (EOA).

These devices offer more benefits than basic airway adjuncts; however, they also carry more risks.

Esophageal obturator airway

Description

The esophageal obturator airway (EOA) is a large-bore plastic tube that is open at the top end and closed at the other end (Fig. 9-48). The closed end has a rounded surface and a cuff. On insertion of the tube into the esophagus, the distal cuff is inflated with 30 to 35 mL of air. This inflation effectively occludes the esophagus and prevents regurgitation. Ventilations are delivered through the open end, which is housed in a removable clear plastic face mask. When a proper seal is maintained between the patient's face and the EOA mask, air exits the tube through 16 holes located along its side at the level of the hypopharynx.

Advantages

- It is easy to insert and does not require visualization of the upper airway.
- It prevents gastric distention and regurgitation.
- It delivers ventilations at the level of the hypopharynx.
- It makes it easier to insert an endotracheal tube (because there is only one passageway remaining).
- A high oxygen concentration can be delivered through the device.

Disadvantages

- It can be accidentally passed into the trachea, resulting in life-threatening airway obstruction.
- It may tear or rupture the pharyngeal or esophageal walls during insertion.
- It requires the EMT–I to maintain an effective seal between the mask and the patient's face. Failure to do so results in inadequate tidal volumes being delivered to the patient.
- It does not keep the patient from aspirating foreign materials (such as blood or vomitus) present in the upper airway.

Contraindications

To reduce risks associated with its use, the EOA should not be employed in patients who:

- Are breathing on their own.
- Are under 16 years of age.
- Are under 5 or over 6 feet 7 inches tall.
- Have swallowed caustic substances.
- Have a history of esophageal disease or alcoholism.
- Have a gag reflex.

Because insertion of the EOA will stimulate the gag reflex, it should only be used in the unresponsive patient. If the patient's responsiveness improves and the gag reflex returns, the EOA must be removed. During insertion or removal of the device, a suction unit should be set up near the patient and checked to make sure it is working properly.

 STREET WISE
The EOA should be used with caution in patients experiencing narcotic drug overdose or hypoglycemia because both conditions can be reversed with medication administration and the patient can regain a gag reflex.

Procedure

To insert the EOA, the EMT–I must:

1. Employ body substance isolation precautions.
2. Open the airway manually using the head-tilt/chin-lift or jaw-thrust.
3. While maintaining ventilatory support, hyperventilate the patient with 100% oxygen.
4. Ask another EMT–I to take over ventilating the patient.
5. Select the proper equipment for EOA insertion and check it.

   - Assemble the airway by connecting the tube to the mask. It will click into place when properly seated.
   - Pull back on the plunger of the syringe and draw in 30 to 35 mL of air. Attach the syringe to the one-way valve of the inflation tube and inflate and deflate the distal cuff of EOA to check for leaks. When inserting the tip of the syringe into the one-way inflation valve, use a twisting action to properly seal the syringe.
   - Inflate the mask through the one-way valve until the mask cushion is firm enough to provide a good seal against the patient's face.
   - Lubricate the EOA tube with a water-soluble lubricant if necessary.

6. Kneel at the top of patient's head, placing it into a neutral or slightly flexed position (if trauma is not suspected).

7. Elevate the tongue by grasping the jaw and tongue between the thumb and index finger of the left hand, lifting it anteriorly.

8. With the mask attached, hold the EOA tube at its midpoint, in a J-shaped position.

9. Insert the tip of EOA tube into patient's mouth and advance the tube following the curvature of the pharynx.

10. Continue inserting the tube until the mask rests on the patient's face. If resistance is met, the tube should be withdrawn and another attempt made. Never use force to insert the tube because pharyngeal or esophageal trauma/laceration can occur. The patient should receive assisted breathing between insertion attempts.

11. Advance the tube until the mask is seated against the patient's face.

12. Seal the mask firmly over the patient's mouth and nose.

13. Attach a ventilatory device (such as bag-valve-mask) to the 15-mm connector and deliver a breath. Look for chest rise and auscultate for breath sounds. If chest rise and lung sounds are absent with assisted breathing, placement of the EOA into the trachea should be suspected and the tube withdrawn.

14. If the chest rises and lung sounds are present, inflate the distal cuff with approximately 30 to 35 cubic centimeters of air (Fig. 9-49 A). The amount of air used to inflate the distal cuff is considered patient-dependent (ie, smaller patients need less). Check the pilot bulb to verify that air is inflating the distal cuff (a filled pilot balloon indicates that the distal cuff is inflated). The abdomen also should be auscultated to ensure proper placement of the EOA tube.

15. Keeping pressure on the plunger and using a reverse twisting action to prevent accidental loss of air, remove the syringe from the one-way valve.

16. Ventilate the patient with the head tilted backward (Fig. 9-49 B). This position helps to maintain an open airway. While ventilating the patient, recheck for proper placement, chest rise, and lung sounds and auscultate over the stomach. Make sure there is a good seal between the patient's face and the EOA mask and that the head is properly positioned.

17. If the patient begins to wake or display gag reflex, turn the patient's head to one side and prepare to suction while deflating the distal cuff and removing the EOA.

CARINA: Bifurcation of the trachea into the right and left mainstem bronchi.

Under normal circumstances the distal cuff of a fully inserted EOA lies below the level of the carina. However, in some patients the cuff may actually lie above the level of the carina. Subsequently, inflation of the distal cuff can obstruct the airway as the posterior membranous portion of trachea is compressed. It is recognized by lung sounds and chest rise that are present prior to inflation of the distal cuff but that disappear after the 30 to 35 mL of air is introduced. To correct this problem, air should be withdrawn from the distal cuff until effective air exchange is restored. It may be necessary to remove the EOA if there is any indication that the obstruction is still present.

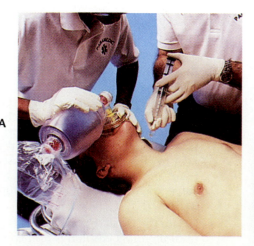
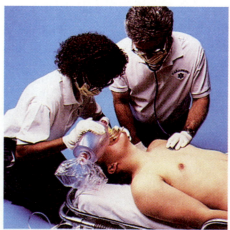

Fig. 9-49   A, Verify placement of the tube and inflate the cuff with 30 to 35 cc of air. B, Ventilate the patient, rechecking for proper tube placement, chest rise, and lung sounds.

Avoiding Incorrect Placement

Great care must be taken when inserting the EOA, because incorrect placement into the trachea will block air flow into the lungs. Before inserting the EOA, the EMT–I must make sure the head and neck are placed in a neutral or flexed forward position. A hyperextended position can cause the tip of the tube to be directed anteriorly into the trachea. When inserting the EOA, the tube should be grasped between its upper and middle thirds in the same way a pencil is grasped. This technique facilitates gentle maneuvering of the tube posteriorly and reduces the risk of pharyngeal trauma. Lastly, the tube must be stored in such a way as to prevent the tube from curling. A curled tube is more likely to drift upward into the trachea during insertion and thus should not be used.

Removal of the EOA

In some cases, it may be necessary to remove the EOA in the field. Given the potential for regurgitation during removal of the device, the patient should be placed on his or her side with suction immediately available. The distal cuff must then be deflated and the tube withdrawn in a steady and gentle manner. Ideally, an endotracheal tube should be in place to protect the airway from aspiration.

Esophageal gastric tube airway
Description

The esophageal gastric tube airway (EGTA) is an improved version of the EOA (Fig. 9-50). Its main advantage is that its tube is open all the way down. This design permits passage of a gastric tube for decompression of the stomach, which alleviates gastric distention and allows suctioning of stomach contents prior to removal of the device. The face mask also is different. Instead of one port, like the EOA, the EGTA has two: one for attachment of the esophageal tube and one for connection to a ventilatory device. During assisted breathing, air is blown into the ventilation port of the mask. With the esophagus blocked, the air has nowhere to go but into the trachea and lungs. The technique for inser-

tion and the complications of the EGTA are the same as those of the EOA.

PHARYNGOTRACHEAL AIRWAYS

Another type of device, the pharyngotracheal airway, is designed to deliver lung ventilation when placed either in the trachea or the esophagus. Several of these devices are available, including the pharyngotracheal lumen airway (PtL) and the esophageal tracheal combitube (ETC). They are designed to be inserted blindly into the oropharynx and esophagus or trachea. Because serious complications with these devices can occur, the EMT–I must receive considerable training and be authorized to use them.

> **CLINICAL NOTES**
> The endotracheal tube is the optimal adjunct to achieve adequate airway protection and ventilation during CPR.

Pharyngotracheal lumen airway
Description

The PtL was developed to address the problems associated with the EOA and EGTA. It is a two-tube, two-cuff system. The first tube is a short, wide tube with a large cuff along its lower portion. When inflated, this cuff seals off the oropharynx and air is introduced through the tube as its proximal end enters the pharynx. A second, longer tube travels through the first, extending past its distal end. Because of its longer length, it can be passed into either the trachea or the esophagus. At the distal end of the longer tube is a cuff that, when inflated, seals off whichever anatomic structure it is in. When the longer tube is in the esophagus, the device acts like an EOA and the patient is ventilated through the first tube. When the longer tube is in the trachea, the device acts like an endotracheal tube and the patient is ventilated through it (Figs. 9-51 and 9-52).

Each tube has a 15/22-mm connector at its proximal end for attachment of a standard ventilatory device. Housed within the second tube is a semirigid plastic stylet that allows the tube to be redirected. On

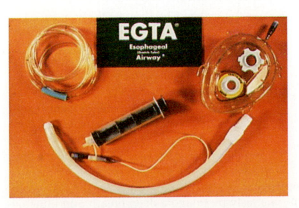

Fig. 9-50 Esophageal gastric tube airway (EGTA).

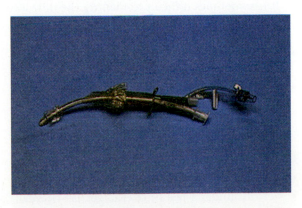

Fig. 9-51 Pharyngotracheal lumen airway (PtL).

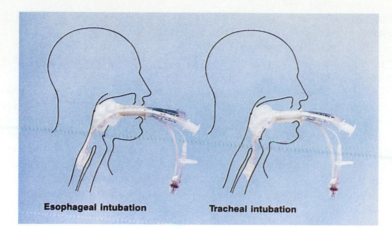

Esophageal intubation   **Tracheal intubation**

Fig. 9-52   Esophageal and tracheal placement of PtL airway.

one side of the cuff inflation valve is a clamp that permits deflation of the oropharyngeal cuff while keeping the other cuff inflated. The device also is equipped with an adjustable cloth neck-strap that keeps the tube in place.

Advantages

- It is inserted blindly, requiring no special equipment or visualization of the upper airway.
- It can be inserted with the patent's head in a neutral position.
- The EMT–I is not required to maintain a face seal because the oropharyngeal cuff eliminates the need for a face mask.
- It can protect the trachea from upper airway bleeding or secretions.

When the longer tube is situated in the esophagus, the oropharynx cuff can be deflated to allow the device to be moved to the left side of the patient's mouth. This action permits endotracheal intubation while continuing esophageal occlusion.

Disadvantages

- It is sometimes difficult to identify the tube location, resulting in ventilation being delivered through the wrong tube.
- The pharyngeal or esophageal walls can be torn or ruptured during insertion.
- The device does not keep the patient from aspirating foreign materials (such as blood or vomitus) present in the upper airway when the longer tube is in the esophagus.

Contraindications

- Persons less than 16 years of age.
- Persons under 5 feet or over 6 feet 7 inches tall.
- When caustic substances have been swallowed.

- When the patient has a history of esophageal disease or alcoholism.
- The presence of a gag reflex.

Procedures

To insert the PtL airway, the EMT–I must:

1. Employ body substance isolation precautions.
2. Open the airway manually using the head-tilt/chin-lift or jaw-thrust.
3. While maintaining ventilatory support, hyperventilate the patient with 100% oxygen.
4. Ask another EMT–I to take over ventilating the patient.
5. Assemble and check the equipment. Close the relief port with the small white cap, open the slide clamp, and blow air into the inflation valve to check the proximal and distal cuffs for proper inflation (Fig. 9-53 A). Once this is done, remove the small white cap and deflate both cuffs fully. Then replace the white cap on the relief port (Fig. 9-53 B).
6. Direct the ventilator to move to the side of the patient's head and kneel above the patient.
7. Place the patient's head into a hyperextended position if there are no suspected spinal injuries. When spinal injury is suspected, the patient's head and neck should be kept in a neutral in-line position. Use the tongue/jaw-lift to move the tongue out of the way.
8. Insert the device into the patient's mouth along the midline. Advance the tube until the flange rests against the patient's teeth (Fig. 9-53 C).
9. Loop the white strap around the patient's head and secure it in place (Fig. 9-53 D).
10. Once in place, inflate both distal cuffs simultaneously by taking a deep breath and blowing into the inflation valve (Fig. 9-53 E).

11. Next, connect a ventilatory device to the green tube (oropharyngeal tube) and deliver a breath. If the chest rises, the longer tube is in the esophagus and ventilations should be continued through the green tube. A gastric tube may be inserted through the long tube into the esophagus and stomach (Fig. 9-53 F, G).

12. If the patient's chest does not rise, the longer tube is in the trachea. The stylet must then be removed from the longer tube and assisted breathing provided through the tube (Fig. 9-53 H).

13. Continue delivering ventilatory support and reassess for proper placement on an ongoing basis.

Esophageal tracheal combitube
Description
The esophageal/tracheal double lumen airway, or Combitube®, is a double lumen tube with two balloon cuffs. It is structurally and functionally similar to the PtL, except for a modified pharyngeal balloon and a simpler basic structure. Two sizes are available for use: a size created for patients between 4 and 5 feet tall, and a size created for patients over 5 feet tall. One cuff is clear in color and located at the tip (distal cuff). The other is a larger, cream-colored cuff located near the halfway point of the tube. The blue lumen is the port used to deliver ventilations when the tube is placed in the esophagus. The clear lumen is the ventilation port if the tube is inserted in the trachea. When inflated, the large cream-colored cuff seals off the oropharynx and nasopharynx. The distal cuff seals off the esophagus or the trachea. A blue pilot balloon and a white pilot balloon correspond to the cream-colored and distal cuffs. Two syringes come in the kit for inflation of the cuffs.

Advantages
Like the EOA and EGTA, the Combitube is inserted without visualization of the vocal cords. Its location is then assessed, and the patient is ventilated through the opening that provides inflation of the lungs. Unlike the EOA and EGTA, there is no need to maintain a constant face mask seal, because the Combitube forms an inflated cuff seal in the oropharynx, and the trachea may be ventilated via a tube rather than a mask. This ease of ventilation is an advantage of the Combitube over the EOA and EGTA.

Other advantages of the Combitube include those listed for the PtL, but because of a difference in design (no stylet in the distal lumen), the ETC allows immediate suctioning of gastric contents. Also, in an undiagnosed tracheal placement, the spontaneously breathing patient may breathe through multiple small ports in the unused lumen. Unlike the PtL, the ETC has a self-adjusting, self-positioning posterior pharyngeal balloon.

Contraindications
Insertion of an Combitube should not be attempted in a responsive or semiresponsive patient who has a gag reflex. Its use also should be avoided in patients under 4 feet tall. Also, it should not be used in patients who are known to have ingested a caustic substance or those who have known esophageal disease.

The following equipment is needed for intubating a patient with the Combitube (Fig. 9-54 A):

- Combitube kit with syringes
- Water-soluble lubricant
- Suctioning unit
- Bag-valve-device or demand valve
- Gloves
- Eye protection

Procedures
To insert the Combitube, the EMT–I must:

1. Employ body substance isolation precautions.

2. If a spinal injury is not likely, open the airway by performing a jaw thrust. In an unresponsive trauma patient, the EMT–I must maintain the neck in a neutral, in-line position during intubation.

3. Next, open and clear the airway of any foreign objects, dentures, vomitus, and/or blood clots. The oropharyngeal airway should be removed if one has been inserted.

4. Assemble and check the proper equipment while the patient is being hyperventilated with 100% oxygen. The Combitube must always be checked to make sure it is working properly before trying to insert it. Connect the blue-tipped syringe (drawn up with at least 100 mL of air) to the blue one-way valve marked tube "No. 1." Then connect the white-tipped syringe (drawn up with at least 15 mL of air) to the white one-way valve marked tube "No. 2." Lubricate the tube with a water-soluble lubricant to facilitate its passage.

5. Direct the ventilator to move to the side of the patient's head and assume a position above the patient. Insert the thumb of the right hand deep into the patient's mouth, grasping the tongue and lower jaw between the thumb and index finger. Lift the tongue and lower jaw anteriorly, away from the posterior pharynx.

6. Hold the Combitube so that it curves in the same direction as the natural curvature of the pharynx. Insert the tip into the mouth along the midline and advance it carefully along the tongue. Gently guide the Combitube along the base of the tongue and into the airway. Do not force the Combitube. If resistance is met, pull back and redirect the Combitube. When the Combitube is at the proper depth, the teeth or alveolar ridge will be between the heavy black lines (Fig. 9-54 B).

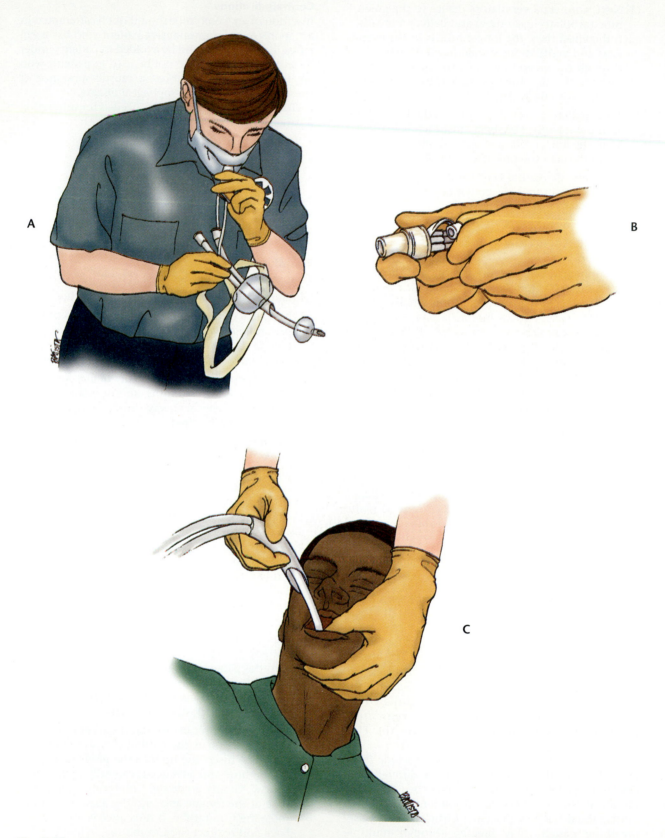

Fig. 9-53 Ventilating a patient using a PtL. *A,* Check the proximal and distal cuffs for proper inflation. *B,* Replace white cap. *C,* Insert the device into the patient's mouth along the midline. *(Continued)*

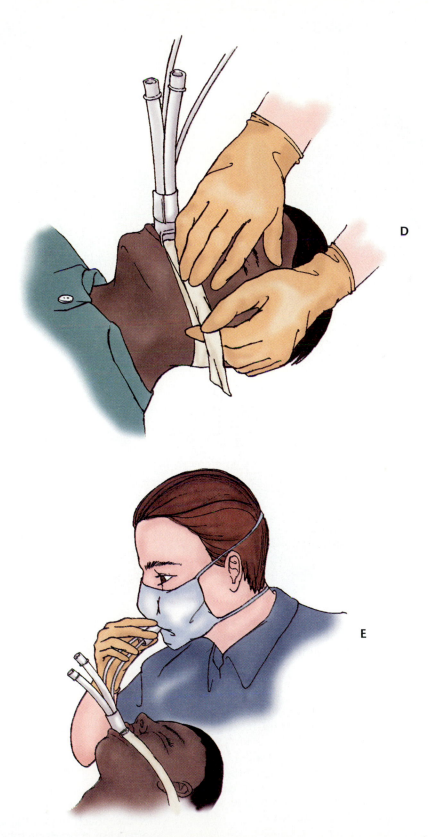

Fig. 9-53 cont'd. D, Loop the white strap around the patient's head and secure the tube in place. E, Inflate both distal cuffs simultaneously.

(Continued)

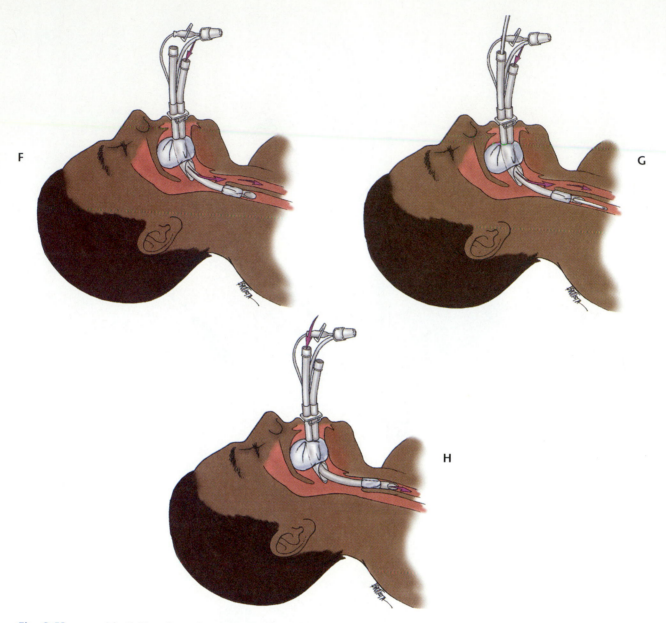

F, Ventilate the patient through the green tube to determine if the longer tube is in the esophagus. G, If the longer tube is in the esophagus, a gastric tube may be inserted into the esophagus and stomach. H, If the longer tube is in the trachea, remove the stylet and proceed with ventilations.

Fig. 9-53 cont'd. F, Ventilate the patient through the green tube to determine if the longer tube is in the esophagus. G, If the longer tube is in the esophagus, a gastric tube may be inserted into the esophagus and stomach. H, If the longer tube is in the trachea, remove the stylet and proceed with ventilations.

7. Next, inflate the blue pilot balloon (and flesh-colored cuff) with the predrawn 100-mL blue-tipped syringe.

8. Once that cuff is inflated and the pilot balloon is tense, immediately inflate the white pilot balloon leading to the smaller distal cuff with the predrawn syringe. The Combitube may move forward slightly, but this is normal.

9. Begin ventilation by attaching the ventilating device to the longer blue connecting tube marked "No. 1."

10. Observe the patient's chest and listen for lung sounds. If the chest rises and falls and breath sounds are heard, the ETC is in the esophagus (Fig. 9-54 C). When this is the case, continue to ventilate through the blue tube.

11. If the chest does not rise and breath sounds are not heard, the Combitube is in the trachea. In this case, attach the ventilation device to the shorter clear connecting tube marked "No. 2" and ventilate the patient through it. Again, listen for breath sounds in all lung fields and in both axillae. Also, listen over the stomach.

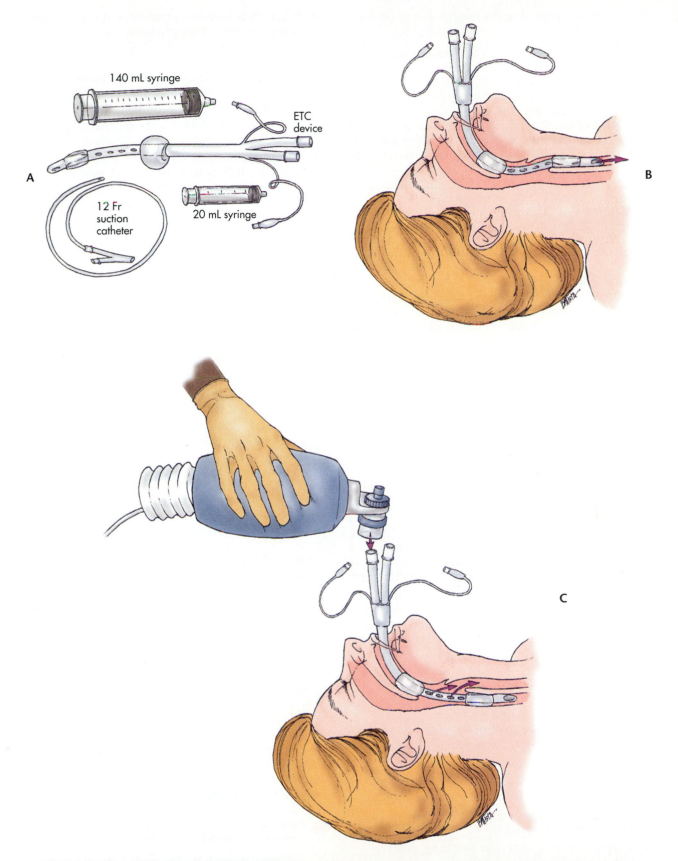

Fig. 9-54   A, Combitube equipment. B, Combitube inserted into trachea. C, Combitube inserted into esophagus.

12. Continue ventilating the patient with a ventilation device.

Throughout placement of the device, the patient should be continuously monitored. Occasionally, the balloon cuffs leak or may be torn by jagged broken teeth, dentures, or bones. Thus, the EMT–I must use special care with this device, especially in the event of facial trauma. The EMT–I should watch for leaks by carefully squeezing the pilot balloon. The syringes can be used to keep the balloon cuffs properly inflated.

STREET WISE
While ventilating a deeply unresponsive patient via the blue tube (No. 1) an endotracheal tube can be inserted around the ETC.

Removing the Combitube

A number of factors may prompt the removal of the Combitube. Removing the device is a fairly simple procedure. First, the patient is turned on his or her side to keep the airway clear of vomitus. When ready, the EMT–I simply deflates the balloon cuffs and gently removes the tube. Because the patient may vomit when the Combitube is removed from the esophagus, a suctioning unit must be readily available.

Endotracheal intubation

ENDOTRACHEAL: Within or through the trachea.
INTUBATION: Passing a tube into an opening of the body.

🍎 Recall the indications, contraindications, and alternatives of endotracheal intubation.

Endotracheal intubation is the insertion of an open-ended tube into the trachea. It is the preferred technique for airway control in patients who are unable to maintain a patent airway in all types of medical and trauma emergencies. Due to the difficulty of the skill, it should only be performed by EMT–Is who are trained and proficient in the procedure.

Indications

- When the EMT–I is unable to ventilate an unresponsive patient with conventional methods.
- When patients cannot protect their airway (coma, respiratory and cardiac arrest).
- When prolonged artificial ventilation is needed.
- In patients experiencing or likely to experience upper airway compromise.
- Unresponsive patients who lack a gag reflex.
- When there is decreased tidal volume due to slow respirations.

- When there is airway obstruction due to foreign bodies, trauma, or anaphylaxis.

Advantages

- Endotracheal intubation seals the trachea, reducing the risk of aspirating blood, vomitus, and other foreign materials into the lungs.
- It facilitates ventilation and oxygenation, because a tight face seal is not required.
- It prevents gastric insufflation, because air is delivered directly into the trachea during positive-pressure ventilation.
- The direct route into the trachea allows for suctioning of the trachea and bronchi.
- It provides an effective route for administration of some medications (epinephrine, atropine, lidocaine, and naloxone). This advantage is particularly beneficial in the presence of peripheral vascular collapse such as often occurs in cardiac arrest.

Disadvantages

- Endotracheal intubation is a complicated skill requiring extensive initial and ongoing training in order to ensure proficiency.
- The procedure requires specialized equipment.
- The vocal cords must be visualized in order to place the tube (when performed orally, using a laryngoscope).

Precautions

- The EMT–I must continually reassess placement of the endotracheal tube; accidental displacement is a common occurrence.

Contraindications

Endotracheal intubation should be avoided in patients who have epiglottitis, because insertion and manipulation of the laryngoscope into the upper airway may precipitate laryngospasm. Rather, in epiglottitis the patient's breathing should be assisted with a bag-valve-mask device until more definitive airway procedures can be performed.

DIGITAL INTUBATION: Intubation using the fingers.

Routes

Endotracheal intubation typically is accomplished using specialized equipment through one of two routes: orotracheal or nasotracheal. It also can be accomplished **digitally** via the orotracheal route.

 Assemble and check the equipment used to perform endotracheal intubation.

List and demonstrate the steps for performing endotracheal intubation.

Equipment

The equipment and supplies used to perform endotracheal intubation include:

- Laryngoscope (handle, blades, and extra batteries and bulb)
- Endotracheal tubes (various size)
- 10-mL syringe for cuff inflation
- Stylet
- Bag-valve-mask device (with supplemental oxygen and reservoir device)
- Suction equipment
- Bite block
- Magill forceps
- Tie-down tape or commercial tube holding device
- Water-soluble lubricant

Laryngoscope

The laryngoscope is used to move the tongue and epiglottis out of the way. This removal allows visualization of the vocal cords and placement of an endotracheal tube. The laryngoscope consists of a handle and blade. The handle holds several batteries that serve as the energy source for the light, which is located in the distal portion of the blade. The light illuminates the airway so the upper airway structures can be seen. On the lower end of the handle is a bar where the hooked indentation of the blade is attached and locked in place (Fig. 9-55).

STREET WISE
The laryngoscope also may be used in conjunction with the Magill forceps to retrieve an upper airway foreign body obstruction.

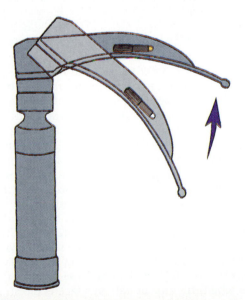

Fig. 9-55   Lock the laryngoscope blade into the handle.

Laryngoscope blades come in a variety of sizes ranging from 1 (for the infant) to 4 (for the large adult patient). There are two types of laryngoscope blades: the curved blade, (Fig. 9-56 A) referred to as the *Macintosh,* and the straight blade, (Fig. 9-56 B) (also referred to as the *Miller, Wisconsin,* or *Flagg*). When used properly, the tip of the curved blade is inserted into the vallecula. In this position, the tongue and epiglottis are raised out of the way when the laryngoscope handle is lifted anteriorly. Two benefits of the curved blade are that it permits more room for visualization of the glottic opening and tube insertion and it is associated with less trauma and reflex stimulation than the straight blade (because many of the sensitive gag receptors are located on the posterior surface of the epiglottis).

In contrast, the straight blade is positioned under the epiglottis. When the handle is lifted anteriorly the epiglottis is lifted out of the way exposing the glottic opening. The straight blade is preferred in infants, because it provides greater displacement of the tongue and better visualization of the glottis, which lies higher and more anterior.

The use of one blade over the other is largely based on user preference because there are advantages to each type of blade. However, the EMT–I should be skilled in the use of both because there are cases in which one blade may be better suited for the patient than the other.

 TRACHEAL LUMEN: Cavity or channel within the trachea.

Endotracheal tube

The endotracheal tube is a flexible, translucent tube that is open at both ends. Its proximal end has a standard 15-mm adapter that can be connected to various devices for delivery of positive-pressure ventilation. Its distal end is beveled to facilitate placement between the vocal cords. It also has a balloon cuff that, when inflated, occludes the remainder of the **tracheal lumen.** This occlusion prevents aspiration around the tube and minimizes air leaks. Attached to the cuff is an inflating tube that has at its end a one-way inflating valve with an inlet port to accept a syringe for inflation. There is a pilot balloon between the one-way valve and the distal cuff, which reveals whether the distal cuff is inflated (Fig. 9-57)

STREET WISE
Some EMT–Is tape the inflation tube to the endotracheal tube to prevent it from being accidentally torn away from the tube. The distal cuff should always be examined for leaks prior to placement in the trachea.

Manufacturers commonly prewrap endotracheal tubes in a curved position to facilitate passage into the trachea. Some endotracheal tubes come with an

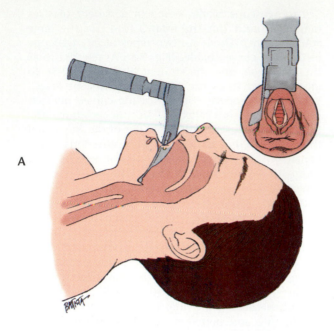

A

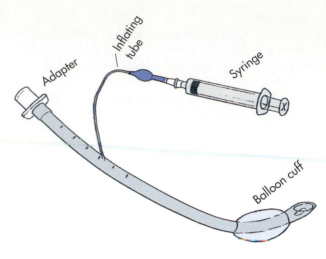

Fig. 9-57   Components of the endotracheal tube.

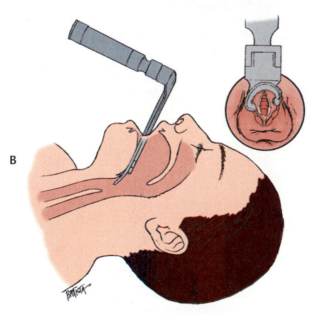

B

Fig. 9-56   A, The Macintosh curved blade is inserted into the vallecula to raise the tongue and epiglottis out of the way. B, The Miller straight blade is positioned under the epiglottis to expose the glottic opening.

O-shaped ring attachment that connects to a plastic wire running the length of the tube and ending distally. Pulling the ring bends the distal end of the tube upward. This bending helps redirect the tube, allowing easier passage into the glottic opening.

Markings on the endotracheal tube indicate its internal diameter (ID). Tubes come in graduated sizes from 3.0 to 9.0 mm. Average sizes for adults are: 7.5 to 8.0 ID for women and 8.0 to 8.5 ID for men. When immediate placement of an endotracheal tube is required, a 7.5 ID tube may be used for both female and male adult patients. Selection of the correct size tube is important—one that is too large can cause tracheal edema and/or damage to the vocal cords. On the other hand, a tube that is too small provides too little airflow and may lead to inadequate ventilatory volumes being delivered. Additionally, it can produce a negative pressure in the lungs, which can lead to pneumothorax and pulmonary edema.

Uncuffed endotracheal tubes are used for infants and children under 8 years of age because the round narrowing of their cricoid cartilage acts as a functional cuff.

Stylet
In cases in which the trachea lies more anterior or the patient has a short, thick neck that makes optimal positioning of the head difficult, the EMT–I may find it difficult to place an endotracheal tube. In cases like this, a bendable plastic-coated wire, called a **stylet**, can be used to shape the endotracheal tube into a "J" or hockey-stick shape, allowing easier manipulation anteriorly. Because the stylet can cause tissue damage it should be recessed at least one-half inch from the distal tip of the endotracheal tube. Although a stylet is not always used, the EMT–I should always keep one close at hand.

Tie-down tape or commercial tube-holding device
To prevent movement or accidental displacement once the tube is in place, it must be secured with tie-down tape or a commercial holding device. Tying is preferred over taping because tape tends to come loose when the tube or patient's face is moist. Alternatively, commercial tube-holding devices work quite well to secure the tube in place.

HELPFUL HINT
The importance of securing the endotracheal tube cannot be understated. Movement of the tube can cause injury to the tracheal mucosa, cardiovascular stimulation, and an elevation in intracranial pressure. During the process of resuscitation, the endotracheal tube can be easily dislodged. This is particularly true when the patient is being moved to the cot or ambulance or into the hospital emergency department. Also, the EMT–I providing ventilatory support may accidentally apply downward pressure on the endotracheal tube, forcing it into the right or left mainstem bronchus. Tying the tube in place prevents accidental movement or displacement.

Magill forceps
The Magill forceps resemble a bent pair of scissors with circle-shaped tips. This device typically is used to remove foreign bodies obstructing the upper airway and redirect the endotracheal tube during nasotracheal intubation.

Other items
During intubation attempts, a suction unit should be on hand to remove secretions and foreign materials from the oropharynx. A water-soluble lubricant should be available to facilitate insertion of the endotracheal tube. Once the endotracheal tube is in place, an oropharyngeal airway can be used as a bite block to prevent the patient from biting and kinking the endotracheal tube.

Use of an airway kit, or intubation wrap ensures that all the equipment and supplies needed to perform endotracheal intubation are readily available. To eliminate potential equipment failure, the airway kit and all the equipment should be inspected at the beginning of each work shift. In volunteer settings in which specific coverage is not provided, the equipment should be checked at least once a week (Fig. 9-58).

Orotracheal route using a laryngoscope

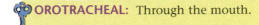
OROTRACHEAL: Through the mouth.

Typically, the **orotracheal** route is used for endotracheal intubation. Its prime advantage over other routes is that it allows the EMT–I to directly observe the endotracheal tube being passed between the vocal cords, which is an essential step for ensuring correct placement. To perform this procedure when no spinal injuries are suspected, the EMT–I should:

1. Employ body substance isolation precautions. At a minimum, gloves and goggles should be worn. A face mask and gown also should be worn when splashing is likely.
2. Use the head-tilt/chin-lift or jaw-thrust to open the patient's airway.
3. While assisting the patient's breathing with 100% oxygen, hyperventilate at a rate of once every 2 to 3 seconds to reduce carbon dioxide levels and increase oxygenation.
4. Direct a partner or first responder to provide ventilatory support of the patient.
5. Assemble and check the equipment (Fig. 9-59A).
- Withdraw the plunger of a 10-mL syringe to pull in 5 to 10 mL of air. Insert the tip of the syringe into the port of the one-way inflation valve, which is connected to the distal cuff. Push the entire contents of the syringe into the distal cuff. It should be firm and have no leaks. Withdraw the air and leave the syringe connected to the inflation valve.

STREET WISE
Use a twisting motion to properly seat the syringe. Otherwise, it may not be inserted deep enough into the one-way inflation valve to allow the introduction of air.

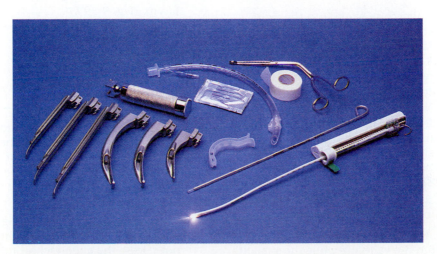
Fig. 9-58 Equipment used in endotracheal intubation.

- Attach the laryngoscope blade to the handle. Once it is properly seated, pull the blade up until it clicks into place and the laryngoscope bulb lights up. The bulb should appear bright white. Move the blade back into its unlocked position until the laryngoscope is required. This action helps to conserve the life of the batteries.

STREET WISE

A yellow, flickering light provides insufficient illumination of the upper airway and suggests the batteries are weak. If the light fails to go on, the EMT–I should suspect that the batteries are dead or the bulb is loose. Infrequently, the problem may lie in the contact point(s) or the wire traveling through the blade to the bulb.

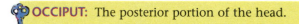

OCCIPUT: The posterior portion of the head.

6. Place the patient's head and neck into a "sniffing position" to align the three axes of the mouth, pharynx, and trachea. The sniffing position is accomplished by flexing the patient's neck forward while, at the same time, tilting the head back. Placing a rolled towel under the patient's shoulders or the **occiput** of the head can facilitate a sniffing position. Accomplishing this task is extremely difficult when the patient has a short, thick neck or when the patient's mobility is limited by arthritis or other such conditions.

7. Using the left hand, grasp the laryngoscope by its handle.

STREET WISE

Most laryngoscopes are designed for right-handed persons. In other words, a right-handed person must hold the laryngoscope in the left hand so that he or she can use the right hand to best manipulate the endotracheal tube.

8. Insert the laryngoscope blade into the right side of the patient's mouth. Using a sweeping motion, displace the tongue to the left. This action pushes the tongue out of the way allowing more room to visualize the upper airway structures and manipulate the endotracheal tube (Fig. 9-59 B).

9. Move the blade slightly toward the midline and advance it until the distal end is positioned at the base of tongue (Figs. 9-59 C, D). Simultaneously, using the index finger of the right hand, push the lower lip away from the blade to prevent injury.

10. Visualize the tip of the epiglottis, then place the laryngoscope blade into the proper position.

   - Remember, the tip of the curved blade is advanced into the vallecula while the straight blade is inserted under the epiglottis.

11. Next, lift the laryngoscope slightly upward and forward to displace the jaw and airway structures without allowing the blade to touch the teeth (Fig. 9-59 E). The epiglottis should come into view unless the blade has been inserted too far, in which case the blade should be withdrawn slowly until the epiglottis is seen (Fig. 9-59 F). Conversely, if the blade is not deep enough into the airway it will need to be advanced. This advancement is facilitated by placing the right thumb into the patient's mouth, grasping the chin, and lifting the jaw up while advancing the laryngoscope.

12. Suction any vomitus or secretions lying in the posterior pharynx. If suctioning fails to resolve the problem, place the patient onto his or her side to facilitate drainage of the secretions. In severe circumstances, it may be necessary to insert an esophageal obturator airway to prevent additional regurgitation of stomach contents.

13. Keeping the left wrist straight, use the shoulder and arm to continue lifting the mandible and tongue at a 45° angle to the ground until the glottis is exposed. Often not all the glottis will be seen, but at least the posterior third or half should be visible.

HELPFUL HINT

If the larynx lies anteriorly, the EMT-I should have a partner or first responder apply firm downward pressure on the patient's neck in the region of the cricoid cartilage. This action pushes the larynx backward allowing better visualization. A stylet may be useful in this situation because the tube can be more easily directed anteriorly.

14. Grasp the endotracheal tube in the right hand, holding it the same way a pencil is grasped. This technique permits gentle maneuvering of the tube. Advance it through the right corner of the patient's mouth, directing the distal end of the tube up or down to pass it into the larynx (Fig. 9-59 G).

STREET WISE

Some clinicians recommend holding the endotracheal tube so it is curved horizontally (bevel sideways). This positioning makes it easier to pass it through the oropharynx.

15. Insert the endotracheal tube into the glottic opening and advance it until the distal cuff disappears slightly ($1/2$ to 1 inch) past the vocal cords. Observe the tube as it enters the glottic opening. This is the first step in ensuring correct placement of the endotracheal tube (Figs. 9-59 H, I).

16. To prevent the tube from being accidentally displaced, hold it in place with the left hand. Do not release the endotracheal tube before it is secured in place.

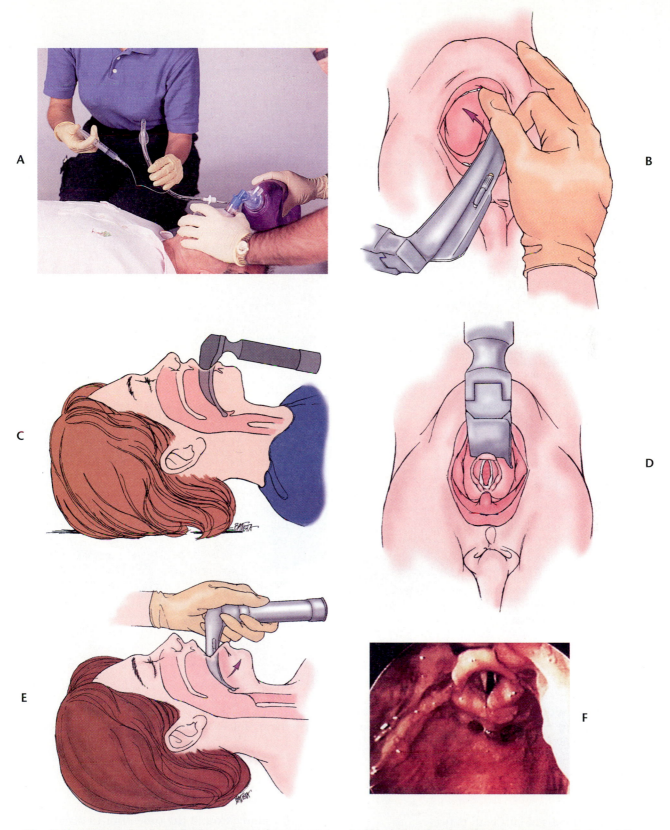

Fig. 9-59 Orotracheal intubation using a laryngoscope. A, Check the distal cuff of the ET tube. B, Insert the laryngoscope blade into the patient's mouth and displace the tongue to the left. C, Move blade toward midline and advance until distal end is positioned at base of tongue. D, An overhead view of laryngoscope placement. E, Lift the laryngoscope upward and forward to displace the jaw and airway structures. F, View of the epiglottis.

(Continued)

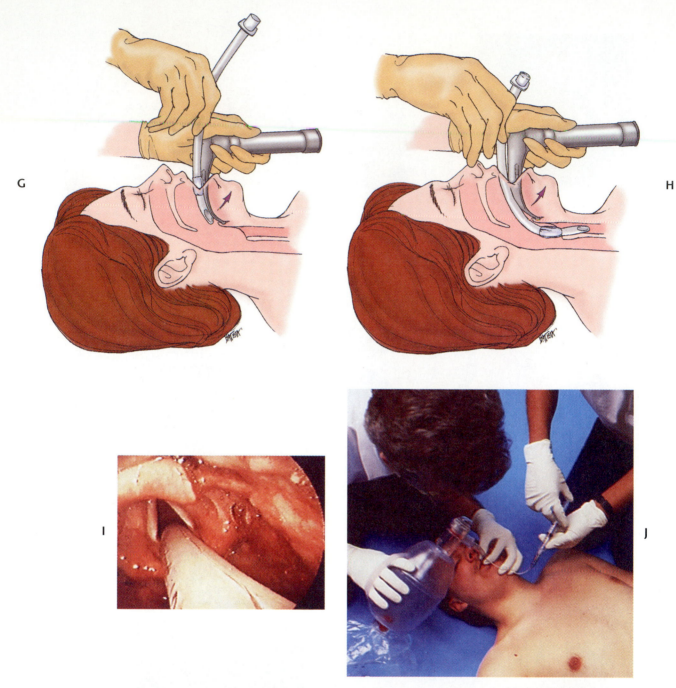

Fig. 9-59 cont'd. **G,** Advance the endotracheal tube into the larynx. **H,** Advance the tube through the glottic opening. **I,** An ET tube passing through the glottic opening. **J,** Inflate the distal cuff while the other rescuer ventilates the patient.

17. Inflate the distal cuff with between 5 to 10 mL of air. Use only the minimum amount of air necessary to create an effective seal. This helps prevent tracheal trauma due to excessive cuff pressure. Determine how much air is needed by listening for the sound of air leaking around the tube prior to distal cuff inflation. The cuff should be inflated only to the point at which air leakage stops (Fig. 9-59 J).

18. Attach a ventilatory device to the 15/22-mm adapter of the tube and deliver several breaths.

19. Recheck for proper tube placement. Auscultate the chest for the presence of equal, bilateral lung sounds. Then listen over the epigastrium to ensure there are no sounds when ventilations are delivered. Next, check the proximal end of the tube for breath condensation during each exhalation. Breath condensation is simply the moisture that is present in exhaled air. It should disappear each time the patient breathes in or a ventilation is delivered. The absence of breath condensation during exhalation suggests improper placement of the tube.

20. Hyperventilate the patient with 100% oxygen and insert an oropharyngeal airway to serve as a bite block.

21. Secure the endotracheal tube in place with umbilical tape or a commercial device while continuing ventilatory support. Loop the tape around the endotracheal tube at the level of the patient's teeth, securing it tightly to the tube without kinking or pinching it. Then wrap the tape around the patient's head and tie it at the side of the neck.

22. Continue supporting the tube manually while maintaining ventilations. Regularly check to ensure proper tube position because it can be easily dislodged during resuscitation efforts or movement of the patient. A pulse oximetry unit should be applied because it provides immediate, ongoing assessment of the oxygen saturation.

Complications

A variety of complications can occur during endotracheal intubation.

Hypoxia

Hypoxia can develop prior to placement of the endotracheal tube if intubation attempts are longer than appropriate or if the EMT–I fails to provide ventilatory support between procedures. For this reason, each intubation attempt should be limited to no more than 30 seconds. It is seldom absolutely necessary to place the endotracheal tube on the first attempt. Unless placement can be easily accomplished, the first attempt may be better used to give the EMT–I an initial view of the patient's anatomy. Subsequent attempts (interspersed between hyperventilation with a bag-valve-mask device and 100% oxygen) then can be used to place the tube.

Injury to teeth and tissue

Injuries to the tissues or teeth can be avoided by gently guiding the laryngoscope blade into place and not allowing it to touch the teeth. When manipulating the jaw anteriorly, the EMT–I should employ upward traction rather than following the natural inclination to rotate and flex the wrist. From that point on, the left wrist should remain straight, with all lifting done from the shoulder and arm.

 Demonstrate the methods used to ensure correct placement of the endotracheal tube.

Misplacement of the tube

Accidental placement of the endotracheal tube into the vallecula, pyriform sinus, esophagus, or mainstem bronchus can have dire consequences.

 SUBCUTANEOUS EMPHYSEMA: Presence of air beneath the skin (in the subcutaneous tissues), giving it a characteristic crackling sensation on palpation.

Vallecula and pyriform misplacement
Vallecula placement occurs when the tube is allowed to slip too far anteriorly and becomes lodged in the space between the epiglottis and base of the tongue. Alternatively, if the tube strays from the midline it can get hung up on either side of the epiglottis in the pyriform sinus (Fig. 9-60 A). This condition is recognized by the skin "bulging out" on either side of the laryngeal prominence (Adam's apple) (Fig. 9-60 B). Forceful efforts to pass the endotracheal tube can perforate these tissues, leading to an absence of ventilation (hypoxia, hypercarbia, death), serious bleeding, and **subcutaneous emphysema.** Vallecula misplacement can be resolved by slightly withdrawing and redirecting the tube posteriorly. Pyriform sinus misplacement can be resolved by slightly withdrawing and rotating the tube to the midline.

Endobronchial misplacement
If the endotracheal tube is inserted too far it will pass into either the right or left mainstem bronchus (Fig. 9-61). Endobronchial intubation results in hypoxia due to one-lung ventilation. Endobronchial intubation is suspected when auscultation of the chest reveals the presence of good lung sounds on one side of the chest but diminished or absent lung sounds on the other side. Poor compliance, felt when delivering ventilations with the bag-valve-mask; cyanosis; and other signs of hypoxia such as cardiac dysrhythmias also suggest endobronchial intubation. The pulse oximetry unit is another useful tool for detecting changes in oxygenation that can help the EMT–I to determine that the tube has been inserted too far.

To correct this problem, the tube should be withdrawn until lung sounds are heard equally on both side of the chest. To prevent the tube from being inserted too far, the EMT–I should:

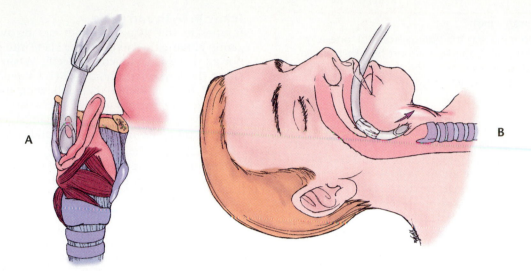

Fig. 9-60   A, A misplaced ET tube in pyriform sinus. B, A characteristic bulge resulting from tube misplacement.

- Advance the distal cuff past the vocal cords no more than 0.5 to 1 inch.
- Once in this position, continue to hold the tube in place with one hand. This prevents the tube from being accidentally inserted any further.
- Firmly secure the tube in place with umbilical tape or a commercial tube holding device to prevent it from being accidentally advanced.
- Mark the side of the endotracheal tube at the level where it emerges from the mouth, which allows quick identification of any changes in tube placement.

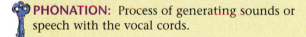

PHONATION: Process of generating sounds or speech with the vocal cords.

Esophageal intubation

Accidental misplacement of the tube into the esophagus has catastrophic results (Fig. 9-62). If left uncorrected, it leads to severe hypoxia and brain death because neither assisted breathing nor oxygen are provided to the patient. Esophageal intubation can be identified by: 1) an absence of chest rise and breath sounds with assisted breathing, 2) gurgling sounds heard over the epigastrium with each breath delivered, 3) an absence of breath condensation collecting inside the endotracheal tube, 4) a persistent air leak despite inflation of the distal cuff of the endotracheal tube, 5) cyanosis and a progressive worsening of the patient's condition, and 6) **phonation.**

A number of commercially available devices also can be used to indicate correct placement of the tube in the trachea. Attached to the proximal end of the tube, some devices are designed to generate a whistlelike sound with expiration when the tube is properly positioned, whereas others change color to

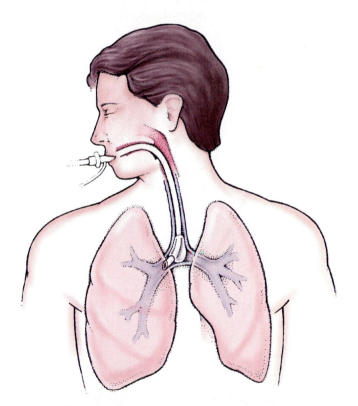

Fig. 9-61   Misplacement of ET tube into right mainstem bronchus.

reflect the amount of carbon dioxide present in the expired air.

If correct placement is uncertain, the location of the endotracheal tube can be checked visually using a laryngoscope. If it is suspected that the tube is in the esophagus, it should be removed.

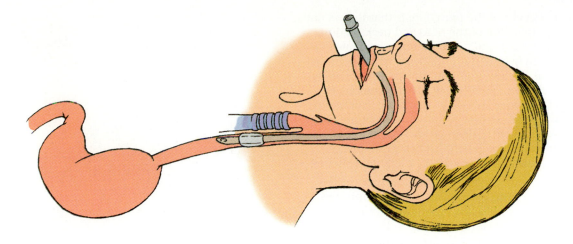

Fig. 9-62   **Misplacement of ET tube into esophagus.**

CLINICAL NOTES

With some cases of esophageal intubation, vomitus will propel from the tube. This occurs due to the high gastric pressures brought about by the resuscitation efforts, particularly because several breaths usually have been delivered as a means of checking for proper tube placement. When this event occurs, the tube should be left in place, because removing it can result in vomitus traveling up into the pharynx and subsequently being aspirated into the trachea. In these cases the tube is essentially functioning as a gastric tube. The EMT–I should simply displace the tube to the side of the mouth and ventilate the patient with a bag-valve-mask device until the trachea can be successfully intubated.

Endotracheal intubation with an EOA in place

There may be situations when the EMT–I is required to place an endotracheal tube in patients who have been intubated with an EOA. Although somewhat cumbersome, endotracheal intubation can be accomplished with the EOA in place.

The steps for performing endotracheal intubation with an EOA in place are basically the same as orotracheal intubation, but, in addition, the EMT–I should:

1. Remove the EOA mask by pinching the obturator tube where it extends through the plastic housing and lifting off the mask

2. Insert the laryngoscope blade into the right side of the patient's mouth. With a sweeping action, displace the tongue and EOA tube to the left. Proceed with intubation in the usual manner.

3. Under direct observation, insert the endotracheal tube into the glottic opening and pass it until the distal cuff disappears past the vocal cords. Then advance the tube slightly ($\frac{1}{2}$ to 1

inch). The appropriate precautions should be used to ensure that the tube has passed into the glottic opening because the distensible esophagus easily can accommodate two tubes–the esophageal obturator and the endotracheal tube.

4. Hold the tube in place with one hand to prevent displacement. Attach a bag-valve-mask to the 15/22-mm adapter of the tube and deliver several breaths.

5. Check for proper tube placement (lung sounds, chest rise, absence of sounds in the epigastrium when ventilations are delivered).

6. Inflate the distal cuff with 5 to 10 mL of air and remove the syringe.

7. Recheck for proper placement of the tube.

8. Hyperventilate the patient with 100% oxygen.

9. Secure the endotracheal tube in place with umbilical tape while continuing to maintain ventilatory support.

10. With suction available, deflate the distal cuff of the EOA. Hold the endotracheal tube firmly in place and remove the EOA tube in a steady manner. The EOA tube must be removed to prevent esophageal or tracheal damage that may result from having two distal cuffs in place at the same time.

11. Maintain ventilatory support, checking periodically to ensure proper tube position.

Digital intubation

Several hundred years ago intubation was performed without the benefit of a laryngoscope and was known as digital (finger) or tactile (touch) intubation. Today, this procedure is useful for a number of prehospital care situations including when the patient is deeply comatose or in cardiac arrest and proper positioning is difficult to achieve (such as the extrication situation).

A primary benefit of the procedure is that it does not require manipulation of the head and neck. Additionally, because this technique does not necessitate visualization, it may be useful in patients who have facial injuries that destroy the anatomy or when copious amounts of blood, vomitus, or other secretions block the EMT–I's view despite adequate suctioning attempts. Two other uses for the procedure are when there is equipment failure or in disaster situations when intubation equipment is in short supply.

To perform digital intubation, the EMT–I should:

1. Employ body substance isolation precautions. At a minimum, gloves and goggles should be worn. A face mask and gown also should be worn when splashing is likely.

2. While assisting the patient's breathing with 100% oxygen, hyperventilate at a rate of once every 2 to 3 seconds to reduce carbon dioxide levels and increase oxygenation. If copious amounts of vomitus, blood, or secretions are present, the patient should be suctioned before intubation is attempted.

3. Direct a partner or first responder to provide ventilatory support of the patient.

4. Assemble and check the equipment:
   - Appropriately sized endotracheal tube
   - Malleable stylet
   - Water-soluble lubricant
   - 5- to 10-cc syringe
   - Bite block
   - Tape or endotracheal tube securing device

5. Insert the stylet into the endotracheal tube and bend the tube and stylet combination into a "J" or hockey-stick configuration.

6. With a fellow crew member or partner stabilizing the patient's head and neck in an in-line position, kneel at the patient's left shoulder, facing the patient. Place the bite block (or other such device) between the patient's teeth to prevent injury to the fingers.

7. Insert the middle and index fingers of the left hand into the patient's mouth. Alternating fingers, "walk" down the patient's tongue, pulling the tongue and epiglottis away from the glottic opening, within reach of the probing fingers (Fig. 9-63 A).

8. Palpate the epiglottis with the middle finger.

9. Press the epiglottis forward and insert the endotracheal tube into the mouth anterior to the fingers.

10. Advance the tube with the right hand (Fig. 9-63 B). Use the index finger of the left hand to maintain the tip of the tube against the middle finger, guiding the tip to the epiglottis.

11. Use the middle and index fingers to manipulate the tube tip until it is between the epiglottis (in

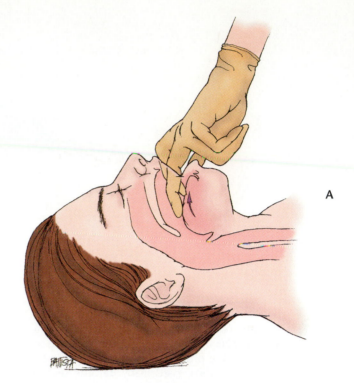

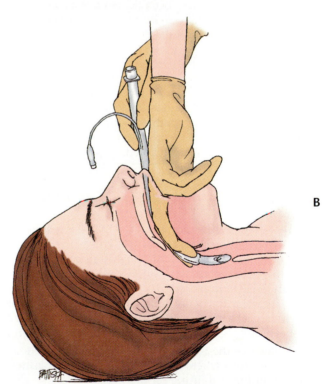

Fig. 9-63 Digital intubation. A, "Walk" down the patient's tongue. B, Insert the endotracheal tube into the mouth anterior to the fingers.

front) and the fingers (behind). Then advance the tube with the right hand through the cords as the index and middle fingers of the left hand press the tube forward to prevent it from falling back into the esophagus.

12. Once the tube is in the trachea, hold it in place with one hand to prevent displacement. Attach a bag-valve-mask to the 15/22-mm adapter of the tube and deliver several breaths.

13. Check for proper tube placement (chest rise when ventilations are delivered).

14. Inflate the distal cuff with 5 to 10 cc of air, remove the syringe.

15. Recheck for proper placement of the tube by listening for lung sounds or absence of sounds in the epigastrium when ventilations are delivered.

16. Hyperventilate the patient with 100% oxygen.

17. Secure the endotracheal tube in place with umbilical tape or a commercial device while maintaining assisted breathing.

18. Maintain ventilation, periodically checking to ensure proper tube position.

Transillumination (lighted stylet) method

An alternative way of performing endotracheal intubation is the transillumination method. With this method, a bright light, introduced into the larynx or trachea, shines through the soft tissues of the neck. This illumination allows the EMT–I to pass an endotracheal tube through the glottic opening without having to directly visualize the structures. As with digital intubation, this procedure permits endotracheal intubation to be performed without manipulating the head and neck. To perform the transillumination technique, a bendable stylet is used. At its distal end is a small high-intensity bulb. Power for the device is supplied by a small battery.

Contraindications

In non-emergency situations, this method is not recommended for patients who have epiglottitis, or when a foreign body is in the airway.

The biggest problem associated with this technique is that outside light can make it difficult to see the light from the stylet. This method works best in a darkened room and with thin patients. In direct sun or bright daylight the patient's neck should be shielded. To use the transillumination technique, the EMT–I must:

1. Employ body substance isolation precautions. At a minimum, gloves and goggles should be worn. A face mask and gown also should be worn when splashing is likely.

2. While assisting the patient's breathing with 100% oxygen, hyperventilate at a rate of once every 2 to 3 seconds to reduce carbon dioxide levels and increase oxygenation.

3. Direct a partner or first responder to provide ventilatory support of the patient.

4. Assemble and check the equipment:
   - Appropriately sized endotracheal tube
   - Lighted stylet
   - Water-soluble lubricant
   - 5- to 10-mL syringe
   - Bite block
   - Tape or endotracheal tube securing device

5. Insert the stylet into the endotracheal tube and bend the tube and stylet combination to form a tight 90° angle.

6. Placing the bend too proximal, or making "too soft" a bend may make proper tube placement difficult.

7. Turn on the stylet light.

8. Grasp the lower jaw and lift it anteriorly. This elevates the tongue and the epiglottis.

9. Introduce the lightwand through the mouth, then use a gentler, rocking motion to place the tube in the glottic opening.

10. When the lightwand enters the glottis, a clearly defined glow transilluminates the cartilage.

11. Hold the tube in place with one hand to prevent displacement and remove the stylet. Attach a bag-valve-mask to the 15/22-mm adapter of the endotracheal tube and deliver several breaths.

12. Check for proper tube placement (lung sounds, chest rise, absence of sounds in the epigastrium when ventilations are delivered).

13. Inflate the distal cuff with 5 to 10 mL of air.

14. Recheck for proper tube placement and continue delivering ventilations while securing the tube in place.

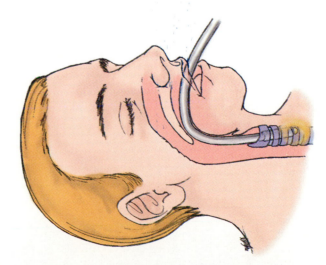

Fig. 9-64   Proper positioning of a transillumination intubation.

CASE HISTORY FOLLOW-UP

EMT–I Simms continues to administer 100% oxygen and assist ventilations en route to the trauma center. The patient's carotid pulse grows stronger and slows from 140 to 90 per minute. His pulse oximetry reading raises from 78% to 92%, and he begins responding with purposeful movement.

In another few minutes, however, he begins to struggle against the straps, fighting EMT–I Simms' attempts to ventilate him. His face becomes flushed, and his neck muscles strain. EMT–I Simms has to extubate him.

EMT–I Simms turns on the suction and places the rigid catheter next to the patient's head as she places a 10-cc syringe in the balloon port and removes the air. She withdraws the tube.

EMT–I Simms watches the patient closely for signs of vomiting or respiratory depression as she places a nonrebreather mask on him with 15 L/min of oxygen. She notes that the patient's speech is slurred as he makes abusive comments to her and her crew. It looks as though he has a good chance of making it.

SUMMARY

Airway management is a critical element of prehospital care. To be effective the EMT–I must practice airway skills on an ongoing basis so that all necessary procedures can be performed automatically.

Airway management centers around maintaining the respiratory system's primary function: moving air in and out of the body and supplying the bloodstream with adequate oxygen. To accomplish this goal, the airway must be patent, there must be adequate oxygen in the inspired air, and the respiratory minute volumes must be sufficient to remove appropriate levels of carbon dioxide.

First, the airway must be secured. Basic maneuvers such as the head-tilt chin-lift can be used to move the tongue and epiglottis away from their obstructing positions. When a cervical spine injury is likely, the chin-lift should be employed without the head-tilt. The EMT–I can use a variety of procedures and devices to support a patient's breathing. Of these procedures, the bag-valve-mask device offers the most advantages. However, it is difficult to use when ventilating the nonintubated patient, so its use must be practiced frequently to ensure proficiency during emergency situations. Inspired oxygen concentrations can be increased using a variety of delivery devices. The nonrebreather mask delivers close to 100% oxygen, making it the preferred device for severely ill or injured patients.

Endotracheal intubation is the preferred technique for securing the airway because it prevents aspiration of foreign materials and allows for efficient delivery of assisted breathing. However, endotracheal intubation has its hazards because accidental misplacement of the tube can result in severe hypoxia and death. When performing endotracheal intubation, care must be taken to prevent injury to the teeth and tissue. Although orotracheal intubation is the most commonly used procedure, there are a number of alternative methods for use in situations when head and neck manipulation must be avoided, including digital intubation and the transillumination method.

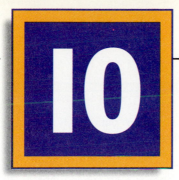

ASSESSMENT AND MANAGEMENT OF SHOCK

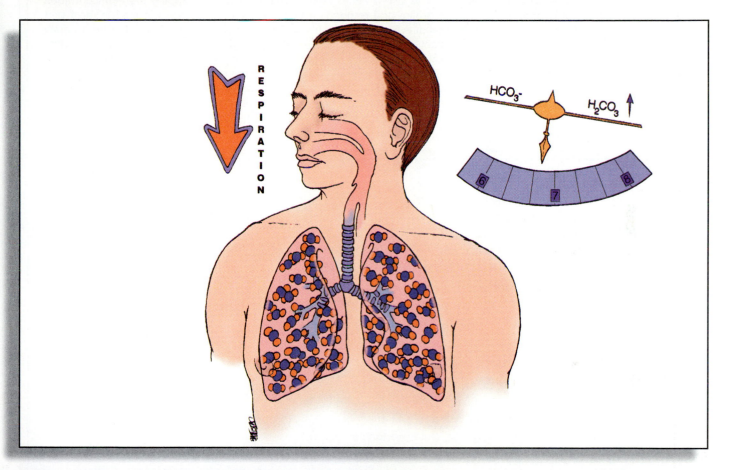

CASE HISTORY

EMT–Intermediates Harris and Peters have been dispatched to a local residence for a medical emergency. En route they are advised that a home-health nurse has requested transport of a patient to a nearby hospital. The patient is reported to be semiresponsive. No other information is available.

As the EMT–Is approach the neighborhood, they notice that all the homes look alike. The neighborhood is in an older, low-income area of town where most of the residents are elderly. The EMT–Is see the nurse waving them down at the front door. They pull into the driveway, gather their gear, and go into the house.

The nurse leads the EMT–Is to a back room where they find a frail, elderly woman lying on a bed. The room is dark and dingy, and the "smell of sickness" is in the air. The nurse tells Harris and Peters that he was recently assigned this patient

Case History, continued

through social services. He knows little about the woman's medical history other than she is a cancer patient who had been treated at the city clinic for the "flu" last week. When he arrived 30 minutes ago, he found her in this condition. At that time, her vital signs were blood pressure 84/50, pulse 110, and respirations 24 and shallow. The patient's lung sounds revealed wheezing and fine crackles. She was hot to the touch with a fever of 101° F.

EMT–I Harris attempts to arouse the patient as EMT–I Peters inserts a nasal airway and applies high-concentration oxygen by nonrebreather mask. The woman groans and responds with purposeful movement, but for the most part "she's out of it." EMT–I Harris contacts medical direction and gives her patient report. The physician orders her to draw a "red top," perform a dextrose stick, and establish an IV line of lactated Ringer's solution. The woman's veins are difficult to see or palpate. EMT–I Harris attempts cannulation with a 16-gauge catheter in the patient's right forearm, but the vein blows and a hematoma quickly develops. A second attempt with an 18-gauge catheter in the left forearm is successful. The patient's serum glucose is normal. The EMT–Is prepare the pneumatic antishock garment, position the patient supine with her legs elevated 10 to 12 inches, package her, and move her to the ambulance. En route to the emergency department, EMT–I Harris sponges the patient's forehead with saline. Although she is not sure the woman can hear her, EMT–I Harris consoles her and tells her that she is in good hands.

LEARNING OBJECTIVES

Upon completion of this chapter, the EMT- Intermediate should be able to:

- EXPLAIN the difference between aerobic and anaerobic metabolism.
- DESCRIBE the importance of tissue perfusion.
- LIST the four elements of the Fick principle.
- LIST the primary components of the cardiovascular system and their roles.
- DISCUSS the role of water in its relationship with body function.
- DISCUSS the fluid compartments of the body.
- IDENTIFY the significant anions and cations in the body.
- EXPLAIN the role of the semipermeable membrane in the function of the cell.
- DISCUSS the concepts of diffusion, facilitated diffusion, osmosis, osmotic pressure, and active transport.
- GIVE EXAMPLES of isotonic, hypotonic, and hypertonic solutions.
- EXPLAIN the function of plasma, erythrocytes, leukocytes, platelets, hemoglobin, and hematocrit in blood.
- DESCRIBE the role of antigens and antibodies in the body.
- EXPLAIN the Rh factor of the blood.
- DESCRIBE acids and bases in relationship to pH.
- EXPLAIN how the buffer systems, respiration, and kidney function help to maintain acid-base balance in the body.
- DESCRIBE the three principal stages of shock.
- LIST the five types of shock.
- DISCUSS the proper assessment and management of the patient in shock.
- DISCUSS the role of the pneumatic antishock garment in the management of shock.
- DESCRIBE fluid replacement in the management of the patient in shock.

KEY TERMS

ACID
ACTIVE TRANSPORT
AEROBIC METABOLISM
AFTERLOAD
ANAEROBIC METABOLISM
ANAPHYLACTIC SHOCK
ANION
ANTIBODY
ANTIGEN
BARORECEPTORS
BASE
CARDIOGENIC SHOCK
CATIONS
CONTRACTILITY
DIFFUSION
ELECTROLYTES
ERYTHROCYTES
EXTRACELLULAR FLUID
FACILITATED DIFFUSION
FICK PRINCIPLE
HEMATOCRIT
HEMOGLOBIN
HISTAMINE
HYPERTONIC SOLUTION
HYPOPERFUSION
HYPOPERFUSION SYNDROME
HYPOTONIC SOLUTION
HYPOVOLEMIC SHOCK

INTERSTITIAL FLUID
INTRACELLULAR FLUID
INTRAVASCULAR FLUID
ISOTONIC SOLUTION
LEUKOCYTES
METABOLIC ACIDOSIS
METABOLIC ALKALOSIS
MILLIEQUIVALENT
NEUROGENIC SHOCK
OSMOSIS
PERFUSION
PERMEABILITY
pH
PLASMA
PLATELETS
PNEUMATIC ANTISHOCK GARMENT
PRELOAD
PSYCHOGENIC SHOCK
RESPIRATORY ACIDOSIS
RESPIRATORY ALKALOSIS
Rh FACTOR
SEMIPERMEABLE
SEPTIC SHOCK
SHOCK
SOLUTES
SOLVENT
STROKE VOLUME

INTRODUCTION

Understanding and caring for the patient in shock is a challenge requiring keen assessment skills and the ability to make rapid, organized decisions. If treatment is performed inadequately or too late, the patient may die immediately from cardiac failure or may survive without brain function. The patient also may die in a few days to a few weeks, due to the failure of organs such as the lung, kidney, or liver.

This chapter addresses the pathophysiology of shock; the basics of cellular physiology, fluids, and electrolytes; acid-base balance; and the assessment and management of shock.

PATHOPHYSIOLOGY OF SHOCK

Shock cannot be defined simply in terms of blood pressure, pulse rate, and respiration nor by superficial symptoms, such as cool and clammy skin. These indicators are some of the signs and symptoms of shock, but they do not indicate what is happening on the cellular level.

 Explain the difference between aerobic and anaerobic metabolism.

Describe the importance of tissue perfusion.

 PERFUSION: The process by which oxygenated blood is delivered to the body's tissue and wastes are removed from the tissue.
SHOCK: The body's response to poor perfusion.
ANAEROBIC METABOLISM: Metabolism without oxygen.

All cells require oxygen to survive. The delivery of oxygenated blood to the tissues is known as **perfusion** (Fig. 10-1). When perfusion falls below a level necessary to sustain life, **shock** occurs. The lack of tissue perfusion leads to **anaerobic** (without oxygen) metabolism and the build-up of toxic waste products in the cells. If left uncorrected, the cells die. Shock is sometimes referred to as **hypoperfusion** (*hypo* means deficient) or **hypoperfusion syndrome.** To understand shock, it is helpful to know the normal processes involved with taking in oxygen and cellular metabolism.

Oxygen in-take

 List the four elements of the Fick principal.

For oxygen to be delivered to the body's cells, four components must be in place. These factors are collectively known as the **Fick principle** (Fig. 10-2).

1. Inspiration of adequate oxygen in the atmospheric air. This process requires adequate ventilation of the lungs, a high concentration of inspired oxygen, and unobstructed passage through the air passageway.

2. On-loading of oxygen to the red blood cells at the lungs. This process requires minimal obstruction to the diffusion of oxygen across the alveolar/capillary membrane (*ie,* no edema) and appropriate binding of oxygen to hemoglobin.

3. Delivery of the red blood cells to the tissue cells. This process requires normal hemoglobin levels, circulation of the oxygenated red blood cells to the tissues in need, adequate cardiac function, an adequate volume of blood flow, and proper routing of blood through the vasculature (blood vessels).

4. Off-loading of oxygen from the red blood cells to the tissue cells. This process requires close proximity of the tissue cells to the capillaries to allow for diffusion of oxygen, and ideal conditions of pH and temperature.

The basic premise of the Fick principle is that the quantity of oxygen delivered to a body organ is equal to the amount of oxygen consumed by that organ plus the amount of oxygen carried away from the organ. For this process to function normally, there must be enough red blood cells available to deliver adequate amounts of oxygen to tissue cells.

Cellular metabolism

The body is made up of billions and billions of cells. These cells require a continuous supply of oxygen and nutrients (*eg,* the simple sugar glucose is the main energy source for the cells) to live. Depending on the workload and needs of the body, physiologic mechanisms ensure that appropriate nutrients and oxygen are available to allow the cells to carry out their life-sustaining functions.

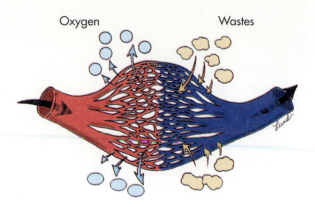

Fig. 10-1 Perfusion is the delivery of oxygenated blood to the tissues.

AEROBIC METABOLISM: Metabolism that occurs with oxygen.

Cellular metabolism begins with food being broken down for energy in a series of reactions, called *cellular respiration.* The first part of this process can occur without oxygen; it is anaerobic. This step yields a very small amount of energy and produces a byproduct called *pyruvic acid.* In low-oxygen states, pyruvic acid is converted to lactic acid. Normally, lactic acid is produced in the muscles during periods of exertion and exercise. Although some small and primitive organisms, such as certain bacteria, can survive using anaerobic metabolism alone, humans cannot survive long with so little energy. A more complete use of food is necessary for survival. **Aerobic** (with oxygen) metabolism allows the human body to use food for energy more completely.

What happens to the body in shock?

In **aerobic metabolism** the combination of oxygen and glucose fuels the individual cells and produces energy (Fig. 10-3). Waste products such as carbon dioxide (CO_2) are produced as a by-product of this reaction and are moved away from the tissues into the blood. Wastes are excreted from the body by the lungs, kidneys, and liver. Oxygen also plays an important role in preventing the accumulation of lactic acid, a waste product that can cause muscle fatigue. Small amounts of lactic acid can be metabolized by the body. In prolonged anaerobic metabolism, however, there is an excess of lactic acid, which the body is unable to handle. This excess causes an increase in hydrogen ions in the blood. As a result, the pH in the blood decreases, and metabolic acidosis occurs. Unresolved acidosis eventually results in cellular death.

A patient in shock experiences **anaerobic metabolism** (Fig. 10-4). The body can continue to function without breathing (therefore without oxygen) for 4 to 6 minutes before irreversible damage is done to the brain. The heart and lungs also

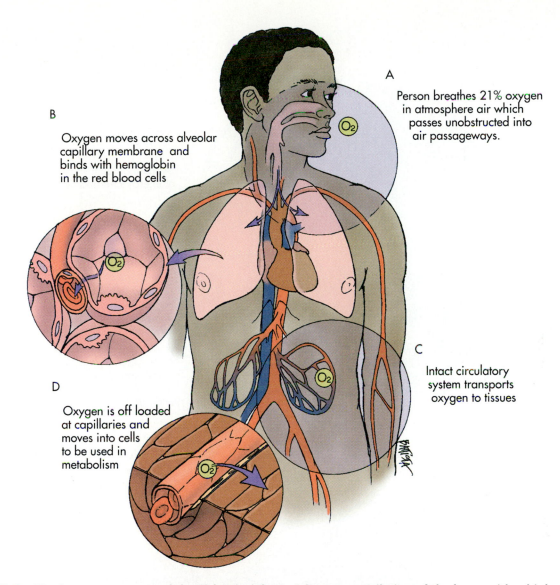

B
Oxygen moves across alveolar capillary membrane and binds with hemoglobin in the red blood cells

A
Person breathes 21% oxygen in atmosphere air which passes unobstructed into air passageways.

D
Oxygen is off loaded at capillaries and moves into cells to be used in metabolism

C
Intact circulatory system transports oxygen to tissues

Fig. 10-2   The four components of the Fick principle. A, Adequate ventilation of the lungs with a high concentration of oxygen. B, Oxygen binds with hemoglobin. C, Oxygen is transported via the circulatory system. D, Oxygen is off-loaded in the capillaries, and is used for metabolism.

are very sensitive to a lack of oxygen during this 4 to 6 minute interval. Other body organs will react in their own time, eg, the abdominal organs may be able to survive from 45 to 90 minutes without oxygen. Skin and muscle may survive for up to 4 to 6 hours. Therefore, death from shock can occur within minutes or hours or may take up to several weeks.

CLINICAL NOTES
An oxygen deficiency does not have to be extreme to cause the body to be less efficient; ie, anaerobic metabolism does not produce as much energy as aerobic metabolism.

When the oxygen concentration of the blood circulating in the body decreases, the body compensates by sending blood to the top priority organs—the heart and lungs. The body does this by shunting

(moving) blood away from less essential systems, such as the liver, intestines, muscle, bone, and skin.

BARORECEPTORS: Sensory nerve endings that adjust blood pressure as a result of vasodilation or vasoconstriction.

Baroreceptors are found in the walls of the atria of the heart, vena cava, aortic arch, and carotid sinus. The baroreceptors (sensory nerve endings) detect a drop in blood pressure and a decrease in blood flow (circulation). The brain receives this information and sends a signal to the sympathetic nervous system. Norepinephrine is released, triggering constriction of the smooth muscles in the peripheral arterioles and venules. Blood is shunted from the peripheral vasculature to the internal organs. The heart rate increases, as does the strength of cardiac contractions. The

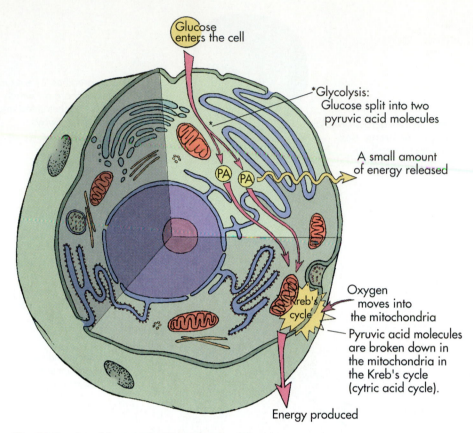

Fig. 10-3 Aerobic metabolism occurs with oxygen and glucose to fuel the cell, and produce energy.

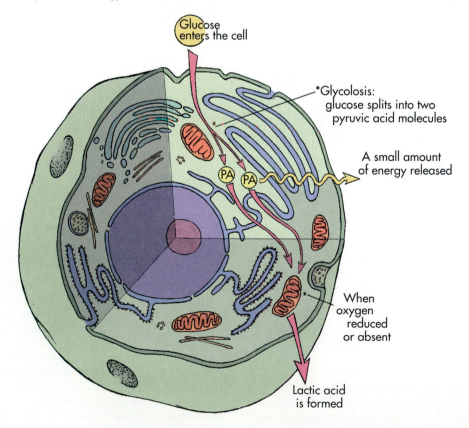

Fig. 10-4 Anaerobic metabolism occurs without oxygen, and produces lactic acid.

result is improved circulation to the vital organs and decreased circulation to the rest of the body.

THE CARDIOVASCULAR SYSTEM

 List the primary components of the cardiovascular system and their roles.

Under normal circumstances, the heart moves blood around inside a closed system of blood vessels (Fig. 10-5). A closed system means that the blood is contained within the system with no opening to the outside. Oxygen is delivered to this system through the alveolar/capillary membrane of the lungs. It is then transported to the tissues. Absent or decreased delivery of oxygen to the body's cells may occur if any of the components of the cardiovascular system are not functioning properly.

Stroke volume

STROKE VOLUME: The amount of blood pumped into the cardiovascular system as a result of one heart contraction.

The amount of blood pumped into the cardiovascular system with each contraction of the heart is called the **stroke volume** (Fig. 10-6). On average, the stroke volume amounts to 70 mL of blood with each contraction of the ventricles. The stroke volume is dependent on contractility, preload, and afterload.

Contractility

CONTRACTILITY: The extent and velocity (quickness) of muscle fiber shortening.

The heart's function as a pump depends largely on its ability to contract. At the onset of contraction the ventricular walls begin squeezing the blood contained in the chamber. Pressure in the ventricle rises quickly and dramatically. When ventricular pressure exceeds pressure in the aorta and the pulmonary artery, the blood is ejected out of the ventricle. The rate at which the pressure rises in the ventricles is determined by how much and how fast the muscle fibers shorten. **Contractility** is the extent and velocity (quickness) of muscle fiber shortening. Myocardial contractility is influenced by oxygen supply and demand, degree of sympathetic stimulation, electrolyte balance, drug effects, and disease.

Calcium, an electrolyte, plays an important role in myocardial contraction. It triggers the action that causes muscle filaments to slide together, one upon another. This action produces a shortening of the muscle fibers and subsequent myocardial contraction. Before the heart can contract, the myocardial cells must take in additional calcium ions through their cell membranes from the extracellular space.

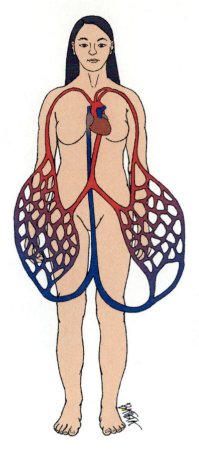

Fig. 10-5 Blood moves throughout the body in a closed system of blood vessels—the cardiovascular system.

Preload

PRELOAD: The passive stretching force exerted on the ventricular muscle at the end of diastole.

The heart muscle is stretched as the heart chambers fill with blood between contractions. This stretching of the muscle fibers before contraction increases the strength of the contraction (Fig. 10-7). **Preload** is affected by the volume of blood returning to the heart. More blood returning increases preload, whereas less blood returning to the heart decreases preload. The more the myocardial muscles are stretched, the more forcefully they contract in systole. In certain pathologic processes there is an optimal point of stretch. If this point is exceeded, a decrease in the contractile state of the heart muscle results.

Afterload

AFTERLOAD: The pressure the ventricular muscles must generate to overcome the higher pressure in the aorta.

Afterload (Fig. 10-8) affects the stroke volume. The greater the afterload, the harder it is for the ventricles

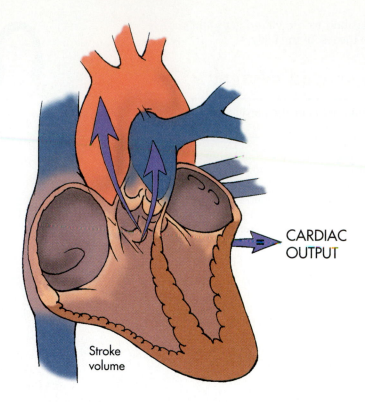

CARDIAC OUTPUT

Stroke volume

Fig. 10-6 Stroke volume is the amount of blood output with each contraction of the heart.

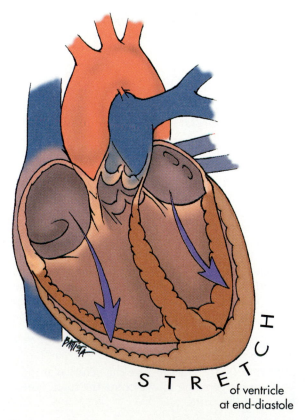

S T R E T C H of ventricle at end-diastole

Fig. 10-7 Preload is the heart's passive stretching force before it contracts.

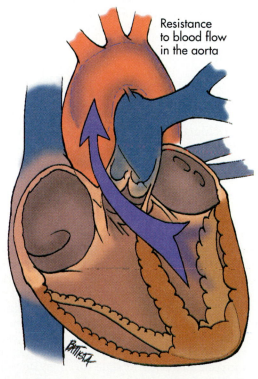

Resistance to blood flow in the aorta

Fig. 10-8 Afterload is the pressure necessary to overcome the pressure in the aorta.

to eject blood into the arteries. To a large degree, afterload is dictated by the arterial blood pressure. Factors that increase afterload include obstruction of the aortic valve and circulatory fluid overload.

Blood pressure

The blood pressure (Fig. 10-9) is the force that blood exerts against the walls of the arteries as it passes through them. The blood pressure is equal to cardiac output times peripheral vascular resistance. Cardiac output is the amount of blood pumped by the heart each minute (*see* Fig. 10-6). It is a product of the heart rate times the stroke volume.

Because the cardiovascular system is a closed system, increasing either cardiac output or peripheral vascular resistance increases blood pressure. Conversely, blood pressure is decreased by decreasing either cardiac output or peripheral vascular resistance. Blood pressure also affects the perfusion of tissues. An abnormally low or high blood pressure can have an adverse effect on perfusion.

Blood vessels

Collectively, the blood vessels are a continuous, closed, and pressurized pipeline moving blood throughout the body. Comprised of arteries, arterioles, capillaries, venules, and veins, the blood vessels make up the delivery system for the circulation (Fig. 10-10).

The intravascular space is a closed system of blood vessels, sometimes referred to as "the container." The blood vessels are elastic, and they change in size, adjusting the fluid volume of the container. The fluid volume of the container is directly related to the diameter of the blood vessels. Any dilation or constriction of the blood vessels will change the volume within the container. This change affects the amount of blood returning to the heart and the amount of tissue oxygenation.

A number of regulatory mechanisms control blood flow to the tissues. First, microcirculation responds to local tissue needs. The blood vessels in the capillary network adjust their diameter to permit the microcirculation (Fig. 10-11) to selectively supply undernourished tissue while temporarily bypassing tissues with no immediate need. The sympathetic nervous system also can directly stimulate the blood vessels to constrict or dilate, thereby redistributing blood to organs in need.

> **CLINICAL NOTES**
> A 70-kg adult man has a blood vasculature container size of about 5 liters. Though the size of any one person's container is relatively constant, the volume of the container is directly related to the diameter of the blood vessels (Fig. 10-12).

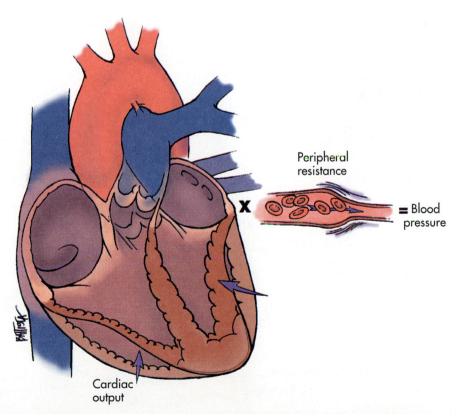

Fig. 10-9 **The elements of blood pressure: bp = cardiac output × peripheral resistance.**

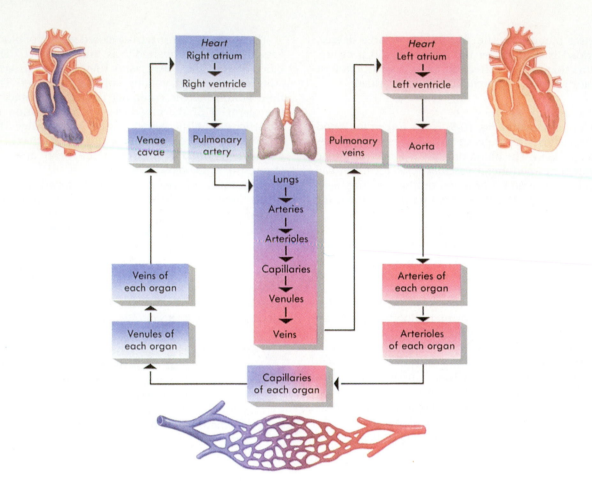

Fig. 10-10   Blood flow through the cardiovascular system.

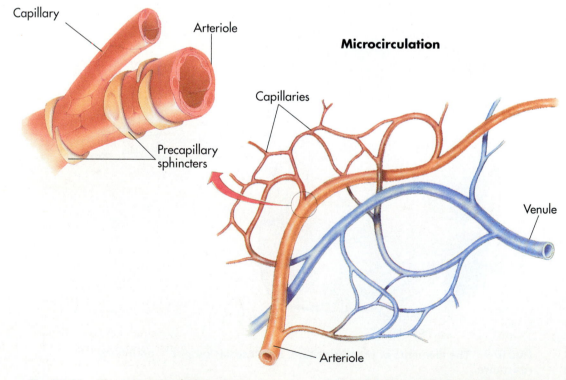

Fig. 10-11   The microcirculation system is composed of arterioles, capillaries and venules.

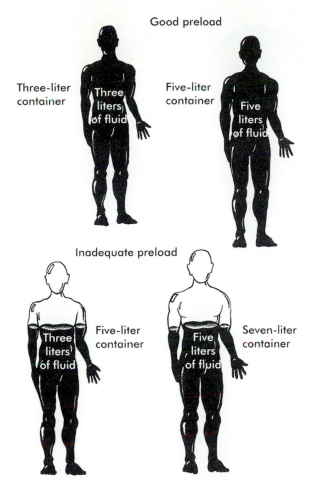

Good preload

Three-liter container — Three liters of fluid

Five-liter container — Five liters of fluid

Inadequate preload

Three liters of fluid — Five-liter container

Five liters of fluid — Seven-liter container

Fig. 10-12   If the size of the human vascular container is greater than the amount of fluid, inadequate preload occurs, which leads to a decrease in cardiac output.

 INTRACELLULAR FLUID: Fluid found within individual cells.
EXTRACELLULAR FLUID: Fluid found outside of the cell membranes.
INTRAVASCULAR FLUID: Fluid found within the vascular system; comprises the fluid portion of blood; plasma.
INTERSTITIAL FLUID: Fluid found outside of the blood vessels in the spaces between the body's cells.

The average adult has a total body water content of approximately 50% to 60% of total body weight. This percentage varies depending on age and sex. In fact, a newborn's total body water may be as high as 75% to 80% of the total body weight. Body fluid is divided into two main compartments (Fig. 10-13):

1. **Intracellular fluid** is found within individual cells and equals approximately 40% to 45% of total body weight. Therefore, the intracellular fluid makes up approximately 75% of all body fluid.

2. **Extracellular fluid** is the fluid found outside of the cell membranes. It equals approximately 15% to 20% of the total body weight, or 25% of all body fluid.

Extracellular fluid is further divided into:

- **Intravascular fluid,** or plasma. This fluid portion of blood is noncellular and is found within the blood vessels. It equals approximately 4.5% of the total body weight.

- **Interstitial fluid** is the fluid located outside of the blood vessels in the spaces between the body's cells. It comprises approximately 10.5% of the total body weight.

FLUID AND ELECTROLYTES

Discuss the role of water in its relationship with body function.

Discuss the fluid compartments of the body.

Fluid

SOLVENT: A dissolving substance, usually a liquid.
SOLUTE: A substance dissolved in a solution.

Water is the most abundant substance in the human body. It plays an important role in the maintenance of homeostasis (constant internal environment of the body) and provides the cells with a life-sustaining environment. It also functions as a universal **solvent** for a variety of **solutes**. These solutes can be classified as either electrolytes or non electrolytes.

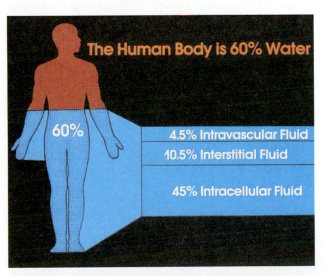

The Human Body is 60% Water

60%

4.5% Intravascular Fluid

10.5% Interstitial Fluid

45% Intracellular Fluid

Fig. 10-13   Body water is divided into intracellular fluid or extracelluar fluid. Extracellular fluid is further divided into intravascular and interstitial fluid.

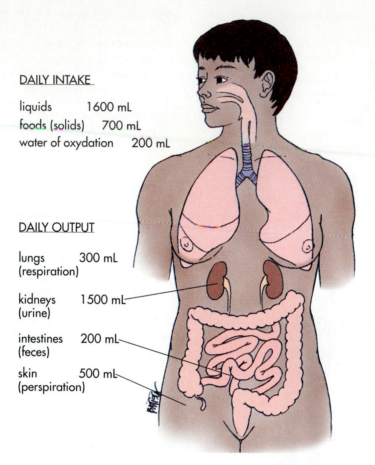

DAILY INTAKE

liquids	1600 mL
foods (solids)	700 mL
water of oxydation	200 mL

DAILY OUTPUT

lungs (respiration)	300 mL
kidneys (urine)	1500 mL
intestines (feces)	200 mL
skin (perspiration)	500 mL

Fig. 10-14 **In order for the body to maintain relative homeostasis, daily fluid intake and output must be relatively equal.**

There is a delicate balance between the various fluid compartments of the body. This balance is essential in maintenance of homeostasis. Loss of fluid volume from any area of the body can lead to disruption of homeostasis and to shock.

Normally the total volume of water in the body as well as its distribution in the three body compartments remains relatively constant, despite wide fluctuations in the amount of water that enters and is excreted from the body on a daily basis. Water coming into the body is referred to as *intake,* whereas water excreted from the body is referred to as *output.* To maintain relative homeostasis, intake must equal output (Fig. 10-14).

Several mechanisms work to maintain a balance between input and output. For example, when the fluid volume drops, the pituitary gland secretes antidiuretic hormone (ADH). ADH causes the kidney tubules to reabsorb more water into the blood and excrete less urine. This action allows fluid volume in the body to build up. Thirst also regulates fluid intake. The sensation of thirst occurs when body fluids become decreased, stimulating the person to take in more fluids. Conversely, when too many fluids enter the body, the kidneys are activated and more urine is excreted, eliminating the excess fluid. The body also maintains fluid balance by shifting water from one compartment to another.

Maintaining a proper balance of fluids and electrolytes within the body is necessary for life. A person may be depleted of fluids and electrolytes for several reasons, such as severe burns or severe dehydration. The patient's chances of survival may depend on how rapidly his or her internal environment is restored.

Electrolytes

 Identify the significant anions and cations in the body.

ELECTROLYTES: Salts, which when dissolved in a solvent break up into ions that are capable of conducting an electrical current.
CATIONS: An ion with a positive charge.
ANION: An ion with a negative charge.

Salts that break up into ions (electrically charged particles) are called **electrolytes.** There are two types of ions: anions and cations. **Cations** have a positive charge. Essential cations include:

- Sodium (Na^+)—A major extracellular cation, sodium is responsible for maintaining fluid balance in the body. When sodium is eliminated from the body, water also is lost. Conversely, when sodium levels in the body rise, water is retained. Sodium is needed for the conduction of nerve impulses and for muscle contraction.

- Potassium (K^+)—A major intracellular cation, potassium is required for growth and is important in conduction of nerve impulses and muscle contraction. It also is responsible for acid-base regulation.

- Calcium (Ca^{2+})—Calcium is the most abundant cation in the body. It is required for blood clotting, bone growth, metabolism, normal cardiac function, and contraction of muscle.

- Magnesium (Mg^{2+})—This cation is required for body temperature regulation, protein and carbohydrate metabolism, and neuromuscular contraction.

An **anion** has a negative charge. Essential anions include:

- Chloride (Cl^-)—A major extracellular anion, chloride's main function is to maintain fluid balance.

- Bicarbonate (HCO_3^-)—This anion is a major buffer of the body. Its main function is to maintain acid-base balance.

- Phosphate (HPO_4^{2-})—This major intracellular anion helps maintain acid-base balance.

Electrolytes are measured in **milliequivalents** per liter (mEq/L). A milliequivalent is the concentration of electrolytes in a certain volume of solution (in this case 1 L) based on the number of available ionic charges.

Body fluid also contains compounds with no electrical charge. These substances are called *nonelectrolytes.* Examples of nonelectrolytes include glucose, protein, urea, and similar substances.

CELLULAR MEMBRANES

 Explain the role of the semipermeable membrane in the function of the cell.

Discuss the concepts of diffusion, facilitated diffusion, osmosis, osmotic pressure, and active transport.

SEMIPERMEABLE: Cell membranes that allow only certain substances to pass through them.
PERMEABILITY: The degree to which a substance is allowed to pass through a cell membrane.

Every healthy cell has an outer membrane that separates the cell contents from the fluid that surrounds it. This membrane must allow nutrients, water, and electrolytes to enter the cell and allow waste products to leave. The membrane also acts as a gatekeeper, preventing valuable proteins and electrolytes from leaving the cell while prohibiting undesirable substances from entering. The term **semipermeable** (Fig. 10-15) is used to classify the cell membrane because it allows some substances to enter or leave, while restricting the passage of others. **Permeability** is the rate at which substances pass through a membrane. Smaller molecules such as water diffuse more easily than larger molecules such as proteins. Other mechanisms also regulate which substances pass through the cell membrane, such as ion pumps (eg, sodium pump), active transport, and diffusion.

Water is the one molecule allowed to pass freely back and forth across the cell membrane. Water (H_2O) is a very tiny molecule made up of two hydrogen atoms (H) and one oxygen ion (O). Small molecules cross the membrane much faster than larger molecules. Other substances may be too large to pass through the membrane. During the process of digestion these substances are broken down into smaller molecules, which are allowed passage. Electrolytes, which are by their nature small, may have difficulty passing through the membrane due to their electrical charge.

Several physical processes are responsible for the exchange of substances across the semipermeable membrane. These transport processes fall into two categories: *passive* and *active.* Passive transport processes do not require the expenditure of energy, whereas active transport processes do. The energy required for active transport is obtained from a chemical substance called *adenosine triphosphate* (ATP). ATP is produced in the mitochondria (located

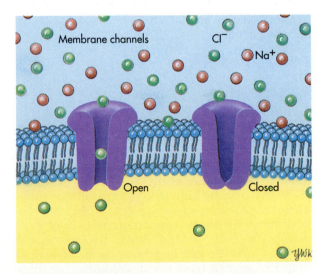

Fig. 10-15 Semipermeable cell membranes allow only certain nutrients to enter or leave the cell.

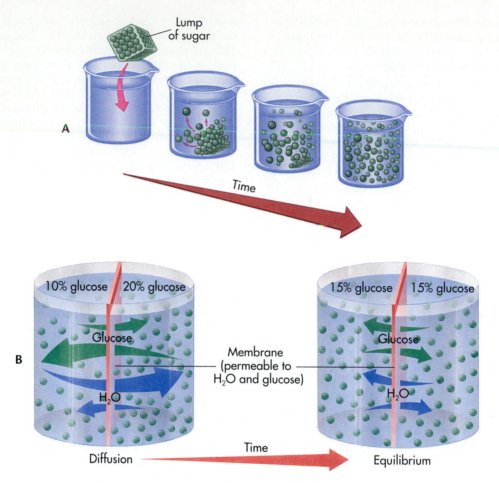

Fig. 10-16   A, The molecules from a lump of sugar spread from an area of high sugar concentration in the water to areas of lower concentration, until the sugar is distributed equally throughout the container. B, The "membrane" allows glucose and water to pass through, creating equilibrium throughout the container.

inside each cell) from nutrients and is capable of releasing energy that enables the cell to work. Active transport is the breakdown of ATP and use of the resulting energy.

Diffusion

> **DIFFUSION:** The movement of particles from an area of higher concentration to an area of lower concentration.

Diffusion (Fig. 10-16 A, B) is the movement of particles from an area of higher concentration to one of lower concentration until the substances scatter themselves evenly throughout an available space. These particles are called *solutes*. When the concentration of a solute is greater on one side of a cell membrane than on the other, the solute will diffuse across the cell membrane from the area of higher concentration to the area of lower concentration. Due to the body's homeostatic mechanism, the natural tendency is to keep a balance of water and electrolytes on each side of the cell membrane. Diffusion is a passive process requiring no energy.

Facilitated diffusion

Many molecules and ions need help diffusing across the cell membrane. In **facilitated diffusion,** a specialized "transport protein" with a binding site specific to one substance binds with a molecule of that substance and moves across the cell membrane. Facilitated diffusion transports molecules of a substance across a cell membrane that would otherwise be impermeable to the substance (Fig. 10-17).

Despite the help of a transport protein, facilitated diffusion is still considered passive transport because the solute is moving down its concentration gradient, *ie,* the molecule or ion is moving from an area of higher concentration to an area of lower concentration. Facilitated diffusion speeds the transport of a solute by providing a specific path through the cell membrane but does not alter the direction of transport. An example of facilitated diffusion is insulin's role in assisting glucose across the cell membrane.

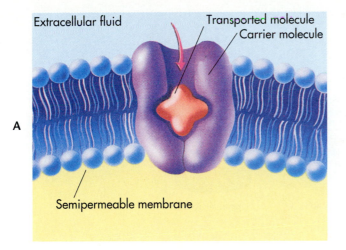
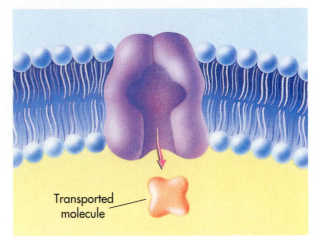

A

B

Fig. 10-17   **A and B, Carrier molecules act as facilitators to the diffusion process, escorting the transported molecule through the membrane into the cell.**

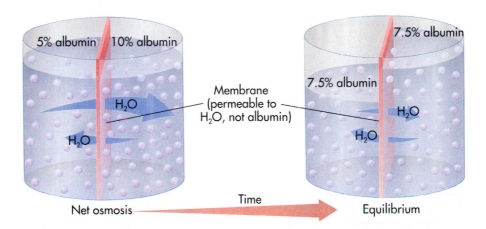

Fig. 10-18   **Osmosis is the movement of water through a semipermeable membrane. The higher concentration of solute (albumin) pulls water from areas of lower concentration, equalizing the concentration on both sides of the membrane.**

Osmosis

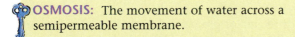**OSMOSIS:** The movement of water across a semipermeable membrane.

Osmosis (Fig. 10-18) is the movement of water across a semipermeable membrane. As previously noted, water moves freely across the cellular membrane. Solutes such as electrolytes may or may not be able to passively pass across the cell membrane. When the concentration of a solute is higher on one side of a membrane than the other, water will cross the membrane until the solute's concentration is equalized. The higher concentration of solute pulls fluid (water) from areas of lower concentration. For example, if there is more sodium inside a cell than outside, water will osmose (move) into the cell. In osmosis, water (the solvent) moves across a semipermeable membrane from an area of lesser solute concentration to an area of greater solute concentration.

Solutions and osmotic pressure

 Give examples of isotonic, hypotonic, and hypertonic solutions.

ISOTONIC SOLUTION: A solution that has an osmotic pressure equal to the osmotic pressure of normal body fluid.
HYPOTONIC SOLUTION: A solution that has an osmotic pressure less than that of normal body fluid.
HYPERTONIC SOLUTION: A solution that has an osmotic pressure greater than that of normal body fluid.

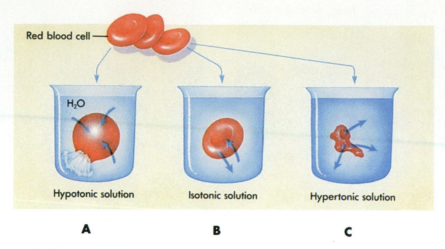

Fig. 10-19 The effects of tonicity on a red blood cell. A, In a hypotonic solution, the cell swells and bursts. B, In an isotonic solution, the cell appears in its normal shape. C, In a hypertonic solution, the cell shrinks.

Solutions are described by their tonicity (the number of particles of solute per unit volume). An **isotonic solution** has an osmotic pressure equal to normal body fluid, meaning that solutions are equal on both sides of the cell membrane. Examples of isotonic intravenous (IV) solutions are 0.9% normal saline and lactated Ringer's solution. A **hypotonic solution** has an osmotic pressure less than that of normal body fluids. When the solute concentration of a given solution is less on one side of the cell membrane than the other, water will be drawn into the solution with a higher solute concentration. A **hypertonic solution** has an osmotic pressure greater than that of normal body fluids. When the concentration of a given solute is greater on one side of the cell membrane than the other it draws water into the solution until the solute-to-solution ratio is equal on both sides (even though the volumes differ) (Fig. 10-19).

Active transport

 ACTIVE TRANSPORT: The movement of a solute across a membrane from an area of lower concentration to an area of higher concentration.

Active transport moves solutes against their concentration gradients, across the cell membrane from the side where they are less concentrated to the side where they are more concentrated. This transport is uphill; it reverses the tendency for substances to diffuse down their concentration gradients and therefore requires work. To pump a molecule across a membrane against its gradient, the cell must expend its own metabolic energy. Active transport is faster than diffusion.

BLOOD

Explain the roles of plasma, erythrocytes, leukocytes, platelets, hemoglobin, and hemocrit.

Blood has three functions: transportation, regulation, and protection. Blood delivers oxygen and nutrients to the cells and carries away waste products such as carbon dioxide. Buffers in the blood regulate the pH of the body. Finally, blood contains cells that protect the body against injury and disease. Blood is composed of cells, formed elements, and water.

PLASMA: The fluid or water portion of the blood.

The fluid, or water, portion of blood is called **plasma** and consists of approximately 55% of the total volume of blood. Plasma contains proteins, carbohydrates, amino acids, lipids, and mineral salts. The three major proteins of the plasma are albumin, globulin, and fibrinogen. Albumin is the most abundant plasma protein.

ERYTHROCYTES: Red blood cells.
LEUKOCYTES: White blood cells.
HEMOGLOBIN: A protein that bonds oxygen to red blood cells.

The cells of the blood include **erythrocytes** (red blood cells) and **leukocytes** (white blood cells) (Fig. 10-20). The erythrocytes are the most numerous of the blood's cells and have the ability to carry oxygen. **Hemoglobin,** a protein that contains iron, bonds the oxygen to the red cells. This oxygen-hemoglobin

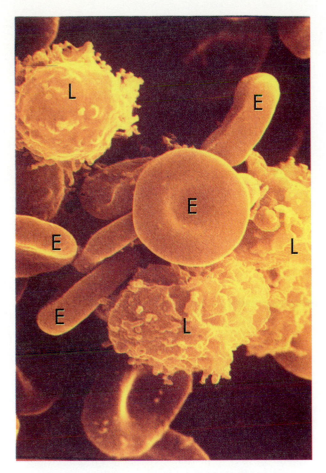

Fig. 10-20   Erythrocytes (E) and leukocytes (L).

Platelets, which are not cells but formed elements, are suspended in the plasma. Platelets are essential for blood clotting. When blood comes into contact with something outside of the blood vessel, such as in an injury, platelets stick together and form a plug that seals the wound. Blood cells and platelets together comprise approximately 45% of total blood volume.

Blood is a viscous fluid, which is thicker and more adhesive than water. Because of this characteristic, it flows more slowly than water. The viscosity (thickness) of the blood is determined by the ratio of plasma to cells and formed elements. The lesser the ratio of plasma to cells and formed elements, the greater the viscosity. Viscosity affects peripheral resistance—the greater the viscosity, the greater the resistance. In shock, when there is a loss of plasma, peripheral resistance can be adversely increased.

The amount of blood in the body varies depending on the size of the individual. Blood accounts for approximately 8% of total body weight. In general, the average adult man who weighs 70 kg (154 lbs) has approximately 5 L (5.2 qt) of blood.

There must be enough blood to fill the container (container = volume within the blood vessels of the cardiovascular system) and to carry oxygenated blood to the body's cells. Because the cardiovascular system is a closed system, the only way blood can escape is through a break in that system, such as in an injury. Even without blood being released from the system, the blood volume can fall due to an increase in the size of the system (increased diameter of the blood vessels).

Blood typing

Describe the role of antigens and antibodies in the body.

ANTIGEN: A protein found on the membrane of red blood cells that triggers the formation of an antibody.
ANTIBODY: A protein developed in the body in response to an antigen.

complex makes it possible for the blood to efficiently transport large quantities of oxygen to the body cells. The combination of hemoglobin and oxygen gives blood its characteristic red color. The more oxygen, the brighter red the blood. Dark red blood has a decreased amount of oxygen.

HEMATOCRIT: The volume percentage of red blood cells in whole blood.

Hematocrit is a term used to identify the volume percentage of erythrocytes in whole blood. A hematocrit of 45 means that every 100 mL of whole blood has 45 mL of erythrocytes and 55 mL of plasma. The average hematocrit for a woman is 42 (+/− 5) and 45 for a man (+/− 7). Leukocytes are outnumbered by erythrocytes 700 to 1 and tend to be colorless. The most important function of leukocytes is to destroy foreign organisms. They may accomplish this goal by producing antibodies or by directly attacking and killing bacterial invaders.

PLATELETS: Formed elements suspended in plasma that are essential to blood clotting.

The term *blood type* (Fig. 10-21) refers to the type of **antigen** present on erythrocyte membranes. The most important antigens when dealing with blood transfusions are AB and Rh. (A person's blood type is determined by heredity.) An antigen is a substance that causes the formation of antibodies. An **antibody** is a protein developed in the body in response to the presence of an antigen that has in some way gained access to the body. Proper blood typing before blood transfusions is very important. The antigen present in the wrong type of blood can cause the formation of antibodies in the recipient's blood, causing the erythrocytes of the donor's blood to become clumped. Blood types are named

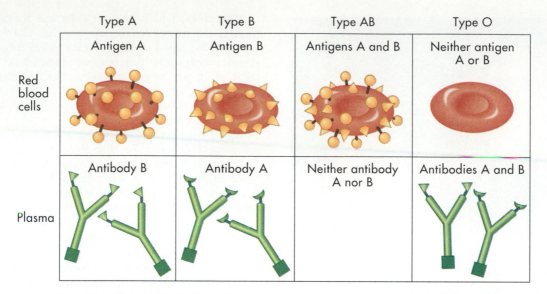

Type A	Type B	Type AB	Type O
Antigen A	Antigen B	Antigens A and B	Neither antigen A or B

Red blood cells

Antibody B	Antibody A	Neither antibody A nor B	Antibodies A and B

Plasma

Fig. 10-21   Blood type is determined by the antigens present on blood cell membranes.

according to the antigens present on the blood cell membranes.

Type A blood has type A surface antigens and anti-B antibodies and will clump in type B blood. Type B blood has type B surface antigens and anti-A antibodies in the plasma and will clump in type A blood. Individuals with type AB blood have both type A and B surface antigens, but neither antibody in the plasma, and are called *universal recipients,* because they can receive blood from most donors. Individuals with type O blood have no surface antigens and both anti-A and anti-B antibodies in the plasma. They are called *universal donors* because their blood can be given to anyone. However, because they have both anti-A and anti-B antibodies they cannot receive any type blood other than type O.

 Explain the Rh factor of the blood.

RH FACTOR: An antigen factor considered during blood typing.

Another antigen considered in blood typing is the **Rh factor.** This antigen is either positive (present) or negative (absent) from the red blood cell membrane. A patient must receive blood from a donor with the same Rh factor. Approximately 85% of people in the United States have Rh-positive blood.

ACID-BASE BALANCE

 Describe acids and bases in relationship to pH.

One function of electrolytes is to combine with each other to form acids or bases (alkalis) to maintain the body's acid-base balance.

pH: A measure of relative hydrogen/ion concentration.

The amount of free hydrogen in the blood is related to whether the blood is acidic, basic, or neutral. The term **pH** means "potential of hydrogen" and is a measurement of hydrogen ion concentration. Because this concentration is so high, hydrogen ion levels are difficult to calculate. To make working with this measurement easier, pH is used. The pH is the inverse logarithm of the hydrogen ion concentration. Therefore, the lower the hydrogen ion concentration, the greater the pH. The pH ranges from 0 (most acidic) to 14 (most basic), with 7.0 being neutral. The pH of pure water is 7.0 (Fig. 10-22).

ACID: A substance that increases the hydrogen ion concentration of water; a substance with a pH less than 7.0.

An **acid** may be defined as a substance that increases the concentration of hydrogen ions in a water solution. The more hydrogen ions, the lower the pH. If the pH is below 7.0, the solution is an acid. Hydrochloric acid (HCl), the acid in the stomach, is a strong acid. The H^+ and Cl^- ions break apart in a water solution.

BASE: A substance that decreases the concentration of hydrogen ions; a substance with a pH greater than 7.0.

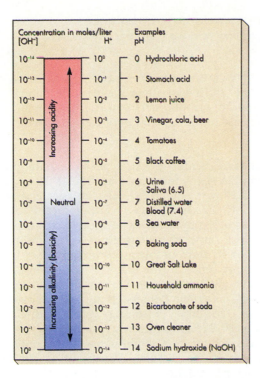

Fig. 10-22   The pH scale. A reading of seven is considered neutral. Values less than seven are considered acidic; values higher than seven are considered basic.

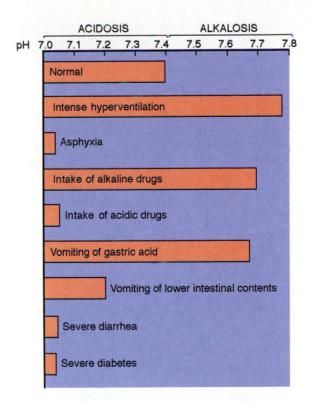

Fig. 10-23   This graph shows the comparative pH levels in the body under various circumstances.

A **base** is a substance that decreases the concentration of hydrogen ions. The fewer hydrogen ions, the higher the pH. If the pH is above 7.0, the substance is a base (alkali).

Acid is a normal waste product of the body's working cells. The pH in the body is a balance between the amount of acid that is produced and the amount of acid that is eliminated from the body. For example, the slightly higher acidity of venous blood (pH 7.36) compared with arterial blood (pH 7.41) is primarily due to carbon dioxide entering venous blood as a waste product of cellular metabolism.

The pH of the human body is normally slightly alkaline, approximately 7.35 to 7.45. Body fluids must stay within this pH range to prevent serious illness. A pH above 7.45 is called *alkalosis,* whereas a pH below 7.35 is referred to as *acidosis.* Even a slight change in pH can be harmful. The acid-base balance of the body is highly dynamic. It varies due to wide fluctuations in the intake and production of acids. The body depends on three principal mechanisms to maintain its pH: buffer systems, the lungs, and the kidneys. These key body systems must continually readjust to maintain the acid-base balance (Fig. 10-23).

Buffer systems

 Explain how the buffer systems, respiration, and kidney function help to maintain acid-base balance in the body.

The buffer systems are the fastest-acting defenses, providing almost immediate protection against changes in the hydrogen ion concentration of the extracellular fluid. The buffer acts as a chemical sponge, absorbing hydrogen ions when they are in excess and donating hydrogen ions when they are depleted. For example, suppose that a small amount of a strong acid, hydrochloric acid, was added to a solution that contains a buffer, such as blood, decreasing the blood pH from 7.41 to 7.27. If the same amount of hydrochloric acid were added to pure water, a solution that contains no buffers, its pH would decrease much more markedly, from 7 to perhaps 3.4. In both instances, pH decreased on addition of the acid, but much less so with buffers present than without them.

The body's major buffer system is the bicarbonate/carbonic acid ($HCO_3^- - H_2CO_3$) buffer system. The carbonic acid can then further break down into water (H_2O) and carbon dioxide (CO_2).

Normally, there are 20 parts of bicarbonate to one part of carbonic acid. This ratio is important because normal cellular metabolism produces an excess of acid. As long as the ratio is maintained, the pH is normal. When a pathologic condition leads to an excess of acid or base, the buffer combines with the excess substance to weaken it and produce water. The buffer system is much more capable of dealing with acidosis than with alkalosis. Twenty buffers are available to combine with excess acid for every one buffer available to combine with excess base. When a strong acid is introduced into the bloodstream, bicarbonate, a weak base, combines with it to form a weak acid, carbonic acid.

Example:

$$H^+ + HCO_3^- \leftrightarrow H_2CO_3 \leftrightarrow H_2O + CO_2$$

Respiration

The respiratory system plays a vital role in maintaining the acid-base balance. It regulates the concentration of carbon dioxide (and subsequently the amount of carbonic acid) in the body. For example, if excess CO_2 builds up, the brain detects the increase in CO_2, which causes the respiratory rate to increase. As the respiratory rate increases, CO_2 is blown off.

Increased ventilation decreases carbon dioxide and carbonic acid (and therefore hydrogen ions) in the blood, thereby increasing blood pH. This process helps restore normal pH in the patient who is acidotic.

Example:

$$\uparrow breathing \rightarrow \downarrow CO_2 \rightarrow \downarrow H_2CO_3 \rightarrow \downarrow H^+ \rightarrow \uparrow pH$$

Decreased ventilation increases carbon dioxide and carbonic acid (and therefore hydrogen ions) in the blood, thereby decreasing blood pH. The additional amount of carbonic acid may provide an additional buffering power in the face of alkalosis by lowering the pH.

Example:

$$\downarrow breathing \rightarrow \uparrow CO_2 \rightarrow \uparrow H_2CO_3 \rightarrow \uparrow H^+ \rightarrow \downarrow pH$$

Patients who are not breathing or who are breathing inadequately are likely to be acidotic due to an inadequate removal of CO_2. In these cases, the treatment must focus on improving ventilation.

However, patients who have metabolic acidosis, as in diabetic ketoacidosis, often hyperventilate to remove CO_2 from the bloodstream and decrease the acidosis. This case is true for the trauma patient. The metabolic acidosis produced by anaerobic metabolism is identified by the respiratory center in the brain. Signals are sent out to increase the respiration and thereby eliminate more CO_2.

Kidney function

The kidney's role in maintaining acid-base balance is complex. Very simply, the kidneys excrete hydrogen ions and form bicarbonate ions in specific amounts as indicated by the pH of the blood. When the plasma pH drops (becomes more acidic), hydrogen ions (acid) are excreted, and bicarbonate ions (base) are formed and retained. Conversely, when the plasma pH rises (becomes more alkaline), hydrogen ions are retained in the body, and bicarbonate ions are excreted.

The kidneys are equally able to deal with alkalosis or acidosis, but there is a limitation. Because it takes at least 10 to 20 hours for kidney function to respond to an alteration in pH, the kidneys are excellent for long-term compensation but are unable to stabilize the pH in critical, rapidly developing conditions.

Primary acid-base imbalances
Respiratory acidosis (carbonic acid excess)

RESPIRATORY ACIDOSIS: An increase in the blood CO_2, a decrease in the blood pH, and a surplus of carbonic acid that results from a decrease in the exhalation of carbon dioxide.

Respiratory acidosis occurs when exhalation of carbon dioxide is inhibited (Fig. 10-24). In addition to increasing the blood CO_2 level and decreasing the blood pH, this imbalance creates a surplus of carbonic acid. Hypoventilation (decreased respiration) is its general cause. Hypoventilation in respiratory acidosis results from problems occurring either in the respiratory center in the brain or in the lungs. Two major conditions that cause hypoventilation are central nervous system depression and obstructive lung disease. Morphine poisoning and anesthesia are examples of central nervous system depression, whereas asthma and emphysema are examples of obstructive lung diseases. Treatment is aimed at improving ventilation.

$$\uparrow PaCO_2 \leftrightarrow \uparrow H^+ \leftrightarrow \downarrow pH = \text{respiratory acidosis}$$

Signs and symptoms of respiratory acidosis:

1. Hypoventilation, seen by shallow respirations or poor exhalation

2. Disorientation and loss of mental alertness progressing to stupor, indicating central nervous system depression

Respiratory alkalosis (carbonic acid deficit)

RESPIRATORY ALKALOSIS: A decrease in the blood CO_2, an increase in blood pH, and a deficiency of carbonic acid that results from an increase in the exhalation of carbon dioxide.

Respiratory alkalosis occurs when exhalation of carbon dioxide is excessive, resulting in a carbonic acid deficit (Fig. 10-25). Its root cause is hyperventilation (rapid respiration), which can be due to fever, anxiety, or pulmonary infections. A hyperventilating patient blows off an increased amount of carbon dioxide, resulting in lowered carbonic acid blood levels. Therefore, the blood pH is increased and the blood CO_2 level is decreased.

$$\downarrow PaCO_2 \leftrightarrow \downarrow H^+ \leftrightarrow \uparrow pH = \text{respiratory alkalosis}$$

Signs and symptoms of respiratory alkalosis:

1. Hyperventilation (deep and/or labored breathing)

2. Sensations of numbness, prickling, or tingling

3. Mental restlessness and agitation progressing to hysteria and finally unresponsiveness

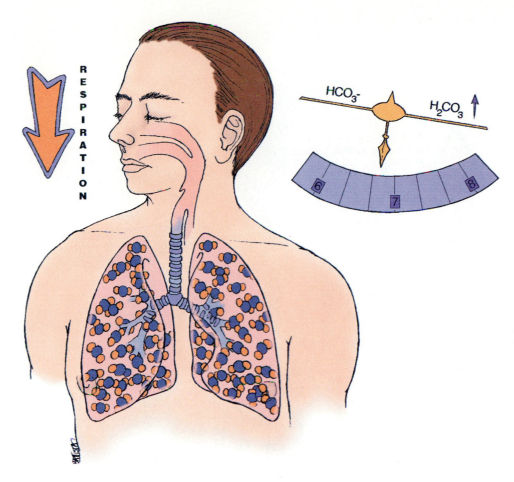

Fig. 10-24   Respiratory acidosis occurs when carbon dioxide exhalation is decreased or inhibited, thereby creating a surplus of carbonic acid.

Metabolic acidosis (base bicarbonate deficit)

METABOLIC ACIDOSIS: A condition in which the level of bicarbonate is low in relation to the levels of carbonic acid.

Metabolic acidosis occurs when the level of bicarbonate (a base) is low in relation to carbonic acid levels (Fig. 10-26). The kidneys normally retain bicarbonate or excrete hydrogen ions in response to altered blood pH. Starvation, renal impairment, and diabetes mellitus are among the conditions that flood the plasma with acid metabolites. With renal impairment, related electrolyte imbalances may develop. Prolonged diarrhea can decrease the level of bicarbonate in the body.

Treatment is aimed at eliminating CO_2 by ventilation. In severe cases, the addition of a bicarbonate, such as sodium bicarbonate, may be required.

Signs and symptoms of metabolic acidosis:

1. Kussmaul breathing (deep rapid respirations), a compensatory mechanism (though absent in infants)

2. Weakness

3. Disorientation

4. Coma

Metabolic alkalosis (bicarbonate excess)

METABOLIC ALKALOSIS: A condition in which the level of bicarbonate is high in relation to the level of carbonic acid.

Metabolic alkalosis occurs when the level of bicarbonate is high (Fig. 10-27). The blood pH is increased, and the blood CO_2 levels are normal. Metabolic alkalosis may be due to excess intake of baking soda or other alkalis, prolonged vomiting, and other conditions that flood plasma with bicarbonate. Prolonged vomiting causes the body to lose chloride and hydrogen ions. Loss of chloride ions causes a proportionate increase of bicarbonate in the blood. Related electrolyte imbalances account for some of the clinical signs. Treatment consists of correcting the underlying cause.

Signs and symptoms of metabolic alkalosis:

1. Slow, shallow respirations (compensatory)

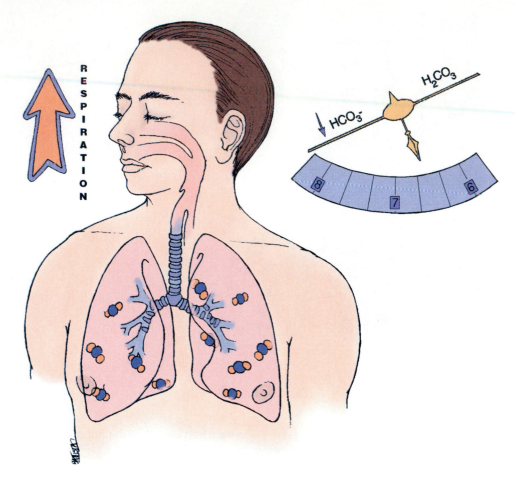

Fig. 10-25 Respiratory alkalosis is hyperventilation, whereby an excessive amount of carbon dioxide is exhaled from the lungs. This results in an increase in blood pH.

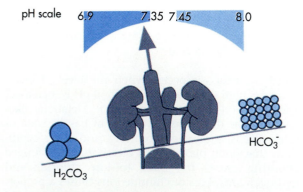

Fig. 10-26 Metabolic acidosis occurs when the levels of bicarbonate are low in relation to carbonic acid.

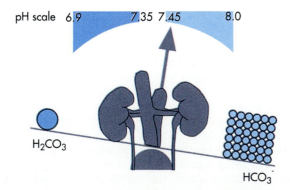

Fig. 10-27 Metabolic alkalosis occurs when there is an excess level of bicarbonate in relation to carbonic acid.

2. Muscular tension
3. Tetany (intermittent spasms that involve the extremities)
4. Mental dullness

STAGES OF SHOCK

 Describe the three principal stages of shock.

The development of shock occurs in three principal stages, which merge with one another. At each stage, certain signs and symptoms are present that may alert the EMT–I to the presence of shock.

Compensated (nonprogressive) shock

The earliest phase of shock is called the *compensated (nonprogressive) stage.* During this stage, the body recognizes the catastrophic event that is occurring and triggers corrective action in an attempt to return cardiac output and arterial blood pressure to normal. Compensatory adjustments begin with the baroreceptors (Fig. 10-28) detecting a drop in arterial blood pressure. Messages are sent to a regulatory center in the brain, which activates the sympathetic nervous system. The sympathetic nervous system stimulates the heart to beat faster and more forcefully in an effort to compensate for the decreased blood flow.

Stimulation of the sympathetic nervous system also causes a release of norepinephrine from sympathetic nerve endings and epinephrine (also called *adrenalin*) from the adrenal glands (Fig. 10-29). The release of these hormones causes constriction of the smooth muscles in the peripheral arterioles and venules (Fig. 10-30). This constriction leads to an increase in blood pressure (by increasing peripheral vascular resistance) and also shunts the blood from the peripheral vasculature to the internal organs. The kidneys act by decreasing urinary output to conserve water. The result is improved circulation to the vital organs and decreased circulation to the rest of the body (Fig. 10-31).

During the compensatory stage, changes in the concentration of oxygen, carbon dioxide, and pH also activate the sympathetic nervous system. A group of specialized receptors, the chemoreceptors (Fig. 10-32), detect these changes in the blood. Like the baroreceptors, the chemoreceptors are located in the walls of the atria of the heart, vena cava, aortic arch, and carotid sinus. Increases in carbon dioxide and/or decreases in oxygen typically initiate a sympathetic response that increases the rate and depth of respirations. The increased respiratory volume brings in more oxygen and removes more carbon dioxide. Initially this compensatory hyperventilation helps to maintain the acid-base balance in early shock by creating a respiratory alkalosis that acts to offset the metabolic acidosis, resulting in a shift of the pH back toward normal.

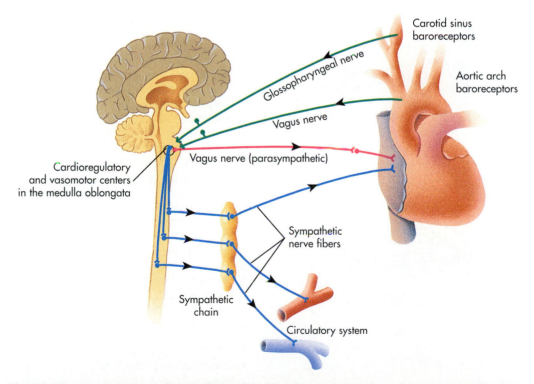

Fig. 10-28 Baroreceptors detect changes in blood pressure and send messages to a regulatory center in the brain. The simple nervous system is then activated, which tells the heart to beat faster or slower.

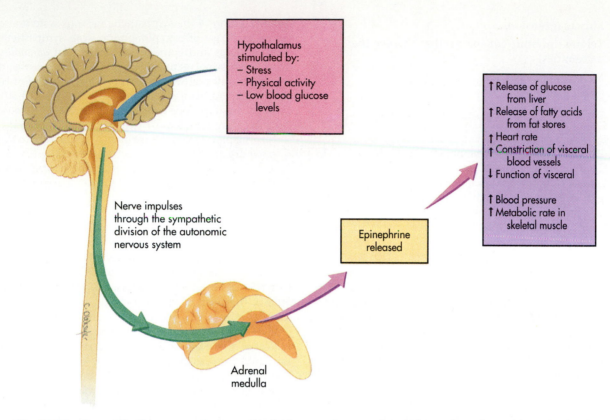

Hypothalamus stimulated by:
– Stress
– Physical activity
– Low blood glucose levels

Nerve impulses through the sympathetic division of the autonomic nervous system

Epinephrine released

↑ Release of glucose from liver
↑ Release of fatty acids from fat stores
↑ Heart rate
↑ Constriction of visceral blood vessels
↓ Function of visceral
↑ Blood pressure
↑ Metabolic rate in skeletal muscle

Adrenal medulla

Fig. 10-29 **Sympathetic nervous system stimulation causes norepinephrine to be released into the body.**

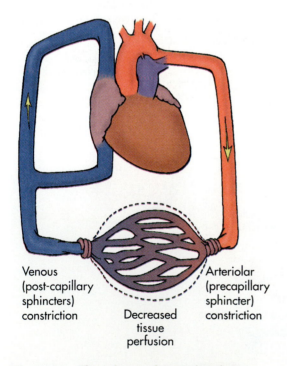

Venous (post-capillary sphincters) constriction

Decreased tissue perfusion

Arteriolar (precapillary sphincter) constriction

Fig. 10-30 **The release of norepinephrine causes the peripheral arterioles and venules to constrict, decreasing tissue perfusion.**

CLINICAL NOTES
Following a small bleed, the heart rate increases, the blood vessels constrict, and the kidneys decrease urinary output to conserve water. These responses help preserve blood volume and maintain blood pressure, cardiac output, and blood flow to the tissues. If the initiating cause (ie, the hemorrhage) does not worsen, a full recovery follows. In an otherwise healthy individual, acute blood loss of as much as 10% of the total blood volume can be handled by compensatory mechanisms.

Signs and symptoms are minimal in this stage of shock and if certain cardiovascular system components compensate, no serious damage will result. It is important that the EMT–I learn to recognize the subtle clues that the body gives off, indicating the development of shock.

- Altered mental status, usually restlessness
- Increased pulse rate
- Increased respiratory rate
- Pale, cool skin

Figure 10-33 shows the body's various reactions to shock during the compensatory stage.

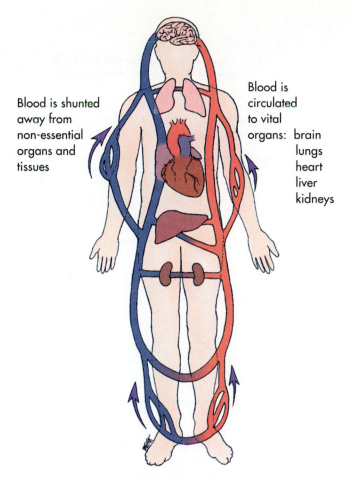

Fig. 10-31 Peripheral vasoconstriction causes blood pressure to increase, and blood is shunted to the internal, more essential organs such as the heart, the lungs, and the brain.

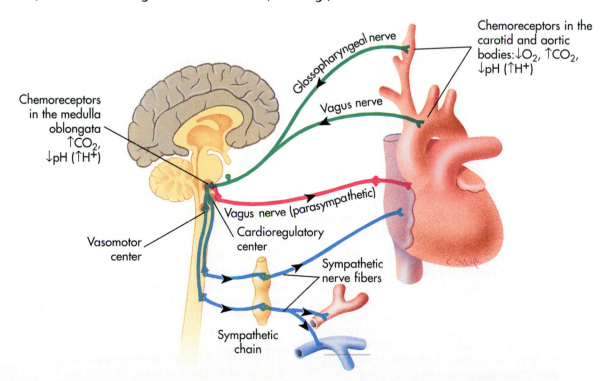

Fig. 10-32 During the compensatory stage of shock, chemorecepters attempt to maintain the body's acid-base balance by stimulating and increasing the rate and depth of respirations, increasing oxygen and decreasing carbon dioxide.

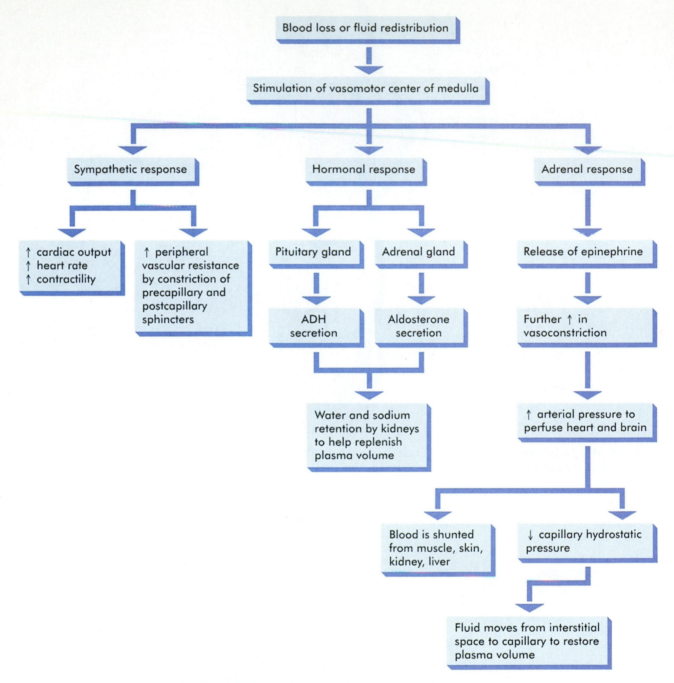

Fig. 10-33 **The body's response to compensatory shock.**

Decompensated (progressive) shock

If blood volume drops more than 15% to 25%, the shock becomes steadily worse because compensatory mechanisms are no longer able to maintain perfusion. As the cardiovascular system progressively deteriorates, cardiac output falls dramatically. This condition can lead to further reductions in blood pressure and cardiac function.

During the decompensated (progressive) stage, the signs and symptoms of shock become more obvious. As epinephrine release continues, constriction of the arterioles and venules shunts blood away from certain nonvital organs (such as the skin, muscles, and gastrointestinal tract) and directs it toward the vital organs (the heart, brain, and kidneys). Although helping to keep the vital organs functioning, this vasoconstriction has a disastrous effect if allowed to continue. The cells in the tissues from which the blood has been diverted become hypoxic, leading to anaerobic metabolism. This condition causes the production of harmful acids, eventually bringing about metabolic acidosis.

As shock progresses, even the cells of the vital organs suffer from the lack of perfusion. For instance, following a severe hemorrhage, cardiac output decreases and the myocardium itself is deprived of blood. The heart weakens, which further decreases cardiac output. Arteries that are deprived of their blood supply cannot remain constricted (Fig. 10-34). As the arteries dilate, venous return decreases, which in turn decreases cardiac output. Immediate medical intervention is required to reverse the changes during the decompensated stage of shock (Fig. 10-35). If this intervention fails, shock progresses to a third stage.

The signs and symptoms of progressive shock include:

- Additional increases in pulse and respirations
- Cool, clammy skin
- Decreased capillary refill
- Thirst (the body's call for increased volume)
- Narrowing of pulse pressure (the difference between systolic and diastolic blood pressure), which indicates an impairment of circulation
- Sweating
- Increased anxiety and confusion

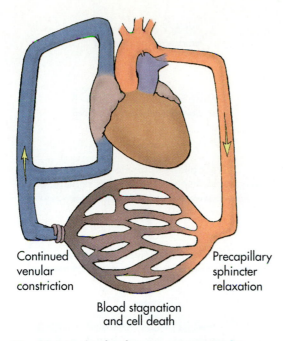

Fig. 10-34　As shock progresses, arteries deprived of their blood supply dilate, decreasing venous return. Decreased cardiac output is the result.

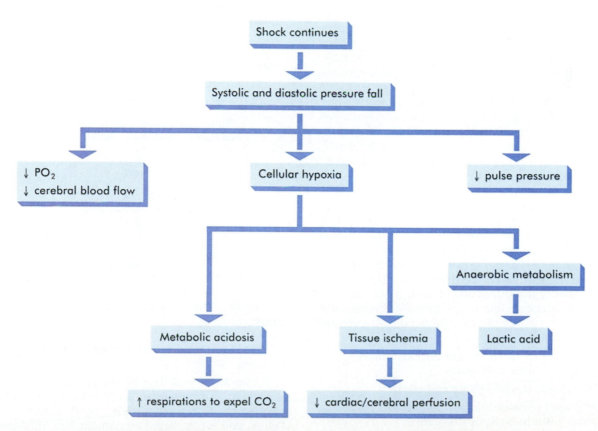

Fig. 10-35　The body's responses to uncompensated (or progressive) shock. This stage of shock is reversible.

- Nausea and vomiting (caused by shunting of blood from the abdominal organs)

 HELPFUL HINT
Decreased blood pressure is a late sign of shock. Children often lose 30% of their blood supply before experiencing a drop in blood pressure.

 CLINICAL NOTES
Hypotension is an abnormal condition in which the blood pressure is too low for normal perfusion and oxygenation of the tissues.

Eventually patients in the uncompensated (progressive) stage of shock will develop hypotension. Hypotension is a late sign of shock. By the time hypotension develops, the body's compensatory mechanisms have failed. Failure to quickly halt the progress of hypotension will lead to irreversible shock.

 HELPFUL HINT
Do not depend on blood pressure measurements alone to determine the presence of shock.

Irreversible shock

In the third stage of shock, a rapid deterioration of the cardiovascular system occurs that cannot be helped by compensatory mechanisms or medical intervention. As the shock cycle continues, the heart deteriorates to the point that it can no longer effectively pump blood and life-threatening reductions in cardiac output, blood pressure, and tissue perfusion occur. The body shunts blood away from the liver, kidneys, and lungs to keep the heart and brain perfused. These organs begin to falter, eventually becoming ineffective. Their malfunction accelerates the overall decline of the body. The cells begin to die and so do the organs (Fig. 10-36).

If the shock syndrome progresses to the point at which the cells in the vital organs begin to die because of inadequate perfusion, the shock syndrome is said to be irreversible. Even if the cause of the shock syndrome was then treated and reversed, the damage to the vital organs could not be repaired, and the patient would eventually die. The "golden hour" theory holds that after 1 hour, the chances of developing irreversible shock increase dramatically. Some signs and symptoms of impending irreversible shock include:

- Marked decrease in level of responsiveness (Glasgow coma scale below 7)
- Decreased respiratory rate and effort
- Profound hypotension and inability to palpate a pulse, even in a responsive patient
- Decrease in the pulse rate from too fast to too slow

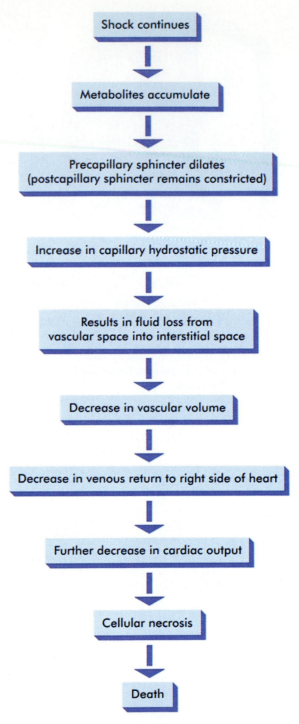

Fig. 10-36 **The body's responses to irreversible shock.**

- Patient communicates a feeling of impending doom

It may be several days before progression to irreversible shock becomes apparent in the form of adult respiratory distress syndrome, renal failure, liver failure, and sepsis. Rapid assessment and immediate transportation are essential to preserve any chance of patient survival.

Shock develops in three successive stages: compensated, decompensated, and irreversible. The keys to the successful recognition and care of the patient in shock include:

1. Have a high level of suspicion. THINK SHOCK!
2. Anticipate the potential for shock from the scene survey.
3. Remember the subtle signs and symptoms of shock that are present in the compensatory stage.
4. The "golden hour" begins at the time of the incident. The guiding philosophy is to get the right person (a patient in shock) to the right place (the appropriate hospital) at the right time (less than 1 hour).
5. Do not rely on any one sign or symptom to judge the degree of shock.
6. Hypotension is a late sign of shock. Other abnormalities indicating poor blood flow (tachycardia, abnormal mental status, or cold/clammy skin) precede hypotension. The EMT–I should be able to recognize shock without having to rely on the presence of low blood pressure.

PATIENTS AT RISK

There are several classes of patients for whom the development of the three stages of shock may be particularly devastating. The trauma patient with multiple injuries may be severely compromised by decreased tissue perfusion, which can lead to hypoxic damage to organs already damaged by the trauma. Elderly patients also are particularly susceptible to the effects of low tissue blood flow. These patients may have previously compromised tissue perfusion secondary to atherosclerotic vascular disease, and even small decreases in perfusion may make the blood flow inadequate to meet their metabolic needs.

Shock poses the greatest danger to pregnant women. During shock, the body sees the fetus as just another piece of peripheral tissue to which the blood flow should be decreased to maintain perfusion of the mother's vital organs. This may be fatal to the fetus if the blood flow is not quickly restored.

TYPES OF SHOCK

 List the five types of shock.

Although shock may have a number of different origins, it is usually caused by one or more of three primary mechanisms:

1. Fluid loss
2. Significant vasodilation
3. Pump failure

Knowing the types of shock allows the EMT–I to anticipate these differences. The EMT–I should know the five major types of shock but should remember that one type may overlap another. The most important point is that all types of shock occur due to an underlying lack of tissue perfusion.

Hypovolemic shock

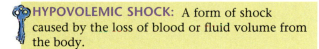
HYPOVOLEMIC SHOCK: A form of shock caused by the loss of blood or fluid volume from the body.

Hypovolemic shock (Fig. 10-37) is caused by the loss of blood or fluid volume from the body. This state commonly occurs after internal or external hemorrhage due to trauma or medical conditions such as gastrointestinal bleeding or a ruptured aortic aneurysm. Hypovolemic shock also results from other conditions associated with fluid volume loss without bleeding, such as burns and severe dehydration. Burns cause the loss of plasma through the damaged skin. Dehydration can occur following severe vomiting, diarrhea, profuse sweating, diabetic ketoacidosis, or inadequate fluid intake.

Hypovolemic shock is the most common type of shock seen in the prehospital setting. It should be suspected in any injured or ill patient whose clinical circumstances suggest the possibility of volume loss (eg, an accident, fall, severe nausea, and vomiting).

ORTHOSTATIC HYPOTENSION: A decrease in blood pressure resulting from a patient being moved to a standing or sitting position from a sitting or supineposition.

 CLINICAL NOTES

A diagnostic test for early hypovolemia is known as the *tilt test*.
Procedure:

1. Place the patient in a supine position and assess vital signs.
2. Sit the patient up and reassess vital signs after 2 minutes of sitting.

An abnormal, or positive, tilt test result is present if the pulse rate increases by 20 beats per minute and/or the systolic blood pressure drops by greater than 10 to 20 mm Hg. The test also is considered positive if the patient complains of dizziness, feels very weak, or faints with the change of position. Positive findings may indicate orthostatic hypotension. The presence of orthostatic changes implies a volume loss of at least 500 mL.
CAUTION: Do not perform the tilt test on patients with suspected spinal injury.

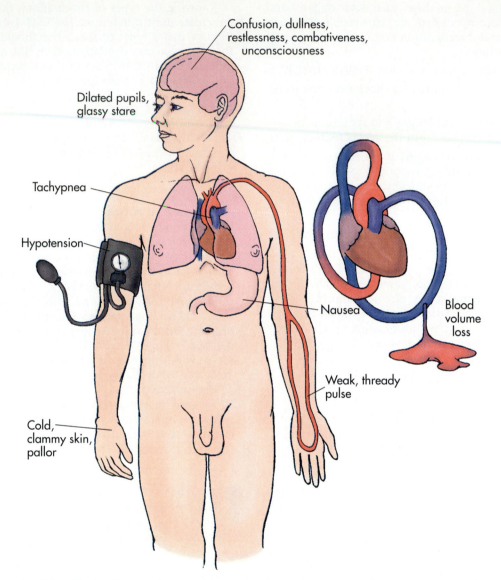

Fig. 10-37 The body experiencing hypovolemic shock, resulting from a large blood or fluid loss in the body.

Cardiogenic shock

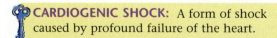 **CARDIOGENIC SHOCK:** A form of shock caused by profound failure of the heart.

Cardiogenic shock (Fig. 10-38) is caused by profound failure of the heart, primarily the left ventricle. When more than 40% of the left ventricle is nonfunctional, the heart loses its ability to efficiently pump blood into the circulatory system. Hence, blood will not be adequately circulated (perfused) to the body. In cardiogenic shock there is good peripheral vascular resistance and adequate blood volume but the heart is not pumping properly.

Cardiogenic shock can be caused by several factors, including:

- Severe myocardial infarction
- Severe heart failure
- Trauma causing excessive pressure on the heart

In a myocardial infarction, for example, there may be damage to the wall of the heart. The heart will not be able to contract as forcefully as it once did, and cardiac output will decrease, leading to shock. Many diseases, if allowed to go untreated, may eventually do enough damage to the heart to cause cardiogenic shock.

In addition to the general signs and symptoms of shock, patients in cardiogenic shock may experience

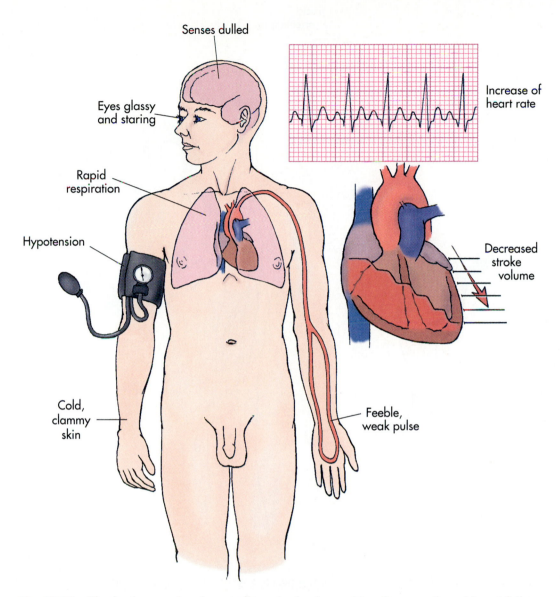

Senses dulled

Eyes glassy
and staring

Rapid
respiration

Hypotension

Cold,
clammy
skin

Increase of
heart rate

Decreased
stroke
volume

Feeble,
weak pulse

Fig. 10-38   **The body experiencing cardiogenic shock, resulting from profound heart failure.**

severe respiratory distress due to a backup of fluid from the right side of the heart into the lungs. They also may have chest pain if there has been an associated myocardial infarction.

Neurogenic shock

> **NEUROGENIC SHOCK:** A form of shock in which the nervous system is no longer able to control the diameter of the blood vessels.

In **neurogenic shock** (Fig. 10-39) the nervous system is no longer able to control the diameter of the blood vessels (as seen in spinal cord injury). Without this control, the blood vessels will dilate, increasing the volume of the cardiovascular system. There is no longer enough blood to fill the

entire system, and blood will pool in the blood vessels in certain areas of the body. Venous return to the heart decreases, and shock results. Neurogenic shock from a spinal injury is sometimes called *spinal shock*. Although no actual blood loss occurs, vasodilation leads to relative hypovolemia. Blood volume is present but not in the necessary places.

Neurogenic shock usually results from severe brain or spinal injury. Damage to the brain or spine prevents nerve impulses from the brain's regulatory center from reaching the vital organs. A disruption in the sympathetic nervous system prevents secretion of epinephrine, resulting in profound vasodilation and shock.

The signs and symptoms of neurogenic shock differ somewhat from those of hypovolemic shock. Due to decreased epinephrine secretion, the patient

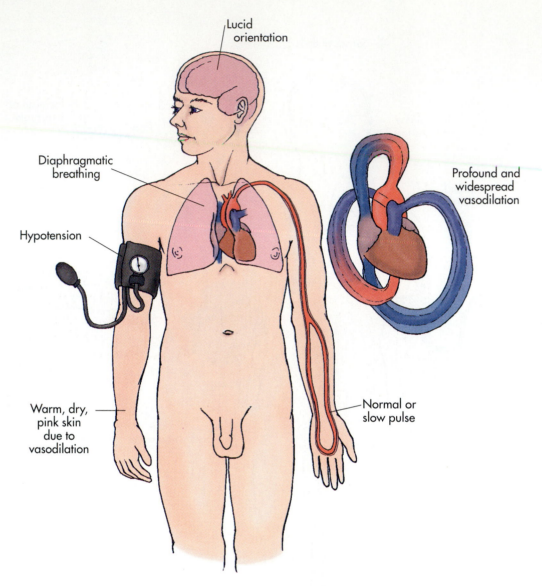

Lucid orientation

Diaphragmatic breathing

Profound and widespread vasodilation

Hypotension

Warm, dry, pink skin due to vasodilation

Normal or slow pulse

Fig. 10-39 Neurogenic shock is caused by the nervous system's inability to control the diameter of blood vessels in the body.

may not exhibit tachycardia, sweating, or a pale skin color. Altered mental status and hypotension may be the only signs of neurogenic shock.

CLINICAL NOTES
Psychogenic shock is simple fainting. The blood vessels dilate, allowing blood pooling. If blood flow falls to the point at which perfusion is momentarily interrupted, the victim will feel faint or pass out. Psychogenic shock usually corrects itself when the victim falls to the ground, restoring circulation to the brain. If the victim is responsive, remaining in the supine position for a few minutes usually returns perfusion to normal.

Anaphylactic shock

ANAPHYLACTIC SHOCK: A form of shock caused by exposure to a substance to which the patient is extremely allergic.
HISTAMINE: A compound released in the body during an allergic reaction.

In **anaphylactic shock** the body reacts to a substance to which the patient is extremely allergic (Fig. 10-40). Anaphylactic shock is a severe response to a foreign substance (antigen) entering the body. Antigens may enter the body through numerous channels:

• Skin contact—poison ivy, poison oak, skin creams

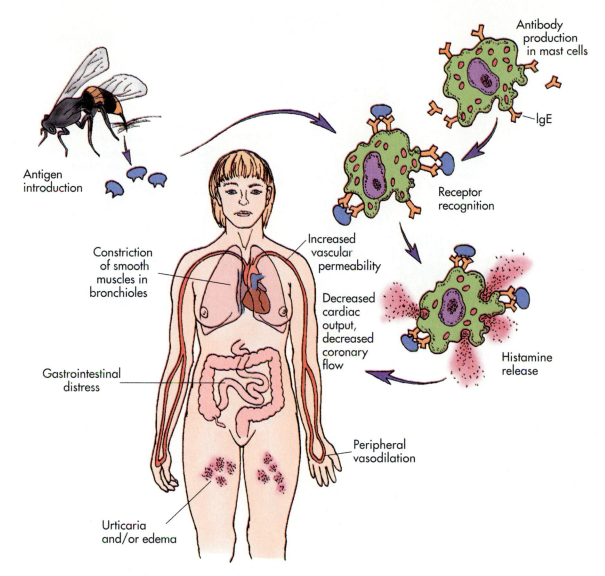

Fig. 10-40   The effects of histamine release in the body.

- Injections—medications given by injection (such as penicillin), insect bites, and stings
- Inhalation—molds, pollen, perfumes
- Ingestion—chocolate, shellfish, peanuts, oral penicillin

When an antigen to which the patient is sensitive enters the body, it is attacked by an antibody. Antibodies function to destroy foreign substances. In the event of anaphylaxis, the antibody does not destroy the antigen. Instead, the reaction between the antigen and the antibody triggers a series of events in the patient's body that leads to shock. After the antibody has reacted with the antigen, there is release of chemicals from a specialized type of leukocyte called a *mast cell*. The most important substance released from mast cells during anaphylactic shock is **histamine**.

The release of histamine causes the following responses:

- Sudden, severe bronchoconstriction, which can cause airway compromise
- Intense vasodilation
- Leaking of fluid from vessels due to a change in permeability

Responses can range from mild to extreme, sometimes causing death.

 HELPFUL HINT

The terms *allergic reaction* and *anaphylaxis* often are used interchangeably. The differences in these terms are not absolute. A guideline to follow is: Allergic

Continued

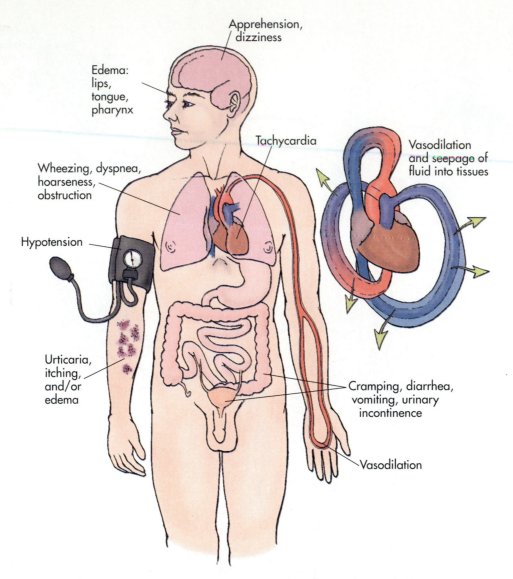

Apprehension, dizziness

Edema: lips, tongue, pharynx

Tachycardia

Vasodilation and seepage of fluid into tissues

Wheezing, dyspnea, hoarseness, obstruction

Hypotension

Urticaria, itching, and/or edema

Cramping, diarrhea, vomiting, urinary incontinence

Vasodilation

Fig. 10-41   **The body experiencing anaphylactic shock.**

HELPFUL HINT, continued

reaction—a systemic response to exposure to an antigen. The symptoms may include rashes, itchiness, a burning sensation of the skin, difficulty breathing, or hypotension.

Anaphylaxis—an extremely severe allergic reaction; includes problems of the airway, breathing, and shock.

The signs and symptoms of anaphylactic shock (Fig. 10-41) differ somewhat from other forms of shock and may develop rapidly or gradually. Anaphylactic shock presents a special problem because profound airway compromise can develop quickly. Signs and symptoms of anaphylactic shock include:

- A sense of uneasiness or agitation. This is often the first symptom noticed by the patient.

- Swelling of the soft tissues such as the hands, tongue, and pharynx. Patients may feel as if their tongue is swelling and their throat is closing up.

- Skin flushing and hives

- Tachycardia

- Coughing, sneezing, or wheezing due to spasms of the upper and lower airway

- Tingling, burning, and itching of the skin

- Abdominal pain

- Profound hypotension (late sign)

- Decreased level of responsiveness

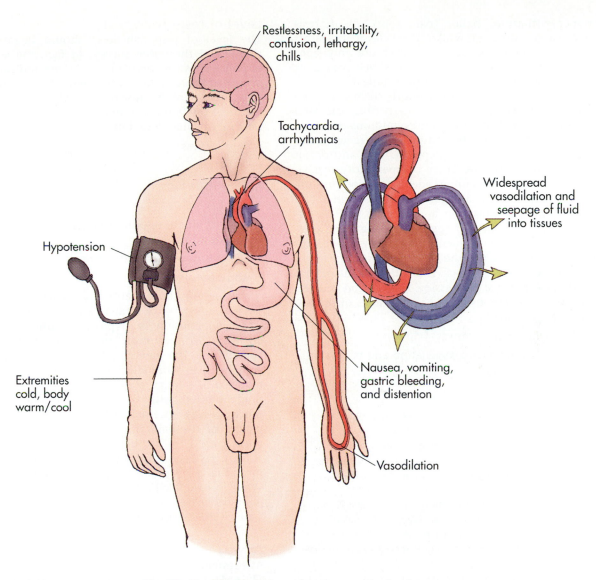

Restlessness, irritability, confusion, lethargy, chills

Tachycardia, arrhythmias

Widespread vasodilation and seepage of fluid into tissues

Hypotension

Nausea, vomiting, gastric bleeding, and distention

Extremities cold, body warm/cool

Vasodilation

Fig. 10-42   The body experiencing septic shock.

Septic shock

 SEPTIC SHOCK: A form of shock caused by an infection resulting in a massive vasodilation of the circulatory system.

Septic shock (Fig. 10-42) is caused by an overwhelming infection (usually bacterial) that leads to massive vasodilation. The blood vessels dilate due to toxins being released into the bloodstream. As in neurogenic shock, the amount of blood available for effective circulation is decreased because it is pooled or trapped in the dilated veins. In addition, blood plasma is lost through blood vessel walls, causing an additional loss in blood volume. Therefore, poor tissue perfusion results.

Until recently, septic shock was rarely seen in the prehospital environment. With expanded long-term care facilities and increased utilization of EMS by the elderly, EMS personnel are beginning to see septic shock more often.

The patient in septic shock may have a fever. The trunk of the body is often warm, but the extremities are cold due to shunting of blood from the skin of the arms and legs. As septic shock progresses, the entire body becomes cool; this is an ominous sign.

ASSESSMENT AND MANAGEMENT OF THE PATIENT IN SHOCK

Discuss the proper assessment and management of patient shock.

The EMT–I must always keep in mind that shock can result from any illness or injury and can present itself in a variety of ways. Hypotension, tachycardia, hyperventilation, pallor (pale skin), diaphoresis (sweating), thirst, and weakness are classic indicators of shock. These indicators, however, are only signs and symptoms. The condition of shock may exist long before any of these indicators appear.

The body's compensatory efforts to maintain an adequate blood pressure and to perfuse the vital organs can mask the signs and symptoms of shock. Shock can be hidden by compensatory mechanisms such as generalized vasoconstriction and/or an increase in heart rate. These compensatory mechanisms work to maintain an adequate blood pressure and to perfuse the vital organs. Rapid assessment and immediate transportation are essential for the survival of the patient. Although measuring blood pressure is the most frequent monitoring device for patient care, it is not the most important factor in the management of shock. Evaluation of the patient in shock is directed at assessing oxygenation and perfusion of the various body organs. Goals of prehospital care include:

1. Ensuring a patent airway

2. Providing adequate oxygenation and ventilation

3. Restoring perfusion

HELPFUL HINT

Some tips for caring for a patient in shock include:

- Conducting the initial assessment (primary survey) and detecting shock early; finding the mechanism of injury may lead the EMT–I to suspect shock.
- Securing and maintaining a patent airway.
- Administering high-flow oxygen. If available, the EMT–I should use a pulse oximeter and adjust the oxygen concentration to raise saturation above 90%.
- Controlling external bleeding.
- Applying and inflating pneumatic antishock garment per local protocols.
- Administering intravenous fluids per local protocols.
- Preserving warmth by covering the patient with a blanket.
- Monitoring the vital signs frequently, at least every 5 minutes.
- Promptly transporting the patient.

The EMT–I's initial approach to the patient often can yield a great deal of information. Before reaching the patient's side, his or her mental status, respiratory effort, and skin color can be observed. In situations in which the patient is obviously in shock, the EMT–I must be aggressive with assessment and management. This chapter addresses only the assessment and management of patients experiencing shock related to volume depletion. Assessment and management of other forms of shock are covered in other chapters in this book.

Level of responsiveness

The level of responsiveness should be assessed throughout the initial survey. In fact, the level of responsiveness is probably a better indicator of decreased tissue perfusion throughout the body than most other signs. Because of the high energy requirements of the brain, any reduction in cerebral blood flow may be manifested by:

- Restlessness
- Agitation
- Disorientation
- Confusion
- An inability to respond to questions or commands appropriately
- Belligerent or combative behavior
- Unresponsiveness

Any significant alteration in the level of responsiveness must be viewed as an indication of critical hypoperfusion or hypoxia. Additionally, with an increased secretion of norepinephrine and epinephrine, the patient often becomes anxious or apprehensive. Mind-altering substances also may be involved in trauma-related shock. When alcohol or drugs interfere with the patient's normal thought processes it is extremely difficult to get an accurate picture of the patient's mental status. The EMT–I must keep in mind, however, that just because a patient has been drinking or taking drugs does not mean that a serious underlying injury does not exist. Whenever the likelihood of serious trauma exists, it is probably best to assume that any altered mental status is due to decreased cerebral perfusion.

Airway
Assessment

The EMT–I begins the assessment by looking for and assuring a patent airway. The airway must be opened and maintained to ensure adequate air movement. This is done using appropriate cervical spine stabilization for any patient who is likely to have suffered a spinal injury. Sounds that point to the presence of upper airway obstruction include:

- Snoring (obstruction by the tongue)
- Gurgling (obstruction by liquids such as blood or vomitus)
- Stridor (obstruction due to foreign body or swelling)

Management

An airway adjunct should be inserted to prevent the tongue from obstructing the airway in any patient with decreased responsiveness and no gag reflex. The EMT–I might use an oropharyngeal airway, nasopharyngeal airway, esophageal obturator airway, or endotracheal tube. When dealing with the patient in shock who is unresponsive, particularly those who are bleeding into the pharynx, endotracheal intubation is the preferred airway technique, because the trachea can be sealed to prevent aspiration of blood.

Blood or fluids should be cleared with appropriate suctioning techniques, taking care not to stimulate the gag reflex or create inadvertent hypoxia. Larger foreign objects such as teeth should be removed using the finger sweep technique. In the presence of ongoing fluid accumulation in the pharynx it may be necessary to place the patient on his or her side. Although this positioning is effective because fluids will seek the lowest point and drain out, it is cumbersome to maintain cervical spine support and assist ventilations while the patient is in this position.

Breathing and oxygenation

Assessment

Once an open airway is assured, the adequacy of air exchange should be checked. The rate and depth of ventilation may be increased to reduce the carbon dioxide content of the blood and to compensate for metabolic acidosis. This condition is referred to as compensatory hyperventilation. Although compensatory hyperventilation tends to occur in early shock, the unresponsive shock patient will often hypoventilate. Hypoventilation occurs when the respiratory center of the brain becomes depressed due to hypoperfusion. When evaluating the ventilatory status, the EMT–I should check both the rate and depth of respirations, watching for patients who exhibit rapid, shallow breathing. This type of breathing is just as ineffective as slow or irregular respirations. Rapid, shallow breathing results in reduced air volume because not enough air is being exchanged.

Management

Any indication of hypoventilation should prompt the EMT–I to assist the patient's breathing with a bag-valve-mask or other ventilatory device. Other conditions that produce respiratory compromise must be managed with the appropriate means as local protocols allow.

Once the airway and breathing have been ensured, the patient should receive 100% oxygen. A nonrebreather mask with an air flow of 10 to 15 L/min should be applied. The EMT–I must be sure to pay attention to the amount of oxygen that remains in the reservoir of the device at the end of each inspiration. Patients experiencing compensatory hyperventilation can deplete the reservoir, in which case a simple face mask should be employed to prevent suffocation. If the patient becomes nauseous or is frightened by the mask, a nasal cannula with a liter flow of 6 to 8 L/min can be employed.

When there is a need to assist ventilation, such as during hypoventilation or when an endotracheal tube has been placed, 100% oxygen should be delivered via a bag-valve-mask or automatic ventilator device. A pulse oximeter will assist the EMT–I in determining the oxygen content of the patient's blood. After patency of the airway and ventilatory effectiveness have been ensured, attention should be turned to evaluating circulation.

Circulation

Assessment

The EMT–I should begin by examining the patient for obvious external bleeding. Usually direct pressure is sufficient to contain blood loss. In cases in which hemorrhage cannot be controlled by direct pressure, other measures must be employed, including using a pressure point over a major artery or, as a last resort, the use of a tourniquet. Application of the pneumatic antishock garment may be helpful in controlling intraabdominal (aorta, liver, spleen, retroperitoneal, pelvic) and lower extremity hemorrhage.

Once major bleeding is controlled, the rate and character of the pulse should be assessed. Compensatory mechanisms can maintain a normal pulse rate even in the presence of a 10% to 15% volume deficit. A fast, weak, or thready pulse suggests decreased circulatory volume. The location of a palpable pulse also will give a rough estimate of the systolic blood pressure. In the case of profound shock in which severe vasoconstriction is present, the EMT–I may not be able to feel a pulse.

The color, appearance, and temperature of the skin also provide useful information about circulatory effectiveness. In early shock, the skin may appear normal. Then, as compensatory mechanisms such as vasoconstriction take effect and blood is routed to the central circulation, the skin becomes pale (decreased perfusion), cyanotic, mottled (combination of pale and cyanotic skin; a late sign of shock), cool to the touch, and diaphoretic (sweaty). Often, the appearance of the skin suggests shock even before there are any noticeable changes in the blood pressure.

Another procedure used to assess the circulation (in children less than years 6 of age) is capillary refill. Capillary refill testing is performed by applying pressure to the nail bed of one of the patient's fingers. This pressure should cause a blanching, or whitening, of the nail bed. When the pressure is released, the nail bed should return to its normal pink color in less than 2 seconds. The EMT–I can approximate this time period by saying "capillary refill." If the normal pink color does not return to the nail bed or the capillary refill is slow, it can be assumed that there is decreased perfusion to this area.

Because the nail bed is the most distal part of the circulation, poor capillary refill is an early indicator of decreased perfusion to the whole body. However, use of the capillary refill test has limited value in the prehospital setting due to poor lighting conditions and other environmental factors. Low skin temperature also may slow capillary refill time. Therefore, as with other signs, delayed capillary refill is just one of the possible signs of shock. See chapter 8, "Patient Assessment," for more information on capillary refill.

Management

Decreased circulation is treated with elevation of the patient's legs, applying and if necessary inflating the pneumatic antishock garment, and placement of intravenous lifelines.

Positioning

The preferred position for the patient in shock is supine with his or her legs elevated 10 to 12 inches. This position promotes increased venous return to the heart and increased cerebral perfusion. In some situations, elevation of the legs alone is enough to raise the blood pressure. However, in cases in which the patient is experiencing respiratory compromise, (*eg*, acute pulmonary edema secondary to cardiogenic shock), an upright, sitting position should be used to ease respirations. If it is necessary to place a patient experiencing respiratory compromise in a supine position, steps must be taken to assure appropriate air exchange. This might include using a bag-valve-mask device to assist the patient's breathing.

Pneumatic Antishock Garment

> Discuss the role of the pneumatic antishock garment in the management of shock.

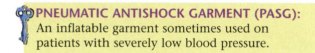
PNEUMATIC ANTISHOCK GARMENT (PASG): An inflatable garment sometimes used on patients with severely low blood pressure.

The **pneumatic antishock garment** (PASG) (Fig. 10-43), is another tool that is sometimes used for the care of hypotension and shock. The PASG consists of three air-containing rubber bladders covered with cloth. Two of the compartments wrap around the patient's legs, and one wraps around the stomach. The bladders are connected by hoses to a manual air pump. Velcro closures hold the sections in place when the PASG is applied to the patient. Initially, only the leg compartments are inflated. If the patient needs additional assistance, the abdominal compartment is then inflated.

Originally, the PASG was thought to increase blood pressure by compressing the vessels of the legs and abdomen, thus squeezing 500 to 1000 mL of blood to the trunk and upper extremities. More recent studies suggest that this "autotransfusion effect" is minimal, less than 250 mL. The PASG probably works by increasing resistance in the blood vessels it encloses, leading to an increase in the blood pressure. It is likely that the mechanism by which hypotension is reversed differs depending on the clinical situation. It is possible that several mechanisms may operate together.

The PASG also helps control bleeding. When the garment is inflated, pressure is exerted on the blood vessels. The same internally transmitted pressure that increases the resistance also serves to decrease blood flow in a bleeding vessel.

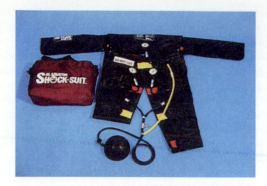

Fig. 10-43   **The PASG can be effective in managing shock patients.**

Indications

The most common indication for the use of the PASG is hypovolemic shock, whether caused by bleeding, trauma, sepsis, a ruptured aneurysm, or ectopic pregnancy. The garment may be of help in hypotension secondary to decreased cardiac output. In cardiac tamponade or tension pneumothorax, PASG inflation may maintain the blood pressure until definitive therapy can be performed.

Another use is stabilization of fractures of the femur, lower leg, and pelvis. A final very helpful role is the PASG's prophylactic placement in air and ground ambulance transfers of potentially unstable patients. If the patient's condition deteriorates, the garment only needs to be inflated.

The criteria for the PASG includes a systolic blood pressure below 90 mm Hg when obvious signs and symptoms of shock are present.

In some EMS systems, the PASG is used based solely on the mechanism of injury and patient presentation rather than blood pressure measurement. Other EMS systems require physician direction for inflation. The EMT–I should check with his or her EMS system for guidelines concerning PASG inflation.

Contraindications

Pulmonary edema is an absolute contraindication to the use of the PASG. Increased venous return (preload) and/or an increase in afterload (arterial resistance) is detrimental to the failing heart. The inflation of the abdominal compartment is contraindicated in pregnancy, respiratory distress of any nature, evisceration, and when there is an impaled object in the abdomen.

Complications

A major complication in the use of the PASG involves chest injuries. Studies have shown that PASG use in the presence of open or closed chest injuries can cause further complications by increasing bleeding into the intrathoracic cavity, thus leading to a tension hemopneumothorax (both blood and air in the chest cavity). It also can cause undue pressure on an injured heart, whether it be a cardiac contusion or pericardial tamponade (blood surrounding the heart). A patient who has a flail segment and is having difficulty breathing will have increased difficulty because the garment is putting added pressure on the diaphragm.

Some other complications may include vomiting, urination, and defecation. If vomiting occurs, the EMT–I must remember to protect the patient's airway.

Techniques for applying and removing the PASG

There are three methods for positioning the PASG under the patient:

1. Spread the garment on top of the long spine board prior to placing the patient on the board. Use this method when anticipating the need for the PASG (Fig. 10-44 A).

2. Slide the garment under the patient.

3. Loosely wrap the garment around your arms and slide it on in a pants-type fashion. Do not use this method when spinal injury is suspected.

STREET WISE

Before positioning the garment, check for wallets, keys, and sharp objects. These can interfere with and damage the PASG.

When positioning the garment ensure that you:

1. Apply it with the inside portion facing toward the patient and the pump connections on the outside. The inside midline is marked to help prevent confusion. Placing the garment on inside-out will not benefit the patient.

2. Position the garment so that the top is just below the rib cage. If placed too high, it will interfere with respirations.

3. Wrap the three sections around the patient. Secure the device by attaching the Velcro pieces together. If they are too tight or too loose they will be less effective.

4. Connect the foot pump to the pump connections on the leg and abdominal sections. Keep the stopcocks closed until ready to inflate.

When you are ready to inflate the PASG:

1. Open both leg compartment stopcocks and ensure that the abdominal compartment is closed (Fig. 10-44 B). Some local protocols call for inflation of all three chambers at the same time.

2. Quickly compress the foot pump until (Fig. 10-44 C):

   A. The vents on the stopcocks begin to leak or

   B. You hear tearing sounds ("crackling") from the Velcro.

3. Close the leg compartment stopcocks and reassess the patient (Fig. 10-44 D).

4. If the systolic blood pressure has not reached 100 to 110 mm Hg systolic or severe shocklike symptoms still exist, inflate the abdominal compartment.

5. Continue inflating the abdominal compartment as you did the leg section.

6. Reassess the patient's vital signs.

HELPFUL HINT

Indications and contraindications for PASG use can vary among EMS systems. The EMT–I should check with his or her instructor, EMS physician, or EMS system concerning local guidelines. Local protocols take precedence over all else.

Although the PASG helps control bleeding under the garment, areas near the femoral artery may require additional manual direct pressure to control bleeding.

Techniques for removing the PASG

Rapid removal of the PASG may cause irreversible shock in some patients. The PASG is rarely deflated in the field. If, however, severe respiratory compromise or pulmonary edema develops, the emergency department physician may order deflation before the patient reaches the hospital.

HELPFUL HINT

Deflation of the PASG in the prehospital setting is done only by direct physician order.

The procedures for PASG deflation are:

1. Ensure that the emergency department physician has ordered PASG deflation.

2. Disconnect the stopcock from the abdominal section tubing of the foot pump. Slowly open the stopcock and allow a small amount of air to escape. Reassess vital signs every 5 minutes.

3. If the blood pressure has dropped by more than 5 mm Hg systolic or the patient's condition has deteriorated, discontinue deflation. After additional intervention (IV fluids) reassess the patient.

4. Continue to slowly deflate the abdominal section. Reassess vital signs every 5 minutes. If the patient's condition quickly deteriorates, the abdominal section may be reinflated.

5. If the patient's condition permits, slowly deflate each leg segment. The deflated garment may be left in place until further stabilization occurs.

STREET WISE

Never remove the PASG by cutting it with a knife or scissors.

The PASG may have to remain in place for several hours. The garments are often left inflated until the patient is in the operating room. Endotracheal intubation, blood gases, radiograph, and Foley catheter (urinary collection bag) placement may be accomplished with the PASG applied and inflated.

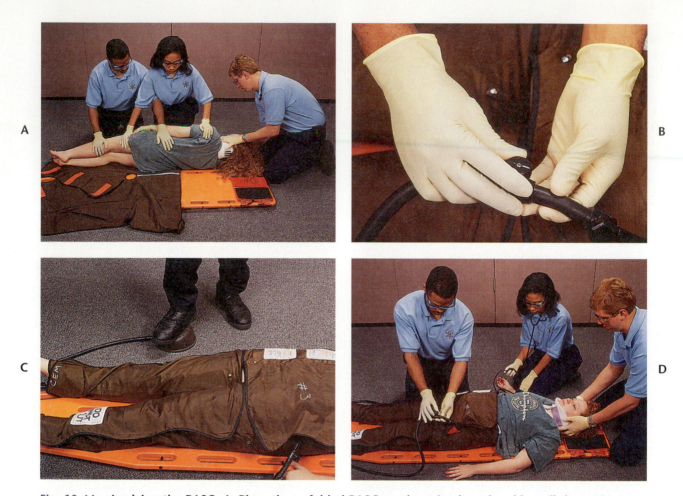

Fig. 10-44 Applying the PASG. **A,** Place the unfolded PASG on the spine board and logroll the patient onto the spine board. **B,** Check all valves to ensure the leg compartments are open and the abdominal compartment is closed. **C,** Inflate the garment. **D,** Close all valves and reassess the patient.

HELPFUL HINT
Pediatric PASG: A smaller pediatric PASG device is used for patients between 2 and 12 years of age. The indication, contraindications, complications, inflation, and deflation procedures are identical to those for the adult with one exception:
The indication for use in these patients is a systolic blood pressure below 60 mm Hg or between 60 to 80 mm Hg with shock–like symptoms.

Pay close attention to respiratory status. When the abdominal section is inflated, the chance of interfering with respiratory effort increases significantly. Some EMS systems have chosen not to use the abdominal section on pediatric patients unless it is absolutely necessary. Prehospital use of the PASG is currently being debated. Some EMS systems have eliminated or restricted the use of the PASG. The information presented in this chapter is meant to explain the actual use of the PASG. The EMT–I should check with his or her instructor, EMS physician, or EMS system on local policies regarding PASG use.

Fluid replacement

 Describe fluid replacement in the management of the patient in shock.

Intravenous lines are used to counter blood loss by introducing fluid into the intravascular space. These fluids act to restore the circulatory volume until the body is able to manufacture more blood. A patient in hypovolemic shock may require at least two IV lines using large bore catheters (14 to 16 gauge).

Three of the most commonly used solutions in prehospital care are lactated Ringer's solution, 0.9% sodium chloride (normal saline), and 5% dextrose in water (D_5W). Lactated Ringer's solution is an isotonic electrolyte solution containing sodium chloride, potassium chloride, calcium chloride, and sodium lactate in water. The lactate of this solution, when metabolized by the liver, is broken down to bicarbonate, a buffer.

Normal saline is an electrolyte solution containing sodium chloride in water, which is isotonic with the extracellular fluid. Both lactated Ringer's solution and normal saline are used to replace fluid volume in patients experiencing shock, because their administration causes an immediate expansion of the circulatory volume. The other solution, 5% dextrose in water, is a hypotonic glucose solution, used to keep a vein open and to supply calories necessary for cell metabolism.

Blood preparations

Blood for transfusion can be processed into packed erythrocytes, plasma, and other products such as platelets, or used as whole blood. Erythrocytes can be stored for approximately 35 days before deterioration, depending on the type of preservative used. Blood is administered to restore circulating red cell volume due to an acute loss of blood from trauma or internal hemorrhage. Plasma, the fluid portion of the blood, is transfused in patients who suffer massive burns or in trauma in which large volumes of red cell replacement is required. Packed erythrocytes used for transfusion are erythrocytes that have been separated from the plasma. Packed erythrocyte transfusion improves the oxygen-carrying capacity of the blood in various types of anemia.

Erythrocytes have no substitutes. Therefore, once the oxygen-carrying capacity is diminished by a massive loss of erythrocytes, only the infusion of additional erythrocytes replenishes the oxygen supply to the body.

For the proper procedures for starting an IV and using necessary equipment and sites for peripheral venous cannulation, *see* Chapter 11, "Intravenous Cannulation."

Maintaining body temperature

When treating the patient in shock the body temperature must be maintained as close to normal as possible. Attention must be paid to factors that affect the body temperature, including environmental/weather conditions, temperature of the oxygen and intravenous fluids, and the location where the patient is found, to name a few. Patients lying on the ground, particularly during inclement weather, may experience hypothermia.

Body temperature can be maintained by protecting the patient from the elements and by removing any wet clothing. Additionally, cover the patient to avoid heat loss but be careful not to over-bundle the patient. Too much heat causes vasodilation, counteracting the body's vasoconstrictive compensatory efforts.

Focus history and physical examination

After completing the initial assessment and initiating necessary treatment modalities, a focused history and physical examination, and detailed assessment should be performed. The thoroughness of the focused history and physical examination, and detailed assessment depends on the severity of the patient's condition. Obvious life-threatening problems that cannot be corrected in the prehospital care setting warrant rapid transportation of the patient to an appropriate definitive care facility. Ideally, when assessing the seriously injured patient, the EMT–I should expose and inspect the head, neck, chest, and abdomen.

Throughout the focused history and physical examination, and detailed assessment and while providing treatment and transporting the patient to the hospital, the EMT–I must continually reassess the patient's level of responsiveness, temperature and moistness of the skin, blood pressure, pulse rate, and respiratory rate. The potential for cardiac arrhythmias exists in shock, and appropriate defibrillation devices should be nearby.

Additional information can be obtained in the detailed assessment by asking the patient appropriate questions to find out how he or she feels. Is the patient thirsty, weak, nauseous, dizzy, etc.? Does the patient have a history of significant medical conditions or take any medications? These answers will give the EMT–I additional information from which he or she can base the treatment modalities.

CASE HISTORY FOLLOW-UP

En route to the emergency department (ED), EMT–I Harris reassesses the patient's vital signs and contacts medical direction. Aside from a slight increase in blood pressure, the patient's condition is unchanged. The EMT–Is deliver the patient to the ED and begin to replenish their supplies. As they are cleaning and restocking the ambulance, they are dispatched to a motor vehicle accident at an intersection near the hospital. This call was the second of what was to be a very busy shift.

Later that evening the EMT–Is stop by the ED to check on a few patients that they had transported that day. They are particularly curious about the elderly woman with the fever. The nurse in charge tells the EMT–Is that the woman was diagnosed with pneumonia and septicemia. According to the nurse, the patient developed shaking chills and began to hyperventilate shortly after arrival in the ED. She was later intubated and placed on a ventilator to manage her respiratory failure. Her blood cultures confirmed bacteremia infection for which she was receiving IV antibiotics. The EMT–Is know that pneumonia is a major cause of death in the elderly and that anti-cancer drugs can markedly reduce normal defense mechanisms to combat illnesses like influenza. But they have never really seen a patient like this before.

The nurse said that the patient was moved to the intensive care unit where she wasn't doing very well. Despite fluid resuscitation and vasopressors, she's still hypotensive. In fact, the doctors don't think she'll make it. So far, they've been unable to locate any family members.

SUMMARY

Long-term survival of the body as a whole is dependent on the delivery of adequate amounts of oxygen and glucose to the individual cells by the blood. Shock is a condition in which there is inadequate perfusion to the tissues and cells of the body. This creates a lack of tissue oxygenation, leading to anaerobic metabolism. Decreased blood flow, which is common in shock syndrome, may occur secondary to hemorrhage, pump failure, or inappropriate system vascular resistance. Because of decreased perfusion, the body's tissues become damaged. Even the cardiovascular system deteriorates, worsening the severity of the shock state. The body tries to compensate for this damage by utilizing several mechanisms. These mechanisms will only work until the body can no longer maintain perfusion to the vital organs: the heart, lungs, and brain.

Shock develops in three successive stages: compensatory, decompensated, and irreversible. The first stage occurs when the body fails to compensate for the insult. Signs and symptoms of shock are more apparent at this stage. Survival often depends on prompt recognition in the field, rapid care, and prompt transport to the hospital. As shock progresses, the oxygen supply to the cells decreases and the cells resort to anaerobic metabolism. This form of metabolism is far less effective than the normal state of aerobic metabolism. Anaerobic metabolism produces several abnormal acids, the best known of which is lactic acid. Accumulation of acids changes the pH of the body, resulting in a condition known as acidosis. Shock progresses to the irreversible stage, when the tissues die.

Evaluation of the trauma victim for shock is begun in the primary survey, during which the most obvious signs of decreased tissue perfusion may be present. It is continued during the secondary survey, when more subtle clues may be found. The patient is then continually assessed for signs of developing shock until he or she is placed in the hands of the receiving medical personnel. Treatment for shock includes adequate ventilation and oxygen and further prevention of the shock process. Rapid transport to the medical facility is imperative.

Low blood pressure (below 90 mm Hg) is a late sign of shock and is therefore not the sole indicator that shock is present. Evaluation begins with the scene survey, mechanism of injury, and history. If any of these factors indicate that shock is or could be present, the EMT–I should already be taking measures to counter the effects of shock.

INTRAVENOUS CANNULATION

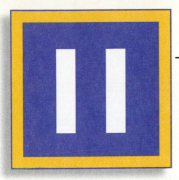

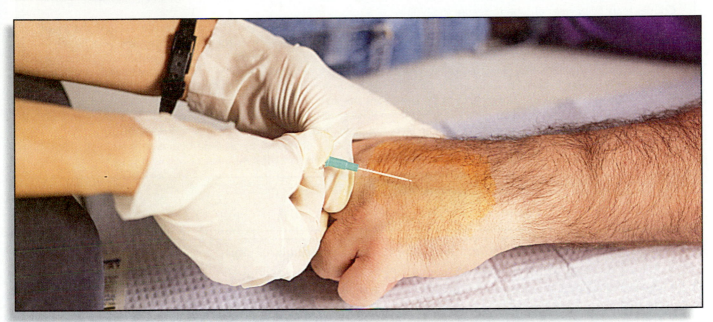

CASE HISTORY

EMT–Intermediate Davis is on duty with Medic 6 when a call comes in for a patient who is bleeding. As EMT–I Davis approaches the scene, a high-rise apartment building, the dispatcher contacts him with additional information. "The patient is an 83-year-old female who's having dark stools and coffee-grounds vomiting, and is cool and clammy."

A home healthcare nurse meets EMT–I Davis at the door. "Hello, I'm Mrs. Brownwell," she says. "The patient's name is Helen Greenley. Her neighbors got concerned about her when she didn't show up for bingo today." She points to a large "coffee-grounds" stain on the bedding and says, "It looks like she's lost a lot of blood."

As EMT–I Davis begins his initial assessment, he notes that the patient is pale and diaphoretic. Her pulse is 142 and thready, and her respirations are 26 and shallow. EMT–I Davis measures her blood pressure at 94/72.

EMT–I Davis leans to the patient's ear and says, "Mrs. Greenley, are you ok?" She just groans.

EMT–I Davis places her on the pulse oximeter and ventilates her with a bag-valve-mask and 100% oxygen. His partner, EMT–I Cooper, places the electrocardiogram electrodes on the patient's chest. Her pulse oximetry reading is 84%, and the electrocardiogram shows sinus tachycardia.

Case History, continued

EMT–I Davis says to the patient, "I'm going to start an IV, Mrs. Greenley," as he places a tourniquet around her left forearm and lowers it over the side of the bed. EMT–I Cooper prepares a 1000-mL bag of normal saline with a macro-drip administration set for EMT–I Davis.

EMT–I Davis palpates a vein on the back of the patient's forearm with his gloved hand and feels confident that he will be able to get it on the first attempt. He prepares the site with Betadine, then wipes it with an alcohol swab. EMT–I Cooper tears five pieces of tape to secure the IV line.

EMT–I Davis holds Mrs. Greenley's skin taut with his thumb as he inserts the 18-gauge needle. He has the bevel pointed up as he penetrates the skin, and then directs the needle into the vein. As the needle enters the vein he sees a small amount of blood flash back into the clear plastic catheter cap. He advances the catheter and withdraws the needle.

EMT–I Cooper holds a red, puncture-proof, container to his partner's side, and EMT–I Davis immediately drops the needle into it. Next, he draws a 3-mL sample of blood using a 5-mL syringe and a red-top tube.

EMT–I Davis connects the administration set and opens the flow control valve. It isn't running.

He checks the insertion site for infiltration, but there is no swelling in the surrounding tissue. He rotates the cannula and pulls it back out approximately 1/16th of an inch, but it still does not run.

EMT–I Cooper quietly leans over and pulls the tourniquet strap loose, and the IV fluid begins to flow freely. EMT–I Davis is embarrassed to have made one of the most common and fundamental mistakes of IV therapy.

LEARNING OBJECTIVES

Upon completion of this chapter, the EMT–Intermediate should be able to:

- DEFINE the term *intravenous cannulation*.
- RECALL the indications and contraindications of intravenous cannulation.
- IDENTIFY the equipment used to perform intravenous cannulation.
- SELECT preferred solutions for use in management of trauma and medical emergencies.
- RECALL the recommended ratio of IV solution replacement to blood loss in patients experiencing hypovolemic shock.
- DESCRIBE the methods used to determine the proper IV flow rate.
- LIST the advantages, disadvantages, and complications associated with use of the peripheral veins.
- IDENTIFY the veins that are commonly used for peripheral intravenous cannulation.
- RECALL the steps used to perform peripheral venous cannulation.
- USE problem-solving skills with IV lifelines that are not functioning properly to determine the cause and correct the problem.
- LIST complications associated with IV therapy.
- DEMONSTRATE the steps for discontinuing an IV lifeline.

KEY TERMS

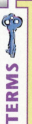

DORSUM

FLEXION

HALF-LIFE

HEPATITIS B VIRUS

HIV

INTRAOSSEOUS

INTRAVENOUS CANNULATION

IPSILATERAL

ISOTONIC SOLUTION

LARGE-BORE CATHETER

NEEDLE

SCLEROTIC

TKO RATE

WIDE OPEN RATE

INTRODUCTION

 Define the term intravenous cannulation.

Definition

Intravenous (IV) cannulation is defined as the placement of a catheter into a vein. It is used to administer blood, fluids, or medications directly into the circulatory system. It also can be used to obtain venous blood specimens for laboratory determinations. **Because IV fluids are drugs, on-line medical direction or standing orders are typically required for the EMT–I to administer IV fluids.**

 Recall the indications and contraindications of intravenous cannulation.

LARGE-BORE CATHETER: Catheter with a large interior diameter (14 to 16 gauge).

Indications

Intravenous therapy is an important adjunct in the management of the seriously ill or injured patient. Some indications for its use include cardiac disease, hypoglycemia, seizures, and shock. As an example, in hypovolemic shock, IV lines are used to counter blood loss by introducing fluid into the circulatory system. This fluid acts to restore the circulatory volume until the body is able to manufacture enough blood to regain control of the circulatory system. In hypovolemia, the patient needs at least two IV lines with **large-bore catheters.** In medical emergencies such as heart problems, IV lines are used to establish a medication administration route. Generally, the IV route is used to administer drugs in the prehospital setting. Giving the drug intravenously places it directly into the bloodstream, resulting in a more rapid onset of action than can be achieved through any other route of administration.

Finally, an IV line can be placed as a precautionary measure in patients who are in stable condition but whose deterioration is anticipated. This treatment could be for the purpose of medication access, volume replacement, or both.

Because time and skill are required to perform venipuncture and establish an IV line, ongoing skill proficiency is required for the EMT–I.

SCLEROTIC: Hardening or thickening of tissues.

Contraindications

Cannulation of a particular site is contraindicated in **sclerotic** veins and burned extremities. **Attempts at IV therapy should not significantly delay transporting critically ill or injured patients to the hospital.**

STREET WISE
When treating a critically ill or injured patient, the EMT–I should not spend a lot of time on the scene trying to start an IV lifeline. Rather, the EMT–I should start the IV en route to the hospital.

BODY SUBSTANCE ISOLATION PRECAUTIONS

HBV: Abbreviation for hepatitis B virus.
HIV: Abbreviation for human immunodeficiency virus.

When performing IV therapy, the EMT–I must employ body substance isolation precautions. All blood and body substances should be regarded as potentially infected with **hepatitis B virus (HBV)** or **HIV.** Next, gloves should be worn whenever the EMT–I is working with IV equipment. After each use, gloves should be disposed of in an appropriate waste receptacle. Hands must be washed before and after working with IV equipment and immediately on coming into contact with blood or other body fluids. If there is any possibility of blood or body fluid splashing, additional barrier protection such as a gown, mask, and eye protection must be worn. Particular attention must be given to proper handling and disposal of needles and sharp instruments as well as the use of barriers. All once-used needles must be placed in a puncture-resistant ("sharps") container as quickly as possible. Needle-stick injuries can be largely avoided by not bending, breaking, or recapping needles; separating them from the syringe; or manipulating them by hand. Another level of protection recommended by the Centers for Disease Control and Prevention is immunization with the HBV vaccine.

This chapter presents information regarding IV therapy in the adult patient. IV therapy in the pediatric patient is discussed in Chapter 17, "Pediatric Emergencies."

EQUIPMENT

 Identify the equipment used to perform intravenous cannulation.

The equipment and supplies needed to establish and maintain an IV lifeline include:

- IV solution
- Administration set
- Extension set
- Needles/catheters (assorted sizes)
- Protective gloves
- Gown and goggles, tourniquet (venous constricting band)

- Tape
- Antibiotic swabs/ointment
- Gauze dressings (2 x 2s, 4 x 4s)
- 10- to 35-mL syringes
- A Vacutainer holder with multisample IV Luer-lock adapter
- Assorted blood collection tubes
- Padded armboards

 Select preferred solutions for use in the management of trauma and medical emergencies.

Intravenous solutions

Intravenous solutions are the fluids that are administered into the venous circulation (Table 11-1). They are typically contained in a clear plastic bag that collapses as it empties. The size of the IV bag varies depending on its use, holding anywhere from 25 to 1000 mL of fluid. Smaller bags (100 to 250 mL) are used in the management of medical emergencies and drug administration, whereas larger bags (1000 mL) are used in the management of trauma emergencies or when the patient has experienced volume loss. The IV bag has two ports at the bottom of the bag: one port has a rubber stopper for the infusion of medications, the other has a plastic tab that is removed in order to insert the spiked piercing end of the IV administration set tubing into the bag (Fig. 11-1).

 Recall the recommended ratio of IV solution replacement to blood loss in patients experiencing hypovolemic shock.

Colloids and crystalloids

There are two major categories of IV fluids: *crystalloids* and *colloids* (Fig. 11-2). Crystalloid solutions are created by dissolving crystals such as salts and sugars in water. They contain no proteins or other high

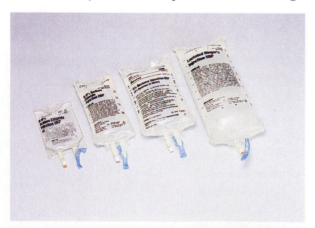

Fig. 11-1 Various sizes of intravenous therapy bags.

molecular-weight solutes. When introduced into the circulatory system, the dissolved ions cross the cell membrane quickly, followed by the IV solution water. For this reason, crystalloid solutions remain in the intravascular space for only a short time before diffusing across the capillary walls into the tissues. Because of this action, it is necessary to administer 3 L of IV crystalloid solution for every 1 L of blood lost (3:1 ratio) when treating patients who have experienced hypovolemic shock. Normal saline and lactated Ringer's solution are examples of crystalloids.

HALF-LIFE: Time required by the body, tissue, or organ to metabolize or inactivate half the substance taken in.

Colloids contain large molecules such as protein that do not readily pass through the capillary membrane. Therefore, colloid solutions remain in the intravascular space for extended periods of time. In addition, the presence of the large molecules in colloids results in an osmotic pressure that is greater than the osmotic pressure of interstitial and intracellular fluid. This difference in pressure causes fluid to move from the interstitial and intracellular spaces into the intravascular space. For this reason, colloids are often referred to as *volume expanders*. Whole blood, plasma, packed red blood cells, and plasma substitutes are examples of colloids. However, because colloids are expensive, have short **half-lives,** and often require refrigeration, they are not commonly used in the prehospital setting.

Normal saline and lactated Ringer's solution

The recommended IV solutions for use in the prehospital setting are normal saline (0.9%) and lactated Ringer's solution. Both are crystalloid **isotonic solutions.**

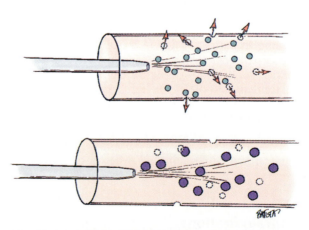

Fig. 11-2 A, Crystalloid solutions move quickly across cell membranes. B, Colloid solutions do not move across cell membranes quickly; therefore, they remain in the intravascular space for longer periods of time.

TABLE 11-1	Characteristics of different IV solutions			
SOLUTIONS	**INDICATIONS**	**ADVANTAGES**	**DISADVANTAGES**	**CONSIDERATIONS**
5% Dextrose in water (D_5W) Hypotonic sugar solution	• To maintain water balance and supply calories necessary for cell metabolism	• Is inexpensive and readily available	• Causes red blood cell clumping so it cannot be given with blood • Is incompatible with some medications • May cause water intoxication, hyponatremia, or hyperglycemia	• Not the solution of choice for shock • Use only to establish an emergency IV line for drug administration
0.9% Sodium chloride solution (normal saline) Isotonic crystalloid solution	• Initial fluid and electrolyte (Na^+, Cl^-) replacement in all types of hypovolemia • Cardiac arrest	• May be used as an emergency plasma expander while whole blood is being typed and crossmatched • Is readily available and inexpensive	• May cause diuresis, hypernatremia, hypokalemia, and acid-base imbalance (following large infusions)	• Use cautiously if patient has CHF or renal dysfunction • Monitor patient for signs of pulmonary edema or fluid overload
Lactated Ringer's solution Isotonic crystalloid solution	• For initial fluid replacement in all types of hypovolemia • Cardiac arrest	• Closely resembles blood plasma • Contains electrolyte content needed for adequate kidney function • Rarely causes adverse reactions • Is inexpensive and readily available • Releases buffer when metabolized	• May lead to volume overload, CHF, or pulmonary edema	• Use with caution in patients with pulmonary edema and impaired lactate metabolism states (liver disease, anoxia) • May induce hypothermia with multiple infusions

CHF = congestive heart failure

HELPFUL HINT
In addition to its volume replacement benefit, lactated Ringer's solution, when metabolized by the liver, releases bicarbonate, which is a buffer.

One liter of lactated Ringer's solution contains 130 mEq of sodium (Na^+), 4 mEq of potassium (K^+), 3 mEq of calcium (Ca^{2+}), 109 mEq of chloride ions (Cl^-), and 28 mEq of lactate. One liter of normal saline contains 154 mEq of sodium ions (Na^+) and 154 mEq of chloride ions (Cl^-).

Five percent dextrose in water

Five percent dextrose in water (D_5W) is a glucose solution that is isotonic in the container but hypotonic after it enters the circulatory system. The reason for this change is that glucose quickly moves from the circulation, leaving free water. In the past, D_5W was a mainstay in the management of medical emergencies. More recently, however, the American Heart Association Advanced Cardiac Life Support Guidelines for cardiac arrest no longer list D_5W as the preferred solution because of neurologic outcomes associated with increased glucose levels in patients who survive. Local protocols will dictate whether or not D_5W is used by an EMT–I's EMS system.

Plasma and dextran

Plasma and dextran are two colloid solutions used for volume expansions in patients with hypovolemia. However, their use is limited to the hospital setting and critical care transport systems (such as helicopters and specialized ground transport units) because they require special storage and are expensive. Dextran

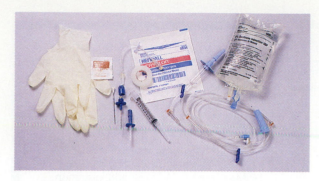

Fig.11-3   An administration set.

also can create type and crossmatch abnormalities and bleeding disorders.

Administration set

The administration set is the clear plastic tubing that connects the IV bag to the catheter (Fig. 11-3). It allows for easy viewing in case of air bubbles or precipitation of certain medications administered through the tubing. There are five primary components to IV tubing with which the EMT–I must be familiar:

- Piercing spike
- Drip chamber
- Flow clamp
- Drug administration port
- Connector end

Piercing spike

The piercing spike is the end of the administration set that is inserted into the tubing insertion port of the IV bag. It comes packaged with a protective cap to prevent it from being contaminated prior to use.

HELPFUL HINT

Great care must be exercised to keep the piercing spike as sterile as possible. The EMT–I only should uncover the piercing spike to insert it into the IV solution bag. The same is true for the connector end of the administration set. The EMT–I should only uncover it just prior to inserting it into the hub of the venipuncture device. This precaution helps avoid the possibility of touching it against something. Also, it is usually not necessary to remove the distal protective cap to drain the administration set of air.

Drip chamber

The drip chamber is the clear, cylindric portion of the tubing where the drops passing through the administration set can be viewed and counted. It is located near the piercing end of the IV tubing where it connects with the IV bag. The number of drops needed to deliver 1 mL of solution is referred to as the *drop factor*. There are two types of administration

sets commonly used in the prehospital setting: the microdrip (mini) and the macrodrip (regular).

The top portion of the drip chamber is called the *drop orifice*. The drop orifice of the microdrip consists of a tiny metal barrel projecting down from the top of the drip chamber. The barrel controls fluid flow through the drip chamber. With the microdrip administration set (Fig. 11-4 A), a smaller amount of fluid is delivered with each drop; 60 drops being equal to 1 mL of IV solution. The microdrip delivers fluid in very precise amounts, making it useful in children and adults who require minimal fluid and when medications are administered via an IV infusion.

The macrodrip is used when a large amount of fluid is needed (Fig. 11-4 B). With this type of drip chamber, the drop orifice consists of a large opening that allows for a bigger drop size. Depending on the manufacturer, the drop size may vary with different types of administration sets. For this reason it is important to read the box or protective wrap in which the administration set is contained.

CLINICAL NOTES

A new IV administration set, the SELEC-3 from Biomedix, recently introduced into the clinical setting, allows EMT–Is the option of three different drop volumes all in one device (Fig. 11-5). By simply turning the selector top, the EMT–I may choose between 10, 15, or 60 drops/mL at any time without breaking the line. This feature allows the EMT–I to respond quickly to a patient's changing needs. It also reduces inventory cost and the risk of contamination and ensures that the right administration set is always available.

Flow clamp

Below the drip chamber is the flow clamp. It has a plastic housing with a roller- or screw-type clamp that is used to control the amount of IV fluid the patient receives. The screw clamp allows the EMT–I greater accuracy. It is controlled by turning the wheel clockwise to close the line and counterclockwise to open the line. The roller clamp, used for standard therapy, is faster and easier to manipulate. By moving the roller up or down, the EMT–I can increase or decrease the flow rate through the IV administration set or turn the IV on or off. A third type, the slide clamp, moves horizontally to start or stop the flow but does not allow fine adjustments and thus cannot regulate the flow rate.

TKO RATE: "To keep open" rate of infusing the IV solution. It is also referred to as KVO (keep vein open). It is equal to approximately 8 to 15 drops per minute.

Describe the methods used to determine the proper IV flow rate.

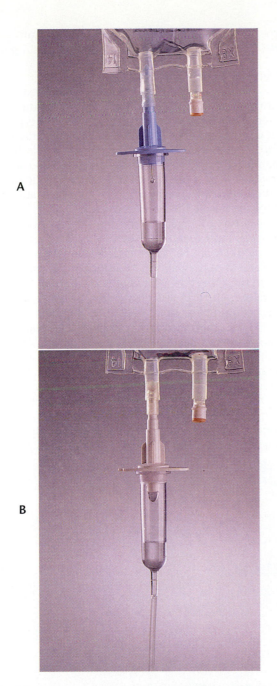

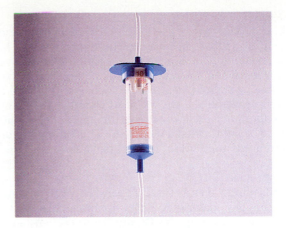

Fig. 11-5   **A SELEC-3 administration set.**

- Capillary refill (in children less than 6 years of age)
- Cerebral function

 WIDE-OPEN RATE: No restriction of fluid flow from the IV bag to the patient.

In the severely hypovolemic patient, the solution should be administered at a rapid or **wide-open rate.** The amount of IV fluid administered in the field setting should be limited to 2 to 3 L. When treating the patient with severe blood loss, the flow rate can be increased three to four times the normal amount by wrapping a blood pressure cuff around the IV bag and inflating it to 300 mm Hg.

Drug administration port
The drug administration port is located below the drip chamber. It is closer to the distal end of the administration set tubing. The port consists of a rubber stopper and a Y-shaped inlet. Medication boluses or an infusion of medication can be delivered through this port.

Connector end
The connector end is the part of the IV administration set that is inserted into the hub of the IV catheter. Like the spiked piercing end, it is packaged with a protective cap to prevent it from being contaminated prior to use.

> **HELPFUL HINT**
> To reduce the amount of IV fluid needed to clear the air from the tubing, the EMT–I should slide the flow control valve toward the spiked end of the tubing until it comes to rest against the drip chamber. Then, the control valve should be opened to flush the air out of the tubing.

Fig. 11-4   **A, A microdrip chamber delivers fluids in very precise amounts. B, A macrodrip chamber.**

In the field setting, there are typically two rates for administering IV fluids. In medical emergencies in which IV lines are placed as a precautionary measure or for the purpose of administering medications, the flow is usually maintained at a **TKO rate.** In trauma or other situations in which IV fluids are being used to replace circulatory volume, the flow rate is based on the patient's response to the IV infusion. Responses include improvement in the patient's:

- Pulse
- Blood pressure

Specialty IV Tubing

Some EMS systems use IV blood tubing instead of macrodrip tubing in patients with hypovolemia. This use reduces the amount of tubing change-over required at the hospital when the patient is switched from a crystalloid solution to blood. Another type of administration set, the Volutrol chamber IV tubing, is commonly used when specific amounts of fluids are to be administered (Fig. 11-6). This tubing is more commonly used for infant and pediatric infusions.

Extension Set

Extra tubing may be used to lengthen the administration set, making it easier to move the patient without disrupting the IV site. However, any extra length of IV tubing may actually slow the IV flow rate. Also, the extra length of tubing may get caught under the stretcher when removing the patient from the ambulance. Appropriate caution must be exercised when choosing a tubing extension set.

> 🔑 **NEEDLE:** Sharp, stainless steel hollow tube that is used to penetrate the skin and blood vessel.

Needle/catheter

The catheter is the tube that remains in the vein to allow the administration of IV fluids or medications. A **needle** is used to facilitate passage of the catheter through the skin and into the vein. The needle has a beveled tip that makes penetration of the skin and vein easier and less painful. The three basic types of IV catheters are plastic catheters inserted over a hollow needle (Angiocath, Quickcath, Jelco, etc.) (Fig. 11-7 A), plastic catheters inserted through a hollow needle or over a guidewire (Intracath) (Fig. 11-7 B), and hollow needles (butterfly type), (Fig. 11-7 C). Plastic catheters are generally preferred over hollow needles in advanced life support.

Over-the-needle catheters

The over-the-needle catheter typically consists of a plastic outer catheter and an inner needle that extends just beyond the catheter. The needle is pulled out after insertion in the vein, leaving the catheter in place. At the proximal end of the needle is a flashback chamber that allows the EMT–I to see blood return when the vein is penetrated. The proximal end of the catheter has a hub where the IV tubing is attached (once the needle has been removed).

Because of their flexibility, over-the-needle catheters most commonly are used in the prehospital setting; they can be better anchored and permit freer movement of the patient. Additionally, the puncture site in the vein is the same size as the plastic catheter, therefore, there is less chance for bleeding around the venipuncture site. Two other benefits of this device are that infiltration occurs less frequently than with steel needle venipuncture devices, and an armboard usually is not necessary after insertion. Because the device has both a catheter and needle, it is more difficult to insert than winged steel needles.

Over-the-needle catheters used to cannulate peripheral veins are commonly available in lengths from 1 inch (2.5 cm) to 2 inch (5 cm), with gauges ranging in size from 14 to 26.

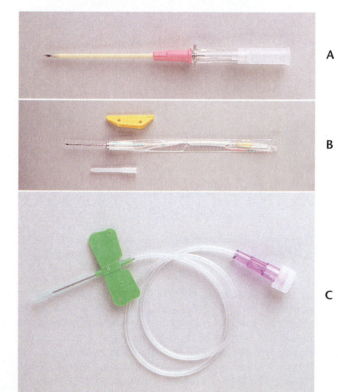

Fig. 11-7 A, An over-the-needle catheter. B, A through-the-needle catheter. C, A hollow needle (Butterfly type).

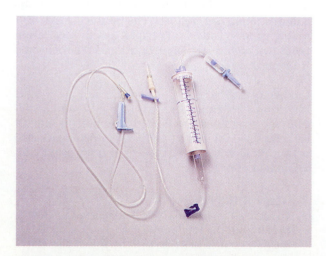

Fig. 11-6 Volutrol chamber IV tubing is commonly used when specific amounts of fluid are to be administered.

IV catheter size

The outside diameter of the venipuncture device is called the *gauge*. The larger the gauge number, the smaller the diameter of the shaft, (*eg*, a 22-gauge catheter is small, whereas a 14-gauge catheter is large). A large diameter catheter (14 gauge) provides much greater fluid flow than does a small diameter catheter (22 gauge). Catheters used for prehospital care come in a variety of sizes, which are listed in Table 11-2.

Choosing the best size over-the-needle catheter for the patient is not always easy; but as a rule, except for when volume replacement is needed, smaller-sized devices are better. A small needle/catheter causes less trauma to the vein. It also allows greater blood flow around the tip, reducing the risk of clotting. Using a catheter that is too big for the vein invites complications. Also, some elderly patients' veins cannot accommodate a large-bore catheter. Large-bore devices (14 to 16 gauge) should be used for patients in shock, cardiac arrest, or other life-threatening emergencies in which rapid fluid replacement is required. At a minimum, an 18-gauge catheter should be used in those patients requiring blood. When employing a large-sized catheter, the EMT–I should be sure to choose a large enough vein to accommodate it. The other variable to consider when selecting an intravenous catheter is its length. **The longer the catheter, the slower the flow rate.** The flow rate through a 14-gauge, 5-cm catheter (approximately 125 mL/min) is twice the flow rate of a 16-gauge, 20-cm catheter. For cannulation of a peripheral vein, a needle and catheter length of 1.5 to 2 inches (5 cm) is adequate. Some over-the-needle catheters are supplied with an attached syringe (Fig. 11-8). The syringe permits an easy check of blood return once the needle is inside the vein and prevents air from entering the vessel on insertion.

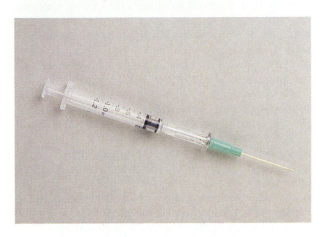

Fig. 11-8 An IV catheter supplied with an attached syringe.

TABLE 11-2	Different sized IV venipuncture devices	
GAUGE	**USED FOR**	**CONSIDERATIONS**
14 to 16	• Adolescents and adults • Volume replacement, as in trauma • When viscous medications such as 50% dextrose are to be administered	• Painful insertion • Requires large vein
18	• Older children, adolescents, and adults • Administration of blood and blood components and other viscous infusions	• Painful insertion • Requires large vein
20	• Older children, adolescents, average-sized adult patients • Suitable for most IV infusions	• Commonly used
22	• Infants, toddlers, children, adolescents, adults (especially elderly) • Suitable for most IV infusions	• Used for fragile and/or small veins • Slower rates must be maintained • More difficult to insert through tough skin
24 to 26	• Neonates, infants, toddlers, children, adolescents, adults (especially elderly) • Suitable for most IV infusions, but flow rates are slower	• For extremely small veins, *eg*, small veins of the fingers or veins of inner arm in elderly patients • May be difficult to insert into tough skin

Supplies and materials

A variety of other supplies are needed to establish and maintain an IV lifeline. Without exception, latex or rubber protective gloves should be worn by the EMT–I when attempting venipuncture. A tourniquet (venous constrictive band), when applied proximal to the IV venipuncture site prior to cannulation, delays venous return and distends the vein making it easier to locate and cannulate. The ideal tourniquet is easily tied, does not roll into a thin band, stays relatively flat, and releases easily. Penrose drain tubing commonly is used as a tourniquet in the prehospital setting. Also, there are a variety of tourniquets commercially available. Some are equipped with a catch mechanism to anchor them. Others have a wide, flat rubber band that is secured with Velcro. Povidone-iodine or alcohol preparations are used to cleanse the IV site prior to venipuncture, reducing the risk of infection. Sterile dressings are applied over the IV site to keep it clean. Adhesive tape is applied over the administration set tubing, sterile dressing, and IV catheter to hold them in place. Armboards stabilize the IV site, preventing the patient from dislodging or causing the catheter to become kinked or positioned against a valve in the vein. A 10- or 35-mL syringe or a Vacutainer holder with a multisample IV Luer-lock adapter fitted to it and assorted blood collection tubes are used to collect blood samples.

SITES FOR PERIPHERAL VENOUS CANNULATION

 List the advantages, disadvantages, and complications associated with use of the peripheral veins.

Structure of veins

Veins have three layers: the tunica intima (inner layer), tunica media (middle layer), and tunica externa (outer layer). The tunica intima is an inner elastic endothelial lining made up of layers of smooth, flat cells that allow blood cells and platelets to flow smoothly through the blood vessels. Unnecessary movement of the venipuncture device can scratch or roughen this inner surface, causing thrombus formation. Semilunar valves, designed to prevent backflow and ensure the flow of blood toward the heart, are located in this layer of the vein. These valves are found in many veins, and are especially common in those of the extremities. The tunica media consists of muscular and elastic tissue. Vasoconstrictor and vasodilator nerve fibers located in this layer stimulate the vein to contract and relax. They are responsible for venous spasm that can occur as a result of anxiety or receiving IV fluids that are too cold. The tunica externa consists of connective tissue that surrounds and supports the vessel, holding it together.

Difference between arteries and veins

Before choosing a vein as an IV site, the EMT–I must make sure the blood vessel is actually a vein, which helps avoid inadvertent arterial puncture (Fig. 11-9). Table 11-3 shows the main characteristics of veins and arteries.

The skin

The skin is made up of two layers: the epidermis and the dermis. The epidermis is the outermost layer. It forms a protective covering for the dermis and varies in thickness in different parts of the body. The thinnest areas of skin are on the inner surface of the limbs. The thickness of the dermis also varies with age. Elderly patients often have such thin skin on the dorsum of the hand that it does not adequately support the vein for venipuncture.

The dermis, or underlayer, is highly vascular and sensitive, containing many capillaries and thousands of nerve fibers, including those that react to temperature, touch, pressure, and pain. The number of nerve fibers varies in different areas of the body, some areas being highly sensitive, others being only mildly sensitive. The insertion of a needle may cause great pain in one area but little pain in another.

 Identify the veins that are commonly used for peripheral intravenous cannulation.

Sites used in routine situations

In noncritical patients, the distal veins on the dorsum of the hand and arms often are used as IV sites. Using these veins permits the patient to freely move his or her arm. Also, the technique is relatively easy to master, and setting the IV in these locations does not interfere with other life-sustaining measures such as airway management (Fig. 11-10). Additionally, if a problem develops with more distal veins, another site higher up on the arm can be selected. The disadvantage of the more distal veins is that they are sometimes fragile and difficult to cannulate. Also, in states of decreased cardiac output, medications administered through these vessels take longer to reach the central circulation. Furthermore, irritating solutions administered through these veins may cause pain and phlebitis. For a summary of IV site locations, advantages, disadvantages, and considerations for uses, see Table 11-4. If available, the EMT–I should use a vein that is:

- Fairly straight
- Easily accessible
- Well-fixed, not rolling
- Feels springy when palpated (Fig. 11-11)

Sclerotic veins, veins near joints (where immobilization will be difficult), areas where an arterial pulse is palpable close to the vein, or veins near injured areas and edematous (swollen) extremities should be avoided as sites of IV cannulation. Circulatory problems in an extremity such as dialysis fistula or a history of mastectomy also should prompt the EMT–I to

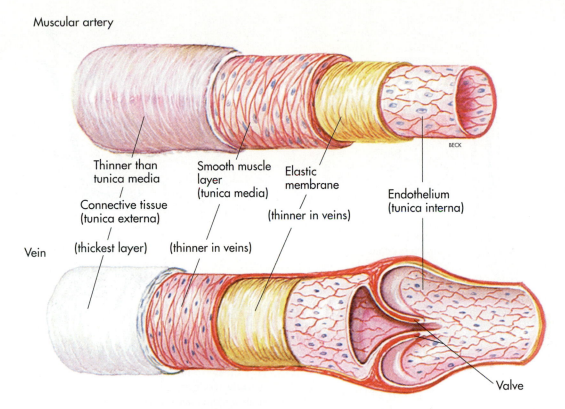

Fig. 11-9   The characteristic differences between veins and arteries.

TABLE 11-3	Differences between arteries and veins	
CHARACTERISTICS	**VEINS**	**ARTERIES**
Location in the body	• Superficial veins lie just under the skin and drain the skin and superficial fascia • Deep veins accompany the principal arteries and take the name of the artery with which they travel	• Arteries run deep and usually are surrounded by muscle. This provides them the protection they need as part of the high pressure portion of the vascular system • Occasionally, an artery is superficially located; this is an aberrant artery
Color of blood	• Dark red due to decreased oxygen concentration	• Bright red due to usually high concentration of oxygen
Pulsation	• Absent	• Present
Valves	• Present; they keep blood flowing toward the heart, counteracting muscular pressure that would make the blood back up • Valves often cause a noticeable bulge in the vein when a tourniquet is applied	• Not present; arteries are under constant pressure because the heart pumps blood through them
Direction of flow	• Toward the heart	• Away from the heart

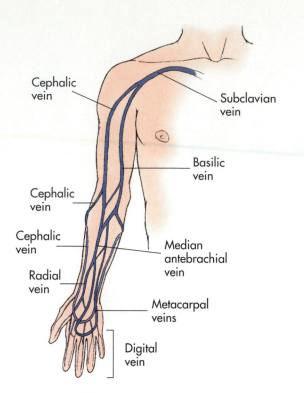

Cephalic
vein

Subclavian
vein

Basilic
vein

Cephalic
vein

Cephalic
vein

Median
antebrachial
vein

Radial
vein

Metacarpal
veins

Digital
vein

Fig. 11-10   **The venous anatomy of the arm.**

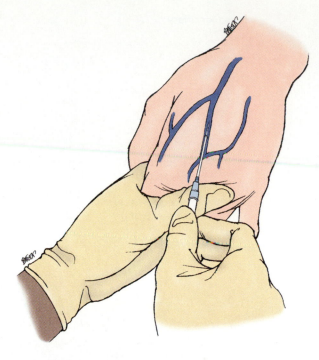

Fig. 11-11   **The ideal vein for delivering IV therapy is fairly straight, easily accessible, well-fixed, and feels springy when palpated.**

select another IV site. If possible, the patient's non-dominant hand should be used, leaving the hand used for writing free.

Sites used in cardiac arrest
In cardiac arrest, the preferred sites for IV cannulation are the peripheral veins of the **antecubital fossa** (the area anterior to and below the elbow), because they are among the largest, most visible, and accessible veins in the arm. The more distal veins are the least preferred IV sites because blood flow from distal extremities is markedly diminished during circulatory collapse, and distal peripheral veins may be difficult or impossible to cannulate.

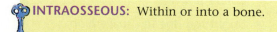

INTRAOSSEOUS: Within or into a bone.

Other sites
Other sites that may be used for intravenous cannulation by the EMT–I include the external jugular vein, peripheral leg veins, and **intraosseous** sites. The external jugular vein is a fairly large vein located in the neck, below the ear and behind the angle of the mandible (Fig. 11-12 A). This vein is clearly visible in the adult but is not as easy to cannulate in the pediatric patient. A disadvantage to using the external jugular vein as an IV site is that the catheter and tubing are hard to tape down and can be displaced with movement of the patient's head. The veins of the

lower leg (Fig. 11-12 B) should be used as a last resort in adults, because use of these veins places the patient at risk for thrombus formation. If the saphenous vein of the leg is used, it should be entered at its most distal point. Intraosseous sites can be used in infants and children and are discussed in Chapter 17, "Pediatric Emergencies."

PROCEDURE FOR PERFORMING IV CANNULATION

 Recall the steps used to perform peripheral venous cannulation.

To perform IV cannulation the EMT–I must do the following:

1. Explain the need for IV cannulation and describe the procedure to the patient. Determine if the patient has any allergies (especially to iodine if using iodine pads to cleanse the skin).

   The EMT–I must keep in mind that the patient may be apprehensive about the procedure and concerned that his or her condition may have worsened. This anxiety can lead to a vasomotor response that can produce syncope or venous constriction. Also, children may have completely unrealistic fears, such as being poisoned or that the IV will never be removed. Hints for preparing the patient for venipuncture include

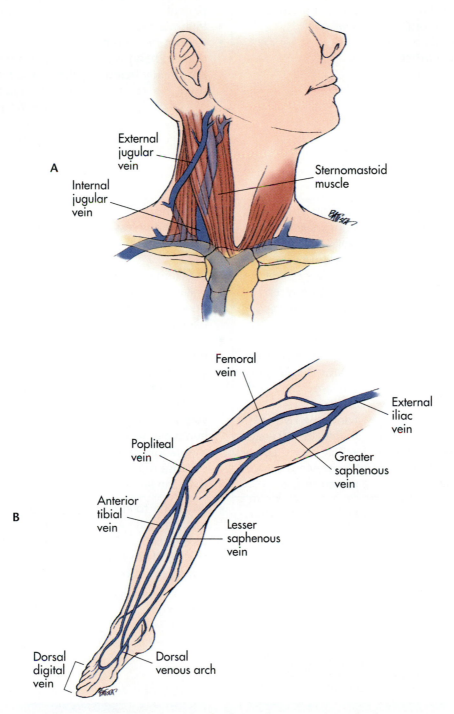

Fig. 11-12   **A, The jugular vein. B, The saphenous vein and other venous anatomy of the leg.**

TABLE 11-4 IV site locations, advantages, disadvantages, considerations for use

SITE	ADVANTAGES	DISADVANTAGES	CONSIDERATIONS
Digital veins Run along the lateral and dorsal portions of the fingers and are joined to each other by communicating branches.	• Can be used when other sites aren't available	• Uncomfortable for patient • Infiltrate easily • Cannot be used if dorsum hand veins are already being used	• In some patients the veins are prominent enough to hold a 21-gauge scalp needle • Adequate immobilization of the fingers with tape can keep the needle from puncturing the posterior wall of the vein
Metacarpal veins Located on dorsum of hand, formed by union of digital veins between knuckles.	• Position of these veins makes them well-suited for IV use • Easily accessible • Lie flat between the joints and metacarpal bones (the bones themselves provide a natural splint) in the large child and adult • Allow the EMT–I to initiate successive venipuncture above the previous puncture site	• Wrist movement is limited unless a short catheter is used • Insertion more painful because of increased nerve endings in hands • Site becomes phlebitic more easily • Veins do not always dilate sufficiently to allow for successful venipuncture; when hypovolemia occurs the peripheral veins collapse more readily than the large veins	• Occasionally, use of the metacarpal veins in the elderly is a poor choice because thin skin and a lack of supportive tissue in this area makes securing the catheter difficult, and small, thin veins may allow extravasation of blood on venipuncture
Cephalic vein Has its source in the radial part of the dorsal venous network formed by the metacarpal veins. Runs along radial side of forearm and upper arm.	• Large vein is excellent for venipuncture • Readily accepts large-bore needles • Does not impair mobility • Its position on forearm creates a natural splint for the needle and adapter	• Proximity to elbow may decrease joint movement • Vein tends to roll during insertion	• May be necessary to shave patient's arm if excessive hair makes taping catheter and tubing in place difficult

TABLE 11-4	Continued		
SITE	**ADVANTAGES**	**DISADVANTAGES**	**CONSIDERATIONS**
Accessory cephalic vein Originates from either a plexus on the back of the forearm or metacarpal veins of the thumb (dorsal venous network). Sometimes it arises from the portion of the cephalic vein just above the wrist and flows back into the main cephalic vein at some higher point. It runs along the radial bone, ascending the arm and joining the cephalic vein below the elbow.	• Large vein is excellent for venipuncture • Readily accepts large-bore needles • Does not impair mobility • Its position on forearm creates a natural splint for the needle and adapter	• Is sometimes difficult to position catheter flush with skin • Usually uncomfortable because venipuncture device is at bend of wrist	
Median antebrachial vein Arises from palm and runs along ulnar side of forearm.	• Vein holds winged needles well	• Many nerve endings in area may cause painful venipuncture or suffer infiltration damage • Infiltration occurs easily in this area	• A last resort when no other means are available
Basilic vein Has its origin in the ulnar part of the dorsal venous network and ascends along ulnar side of forearm and upper arm. It diverges toward the anterior surface of the arm just below the elbow, where it meets the median cubital vein.	• Can take a large-gauge needle easily • Straight, strong vein suitable for large-gauge venipuncture devices	• Patient must be in uncomfortable position during insertion • Penetration of dermal layer of skin where nerve endings are located causes pain • Vein tends to roll during insertion	• This vein is often overlooked because of its inconspicuous position on the ulnar border of the hand and forearm; when other veins have been exhausted, this vein may still be available • The vein can be brought into view by flexing the elbow and bending the arm up

TABLE 11-4 Continued

Site	Advantages	Disadvantages	Considerations
Antecubital veins Located in antecubital fossa (median cephalic is located on radial side, median basilic is on ulnar side, and median cubital rises in front of elbow joint)	• Readily accessible • Large veins facilitate placement of large catheter • Often visible or palpable in children when other veins will not dilate • May be used numerous times without damage to the vein, provided good technique and sharp needles are used • Because of muscular and connective tissue supporting them, they have little tendency to roll	• Difficult to splint area with armboard • Median vein crosses in front of brachial artery, increasing risk of accidental puncture of artery • Veins may be small and scarred if blood has been drawn frequently from this site • May be uncomfortable for patient because arm must be kept straight, otherwise the catheter could kink or slide in and out of the vein, damaging it	• Location is over an area of joint flexion where any movement can dislodge catheter and cause infiltration or result in mechanical phlebitis • If these large veins are impaired or damaged, thrombophlebitis may occur, which then limits use of many available hand veins
Great saphenous vein Located at internal malleolus	• Large vein excellent for venipuncture	• Circulation of lower leg may be impaired • Walking difficult with catheter in place • Increased risk of deep vein thrombosis	
Dorsal venous network Located on dorsal portion of foot	• Suitable for infants and toddlers	• Veins may be difficult to see or find if edema present • Walking difficult with device in place • Increased risk of deep vein thrombosis	
External jugular vein Runs from behind the angle of the jaw downward superficially across the sternocleidomastoid muscle (lateral portion of the neck) to pierce the fascia above the middle third of the clavicle. It joins the subclavian vein just behind the clavicle	• Easy to cannulate • Is considered a peripheral vein • Provides rapid access to the central circulation	• Difficult to keep dressing in place • IV may be easily dislodged and positional with head movement	• May not be readily accessible during arrest situation due to EMT–Is working to manage airway

asking the patient if he or she has ever had an IV before and being supportive if the patient is fearful. The EMT–I should explain to the patient:

- The need for the IV
- How venipuncture is performed
- How much discomfort will be felt
- How therapy will limit his or her activities

2. Next, select the IV fluid to be used and check to make sure it is:

- The proper solution
- Clean, without particulate matter
- Not outdated
- Not leaking

3. Select an appropriately sized catheter (14 to 16 gauge for trauma, volume replacement, or cardiac arrest, 18 to 20 gauge for medical conditions).

4. Select the proper administration set (macro for trauma, micro for medical conditions and drug administration).

5. Prepare the IV bag and administration set using an aseptic technique to prevent contamination, which can cause local or systemic infection.

- Remove the IV bag from its protective envelope and gently squeeze it to detect any punctures or leakages.
- Steady the port of the IV bag with one hand, and remove the protective cap by pulling smoothly to the right.
- Remove the administration set from its protective wrapping or box.
- Slide the flow control valve close to the drip chamber.
- Close off the flow control valve.
- Remove the protective cap from the spiked piercing end of the administration set.
- Invert the IV bag.
- Using sterile technique, insert the spiked piercing end of the administration set into the tubing insertion port of the IV bag. Use one quick, smooth motion (Fig. 11-13 A).
- Turn the IV bag right side up, and squeeze the drip chamber two or three times to fill it half-way (Fig. 11-13 B).
- Open the control valve to flush IV solution through the entire tubing, which should force out all the air.

> **STREET WISE**
> The plastic wrapper in which the IV bag is packaged can be used to collect miscellaneous trash and the IV solution that is used to flush the IV tubing of air bubbles.

> **STREET WISE**
> One way to shorten the time it takes to set up the IV bag and administration set is to do it en route to the scene. The benefit is obvious–the IV bag and administration set are ready for immediate use when arriving at the scene. However, the bag and set are wasted if the patient does not need an IV after all.

6. Cut or tear several pieces of tape of different lengths.

7. Employ body substance isolation precautions (at a minimum, apply gloves).

8. If possible, place the patient into a suitable position with the selected extremity lower than the heart. This positioning helps distend the distal veins.

9. Apply a tourniquet. To tie it, follow these steps:

- Place the tourniquet under the patient's arm, about 6 inches above the venipuncture site. Position it so that it is in the middle of the arm with an equal distance from either end to the patient's arm (Fig. 11-13 C).
- Bring the ends of the tourniquet together, placing one on top of the other (Fig. 11-13 D).
- Holding one end on top of the other, lift and stretch the tourniquet and tuck the top tail under the bottom tail. Do not allow the tourniquet to loosen (Fig. 11-13 E).
- Tie the tourniquet smoothly and snugly, being careful not to pinch the patient's skin or pull arm hair.

To reduce the risk of pain and discomfort when using a tourniquet, avoid keeping it in place for more than 2 minutes. Also, the tourniquet should be kept as flat as possible. It should be snug but not uncomfortably tight. A tourniquet that is too tight impedes arterial as well as venous blood flow. Palpate the patient's radial pulse. If it cannot be felt, the tourniquet is too tight and must be loosened. Also, the tourniquet should be loosened and retightened if the patient complains of severe tightness.

A tourniquet that is applied too tightly or kept in place too long may cause increased bruising, especially in the elderly patient whose veins are fragile. Therefore, the tourniquet should be released as soon as the venipuncture device has been placed into the vein and blood samples have been drawn (if applicable).

10. Select a suitable vein by palpation and sight. Avoid areas of the veins where a valve is situated. If the vein rolls, or feels hard or ropelike, select another vein. Veins can be distended for easier cannulation by:

- Having the patient open and close his or her fist tightly five or six times

- Flicking the skin over the vein with one or two sharp snaps of the fingers
- Rubbing or stroking the skin upward toward the tourniquet

If a suitable vein can not be found, or if the vein still feels small and uniform, release the tourniquet and apply it closer to the IV site. If that fails to resolve the problem, apply the tourniquet to the other arm.

11. Cleanse the site thoroughly with povidone-iodine or alcohol wipe, using a firm circular motion (Fig. 11-13 F). The area should be allowed to dry before penetrating the skin. It may be necessary to shave the hair around the selected insertion site to provide better adherence of the tape that is used to secure the catheter and administration set tubing.

12. Stabilize the vein by anchoring it with the thumb and stretching the skin downward. This action makes the venipuncture site taut. Stabilizing the vein helps ensure successful cannulation the first time and decreases the chance of bruising. Bruising occurs when the tip of the needle repeatedly probes a moving vein wall, nicking the vein and causing it to leak blood. When this injury occurs, the vein can not be immediately reused and another site must be found. This event requires the patient to endure the discomfort of another needle puncture. If the vein is in the hand, it may be helpful to have the patient flex his or her wrist.

13. Perform the venipuncture without contaminating the equipment or site.

    - Tell the patient there will be a small poke or pinch as the needle enters the skin.

    - Hold the end of the venipuncture device between the thumb and index/middle fingers—much the same as holding a pool cue. This technique allows easy visualization of the flashback chamber. Avoid touching any portion of the catheter, because a contaminated device is not usable.

    - Depending on the type of venipuncture device and manufacturer recommendations, hold the needle at a 15°, 30°, or 45° angle to the skin.

    - Penetrate the skin with the bevel of the needle pointed up (Fig. 11-13 G). If significant resistance is felt, do not force the catheter. Instead, withdraw the needle and catheter together as a unit.

    - If possible, penetrate the vein at its junction or bifurcation with another vein, because it is more stable at this location (Fig. 11-13 H).

    - Enter the vein with the needle from either the top or side (Fig. 11-13 I).

Normally, a slight "pop" or "give" is felt as the needle passes through the wall of the vein. Be careful not to enter too fast or too deeply, because the needle can go through the back wall of the vein.

- Note when blood fills the flashback chamber of the needle (Fig. 11-13 J).

HELPFUL HINT

If the vein is not entered with the initial penetration, it is necessary to continue advancing the venipuncture device until the vein is penetrated. However, the EMT–I should not insert the device so that less than half the catheter is outside the skin. The reason is that, in this position, only a small portion of the catheter will enter the vein itself. If the vein is still not located after advancing the needle, the EMT–I should withdraw both the needle and catheter slightly and attempt to advance it into the vein again. The EMT–I should avoid pulling the needle entirely out of the skin. However, if it is accidentally withdrawn, a new venipuncture device must be used to reattempt the IV cannulation.

- Lower the venipuncture device and advance it another 1 to 2 cm until the tip of the catheter is well within the vein (Fig. 11-13 K). The reason for this is that the catheter is slightly shorter than the needle. As a result, blood backflow sometimes occurs when only the needle is in the vein. Advancing the venipuncture device a bit more ensures that the catheter is correctly situated in the vein.

- While holding the needle stable between the first and middle fingers and thumb, use the first finger and thumb of the other hand to slide the catheter into the vein until the hub is against the skin (Fig. 11-13 L).

- Once the catheter is within the vein, apply pressure to the vein beyond the catheter tip with the little finger to prevent blood from leaking out of the catheter hub once the needle is completely withdrawn (Fig. 11-13 M).

14. Draw a blood sample (Fig. 11-13 N). The tourniquet should be left in place while drawing blood samples.

    - Stabilize the catheter with one hand, and attach a Vacutainer holder with a multi-sample IV Luer-lock adapter or a syringe to the hub. Be careful not to disrupt the catheter placement while connecting the Vacutainer or syringe. Once the device is connected, release the finger pressure at the distal tip of the catheter.

    - If using a Vacutainer device, insert the blood collection tube fully into the holder and allow its internal vacuum to draw blood out of the vein. If using a syringe, slowly withdraw the plunger to fill the syringe with blood. If blood flow into the syringe stops, it usually means that the vein is being collapsed by the sucking pressure of the syringe. To correct this problem, slow the rate at which the plunger is being withdrawn.

15. Once enough blood collection tubes have been filled or the syringe is completely full, release the tourniquet from the patient's arm (Fig. 11-13 O). Next, reapply pressure to the vein beyond the catheter tip with the little finger to prevent blood from leaking out of the catheter hub once the blood drawing device is disconnected. Disconnect the syringe or Vacutainer device from the hub of the catheter by holding the hub between the first finger and thumb and pulling the device free with the other hand.

16. Connect the IV tubing to the catheter hub. Be careful not to contaminate either the hub or connector prior to insertion.

17. Open the IV flow control valve and run the IV for a brief period of time to ensure the line is patent (Fig. 11-13 P). To ensure proper IV flow rates, the IV container must hang at least 30 to 36 inches above the insertion site.

18. Cover the IV site with povidone-iodine ointment and a sterile dressing or a bandage.

19. Secure the catheter, administration set tubing, and sterile dressing in place with tape (Fig. 11-13 Q) or a commercial device (Fig. 11-13 R). The tubing should be looped and secured with tape above the IV cannulation site. The loop gives the tubing more play, making the catheter less likely to be dislodged by accidental pulls on the tubing. However, do not make the loop so small that it kinks the tubing and restricts fluid flow.

20. Adjust the appropriate flow rate for the patient's condition.

21. Dispose of the needle(s) in a proper biomedical waste container (Fig. 11-13 S).

STREET WISE

In some cases it is hard to get the tape to stay in place. Common problems include hairy arms and moist or wet skin. Excess hair can be shaved away from around the insertion site. However, care should be taken to prevent contamination of the venipuncture site. Moist skin can be dried before the application of tape. However, if the skin remains moist or wet, it may be necessary to wrap the tape around the entire arm and tape it to itself. The EMT–I should careful not to wrap it so tight that blood flow is restricted.

The EMT–I should attach one piece of tape to the catheter hub and another piece to the administration set tubing, not one piece to both. This way, if the administration set is pulled on, it will only separate the connector from the IV catheter hub and not pull the catheter out. Additionally, if the tubing requires changing, the EMT–I will not have to waste time and energy trying to separate the two.

CLINICAL NOTES

A variety of commercial transparent semi-permeable dressings are available for use in the prehospital setting. These dressings allow air to pass through them but are impervious to microorganisms. Among the benefits of these dressings:
- They cause fewer adverse reactions than medical tape.
- The insertion site is clearly visible (allowing detection of early signs of phlebitis and swelling).
- Because the tape is waterproof, it protects the site should it become wet.
- Because the dressing adheres well to the skin, there is less chance of accidentally dislodging the venipuncture device.

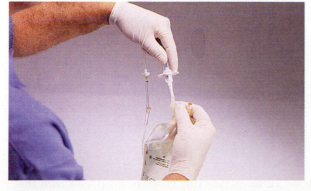

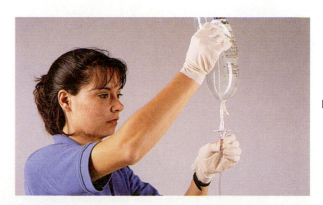

A

B

Fig. 11-13　**A, Insert the spiked piercing end of the administration set into the tubing of the IV bag. B, Squeeze the drip chamber to fill it half-way.**

(Continued)

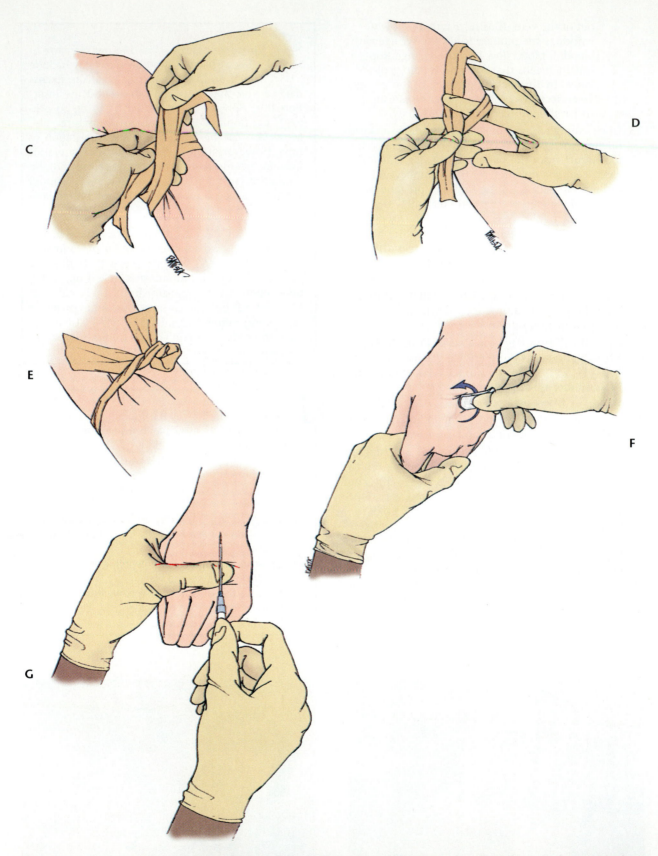

Fig. 11-13 cont'd. C, Place the tourniquet 6 inches above the venipuncture site. D, Make a slip knot with the tourniquet. E, Complete band placement. F, Use povidone-iodine or an alcohol wipe to cleanse the site. G, Pull the skin taught; the bevel of the needle should be facing up when penetrating the skin.   *(Continued)*

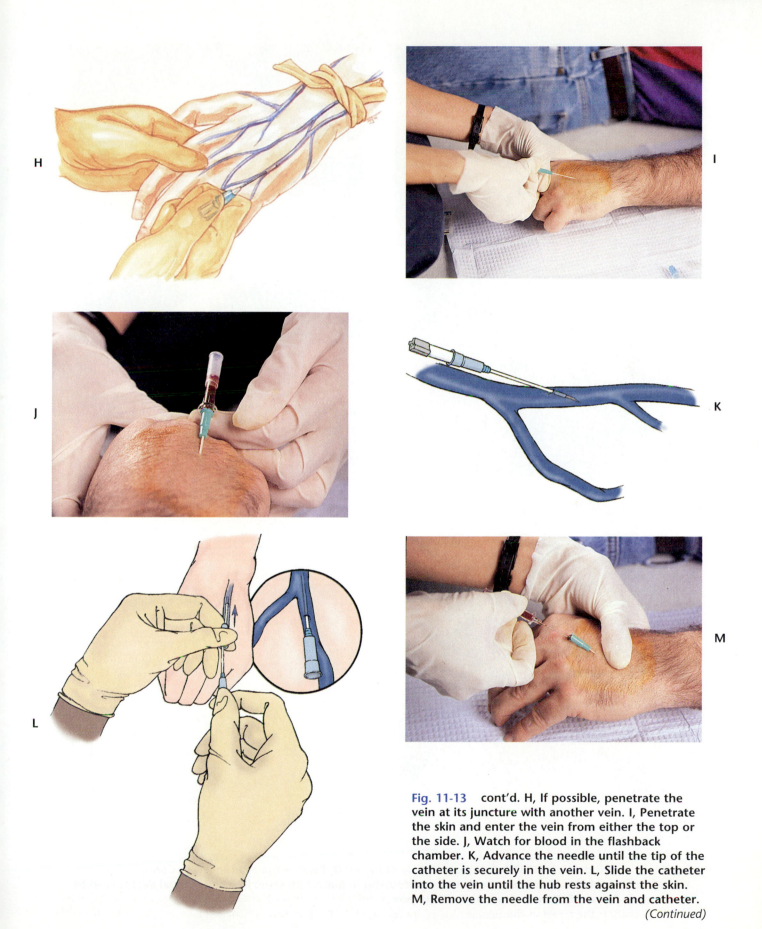

Fig. 11-13 cont'd. H, If possible, penetrate the vein at its juncture with another vein. I, Penetrate the skin and enter the vein from either the top or the side. J, Watch for blood in the flashback chamber. K, Advance the needle until the tip of the catheter is securely in the vein. L, Slide the catheter into the vein until the hub rests against the skin. M, Remove the needle from the vein and catheter.

(Continued)

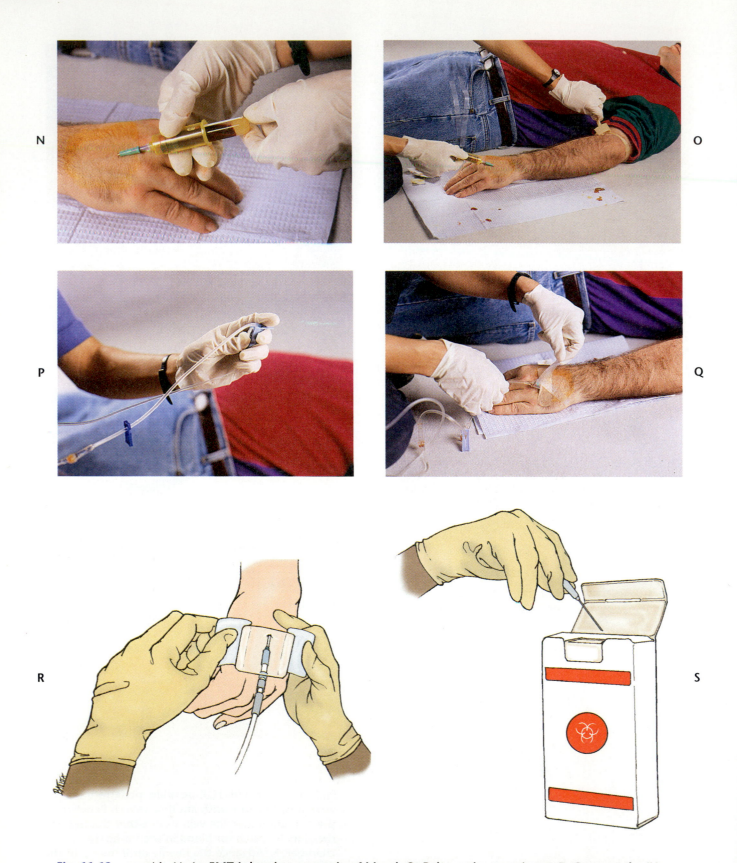

Fig. 11-13 cont'd. N, An EMT-I drawing a sample of blood. O, Release the tourniquet. P, Connect the IV tubing to the catheter. Q, Secure the catheter and tubing in place with tape. R, A commercial device used to secure the catheter. S, Proper disposal of used needle.

22. If a syringe was used to draw the blood, the necessary blood collection tubes must be filled by attaching a needle to the syringe and inserting it into each blood tube. The tubes should then be labeled and stored in a safe location.

STREET WISE

In normal situations, a family member or bystander can be asked to hold the IV bag while the EMT–I is on the scene taking care of the patient. It gives them something to do and frees the EMT–I to do other tasks. When moving the patient to the ambulance, the IV bag typically is placed in an IV holder. This device is attached to the stretcher, looks like a pole, and has one to two hooks along with a Velcro strap that holds the IV bag in place. The IV holder folds down for easy storage when not in use. When carrying the patient out in a stair chair, Reeves stretcher, or backboard, the plastic IV bag can be kept running by placing the bag under the patient's shoulder. Placing the IV bag under the patient's shoulder also is useful in frigid temperatures when the EMT–I needs to keep the IV solution warm. Additionally, the IV tubing should be kept under the blankets and close to the patient, to prevent it from becoming chilled. An alternative method is to employ an intermittent infusion device.

The number of attempts (or "sticks") the EMT–I should make to place an IV line depends on local protocol. However, a good rule of thumb is to limit the number of attempts to three.

Although the EMT–I's IV skills will improve with practice, some veins are particularly difficult to cannulate. Obese patients, patients in shock and cardiac arrest, chronic mainline drug users, elderly patients with fragile rolling veins, and small children may each pose a challenge. In shock and cardiac arrest, the patient's veins can constrict and disappear from sight. The EMT–I should not waste time searching for a vein in one arm. If one is not found easily, the EMT–I should go to the patient's other arm or external jugular vein.

HELPFUL HINT

To cannulate a rolling vein, the EMT–I should pull the skin tight. The EMT–I must be careful not to pull too tightly or the vein will flatten. The EMT–I should pass the needle through the skin, pausing for a second to line up the needle in the same direction as the vein. Then, the EMT–I penetrates the vein from the side rather than the top. He or she should try to insert the needle into the center of the vein to keep it from moving. Sometimes the EMT–I has to "chase the vein" as it moves from side to side.

To cannulate a fragile vein the EMT–I should use a smaller needle and insert it into the vein carefully. The gentler the EMT–I is, the better chance he or she has of successfully placing the IV cannula.

After venipuncture is performed

When it appears the needle has penetrated a vein, the EMT–I should try to confirm proper needle placement. Sometimes blood may not flow back into the flashback chamber of the needle (eg, during severe hypovolemia). When this happens, if the EMT–I is sure of correct placement, he or she should start the IV infusion cautiously and watch the site carefully for signs of infiltration (eg, coolness and swelling around the site). If infiltration occurs, the EMT–I should remove and discard the catheter and place a dressing on the venipuncture site. Then, using sterile equipment, the EMT–I should attempt venipuncture at another site.

Other methods of determining proper placement of the catheter include:

- Lowering the IV bag below the IV site. If it is correctly positioned, blood backflow should be seen in the IV tubing.
- Palpating the vein above the IV site. It should be cool or the same temperature as the IV solution being infused.
- Palpating the tip of the catheter in the vein.
- Aspirating blood with a 10-mL syringe, then discarding the syringe in an approved container.

FLEXION: The act of bending, especially at the joint.

Using an armboard

The EMT–I usually can avoid using an armboard simply by choosing a venipuncture site well away from any **flexion** areas. However, an armboard may be necessary when a venipuncture device is inserted near a joint or in the dorsum of the hand, or it may be used along with restraints in confused or disoriented patients (Fig. 11-14).

The patient should be asked to flex his or her arm while the EMT–I watches the IV flow rate. If the flow stops during movement, an armboard is needed. Because armboards do not prevent rotation, they cannot always prevent infiltration. The armboard must be long enough to prevent flexion or extension at the tip of the venipuncture device. It should be covered with a soft material and applied with tape that is padded with folded gauze or tissue. Use caution when using an armboard because one that is applied too tightly can cause nerve and tendon damage. Also, the EMT–I must make sure that the tape that keeps the venipuncture device in place is in no way attached to the armboard. This precaution will prevent any motion of the arm on the armboard from pulling on and potentially displacing the venipuncture device.

Regulating fluid flow rates

The IV flow rate should be adjusted as ordered by medical direction. The EMT–I must know the volume to be infused, the period of time over which the fluid

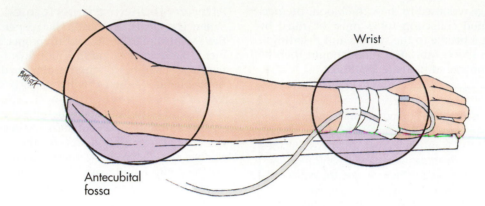

Fig. 11-14   **Common puncture sites that may require the use of an arm board.**

is to be infused, and the number of drops per milliliter the infusion set delivers. The formula below can be used to calculate IV solution drip rates per minute.

drops/min = volume to be infused × drops/mL of
administration set ÷
total time of infusion in minutes

Example: The EMT–I is instructed to administer 35 mL of IV fluid over 40 minutes using a microdrip administration set. The formula is 35 mL x 60 drops/mL = 2100 drops divided by 40 minutes = 52.5 drops/min (rounded to 50 drops/min) to be administered.

After determining the rate, setting the flow is easy. When the IV line has been established, the clamp should be slowly opened to start fluid dripping into the drip chamber. The EMT–I should hold a watch close to the chamber and count the drops for 1 minute (or count for 30 seconds and multiply the number by 2). The clamp should be opened or closed as needed to adjust the drip rate. If at any time the clamp slips or the patient makes a sudden move, the drip rate may be affected. The EMT–I should check it periodically, using the method described previously. However, the EMT–I should avoid spending excessive time at the scene counting for small discrepancies.

Documenting IV cannulation

Depending on local protocol, when an IV is started, the following must be documented on the run report:

- Date and time of the venipuncture
- Type and amount of solution
- Type of venipuncture device used, including the length and gauge
- Venipuncture site
- Number of insertion attempts (if more than one)
- IV flow rate
- Any adverse reactions and the actions taken to correct them
- Name or identification number of the EMT–I initiating the infusion

In addition to documenting correct IV placement, unsuccessful attempts also should be documented.

Some local protocols call for the EMT–I to document the following information directly on the tape that is used to secure the venipuncture device and administration set tubing in place:

- Date and time of insertion
- Type and gauge of needle or catheter
- Initials of the EMT–I who placed the device

To do this procedure properly, the EMT–I should cut a piece of tape and place it on a flat surface. He or she should write the information on it, then apply it over the dressing. The tape should never be labeled after it has been applied over the dressing. Doing so will irritate the venipuncture site (Fig. 11-15).

When the IV does not flow

 Use problem-solving skills with IV lifelines that are not functioning properly to determine the cause and correct the problem.

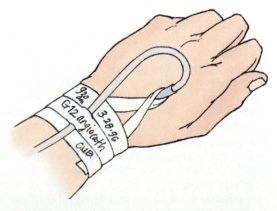

Fig. 11-15   **Document the IV cannulation by writing the necessary information on a piece of tape and applying it over the dressing.**

In some cases the IV will not flow as it should. In those situations the EMT–I should consider the following (Fig. 11-16):

Was the venous tourniquet (constricting band) removed? Not releasing the tourniquet after cannulating the vein is probably the most common mistake made in both the hospital and field settings. Additionally, the EMT–I should check to make sure that the patient is not wearing restrictive clothing that is interfering with venous flow or that a shirt sleeve has not been pushed up too high on the arm.

Is there swelling at the cannulation site? This swelling indicates that the catheter is displaced and there is infiltration into the tissues.

Is the flow regulator in an open position? If it is turned off, no flow will occur. The EMT–I should be sure to check both the primary and secondary control valves that are part of the administration set.

Is the tip of the catheter positioned against a valve or wall of the vein? This problem can be checked by slightly twisting or withdrawing the catheter. It may be necessary to untape the catheter and retape it after a good flow rate has been achieved by repositioning the catheter. Additionally, a padded armboard can be used to keep the patient's hand or arm in an appropriate position.

Is the IV bag high enough? Sometimes when moving the patient, the cannulation site is raised higher than appropriate. This problem interferes with the gravity that is required to move the IV fluid. To correct this problem, the EMT–I should lower the extremity, raise the IV bag, or consider a pressure infuser.

Is the drip chamber completely filled with IV solution? This problem can be corrected easily by inverting the bag and squeezing the drip chamber to return some of the fluid to the bag.

If the flow is still slow or absent, the EMT–I should lower the IV bag below the level of the insertion site. If blood return is seen in the IV tubing at the connection point with the catheter, the site is patent. If problems still persist, the IV should be removed and reestablished in another extremity.

Complications

 List complications associated with IV therapy.

All IV techniques share both local and systemic complications, including pain, catheter shear, circulatory overload, cannulation of an artery, infiltration/hematoma, local infection, pyrogenic reaction, air embolism, and thrombosis, phlebitis, sepsis, and pulmonary thromboembolism. Those complications that are most likely to occur in the prehospital setting are described below.

Pain
Pain at the puncture site is a common complication. It typically is due to penetration of the skin with the

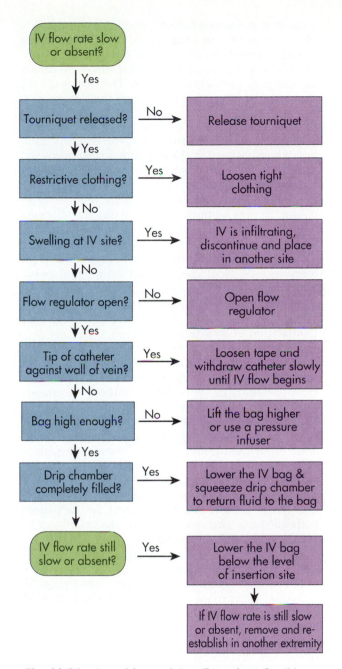

Fig. 11-16   A problem-solving flow chart for IV therapy.

needle or extravasation of IV fluid into the tissue. Pain can lead to increased anxiety and worsening of the patient's condition. The pain associated with venipuncture can be reduced by using a smaller-gauge catheter or the sharp tip of a smaller needle to make an incision in the skin through which a larger catheter can pass more easily.

Catheter shear
A catheter shear can occur when the catheter is pulled back through (through-the-needle catheter) or over (over-the-needle catheter) the needle after

it has been advanced forward. Because the catheter is plastic, it easily can snag on the sharp edge of the needle and be sheared off, becoming a plastic emboli. For this reason the catheter must never be drawn back over or through the needle. The needle always should be withdrawn first and then the catheter.

Circulatory overload

Circulatory overload occurs when too much IV solution is administered or the IV solution is administered too rapidly for a given patient's condition. To prevent circulatory overload the EMT–I must closely monitor the IV flow rate, particularly in patients prone to heart failure. The EMT–I must constantly watch all patients receiving IV fluids for signs of developing congestive heart failure, in which case the IV flow rate should be significantly reduced or terminated. Signs and symptoms include headache, flushed skin, rapid pulse, increased blood pressure, rales, dyspnea, tachypnea, coughing, and external jugular vein distention.

Cannulation of an artery

Veins tend to lie superficially, whereas arteries are found deeper in the skin. Despite this difference, an artery can be inadvertently punctured because of its close proximity to veins. Arterial puncture is characterized by the appearance of spurting bright red blood (or darker red blood in hypoxic patients). If bright red blood suddenly appears in the syringe (with over-the-needle catheters equipped with a syringe) and pushes the plunger up, the device should be completely removed. Direct pressure is then applied to the puncture site for at least 10 minutes, until the bleeding has stopped. In the patient with adequate circulatory output, the artery can be detected by checking for a pulse.

Hematoma or infiltration

A hematoma or infiltration at the puncture site can be caused by injury to the blood vessel, inadvertent puncture during IV cannulation, or a cannula that becomes dislodged from the vein. Fluid then accumulates in the tissues. Signs and symptoms include edema, blanching of the skin, discomfort, infiltration site that feels cool to touch, IV fluid flowing more slowly, and an absence of blood flashback. When a hematoma or infiltration occurs at the puncture site, the catheter should be removed and the IV reestablished at another site.

Local infection

A local infection can occur when appropriate cleansing techniques are not used and bacteria are introduced into the venipuncture site. Swelling and tenderness at the IV site are common signs. This infection is not seen in the prehospital setting but occurs several days following initial treatment.

Air embolism

An air embolism occurs when air is allowed to enter the vein. It can occur during central vein cannulation, when air is not cleared from the IV administration set appropriately, or when the IV tubing becomes dislodged from the hub of the catheter. Signs and symptoms include hypotension, cyanosis, tachycardia, increased venous pressure, and loss of responsiveness.

Pyrogenic reaction

This type of reaction occurs when foreign proteins, capable of producing fever, are present in the administration set or IV solution. It is characterized by the abrupt onset of fever (100° to 106° F), chills, backache, headache, nausea, vomiting, face flushing, and sudden pulse change. Cardiovascular collapse also may result. The reaction usually occurs within 30 minutes of the initiation of IV therapy. If a pyrogenic reaction is suspected, the IV should be immediately terminated and established in the other arm, using a new administration set and solution. This complication emphasizes the need to discard any IV bag that shows leakage or cloudiness.

DRAWING BLOOD

Drawing blood from a vein is done to acquire blood samples from a patient for analysis. These blood samples can reveal a great deal of information about the patient, including the blood glucose level, hemoglobin and hematocrit levels, clotting time, presence of medications, cardiac enzyme evaluation, and more. The most commonly used venous blood assessment in the field setting is the evaluation of blood glucose levels. Information that reveals the presence of hypoglycemia will prompt the administration of 50% dextrose to resolve the glucose deficiency. Although blood samples can be drawn as a separate procedure from starting an IV, it is more common for the EMT–I to draw them immediately after placing the venipuncture device (but before attaching the administration tubing). This method reduces the number of painful sticks to which the patient is subjected. However, when the quality of the patient's veins is extremely fragile and drawing blood may jeopardize the IV line, blood should be drawn from another vein using a needle and syringe or a Vacutainer device.

Blood drawing equipment

A variety of sizes and types of blood tubes are available to collect and store blood samples (Fig. 11-17). The rubber caps on the tubes come in several colors and patterns, denoting the specific tests that are conducted with the blood that is stored in them. Most commonly used in the field setting are the red, purple, green, or "jungle" blue, and gray tops. Some of these tubes have small amounts of liquids or agents inside the tube to prevent blood coagulation or to aid in preserving the blood in a way necessary for a particular type of test. During the manufacture of blood tubes, a vacuum is created in the tube that acts

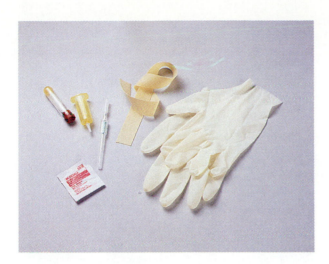

Fig. 11-17   Equipment used to draw blood.

to "suck blood" into the tube. Blood tubes can be filled by drawing blood from the vein with a syringe and then using at least a 19-gauge needle to introduce it into the blood tube or using a special holder that has a multisample IV Luer-lock adapter.

CLINICAL NOTES

The Vacutainer holder looks like the barrel of a large syringe and contains a threaded tip that is used to hold the multisample IV Luer-lock adapter. On the inside end of the adapter is a needle that is used to puncture the rubber cap of the blood collection tube. The other end of the adapter attaches to the hub of the IV catheter. To draw a blood sample once the adapter is connected to the IV catheter, the blood collection tube is inserted (rubber cap first) into the holder and pushed downward with the thumb until the needle punctures the cap and blood is sucked into the tube. Sometimes using a Vacutainer device to withdraw blood in a fragile vein will cause it to collapse. If this occurs, the Vacutainer device should be removed and a syringe used to collect the blood sample. This way, the EMT–I can control the amount of pressure used to withdraw the blood sample by applying slower, more delicate, upward pressure on the plunger of the syringe.

When drawing blood, each tube should be filled completely. Once the blood is obtained, the outside of the tube should be labeled with the patient's name, date, time drawn and by whom, and any information that may be useful such as: "drawn before the administration of 50% dextrose." During transportation of the patient to the hospital, the filled blood collection tubes can be stored in a plastic "zip-lock" bag to prevent contamination of the EMT–I should one or more of the blood collection tubes be accidentally broken.

DISCONTINUING THE IV LIFELINE

 Demonstrate the steps for discontinuing an IV lifeline.

Occasionally, it may be necessary to discontinue an IV lifeline in the prehospital setting. To perform this task, the EMT–I needs protective gloves, a sterile gauze pad, and an adhesive bandage. The EMT–I should begin by closing the flow control valve completely. Then, taking care not to disturb the catheter, he or she should carefully untape and remove the dressing. Next, the EMT–I gently holds a 2 x 2 sterile gauze dressing just above the site to stabilize the tissue and withdraws the catheter by pulling straight back until the catheter is completely out of the vein. To prevent blood loss, the EMT–I should immediately cover the IV site with the 2 x 2 sterile dressing and hold it against the puncture site until the bleeding has stopped. Then, the dressing is taped in place or covered with an adhesive bandage.

CLINICAL NOTES

Another device that is becoming popular in the field and hospital settings is the intermittent infusion device. This device commonly is called a heparin lock because a heparin flush is instilled into the cap to keep blood from backing up into the venipuncture device and clotting. It is available as a winged needle set or over-the-needle catheter, and each has an attached latex cap. However, any type of venipuncture device can be converted into an intermittent device by placing a latex cap over the proximal end of the catheter. Typically, a Luer-lock tip is used to prevent accidental loosening of the cap.

The benefits of using the intermittent infusion device are that it creates a route for administering medications without necessitating a TKO infusion of IV fluids, which can be harmful to patients experiencing circulatory overload; it is cost effective (because the administration set and IV solution are not used); and it makes it easier to move the patient (because there is no IV bag and administration set). Once in place, the device should be flushed with saline or heparin before or after medication administration or at least once a day.

EXTERNAL JUGULAR VEIN CANNULATION

 IPSILATERAL: On the same side of the body.

As identified earlier, the external jugular vein is considered an appropriate site for cannulation in a wide range of medical emergencies. To cannulate the external jugular vein, the EMT–I should do the following (Fig. 11-18):

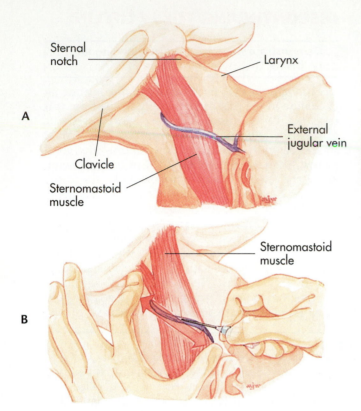

Fig. 11-18 **A, Anatomy of the area surrounding the external jugular vein. B, Proper IV cannulation of the external jugular vein.**

1. Place the patient into a supine, head-down position to fill the vein.
2. Turn the patient's head away from the EMT–I.
3. Locate the vein and cleanse the overlying skin with alcohol or povidone-iodine.
4. Hold the vein in place by applying pressure on the vein distal to the point of entry at the angle of the mandible.
5. Align the venipuncture device in the direction of the vein with the point aimed toward the **ipsilateral** nipple.
6. Tourniquet the vein lightly with one finger above the clavicle.
7. Make the venipuncture midway between the angle of the jaw and the midclavicular line.
8. Puncture the skin with the bevel of the needle upward, approximately 0.5 to 1.0 cm from the vein.
9. Enter the vein from the top or side.
10. Note the return of blood and advance the catheter.
11. While holding the catheter steady, withdraw the needle and attach the administration set tubing to the catheter hub.

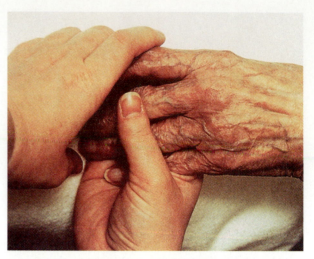

Fig. 11-19 **The skin of a geriatric patient will necessitate extra care during IV cannulation.**

12. Cover the site with povidone-iodine and a sterile dressing.
13. Tape the dressing and catheter in place.

ELDERLY PATIENTS

Elderly patients have more prominent veins and less-resistant skin, which makes venipuncture easier (Fig. 11-19). However, because the tissues are looser, it is more difficult to stabilize the vein. Because the veins are more fragile, the venipuncture must be done carefully and efficiently to avoid excessive bruising. It also is necessary to remove the tourniquet quickly after venipuncture, because increased vascular pressure can cause bleeding through the vein wall around the insertion site. Usually, smaller, shorter venipuncture devices work best with an elderly patient's fragile veins.

CASE HISTORY FOLLOW-UP

EMT–I Davis makes certain that the IV is secure by placing a 0.5-inch strip of tape under the cannula and crossing it over into a "V" shape to keep it from pulling out. He then loops the line and secures it with the pieces of tape, being certain not to encircle the arm completely and possibly creating a restrictive tourniquet.

After securing the line, EMT–I Davis places the patient's hand and wrist on a padded splint and secures them with roller gauze. He is careful not to wrap the gauze too tightly. He opens a Betaine packet and squeezes the contents on the insertion site, then covers it with a small gauze pad and tape.

Mrs. Greenley is beginning to talk and have meaningful movements with her hands when the ambulance arrives at the emergency department and after only 250 mL of normal saline has been administered.

SUMMARY

Intravenous cannulation is the placement of a catheter into a vein for the purpose of administering blood, fluids, or medications into the circulatory system and/or obtaining venous blood specimens. Although its use is beneficial in a wide variety of situations, placement of an IV lifeline should not significantly delay transporting critically ill or injured patients to the hospital.

The recommended IV solutions for use in the prehospital setting are normal saline (0.9%) and lactated Ringer's solution. Both are isotonic crystalloid solutions. Crystalloid solutions quickly diffuse out of the circulatory system, therefore at least 3 L of IV solution must be administered for every 1 L of blood lost. The two most common types of administration sets are the micro (delivering 60 drops/mL) and the macro (delivering 10 to 20 drops/mL). Plastic over-the-needle catheters most commonly are used in the prehospital setting because they can be better anchored and permit freer movement of the patient.

In noncritical patients, the distal veins of the dorsal aspect of the hand and arms are preferred IV sites. The veins on the back of the hand allow the patient to freely move his or her hand, the technique is relatively easy to master and does not interfere with other life-sustaining measures such as airway management. During cardiac arrest, the preferred sites for IV placement are the veins of the antecubital fossa, because they are among the largest in the arm. There are some patients in which cannulating a vein is particularly difficult, including obese persons, patients in shock and cardiac arrest, chronic mainline drug users, elderly patients with "fragile" or "rolling veins," and small children.

When selecting the equipment for IV therapy, the IV fluid must be checked to ensure that it is not outdated, is clear, and the bag has no leaks. When setting up the administration set, cannulating the vein, and attaching the IV solution to the catheter, the EMT–I must be sure to continually employ infection control procedures. Needles should always be discarded appropriately in a sharps container. The EMT–I must remember to release the tourniquet once the IV tubing is connected to the catheter. Once the IV is successfully established, the EMT–I must continually monitor the patient for signs of improvement and also for signs of circulatory overload.

All IV techniques share a number of complications including pain, catheter shear, circulatory overload, cannulation of an artery, infiltration/hematoma, local infection, and air embolism.

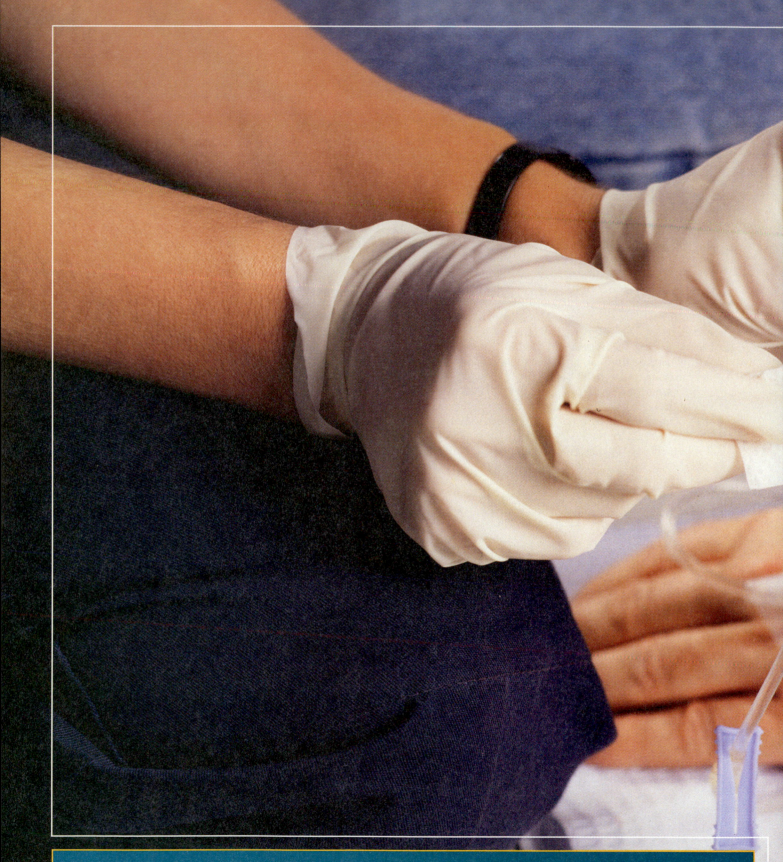

ENRICHMENT

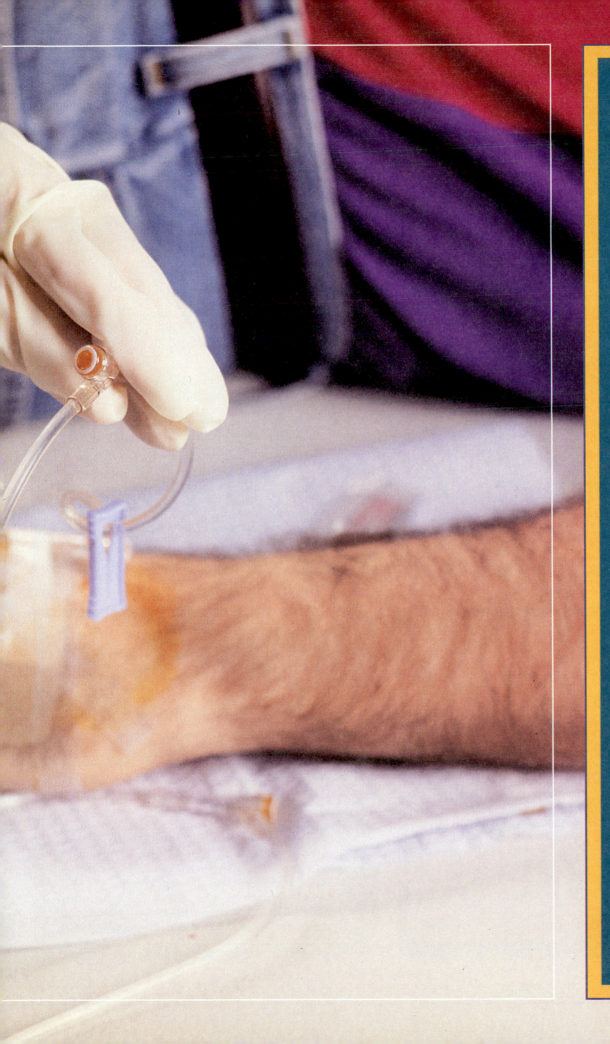

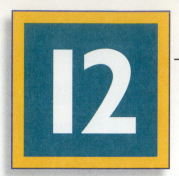

12

PHARMACOLOGY

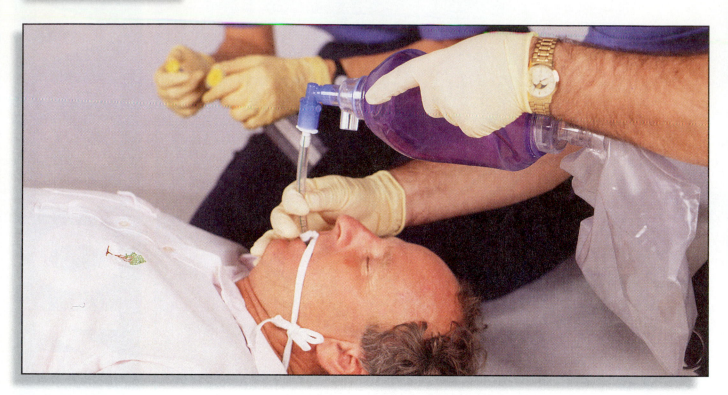

CASE HISTORY

It is 11:00 Thursday morning when EMT–Intermediate Maloney receives a call to the local elementary school for a patient "having trouble breathing, history of asthma." She arrives in approximately 4 minutes and finds the patient, Rosy, aged 8, sitting upright and struggling to breathe. She has inspiratory wheezes and diminished breath sounds in all her lung fields.

EMT–I Maloney takes Rosy's pulse with her gloved hand, and checks her blood pressure and pulse oximetry reading as her partner applies 100%

Case History, continued

oxygen via a nonrebreather mask. The school nurse says to the EMT–Is, "Rosy has used her inhaler about four times since she came in here today, but she hasn't been getting better. It usually works faster than this."

EMT–I Maloney prepares a nebulizer dosage of albuterol while her partner takes off his gloves and calls medical direction for orders. The medical direction physician confirms the order, and EMT–I Maloney proceeds with treatment.

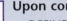

LEARNING OBJECTIVES

Upon completion of this chapter, the EMT–Intermediate should be able to:

- DEFINE the terms *drug* and *pharmacology*.
- RECALL the four names given to a drug.
- IDENTIFY the various laws and regulatory agencies that regulate drug administration.
- DESCRIBE the five schedules of drugs established by the DEA.
- LIST the various references for drug information available to the EMT–I.
- DESCRIBE the different sources of drugs.
- LIST the common packaging of drugs used in the prehospital setting.
- DEFINE the terms *drug action, drug effect,* and *pharmacokinetics*.
- RELATE the factors that influence drug action on the body.
- DESCRIBE the different components of the autonomic nervous system.
- DEMONSTRATE how to use decimals with basic math problems.
- CALCULATE dosages for various medications.
- DESCRIBE the various drug administration routes and recall the indications for each.
- RECALL the characteristics and indications for the various types of drug administration devices.
- DEMONSTRATE the techniques used to administer drugs in the prehospital setting.
- LIST the common drugs administered by the EMT–I.
- RECALL the indications, dosages, and administration routes of the primary drugs administered by the EMT–I.

KEY TERMS

ABSORPTION	DRUG ACTION
ADVERSE REACTIONS	DRUG ALLERGY
AEROSOL	DRUG EFFECT
AMERICAN HOSPITAL FORMULARY SERVICE	DRUG ENFORCEMENT AGENCY
AMPULE	DRUG TOLERANCE
ANAPHYLACTIC REACTION	DRUG TOXICITY
ANTAGONIST	ELIXIR
APOTHECARY SYSTEM	EMULSION
CHEMICAL NAME	ENTERIC-COATED TABLET
COMPENDIUM OF DRUG THERAPY	EXCRETION
CONTRAINDICATIONS	FEDERAL FOOD, DRUG, AND COSMETIC ACT
CONTROLLED SUBSTANCES ACT	FEDERAL TRADE COMMISSION
CUMULATIVE EFFECT	FIGHT OR FLIGHT
DISTRIBUTION	FLUID EXTRACT
DRUG	FOOD AND DRUG ADMINISTRATION

KEY TERMS

GENERIC NAME

HARRISON NARCOTIC ACT OF 1914

HYPERSENSITIVITY

IDIOSYNCRATIC REACTIONS

INDICATIONS

INHALATION

INTRAMUSCULAR

INTRAOSSEOUS

INTRAVENOUS

LINIMENT

LOCAL EFFECT

METABOLISM

METRIC SYSTEM

NARCOTIC CONTROL ACT

OFFICIAL NAME

PARASYMPATHETIC DIVISION

PARENTERAL DRUGS

PHARMACOKINETICS

PHARMACOLOGY

PHYSICIANS' DESK REFERENCE

POTENTIATION

PREFILLED SYRINGE

PUBLIC HEALTH SERVICE

PURE FOOD AND DRUG ACT

SIDE EFFECT

SUBCUTANEOUS

SUBLINGUAL

SUPPOSITORY

SUSPENSION

SYMPATHETIC DIVISION

SYNERGISM

SYSTEMIC EFFECT

THERAPEUTIC EFFECT

TRADE NAME

TRANSDERMAL

UNITED STATES PHARMACOPEIA

VIALS

INTRODUCTION

Quick decisions on the part of the EMT–I can mean the difference between life and death, especially when administering drugs. Carrying, preparing, and administering drugs carry a tremendous professional and legal responsibility. If the wrong drug or the incorrect dose of the appropriate drug is given, the results can be fatal.

EMT–Is may administer certain emergency drugs via local protocol or standing orders, with or without contacting medical direction. This chapter includes information on certain emergency drugs and their uses, range of dosages, methods of administration, and side effects. Administration of drugs is an exacting science and can be harmful to the patient when errors are made. It is important for the EMT–I to understand the safety precautions and legal aspects of drug administration.

PHARMACOLOGY AND DRUG NOMENCLATURE

 Define the terms *drug* and *pharmacology*.

 DRUG: A substance taken into the body to affect change to one or more body functions, often to prevent or treat a disease or condition.

 PHARMACOLOGY: The study of drugs and their effects and actions on the body.

A **drug** is any substance that, when taken into the body, changes one or more of the body's functions. For example, a particular drug may raise or lower blood pressure or increase or decrease the heart rate. Drugs are most commonly used in medicine to treat or prevent disease. Drugs are available in many forms and are administered in a variety of ways. **Pharmacology** is the term given to the study of drugs and their actions, dosages, and side effects. Pharmaceutical companies are required to list, in the drug inserts, the chemical compounds, actions, dosages, side effects, indications, and contraindications of the drugs they manufacture.

Recall the four names given to a drug.

The written direction for the preparation and administration of a drug is called a *prescription*. In the United States, drugs are usually dispensed on the order of a physician. In some states, specially qualified nurse practitioners or physician assistants also may prescribe drugs.

A drug may have as many as four names: chemical, generic, official, and trade. The **chemical name** is the first name given to any drug. It gives the exact description of the chemical structure of the drug. The **generic name** is often related to the chemical name of a drug, but is completely independent of the man-

Drug Names

Chemical name:	glyceryl trinitrate
Generic name:	nitroglycerin
Trade name:	Nitro-Bid
Chemical name:	7-chloro-1, 3-dihydro-1-methyl-5-phenyl-2H-1, 4-benzodiazepin-2-One
Generic name:	diazepam
Trade name:	Valium
Chemical name:	2-(diethylamino-N= (2, 6-dimethylpenyl) acetamide monohydrochloride monohydrate
Trade name:	Lidocaine HCL

ufacturer(s); the generic name is the nonproprietary designation of a drug. The **official name** is the name under which it is listed in one of the official publications (*eg*, the *United States Pharmacopeia*). When the drug is available for commercial distribution by the original manufacturer a trade name (also called the *brand name* or *proprietary name*) is given. The **trade name** is registered by the United States Patent Office and has the official mark of the Patent Office after its name. For 17 years, the original manufacturer of the drug has the exclusive rights to production of the drug. After that time, other companies may combine the same chemicals and produce their own equivalent (generic) of the drug. Each company marketing the generic form of the trade name drug then assigns its own trade name to its generic equivalent.

DRUG LEGISLATION

 Identify the various laws and regulatory agencies that regulate drug administration.

Prior to 1906, there was little regulation of the use of drugs in the United States. In 1906 the **Pure Food and Drug Act** was passed. It was amended in 1938. The original law was enacted to prevent the manufacture and trafficking of mislabeled, poisonous, or harmful food and drugs. The amended law, called the **Federal Food, Drug, and Cosmetic Act**, required that the safety of a drug must be proven before it could be distributed to the public. It also required that labels be used to list the possible habit-forming properties and side effects of drugs.

The **Harrison Narcotic Act of 1914** was the first federal legislation designed to stop drug addiction or dependence. It established federal control over the importation, manufacture, and sale of the opium and coca plants and all their compounds and derivatives. This law has been revised many times to include new and synthetic forms of potentially addictive drugs.

In 1956 the **Narcotic Control Act** was passed to amend the Harrison Act and increase penalties for the law's violation. This act also made the possession of heroin and marijuana illegal. The Bureau of Narcotics and Dangerous Drugs was an agency of the Department of Justice, which kept a registry of physicians who were permitted to give out or prescribe controlled substances.

In 1970 the **Controlled Substances Act,** which regulates the manufacture and distribution of drugs whose use may result in dependency, was passed. It went into effect on May 1, 1971. This act requires that anyone who manufactures, prescribes, administers, or dispenses such controlled substances must register annually with the United States Attorney General under the Drug Enforcement Administration. The following five schedules of controlled substances were established by the Drug Enforcement Administration and may be revised annually:

 Describe the five schedules of drugs established by the DEA.

Schedule I: Drugs that have the highest potential for abuse and have no currently accepted medical use in the United States. There is a lack of accepted safety for use of these drugs or substances even under medical supervision. Examples of such drugs include opium, marijuana, LSD, peyote, and mescaline.

Schedule II: Drugs that have a high potential for abuse. These drugs have a current accepted medicinal use in the United States, but with severe restrictions. Abuse of a Schedule II drug can lead to either psychologic or physiologic dependence. A Schedule II drug requires a written prescription that must be filled within 72 hours of when it was written. A Schedule II drug cannot be refilled or called into the pharmacy by a medical office. Examples of such drugs include morphine, codeine, Seconal®, cocaine, amphetamines, Dilaudid®, and Ritalin®.

Schedule III: Drugs that have a limited potential for psychologic or physiologic dependence. The prescription may be called in to the pharmacist by the physician and refilled up to five times in a 6-month period. Schedule III drugs have a limited amount of opium, codeine, and morphine. Examples include paregoric, Tylenol with codeine, and Fiorinal.

Schedule IV: Drugs that have a lower potential for abuse than those in Schedules II and III. Schedule IV drugs can be called in to the pharmacist by the medical office and may be refilled up to five times in a 6-month period. Examples include Librium, Valium, Darvon, and phenobarbital.

Schedule V: Drugs that have a lower potential for abuse than those in Schedules I, II, III, and IV. These drugs are used for relief of coughs or diarrhea and contain limited amounts of certain narcotics. Examples include Lomotil, Dimetane expectorant-DC, and Robitussin-DAC.

REGULATING AGENCIES

Because the administration of drugs in the United States is controlled by law, several agencies have a role in monitoring and enforcing drug legislation. The **Federal Trade Commission** regulates drug advertising. The **Food and Drug Agency** (FDA) was established to review drug applications and petitions for food additives; inspect factories where drugs, cosmetics, and foods are made; and to remove unsafe drugs from the market. The FDA also ensures that the labels on food, drugs, and cosmetics are correct.

In 1970 the **Drug Enforcement Administration** (DEA) was established to oversee the control of dangerous drugs. The DEA is concerned with controlled substances only and enforces laws against the manufacture, sale, and use of illegal drugs. The DEA also is responsible for revising the list of drugs included in the schedules of controlled substances. The United States **Public Health Service** inspects and licenses establishments that manufacture drugs.

All drugs sold in the United States must meet and maintain high standards for therapeutic results, patient safety, and packaging safety. To meet these standards, drugs must go through strict and accurate testing, which may take several years to complete. The FDA is responsible for final approval of all drugs.

REFERENCES FOR DRUG INFORMATION

 List the various references for drug information available to the EMT–I.

There are several references of drug information. The **Physicians' Desk Reference** (PDR) is widely used as a reference for drugs in current use. It contains such information as each drug's indications, therapeutic effects, dosages, administration, warnings, contraindications, precautions, side effects and drug interactions. It also includes photographs of various drugs. The information is essentially the same as that included in the package insert required by the FDA in prescription medications. The book is written to be used by physicians but is readily available to the general public in offices, libraries, and bookstores.

The **United States Pharmacopeia** (USP) consists of two paperback volumes of drug information for the healthcare provider. It defines drugs with respect to sources, chemistry, physical properties, tests to identify, storage, and dosage. It also provides directions for compounding and general use. The USP does not contain photographs of the drugs and, unlike the PDR, which is sometimes distributed to physicians at no charge, must be purchased. Some other sources of drug information include:

1. **American Hospital Formulary Service** is distributed to practicing physicians and contains concise information that is arranged according to drug classifications.

2. **Compendium of Drug Therapy** is published annually and is distributed to practicing physicians. It includes photographs of the drugs and phone numbers of major pharmaceutical companies and poison control centers. It also includes copies of some package inserts.

SOURCES OF DRUGS

 Describe the different sources of drugs.

Drugs may be derived from natural sources such as plants, minerals, or animals, or they may be synthesized in the laboratory. For example, digitalis, morphine sulfate, and atropine are plant-derived; iron, iodine, sodium bicarbonate, and calcium chloride are minerals; insulin, epinephrine (adrenalin), and vaccines have animal or human sources; and the sulfonamides, propoxyphene hydrochloride (the analgesic Darvon), lidocaine (Xylocaine), bretylium tosylate (Bretylol), and diazepam (Valium) are the products of laboratory synthesis.

FORMS OF DRUGS

 List the common packaging of drugs used in the prehospital setting.

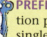 **PREFILLED SYRINGE:** A syringe and drug solution packaged together, to be used to deliver a single dose of a drug.
AMPULE: A glass container containing a drug; the bottle must be broken at the neck to retrieve the medication.

Most of the drugs that the EMT–I will use are given by injection and are in liquid form. Liquid drugs administered into the body by subcutaneous, intramuscular, or intravenous routes are called **parenteral drugs**. Drugs administered through the parenteral route are packaged in several ways, including prefilled syringes, ampules, and vials.

Prefilled syringes

Prefilled syringes are used for administration of intravenous, intramuscular, or subcutaneous drugs (Fig. 12-1). They are usually packaged in tamperproof containers, and the drug solution component and syringe often must be assembled. They are intended for single dose use.

Ampules

Ampules are breakable glass containers from which drugs must be drawn with a syringe (Fig. 12-2). They are intended for single dose use. Ampules must be

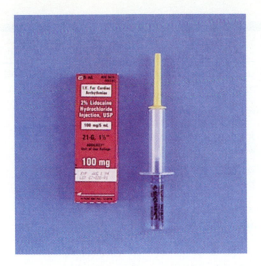

Fig. 12-1   A prefilled syringe for medication injection.

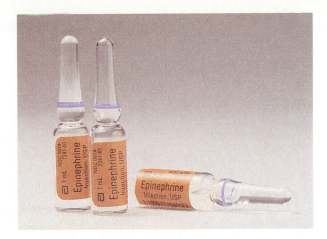

Fig. 12-2   Ampules are breakable glass containers from which drugs are drawn into the syringe.

broken at the neck to aspirate the solution into the syringe. Once the ampule is opened, all contents from it must be either used or discarded; it must not be saved for later use, because there is no way to maintain the sterility of the solution.

Vials

Vials are glass or plastic containers that have a self-sealing rubber stopper in the top, from which multiple doses may be drawn (Fig. 12-3). The contents of vials may be in solution, powder, or crystal form, which require reconstitution with a specific diluent, usually sterile water or saline.

The EMT–I also may be called on to administer medications via tablet form, such as nitroglycerin, administered sublingually; or bronchodilators, administered by aerosol, or through a nebulizer mask. The different forms in which drugs might be found are listed in Tables 12-1 and 12-2.

DRUG ACTIONS AND EFFECTS

 Define the terms *drug action*, *drug effect*, and *pharmacokinetics*.

DRUG ACTION: The cellular change effected by a drug.
DRUG EFFECT: Degree of a drug's physiologic change.
PHARMACOKINETICS: The movement of drugs through the body; including absorption, distribution, metabolism, and excretion.

Drugs are commonly categorized by their effects on body function. All drugs cause cellular change, which is their **drug action**, and a degree of physiologic change, which is their **drug effect**. Drug actions are

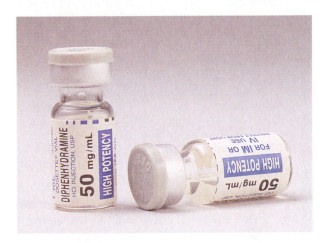

Fig. 12-3   Vials have a self-sealing rubber stopper in the top.

achieved by a biochemical interaction between the drug and certain tissue components in the body (usually receptors). Drugs do not confer any new functions on a tissue or organ; they only modify existing functions. The movement of drugs in the body as they are absorbed, distributed, metabolized, and excreted is called **pharmacokinetics**.

An action of a drug administered for a **local effect** is limited to the area where it is administered. An example is Xylocaine 2% jelly, which acts as a local anesthetic agent for skin disorders. A drug administered for a **systemic effect** (pertaining to the whole body rather than to one of its parts) is absorbed into the blood and then carried to the organ or tissue on which it will act. A systemic effect can be produced by administering drugs orally, sublingually, rectally, parenterally, or by inhalation. In addition, there are topical drugs that will produce a systemic effect, such as drugs that are applied to the mucous membranes in the vagina, eyes, or nose. Because mucous membranes are bathed in watery solutions and are very vascular, they are more permeable than the skin.

TABLE 12-1 Solid Forms of Drugs

FORM	DESCRIPTION
Capsule	A powdered or granulated drug enclosed in a gelatin capsule designed to dissolve quickly in the stomach.
Cream	A nongreasy, semisolid preparation used on the skin.
Enteric (coated tablet)	A compressed dry form of a drug coated to withstand the stomach acidity and dissolve in the intestines. These tablets may be drugs that would be destroyed by the stomach enzymes or might be damaging to the stomach lining. These tablets are never to be crushed or broken.
Lozenge	A firm, compressed form of a drug, usually for a local effect in the mouth or throat. Patients should be cautioned to let lozenges dissolve slowly and avoid drinking any fluids for a period of time after using the lozenge.
Ointment	A semisolid preparation of one or more drugs for prolonged contact with the skin. Intended to be difficult to wash off.
Pill	One or more drugs mixed with a cohesive material in oval, round, or flattened shapes.
Powder	A drug ground into fine powder.
Suppository	One or more drugs mixed in a firm base that dissolves gradually at body temperature. It is shaped for insertion into the body.
Time-release capsule	A gelatin capsule filled with forms of the drug that will dissolve over a period of time rather than all at once.
Tablet	A powdered drug compressed into a hard, small disc. Tablets may be found in many colors for easy identification. They will usually dissolve high in the gastrointestinal tract. These may be broken into halves or quarters only if they have been scored for that purpose.

The **therapeutic effect** of a drug is the drug's desired effect and the reason the drug is prescribed. For example, the therapeutic effect of morphine is the relief of pain. The **side effect** of a drug is any effect that is unintended. Side effects usually are predictable and may be either harmless or potentially harmful. For example, albuterol, which relaxes bronchial smooth muscle, results in bronchodilation and may have a side effect of nausea and vomiting.

A **drug allergy** occurs in a person who has been previously exposed to the drug and has developed antibodies. Drug allergies can manifest in a variety of signs and symptoms, ranging from minor to serious. The reaction can occur immediately after the patient has received the drug or may be delayed for hours or days. Signs and symptoms of a drug allergy are skin rash, fever, diarrhea, nausea, and vomiting. A life-threatening immediate reaction is called an **anaphylactic reaction** and results in respiratory distress, sudden severe bronchospasm, and cardiovascular collapse. In gathering the patient's history, the EMT–I must always ask about allergies of any sort, particularly allergies to drugs. If the patient is aware of existing allergies, these must be noted on the patient run report.

Drug toxicity results from overdosage, ingestion of a drug intended for external use, or buildup of the drug in the blood due to impaired metabolism or excretion. Like a drug allergy, some effects are realized immediately, but others may be delayed and not be apparent for weeks or months. Most drug toxicity is avoidable if careful attention is paid to dosage and monitoring for toxicity.

When the human body becomes accustomed to a particular drug over a period of time, the body is said to have gained a **drug tolerance.** Larger doses of the drug must be given to the patient to produce the desired effect. Drugs that commonly produce tolerance are opiates, barbiturates, ethyl alcohol, and tobacco.

Factors influencing drug action

 Relate the factors that influence drug action on the body.

TABLE 12-2 Liquid Forms of Drugs

FORM	DESCRIPTION
Aqueous solution	One or more drugs dissolved in water.
Liniment	An oily liquid used on the skin.
Lotion	An emollient liquid that may be used on irritated or inflamed skin with a minimum of rubbing.
Aerosol spray or foam	A liquid, powder, or foam deposited in a thin layer on the skin by air pressure.
Elixir	A drug dissolved in alcohol and added flavoring. These are less sweet than syrups and are usually preferred by adults. They should not be used for patients with alcoholism or diabetes.
Emulsion	A drug combined with water and oil. Emulsions must be thoroughly shaken to disperse the medication evenly.
Extract	A very concentrated form of drug made from vegetables or animals. Extracts may be administered as drops and usually are given in a liquid to disguise the very strong taste.
Fluid extract	An alcohol solution of a drug from a vegetable source. This form is the most concentrated of all fluid preparations.
Gel or jelly	A drug suspended in a thin gelatin or paste base.
Spirit	A concentrated alcohol solution of a volatile substance.
Suspension	Finely ground drugs that are dissolved in a liquid, such as water. Suspensions must be shaken well before administering.
Syrup	A very sweet form of medication, due to a high sugar content. Syrups frequently are used for children's medications and are usually flavored to disguise unpleasant-tasting drugs.
Tincture	An alcohol or water and alcohol solution prepared from drugs derived from plants.

A number of factors influence the actions of drugs on the body. Among these factors are age, weight, sex, existing pathology, and drug tolerance.

Age

Elderly people have slower metabolic processes. Age-related kidney and liver dysfunction will extend the breakdown and excretion times in these patients. It is very important to monitor the cumulative effects of drugs in elderly patients.

Infants and children are not simply small adults. Infants have immature livers and kidneys, so it is difficult for them to metabolize and eliminate the same dosages of drugs as adults. A child's body and chemistry is affected by adolescence, body proportion, and an inability to metabolize medications as effectively as adults.

Weight

Many medications have an effect on the body only within a specific concentration. To achieve a concentration of medication per unit of body water, the patient's body weight frequently serves as a guide to dosage determinations.

Gender

Women and men may have different reactions to some drugs because of different body compositions and hormone levels. A woman's hematocrit (concentration of red blood cells per unit of volume) measurements are lower than a man's. Men have a lower proportion of subcutaneous fat than women. Men and women also have differences in the proportion of water volume per body weight.

A woman's ability to receive medication is affected by pregnancy and considerations of the medication's effect on an unborn fetus. The use of some medications by pregnant women may cause birth defects in their children.

Existing pathology

If the body is compromised by a disease process, absorption, distribution, metabolism, and excretion of a drug may be altered.

Tolerance

Tolerance is an individual's capacity to endure medications. Some drugs given over a long period of time may cause the body to become resistant to their effect, requiring larger dosages to achieve the desired response.

Pharmacokinetics

The movement of drugs in the body as they are absorbed, distributed, metabolized, and excreted is pharmacokinetics (Fig. 12-4). Drugs undergo numerous changes during their movement from the administration site to the point at which they are inactivated and excreted.

Absorption gets the drug into the bloodstream. Absorption usually takes place in the mouth, dermal layers of the skin, subcutaneous tissue, blood vessels in the muscles, the lining of the stomach and small intestines, or the rectum. It is important that administration of drugs be done correctly, or the drug may be destroyed before it reaches its site of action.

Distribution moves the drug from the bloodstream into the tissues and fluids of the body.

Metabolism is the physical and chemical alterations that the drug undergoes within the blood. During the process of metabolism the liver breaks down the drug and alters it to more water-soluble by-products that can be excreted by the kidneys. In the

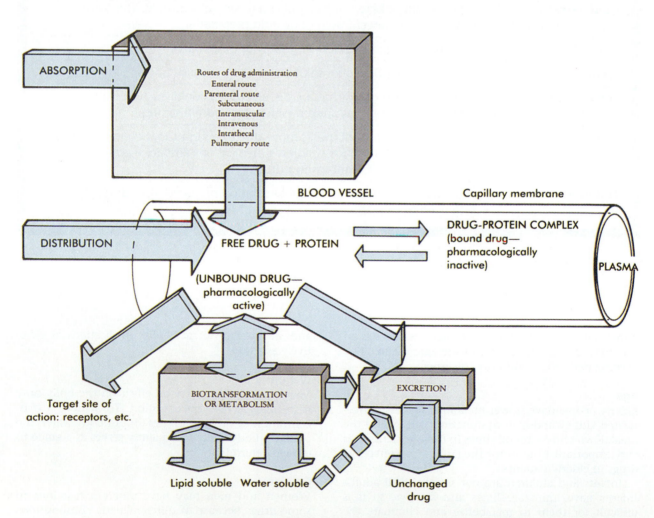

Fig. 12-4 Pharmacokinetics—the absorption, distribution, metabolism, and excretion of a drug through the body.

presence of hepatic disease, the liver may not be able to break down the drug properly for excretion by the kidneys. In this case, the patient may experience toxic effects due to an accumulation of the drug in the liver. In some instances, drugs may bypass the metabolic processes. Some drugs reach the kidneys unchanged; these drugs can be detected in the urine.

Excretion eliminates the waste products of drug metabolism from the body. Most drugs are excreted by the kidneys. Unless the drug is excreted before a repeat dose is given, a cumulative effect can occur. A **cumulative effect** may be dangerous and result in toxic levels of drugs in the body. In some instances, the accumulation of the drug in the body may be the desired effect. Digoxin, which is a cardiac drug, has the potential for causing a toxic cumulative effect. If digoxin accumulates, the patient's heart rate may slow to a dangerously low level. It is for this reason that patients taking digoxin must be monitored. Digoxin levels in the blood are checked periodically to avoid digoxin toxicity.

Drug interactions

When two or more drugs are taken simultaneously, one drug may increase, decrease, or cancel the effects of the others. The following terms describe drug interactions:

Synergism

Two drugs working together. One drug helps the action of the other to produce an effect that neither produces alone. For example, small doses of phenergan (a nonnarcotic sedative) and Demerol (a synthetic narcotic analgesic) are more effective for pain relief than the same dose of Demerol alone.

Potentiation

One drug prolongs or multiplies the effect of another drug. For example, Benemid (an antigout drug) is given with penicillin (an antibiotic) to delay the excretion of penicillin and to build up a high level of penicillin in the blood.

Antagonist

A drug that prevents receptor stimulation. An antagonist drug has an affinity for a cell receptor, and, by binding to it, the cell is prevented from responding. For example, Naloxone is a commonly used narcotic antagonist used to treat suspected narcotic overdose and unresponsiveness with unknown etiology. Naloxone binds to the receptor sites, blocking the action of the toxic drugs.

All of these examples of drug interactions are desirable interactions. There are, however, occasions when drug interactions produce undesirable effects.

Examples of undesired effects:

Synergism

Sedatives and barbiturates given together can cause central nervous system depression.

Potentiation

Tagamet (a gastric antisecretory) given with Tofranil (an antidepressant) will increase the levels of Tofranil in the blood.

Antagonist

Antacids taken with tetracycline (an antibiotic) prevent the absorption of tetracycline.

Other terms relating to the effects of drugs in the body include:

Indications

Disease states or reasons for which a drug is prescribed.

Contraindications

Conditions or instances for which a drug should not be used.

Adverse reactions

Undesirable side effects of a drug.

Hypersensitivity

Also known as *drug allergy*. The body must build this response; the first exposure may or may not indicate that a problem is developing.

Idiosyncratic reactions

An abnormal or unexpected reaction to a drug peculiar to a certain patient. This is not technically an allergy.

AUTONOMIC NERVOUS SYSTEM

Many of the drugs used in the field of emergency medical services affect tissues and organs that receive their nerve impulses from the autonomic nervous system. This discussion of the autonomic nervous system will help explain the effects of various drugs on the human body.

The nervous system is divided into two basic components: the voluntary and the involuntary (autonomic) systems. The voluntary system is under the control of conscious thought and controls voluntary movement. The involuntary, or "autonomic," nervous system controls "vegetative" functions of life by affecting vital organ functions.

The autonomic system is further broken into two divisions, which tend to act in a reciprocal manner. Most organs are dominated by one component or the other. The two divisions are the sympathetic and parasympathetic (Table 12-3).

 Describe the different components of the autonomic nervous system.

Sympathetic division

The **sympathetic division** (sometimes called the *adrenergic division*) originates in the brain. Messages are sent out to the organs by two "sympathetic chains"

TABLE 12-3 | **Autonomic Innervation of Target Tissues**

ORGAN	EFFECT OF SYMPATHETIC STIMULATION	EFFECT OF PARASYMPATHETIC STIMULATION
Heart		
Muscle	Increased rate and force *	Slowed rate †
Coronary arteries	Dilation *‡, constriction *§	Dilation †
Systemic blood vessels		
Abdomen	Constriction §	None
Skin	Constriction §	None
Muscle	Dilation *†, constriction §	None
Lungs		
Bronchi	Dilation *	Constriction †
Liver	Release of glucose into blood *	None
Skeletal muscles	Breakdown of glycogen to glucose *	None
Metabolism	Increase of up to 100% §	None
Glands		
Adrenal glands	Release of epinephrine and norepinephrine †	None
Salivary glands	Constriction of blood vessels and slight production of thick, viscous secretion §	Dilation of blood vessels and thin, copious secretion †
Gastric glands	Inhibition §	Stimulation †
Pancreas	Inhibition §	Stimulation †
Lacrimal glands	None	Secretion †
Sweat glands		
Merocrine glands	Copious, watery secretion †	None
Apocrine glands	Thick, organic secretion †	None
Gut		
Wall	Decreased tone *	Increased motility †
Sphincter	Increased tone §	Decreased tone †
Gallbladder and bile ducts	Relaxation *	Contraction†
Urinary bladder		
Wall	Relaxation *	Contraction †
Sphincter	Contraction §	Relaxation †
Eye		
Ciliary muscle	Relaxation for far vision *	Contraction for near vision †
Pupil	Dilation §	Constriction †
Arrector pili muscle	Contraction §	None
Blood	Increased coagulation §	None
Sex organs	Ejaculation §	Erection †

*—Mediated by beta receptors.
†—Mediated by cholinergic receptors.
‡—Normally there is increased blood flow through coronary arteries as a result of sympathetic stimulation of the heart because of increased demand by cardiac tissue for oxygen. In experiments that isolate the coronary arteries, however, sympathetic nerve stimulation, acting through alpha receptors, causes vasoconstriction. The beta receptors are relatively insensitive to sympathetic nerve stimulation but can be activated by drugs.
§—Mediated by alpha receptors.

that leave the spinal cord at approximately the first thoracic vertebra and end at approximately the second lumbar vertebra.

> **CLINICAL NOTES**
> The term adrenergic comes from "adrenaline," a synonym for epinephrine.

The primary effect of sympathetic stimulation is increased heart rate, bronchiole dilation, and increased metabolism and strength. These responses prepare the body for **fight or flight** when in a dangerous situation. When the sympathetic division is stimulated, impulses are transmitted electrically along the nerve fibers until they reach a synapse, or nerve junction. At this point, the transfer of the impulse across the synapse is carried by a chemical neurotransmitter called *norepinephrine*. This transfer also occurs at the organ to be affected.

Norepinephrine is stored and manufactured at the presynaptic neuron. When an impulse crosses, norepinephrine is secreted into the synapse. Then it is free to act on the organ or postsynaptic neuron. The effect of norepinephrine lasts only a few seconds. Any remaining norepinephrine is either absorbed by the presynaptic neuron or destroyed by an enzyme known as *monoamine oxidase*. In addition, whenever the sympathetic division is stimulated, epinephrine is released from the adrenal medulla, causing a more prolonged response.

Sympathetic receptors
The two different types of receptors in the sympathetic division are the α-adrenergic and β-adrenergic receptors. Beta receptors are separated into β-1 and β-2 receptors.

When α-adrenergic receptors are stimulated, vasoconstriction results. The effect of an alpha agonist on any organ depends on the type and quantity of receptors. The heart is not directly affected by alpha agonists because it has few α-adrenergic receptors.

When β-1 adrenergic receptors are stimulated, they cause an increase in the heart's contractility and force (inotropic effect), rate and automaticity (chronotropic effect), and conduction of impulses (dromotropic effect). They also cause slight vasodilation in skeletal muscle. Stimulation of β-2 adrenergic receptors results in bronchodilation.

Drugs that are sympathetic division agonists usually are described by their effect on α-adrenergic and β-adrenergic receptors. For example, a group of drugs commonly used in the treatment of asthma because of their bronchodilation effects are called β-2 agonists. Specific examples include metaproterenol and albuterol.

Drugs that affect the sympathetic division
Several drugs encountered in prehospital care are sympathetic agonists or activators. Although a few are pure alpha or beta, most have both alpha and beta effects, usually with one or another being predominant. Some drugs, such as dopamine, have dose-related effects and may act as alpha or beta receptors depending on the dosages given. Some drugs are even selective in a beta category, affecting β-2 adrenergic receptors only.

Another commonly encountered class of drugs is the β-blockers. They are prescribed for hypertension, angina, and arrhythmias because of their beta antagonistic actions. They occupy β-adrenergic receptors and prevent agonists, such as some of those previously discussed, from activating receptors. One of the most common β-blockers is Propranolol.

Parasympathetic division
The **parasympathetic division** of the autonomic nervous system (also called the *cholinergic division*, derived from "acetylcholine") originates in the brain and sends messages to affect organs by the cranial nerves. Pairs of cranial nerves exit directly from the brain and travel to organs without using the spinal cord as a conduit. The tenth cranial nerves, or vagus nerves, are the primary nerves of the parasympathetic division and account for approximately 75% of actions caused by parasympathetic stimulation, which affects the heart, stomach, and gastrointestinal tract.

Parasympathetic stimulation also causes increased activity in the gut for digestion. Its effects on the lungs are slight, causing only minimal bronchoconstriction. Blood vessels are not affected by parasympathetic stimulation.

When the parasympathetic division is stimulated, impulses travel along the cranial nerves. At neuron synapses and at the junction between the nerve and effector organs, the primary neurotransmitter substance is acetylcholine. However, no indirect effect is produced in the parasympathetic division, because adrenal glands produce in the sympathetic division.

Acetylcholine crosses the synapse to reach a postsynaptic neuron or effector organ. It then occupies receptor sites and is broken down by the enzyme cholinesterase. This action only lasts a few seconds at most. Cholinesterase breaks acetylcholine into acetic acid and choline. Choline is then transported back and reused in the manufacture of new acetylcholine.

Atropine, a drug commonly used in prehospital care, is an acetylcholine antagonist or blocker. It occupies receptor sites and prevents a parasympathetic response. It commonly is used to increase the heart rate by increasing the discharge rate of the sinoatrial node and to increase conduction through the atrioventricular node.

It is not possible to administer acetylcholine as a drug because it is broken down by cholinesterase in the blood and at synapses before it can occupy receptors. Some drugs mimic its actions, however, and can cause parasympathetic stimulation. Muscarine, a poison found in mushrooms, and pilocarpine, a drug used to treat glaucoma, are examples of these drugs.

Other drugs inhibit the breakdown of acetylcholine by cholinesterase, potentiating the parasympathetic response. Poisons such as organophosphates are such inhibitors. Accidental exposure to these poisons results in severe parasympathetic overstimulation. This condition is counteracted by using atropine as an antagonist to acetylcholine. Other drugs, such as physostigmine, neostigmine, and edrophonium, are also cholinesterase inhibitors. All these drugs can be counteracted by the administration of atropine.

REVIEW OF BASIC ARITHMETIC

The following is a review of basic arithmetic including converting fractions to decimals and adding, subtracting, multiplying, and dividing decimals. Also included is a section on how to round off decimals. For help or a review of addition, subtraction, and division please refer to a basic math book.

 Demonstrate how to use decimals with basic math problems.

Decimals

A decimal is a fraction whose denominator is a power of 10 expressed by placing a point at the left of the numerator.
Recall:
2/10 = numerator/denominator
Examples:

2/10	=	0.2
25/100	=	0.25
2/100	=	0.02
3/100	=	0.03

Changing fractions to decimals

To change fractions to decimals, divide the numerator by the denominator. Place a decimal point the same number of places to the right as the numerator.
Examples:

1/4	=	0.25
3/8	=	0.375
2/3	=	0.6666
1/12	=	0.08333

Adding decimals

To add decimals, align all the decimal points in a column and then add all the numbers. The decimal point will stay in the same place after all the numbers are added.
Examples:

```
  2.33        1.50        3.20
  1.25        3.00       +2.00
  3.22       +1.55        5.20
 +1.23        6.05
  8.03
```

Subtracting decimals

To subtract decimals, align the decimal points in a column and then subtract the numbers. The decimal point will stay in the same place after the numbers are subtracted.

```
  2.33        1.55        4.23
 -0.44       -1.33       -2.33
  1.89        0.22        1.90
```

Multiplying decimals

Multiply decimals the same as whole numbers. After multiplying the numbers:

a. Count the number of decimal places in the multiplier and the multiplicand.

b. Count that number from right to left in the product and place the decimal point.

Examples:

```
   1.45 (multiplicand)            2.33
 × 0.33 (multiplier)            × 0.04
    435                           932
  +435                           000
 0.4785 (product)               +000
                               0.0932
```

Dividing decimals

To divide decimals:

a. Convert the divisor to a whole number by moving the decimal point to the right.

b. Move the decimal point in the dividend the same number of places to the right as in the divisor.

c. Divide.

d. Place the decimal point in the answer (quotient) directly above the decimal point in the dividend.

e. Carry out the answer to three decimal places before rounding off to two places.

Example:

```
                     1.277
.75 |.95800  = 75 |95.800  = 1.27
                     75.
                     208
                     150
                     580
                     525
                     550
```

Rounding off decimals

To round off a decimal, first determine how many significant digits are required after the decimal point. Then, look at the number to the right of the last number wanted. For example, to round off 4.113 to two digits to the right of the decimal point, look at the number 3. If 3 (in this example) is 5 or greater, the preceding point is rounded up to the next digit. If it is less than 5, the preceding digit is left as it is. The last decimal place is then dropped from the number. In this example, 4.113 would be rounded off to 4.11.

Examples:

2.247	is rounded to 2.25
3.144	is rounded to 3.14
5.26	is rounded to 5.3
7.24	is rounded to 7.2
3.24	is rounded to 3.2

SYSTEMS FOR MEASURING DRUGS

 Calculate dosages for various medications.

APOTHECARY SYSTEM: System for measuring drug dosages; the system is gradually being replaced by the metric system.

There are two systems of measuring drug dosage: the metric system and the **apothecary system**. Although the apothecary system will be discussed, the primary system of measuring drug dosages is the metric system.

Although many drugs are supplied in various dosages and packaged in unit packs of the dosages most often ordered, occasionally the EMT–I may be required to calculate a dosage by using mathematical equations. It is necessary to master the elements of the metric system before calculations can be attempted.

The metric system

The **metric system** is used throughout the world. Because the system is based on multiples of 10, decimals are often used, but never fractions. In the metric system, the base unit of length is the meter (m), the base unit of weight is the gram (g), and the base unit of volume is the liter (L). Prefixes show which fraction of the base is being used. Prefixes often used are:

micro = (0.000001)	milli = (0.001)
centi = (0.01)	kilo = (1000.0)

Symbols for the metric system

gram	=	g
liter	=	L
kilogram	=	kg
milliliter	=	mL
milligram	=	mg
cubic centimeter	=	cc
microgram	=	µg

Metric units and equivalents

1 L	=	1000 mL
1 mL	=	1 cc
1 g	=	1000 mg
1 mg	=	1000 µg
1 cc	=	1 mL
1 µg	=	0.001 mg
1 mg	=	0.001 g

The apothecary system

The **apothecary system** is used less frequently today and is gradually being replaced by the metric system. The liquid measurements include the minim, fluid dram, fluid ounce, pint, quart, and gallon. The system for measuring solid weights includes the grain, dram, ounce, and pound. Roman numerals may be used for smaller numbers, such as gr V or gtt II. Fractions may be used when necessary, but never decimals.

Symbols for the apothecary system

grain	=	gr
dram	=	dr
minim	=	m, min
drop (s)	=	gtt (s)
ounce	=	oz
pint	=	pt
quart	=	qt

Apothecary units and equivalents

60 grains	=	1 dr
1 dr	=	1 tsp
8 dr	=	1 fluid ounce
60 gtt	=	1 teaspoon (tsp)
3 tsp	=	1 tablespoon (tbsp)

MATH FOR PHARMACOLOGY AND DRUG CALCULATIONS

In the metric system, it is sometimes necessary to convert measurements to the same unit of measure. For example, the physician may order 0.5 g of a drug, and the drug container label reads 500 mg. To convert within the metric system the following rules are used:

1. To change grams to milligrams multiply grams by 1000 or move the decimal point three places to the right.

    5 g = ? mg
    5 × 1000 = 5000 milligrams
    2 g = ? mg
    2 × 1000 = 2000 milligrams

2. To change milligrams to grams divide the milligrams by 1000 or move the decimal point three places to the left.

    100 mg = ? g
    100 ÷ 1000 = 0.1 g
    500 mg = ? g
    500 ÷ 1000 = 0.5 g

3. To change milligrams to micrograms multiply the milligrams by 1000 or move the decimal point three places to the right.

    5 mg = ? µg
    5 × 1000 = 5000 µg
    8 mg = ? µg
    8 × 1000 = 8000 µg

4. To change micrograms to milligrams divide the micrograms by 1000 or move the decimal point three places to the left.

3000 μg = ? mg
3000 ÷ 1000 = 3 mg
2000 μg = ? mg
2000 ÷ 1000 = 2 mg

5. To change liters to milliliters multiply the liters by 1000 or move the decimal point three places to the right.

5 L = ? mL
5 × 1000 = 5000 mL
1 L = ? mL
1 × 1000 = 1000 mL

6. To change milliliters to liters divide the milliliters by 1000 or move the decimal point three places to the left.

500 mL = ? L
500 ÷ 1000 = 0.5 L
1500 mL = ? L
1500 ÷ 1000 = 1.5 L

There is no conversion necessary when changing milliliters to cubic centimeters, because they are approximately the same.

Examples:
1 mL   =   1 cc
3 mL   =   3 cc
5 mL   =   5 cc

Calculating drug dosages

Administration of drugs is an exacting science; errors in calculation could prove fatal to the patient. Many of the drugs used in the field are premixed and premeasured and ready to deliver to the average adult patient. This convenience decreases both preparation time and the likelihood of error. However, when giving certain drugs, calculation of volume of delivery is often necessary.

Calculation of volume

Most calculations are based on the following volume calculation formula:

$$\text{Volume to administer} = \frac{\text{Dose desired} \times \text{Volume on hand}}{\text{Dose on hand}}$$

The dose desired equals the amount of drug ordered (usually in mg). The volume on hand equals the quantity of fluid in the drug container (usually expressed in mL). The dose on hand equals the total amount of drug present in the drug container (usually expressed in mg).

Example 1:

Give atropine, 0.5 mg, from a prefilled syringe that contains 1 mg in 10 mL of fluid:

$$\text{Volume} = \frac{0.5 \text{ mg} \times 10 \text{ mL}}{1 \text{ mg}} = \frac{5}{1} = 5 \text{ mL}$$

A slight variation is to calculate the drug present per mL of solution:

$$\frac{1 \text{ mg}}{10 \text{ mL}} = 0.1 \text{ mg/mL}$$

and insert this value into the previous formula:

$$\text{Volume} = \frac{0.5 \text{ mg} \times 1 \text{ mL}}{0.1 \text{ mg}} = 5 \text{ mL}$$

Example 2:

An adult patient weighs 260 lbs and is in a coma due to a narcotic overdose. The physician orders an initial dose of naloxone at 1.5 mg intravenous (IV) push. The EMT–I has a 5-mL glass ampule containing 2.0 mg. How many mL would the EMT–I give this patient?

Calculate the volume of the dose by using the volume calculation formula:

$$\text{Volume to administer} = \frac{\text{Dose desired} \times \text{Volume on hand}}{\text{Dose on hand}}$$

$$X = \frac{1.50 \text{ mg} \times 5 \text{ mL}}{2.0 \text{ mg}}$$
$$X = 3.75 \text{ mL}$$

Calculation of volume based on weight

Some drug dosages are based on the patient's weight. Normally, body weight will be expressed in pounds (lbs) and must be converted to kilograms (kg).

Example 1:

An adult patient weighs 176 lbs and is in cardiac arrest from ventricular fibrillation. At some point during the code, the physician orders an initial dose of lidocaine at 1.5 mg/kg IV push. The EMT–I has a prefilled 5-mL syringe with 20 mg/mL. How many mL would the EMT–I give this patient?

Step 1. Calculate the patient's weight in kilograms. The symbol "X" indicates for what is being solved. (Note that 1 kg = 2.2 lbs)

$$\frac{X}{176 \text{ lbs}} = \frac{1 \text{ kg}}{2.2 \text{ lbs}}$$
$$2.2 X = 176$$
$$X = 80 \text{ kg}$$

Step 2. Calculate the mass (in this case, mg) of the dose.

$$\frac{X}{80 \text{ kg}} = \frac{1.5 \text{ mg}}{1 \text{ kg}}$$
$$X = 1.5 \times 80$$
$$X = 120 \text{ mg}$$

Step 3. Calculate the volume of the dose by using the volume calculation formula:

$$\text{Volume to administer} = \frac{\text{Dose desired} \times \text{Volume on hand}}{\text{Dose on hand}}$$

$$X = \frac{120 \text{ mg} \times 5 \text{ mL}}{100 \text{ mg}}$$
$$X = 6 \text{ mL}$$

Step 4. Administer 6 mL of lidocaine to the patient.

Example 2:

A pediatric patient weighs 66 lbs and is in acute bronchospasm. The physician orders an initial dose of epinephrine, 1:1000 solution, at 0.01 mg/kg sub-cutaneously. The EMT–I has a 1-mL glass ampule containing 1 mg/mL of the 1:1000 solution. How many mL would the EMT–I give this patient?

Step 1. Calculate the patient's weight in kilograms. The symbol "X" indicates for what is being solved. (Note that 1 kg = 2.2 lbs.)

$$\frac{X}{66 \text{ lbs}} = \frac{1 \text{ kg}}{2.2 \text{ lbs}}$$

$$2.2 \, X = 66$$

$$X = \frac{66}{2.2}$$

$$X = 30 \text{ kg}$$

Step 2. Calculate the mass (in this case, mg) of the dose.

$$\frac{X}{30 \text{ mg}} = \frac{0.01 \text{ mg}}{1 \text{ kg}}$$

$$X = 0.01 \times 30$$

$$X = 0.30 \text{ mg}$$

Step 3. Calculate the volume of the dose by using the volume calculation formula.

$$\text{Volume to administer} = \frac{\text{Dose desired} \times \text{Volume on hand}}{\text{Dose on hand}}$$

$$X = \frac{0.30 \text{ mg} \times 1 \text{ mL}}{1 \text{ mg}}$$

$$X = 0.30 \text{ mL}$$

Step 4. Administer 0.30 mL of epinephrine to the patient.

ROUTES FOR DRUG ADMINISTRATION

 Describe the various drug administration routes and recall the indications for each.

There are many routes by which a drug can be administered. The route of administration is chosen after considering many factors. Sometimes a given route is selected because of cost, safety, or speed with which the drug will be absorbed into the system. In other cases, certain drugs:

- May be administered by only one route
- May be toxic if given by a particular route
- May not be effective if given by a certain route
- Can only be absorbed by a certain route

The routes chosen by the EMT–I to administer drugs in the prehospital setting include sublingual, intravenous, subcutaneous, intramuscular, inhalation, endotracheal, transdermal, or intraosseous.

Drug Routes

Sublingual

The drug is placed under the patient's tongue and must not be swallowed. The drug is dissolved by the saliva in the mouth and is absorbed into the bloodstream through the vascular oral mucosa. The number of drugs administered sublingually is limited. Nitroglycerin is the most frequently prescribed sublingual drug and it is used to treat angina pectoris. To administer the drug, the EMT–I places the tablet under the patient's tongue, where it is dissolved. The patient should avoid drinking fluids while the drug is being absorbed. Swallowing the drug may diminish or delay the effects.

Intravenous

A sterile solution of a drug is injected into the body by venipuncture. This method allows for an infusion of larger amounts of the drug. IV drugs have the quickest action because they enter the bloodstream immediately. Only drugs intended for IV administration should be given by this route.

Subcutaneous

Injections are given into the fatty layer of tissue below the skin by positioning the needle and syringe at a 45° angle to the skin. The subcutaneous route is chosen for the drugs that should not be absorbed as rapidly as through the intramuscular or IV route.

The best sites for subcutaneous injection are areas where the skin is loose and easily pinched, such as the upper arms and thighs. By this method of injection, a drug is absorbed into the body in a slow but steady rate.

Intramuscular

Small quantities of a drug are injected into a muscle. Absorption is limited by the type of drug and circulation to the muscle used for injection. If a drug is injected into poorly perfused muscle, absorption is limited.

Although it is possible to give some emergency drugs by this route, it is generally avoided in favor of routes of more predictable absorption.

Inhalation or endotracheal

Administration of drugs, water vapors, or gases by inspiration of the substance(s) into the lungs. A drug is absorbed quickly through the alveolar walls into the capillaries. Existing pathology may make absorption difficult to predict. Patients with chronic pulmonary conditions may self-administer the medication with a hand-held nebulizer, an apparatus for producing a fine spray of medicated mist. In a cardiac arrest patient the EMT–I may administer certain drugs through the endotracheal tube.

Transdermal

A drug is delivered to the body by absorption through the skin. Delivery is slow and maintains a steady, stable level of the drug. Dermal patches are placed on the skin, usually on the chest, upper arm, or behind the ear. Antiangina medications placed anywhere on the chest wall are very effective by this route.

Intraosseous

Administration of medication directly into the bone marrow of a long bone. This technique provides rapid vascular access in the critically-injured infant or child. It is not considered a replacement for IV access but is reserved for emergencies.

Many drugs are available in unit-dose packages that contain the amount of the drug for a single dose, in the proper form for administration. Unit-dose packages are labeled with the trade name, generic name, precautions, instructions for storage, and an expiration date.

The parenteral route is the most frequently used route in the prehospital setting. Parenteral refers to all the ways in which drugs are administered other than oral. In the prehospital setting, the IV route is the most commonly used because it is the quickest acting. The intramuscular route is commonly used in a nonemergency setting in the hospital because the muscles are highly vascular and absorption is fairly rapid.

Parenteral administration is the most efficient method of drug administration, but it also can be the most hazardous. The effects may be quite rapid because the drug cannot be retrieved, and if the skin is broken it is possible for infections to develop. The EMT–I must use aseptic technique whenever administering medications by the parenteral route. If an injection is placed incorrectly, nerve damage could occur or the penetration of blood vessels could cause formation of a hematoma. Incorrect placement of the needle during an intramuscular injection could cause the medication to be delivered intravenously.

DRUG ADMINISTRATION

 Recall the characteristics and indications for the various types of drug administration devices.

Needles and syringes

There are a variety of needles and syringes used for injections. The 3-mL hypodermic syringe is the most common type used for injections. The syringe consists of a plunger, body or barrel, flange, and tip. The other types of syringes used for parenteral administration are tuberculin and insulin. Needle lengths vary from 3/8 to 1 inch or 1 1/2 inches for standard injections. "Gauge" refers to the diameter of the needle lumen. Needle gauge varies from 18 (large) to 27 (small); the higher the number, the smaller the gauge (Fig. 12-5).

Most companies prepackage hypodermic syringes in color-coded envelopes with the needle attached. Separate needles and syringes may be purchased as needed. This type of syringe may be used for either subcutaneous or intramuscular injections. It is necessary to choose the package with a needle length and gauge appropriate for the route of the injection and medication to be given (Fig 12-6). For example, an intramuscular injection requires a needle length of at

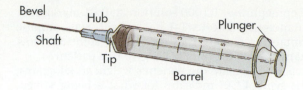

Fig. 12-5   The components of a syringe.

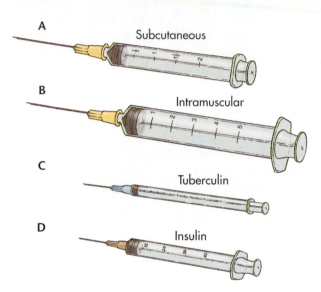

Fig. 12-6   Various types of syringes. A, A subcutaneous syringe. B, An intramuscular (or intravenous syringe). C, A tuberculin syringe. D, An insulin syringe.

least 1 inch. The needle will vary from 20 to 25 gauge, again depending on the drug to be administered. Some drugs, such as penicillin, cannot be drawn into a syringe using a small-gauge needle.

Subcutaneous injections generally are given using a short, small-gauge needle—25 gauge, 5/8 inch or 23 gauge, 1/2 inch.

All hypodermic syringes are marked with 10 calibrations per mL on one side of the syringe. Each small line represents 0.1 (one-tenth) mL. The other side of the syringe is marked in minims.

The tuberculin syringe is narrow and has a total capacity of 1 mL. There are 100 calibration lines marking the capacity. Each line represents 0.01 mL. Every tenth line is longer than the others to indicate 0.1 mL. TB syringes are used for newborn and pediatric doses and for intradermal (eg, TB) skin tests.

The insulin syringe is used strictly for administering insulin to diabetics. It has a total capacity of 1 mL. The 1 mL volume is marked as 100 units (U) indicating the strength of 100 U of insulin per mL when full. Each group of 10 U is divided by five small lines. Each line represents 2 U. A smaller insulin syringe with a capacity of 0.5 mL can be used when less than 50 U of insulin is ordered. The smaller insulin syringe has 50 small calibration lines, each representing 1 U of insulin. Most of the insulin used today is U-100, which means that there are 100 U of insulin in each mL. It is important to remember that the insulin syringe must be marked U-100 to match the insulin used.

Prefilled syringes contain a premeasured amount of a medication in a disposable cartridge with a needle attached. The prefilled cartridge and needle are placed in a holder.

Guidelines for administering drugs

To ensure safety when administering drugs, the EMT–I should do the following:

1. Know the policies of the medical director regarding the administration of drugs.
2. Know the local protocols or standing orders.
3. Give only the drugs that the medical director or protocols have ordered.
4. Check with the medical director or medical direction if there is any doubt about a drug.
5. Do not talk while drawing up and administering a drug. It is important to remain attentive during this task.
6. Read drug labels carefully. Check the expiration date.
7. If the order is received over the radio, repeat the instructions back to medical direction.
8. Know the drugs. Be alert for color changes, precipitation, odor, or any indication that the drug has changed its properties.
9. Make sure to ask about any allergies that the patient may have to the drug. If the patient is unresponsive, attempt to elicit information from family members or friends.
10. Stay with the patient while the drug is being taken or administered. Watch for any reaction and record the patient's response.
11. Check the strength of the medication (eg, 250 mg versus 500 mg) and the route of administration.
12. If using a syringe, measure the amount exactly; make sure there are no bubbles in the liquid.
13. Never return a drug to its container.
14. Have "sharps" containers as close to the area of use as possible.
15. Never recap, bend, or break a used needle.
16. Wear gloves for all procedures that might result in contact with blood or body fluids.

Techniques of measuring drugs

Demonstrate the techniques used to administer drugs in the prehospital setting.

Drugs may be packaged in a variety of ways, depending on the form of drug and the manufacturer. Some of the common packaging that the EMT–I will use are vials, ampules, and prefilled syringes.

Vials
Vials are packaged in either single- or multidose amounts. When using a vial, the EMT–I should take the following steps:

1. Confirm the drug type, concentration, and dose.
2. Check for cloudiness and the expiration date.
3. Clean the rubber stopper with alcohol.
4. Determine the volume of drug to be withdrawn and draw that amount of air into the syringe.
5. Invert the vial, insert the needle through the rubber stopper and inject the air into the vial.
6. Withdraw the desired amount of solution (Fig. 12-7). Remove the needle from the vial.
7. Invert the syringe and expel any trapped air.
8. Reconfirm the drug type, concentration, and dose.
9. Recap the needle, being careful not to contaminate it.

Ampules
Glass ampules are typical containers for inexpensive single-dose packaging. When using an ampule, the EMT–I should take the following steps:

1. Confirm the drug type, concentration, and dose.
2. Check for cloudiness and the expiration date.
3. Shake the ampule or tap the stem and top to shift the fluid to the bottom.
4. Place a gauze square or alcohol wipe over the bottle neck and snap the top off (Fig. 12-8 A).

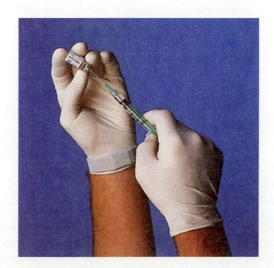

Fig. 12-7 **Withdrawing medication from vial.**

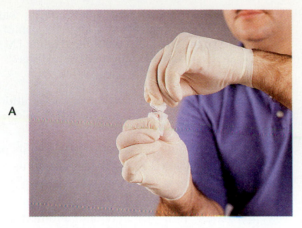
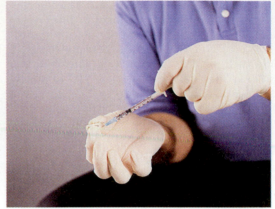

Fig. 12-8 A, Break the glass top. B, Draw solution into the syringe and invert the needle.

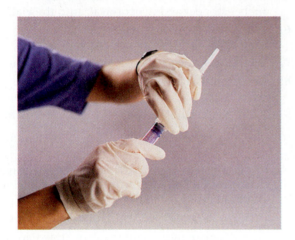

Fig. 12-9 Screw the syringe and drug cartridge together.

5. Insert the needle into the solution without touching the sides.

6. Draw the solution into the syringe (Fig. 12-8 B).

7. Invert the syringe (needle pointing up) and tap the syringe barrel to get the air bubbles to the top.

8. Push on the plunger to expel any trapped air.

9. Draw in more medication and repeat the procedure if necessary to have the correct amount of medication in the syringe.

10. Recap the needle, being careful not to contaminate it.

Prefilled syringes

Prefilled syringes are a convenient form of packaging for emergency drugs. Some are preassembled and require no preparation, whereas others must be assembled before administration. When using a prefilled syringe, the EMT–I should take the following steps:

1. Confirm the drug type, concentration, and dose.

2. Check for cloudiness and the expiration date.

3. If assembly is required, pop the caps off the syringe and drug cartridge and screw both together (Fig. 12-9).

4. Invert the syringe and expel any excess air.

5. Reconfirm the drug type, concentration, and dose.

6. Administer the drug by the desired route.

To administer drugs via various routes, specific procedures must be used.

Sublingual administration

To administer a medication through the sublingual route, the EMT–I should do the following:

1. Identify the need for medication based on patient history and presenting signs and symptoms.

2. Contact medical direction for permission to administer medication or follow off-line standing orders.

3. Confirm the order, repeating to medical direction the name of the medication, dosage, and route.

4. Write down the order.

5. Reassure the patient and check for allergies.

6. Select the appropriate medication container, checking the name, dosage, and expiration date.

7. Uncap the container and remove the indicated number of tablets.

8. Direct the patient to place the tablet underneath the tongue so that it does not get swallowed or chewed (Fig. 12-10 A).

9. Confirm the medication administration with medical direction, record the administration time, and watch for patient response to the medication administration (Fig. 12-10 B).

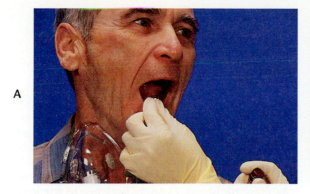
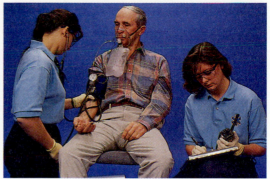

Fig. 12-10   A, Have the patient place the tablet underneath the tongue. B, Record the administration time and reconfirm the medication administration with medical direction.

Subcutaneous administration

To administer a medication through the subcutaneous route, the EMT–I should do the following:

1. Use body substance isolation precautions.
2. Identify the need for medication based on patient history and presenting signs and symptoms.
3. Contact medical direction for permission to administer medication or follow off-line standing orders.
   - If orders are obtained from medical direction, repeat orders back to the medical direction physician and write down the information on the run sheet.
4. Reassure the patient and check for allergies.
5. Expose and cleanse the area to be used for medication administration (Fig. 12-11 A). Usually the lateral aspect of either an upper arm or thigh is selected.
6. To make sure the needle does not go in too deeply, pinch the skin and dart the needle in rapidly at a 45° angle (Figs. 12-11 B, C).
7. Pull back on the syringe plunger to aspirate for blood (Fig. 12-11 D). If blood is seen in the syringe, withdraw the needle and apply firm pressure over the site with a sterile dressing. Select another site for administering the medication.
8. Inject the medication and remove the needle from the skin.
9. Apply circular pressure to the injection site to disperse the medication throughout the tissue (Fig. 12-11 E).
10. Dispose of the needle/syringe in an appropriate "sharps" container (Fig. 12-11 F). Do not recap the needle.
11. Store any unused medication appropriately.
12. Confirm the medication administration with medical direction, record the administration

time, and watch for patient response to the medication administration (for both desired effects as well as adverse effects).

Intramuscular administration

To administer a medication through the intramuscular route, the EMT–I should do the following:

1. Use body substance isolation precautions.
2. Identify the need for medication based on patient history and presenting signs and symptoms.
3. Contact medical direction for permission to administer medication or follow off-line standing orders.
   - If orders are obtained from medical direction, repeat orders back to the medical direction physician and write down the information on the run sheet.
4. Reassure the patient and check for allergies.
5. Expose and cleanse the area to be used for medication administration. Use either the deltoid muscle in the shoulder or the upper outer quadrant of the gluteal area.
6. To make sure the needle goes into the muscle and not the subcutaneous layer, stretch the skin over the injection site and insert the needle at a 90° angle to the skin (Fig. 12-12).
7. Pull back on the syringe plunger to aspirate for blood. If blood is seen in the syringe, withdraw the needle and apply firm pressure over the site with a sterile dressing. Select another site for administering the medication.
8. Inject the medication and remove the needle from the skin.
9. Apply circular pressure to the injection site to disperse the medication throughout the tissue.
10. Dispose of the needle/syringe in an appropriate "sharps" container. Do not recap the needle.

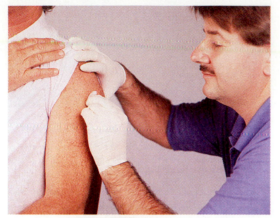

A

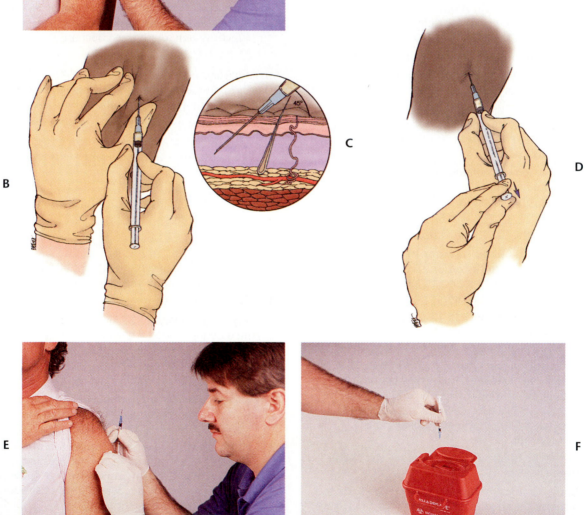

B

C

D

E

F

Fig. 12-11 Subcanteous administration. A, Cleanse the area. B, Pinch the skin and inject the needle at a 45° angle to the skin. C, A cross-section view of the skin showing proper subcutaneous injection. D, Aspirate for blood. E, Apply pressure to the injection area to disperse the medication. F, Dispose of all used sharp objects in a proper waste container.

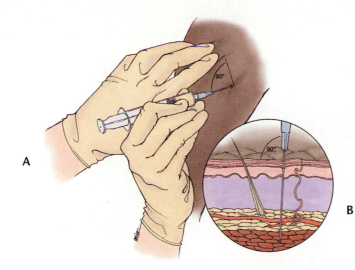

Fig. 12-12 **Intramuscular injection. A, For intramuscular injections, stretch the skin across the site and inject the needle at a 90° angle to the skin. B, A cross-section view of the skin showing proper intramuscular injection.**

11. Store any unused medication appropriately.

12. Confirm the medication administration with medical direction, record the administration time, and watch for patient response to the medication administration (for both desired effects as well as adverse effects).

Intravenous medication administration

To administer a medication through an IV infusion, the EMT–I should do the following:

1. Use body substance isolation precautions.

2. Identify the need for medication based on patient history and presenting signs and symptoms.

3. Contact medical direction for permission to administer medication or follow off-line standing orders.
   - If orders are obtained from medical direction, repeat orders back to the medical direction physician and write down the information on the run sheet.

4. Reassure the patient and check for allergies.

5. Cleanse the medication injection site (Y-port or hub) of the IV tubing (Fig. 12-13 A).

6. Penetrate the injection site with the needle (Fig. 12-13 B).

7. Stop the IV flow by pinching the IV tubing above the injection site (Fig. 12-13 C). This can be done by using the stop-cock device on the tubing. Closing the tubing leading to the IV bag prevents the medication from flowing up into the IV bag instead of into the patient.

8. Administer the correct dose of medication at the correct push rate (Fig. 12-13 D).

9. Flush the IV tubing by briefly running it wide open or following the drug bolus with a 20-mL bolus of IV fluid.

10. Adjust the IV flow rate to a keep open rate.

11. Dispose of the needle/syringe in an appropriate "sharps" container. Do not recap the needle.

12. Store any unused medication appropriately.

13. Confirm the medication administration with medical direction, record the administration time, and watch for patient response to the medication administration (for both desired effects as well as adverse effects).

Endotracheal administration

To administer a medication through the endotracheal tube, the EMT–I should do the following:

1. Ensure adequate oxygenation and ventilation of the patient.

2. Prepare the medication per medical direction. Also check the drug inserts at the end of this chapter.

3. Hyperventilate the patient's lungs (Fig. 12-14 A).

4. Remove the ventilatory device from the endotracheal tube and inject the medication through a catheter deep into the tube (Fig. 12-14 B).

 CLINICAL NOTES
ET tubes with separate injection ports are commercially available.

HELPFUL HINT
If cardiopulmonary resuscitation is being delivered at the time of endotracheal medication administration, the EMT–I should stop chest compressions momentarily during endotracheal drug injection until several ventilations are given. Otherwise, the drug may be forced back up and out of the endotracheal tube.

5. Reconnect the ventilatory device and resume assisted breathing with several large ventilations to help enhance absorption of the medication.

6. Confirm the medication administration with medical direction, record the administration time, and watch and record patient response to the medication administration (for both desired effects as well as adverse effects).

7. Dispose of the needle/syringe in the appropriate "sharps" container. Do not recap the needle.

8. Monitor the patient for the desired therapeutic effect and any possible undesired side effects.

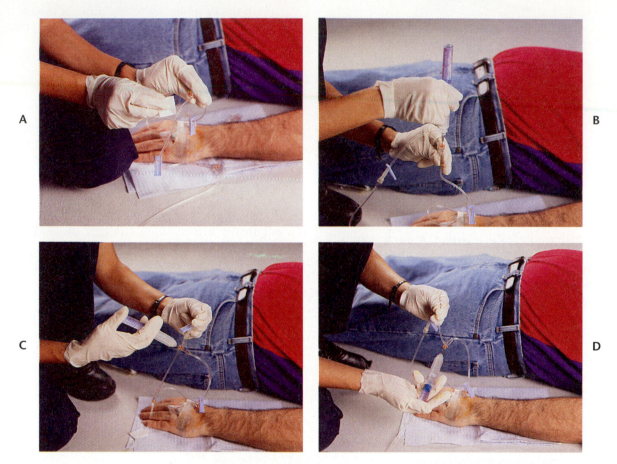

Fig. 12-13 IV medication administration. A, Cleanse the medication injection site of the IV tubing. B, Insert the needle into the injection site. C, Pinch the IV tubing above the infection site to stop the flow of the IV. D, Administer the correct dosage.

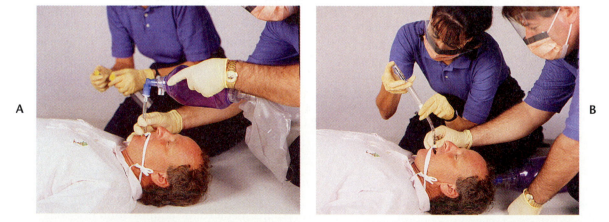

Fig. 12-14 Endotracheal administration. A, Hyperventilate the patient. B, Inject the medication through a catheter into the ET tube.

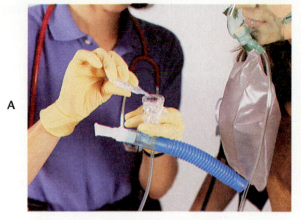
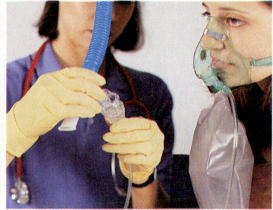

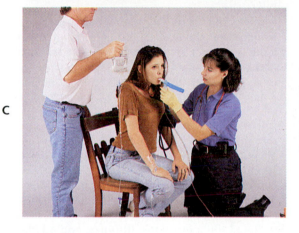

Fig. 12-15 Aerosol administration. A, Mix the drug with an appropriate amount of normal saline. B, Connect the nebulizer to a T-piece and mouth piece and connect to an oxygen regulator. C, Have the patient inhale the aerosol slowly, exhaling after 3-5 seconds.

Aerosol administration

To administer a medication by aerosol, the EMT–I should do the following:

1. Use body substance isolation precautions.

2. Identify the need for medication based on patient history and presenting signs and symptoms.

3. Contact medical direction for permission to administer medication or follow off-line standing orders.

   • If orders are obtained from medical direction, repeat orders back to the medical direction physician and write down the information on the run sheet.

4. Reassure the patient and check for allergies.

5. Mix the prescribed drug (using aseptic technique) with a specified amount of normal saline and pour it into the nebulizer (Fig. 12-15 A). Some medications are available in a packaged unit dose and contain a fixed amount of diluent (usually 0.9% normal saline).

6. Attach the nebulizer to a T-piece and mouthpiece (Fig. 12-15 B) and connect it to the oxygen regulator with oxygen connecting tubing. Alternatively, a nebulizer face mask may be used instead of a mouthpiece.

7. Adjust the oxygen flowmeter to 4 to 6 L/min to produce a steady, visible mist.

> **HELPFUL HINT**
> If an aerosol mask is used, the flow rate of oxygen should be maintained at 6 to 10 L/min to prevent potential buildup of exhaled carbon dioxide in the mask.

8. When the mist is visible, treatment should be started.

9. Instruct the patient to inhale slowly and deeply through the mouth and to hold the breaths 3 to 5 seconds before exhaling (Fig. 12-15 C). Inhalation and exhalation should be continued until the aerosol canister is depleted of the medication.

> **HELPFUL HINT**
> Nebulization requires a cooperative patient who can be instructed to breathe deeply so that the drug can be absorbed. If a patient cannot inhale the drug or if bronchospasm is severe, the administration of another drug via a different route should be considered.

10. Confirm the medication administration with medical direction, record the administration

time, and watch for patient response to the medication administration (for both desired effects as well as adverse effects).

11. If changes in heart rate or dysrhythmias are noted, nebulization should be stopped and medical direction contacted for further orders.

DRUGS ADMINISTERED BY THE EMT–I

 List the common drugs administered by the EMT–I.

An EMT–I delivers drugs that can be given to the patient under certain conditions. The EMT–I also should be able to assist the patient in taking his or her prescribed medication. The 1994 DOT EMT–Basic curriculum includes the delivery of the following six medications:

Activated charcoal
Activated charcoal is used because it absorbs toxic substances from the gastrointestinal tract. It is used for oral poisonings and overdoses. The adult and pediatric dosages: 1 to 2 g/kg; if not in a premixed slurry, mix one part charcoal with four parts water. The solution is given to the patient orally. It is important that the patient is conscious and alert to avoid aspiration.

Oral glucose
This type of glucose is taken by mouth. It is indicated in a patient with a history of diabetes or in a patient with an altered level of responsiveness. The patient must be alert enough, however, to be able to take the glucose easily without aspiration.

Oxygen
Oxygen is used to treat patients with conditions that cause the oxygen content to be low. These conditions may be caused by a medical or trauma condition.

Prescribed inhalers
There are various types of drugs given by an inhaler device. Most commonly the patient will present with diseases such as chronic bronchitis, emphysema, or asthma. The drug contained in the inhaler will relax bronchial muscles and make breathing easier.

Nitroglycerin
Nitroglycerin is a smooth muscle relaxant. It reduces the workload on the heart and dilates the coronary arteries. It is used for angina and congestive heart failure. It may be given sublingually as a 1/150 gr (0.4 mg) tablet, topical as a one patch of paste, or by aerosol in 1 to 2 metered doses. It is not used for the pediatric patient.

Epinephrine auto injector
An epinephrine auto injector is used for severe allergic reaction (and phoylaxis). An autoinjector is a syringe with a spring-loaded needle that will release and inject the drug into the muscle. The large muscle in the thigh is the place of choice for administration.

 Recall the indications, dosages, and administration routes of the primary drugs administered by the EMT–I.

Additional drugs that may be administered by the EMT–I are included in Table 12-4.

TABLE 12-4	Additional Drugs Used by the EMT–I
Generic name:	**Albuterol sulfate**
Brand name:	Proventil, Ventolin
Class:	Sympathomimetic
Mechanism of action:	Relaxes bronchial smooth muscle, resulting in bronchodilation
Indications and field use:	Bronchospasm from emphysema or asthma
Contraindications:	Synergistic with other sympathomimetics. Use with caution in patients with diabetes, hypertension, hyperthyroidism, and cerebrovascular disease.
Adverse reactions:	Excessive use may cause arrhythmias, tachycardia, tremors, nervousness, nausea, and vomiting.
Incompatibilities/drug interactions:	Cyclic antidepressants, monoamine oxidase inhibitors
Adult dosage:	2.5 mg; dilute 0.5 mL of the 0.5% solution for inhalation with 2-4 mL normal saline in nebulizer over 5-15 min 1-2 inhalations (90 µg each) with metered-dose inhaler, may be repeated every 15 min as needed.

TABLE 12-4 Continued

Pediatric dosage:	Age younger than 12 yrs, 0.03 mL/kg of a 0.5% solution up to 1.0 mL over 5-10 min. Age older than 12 yrs, use full adult dose
Routes of administration:	Nebulized inhaler, also in a metered-dose inhaler
Onset of action:	5-15 min
Peak effects:	30 min–2 h
Duration of action:	3-4 h
Dosage forms/packaging:	Aerosol inhaler: 90µg/metered spray, 100µg/metered spray. Solution for inhalation: 0.083% or 0.5%.
Generic name:	**Atropine sulfate**
Brand name:	None
Class:	Parasympatholytic
Mechanism of action:	Inhibits acetylcholine in smooth muscle and glands, blocking parasympathetic response and allowing sympathetic response to take over. Small doses cause sedation, and high doses cause stimulation. The systemic effect is depressed salivary and gastrointestinal secretions and bronchodilation. Heart rate will increase and there will be an increase in AV conduction.
Indications and field use:	First drug for symptomatic bradycardia. Second drug (after epinephrine) for asystole or bradycardial pulseless electrical activity. Poisonings by certain mushrooms, insecticides, and nerve gas.
Contraindications:	Use with caution in presence of myocardial ischemia and hypoxia. Use with caution in AV block at the His-Purkinje level (type II AV block and third-degree AV block with new wide-QRS complexes). Glaucoma, myasthenia gravis.
Adverse reactions:	Pupil dilation, increases myocardial oxygen demand, dry mouth
Incompatibilities/drug interactions:	Antihistamines, phenothiazine antipsychotics, and tricyclic antidepressants enhance the effects of atropine.
Adult dosage:	Asystole or PEA: 1 mg IV push; repeat every 3-5 min (if asystole persists) to a maximum dose of 0.04 mg/kg. Bradycardia: 0.5-1.0 mg IV push every 3-5 min as needed; not to exceed total dose of 0.03-0.04 mg/kg. Use shorter dosing interval (3 min) and higher doses (0.04 mg/kg) in severe clinical conditions. In poisonings: larger doses are required; usually initial dose of 2.0 mg. Endotracheal: 1-2 mg diluted in 10 mL sterile water or normal saline
Pediatric dosage:	0.02 mg/kg (minimum of 0.1 mg) rapid IV push Maximum single dose: 0.5 mg in child, 1.0 mg in adolescent.
Routes of administration:	IV, ET, IO.
Onset of action:	1 min.
Peak effects:	2-5 min.
Duration of action:	2 hrs.
Dosage forms/packaging:	0.1 mg/mL in 10-mL prefilled syringe (total = 1 mg).

TABLE 12-4	Continued

Generic name:	**Dextrose 50% solution**
Brand name:	None
Class:	Hyperglycemic
Mechanism of action:	Increases blood glucose levels
Indications and field use:	Hypoglycemia, coma of unknown origin, altered level of responsiveness, seizure of unknown origin
Contraindications:	Intracranial hemorrhage, cerebral vascular accident, delirium tremens
Adverse reactions:	If IV is not properly in vein, necrosis of tissue surrounding IV site could occur.
Incompatibilities/drug interactions:	None
Adult dosage:	25-50 g IV bolus (50-100 mL of a 50% solution)
Pediatric dosage:	25% dextrose at 0.5-1.0 g/kg IV bolus A 50% solution may be diluted 1:1 with normal saline or sterile water
Routes of administration:	IV bolus
Onset of action:	Immediate
Peak effects:	Variable
Duration of action:	Variable
Dosage forms/packaging:	Prefilled syringe, 25 g in 50 mL
Special considerations:	Draw blood sugar to confirm hypoglycemia before administering medication.
Generic name:	**Epinephrine**
Brand name:	Adrenalin
Class:	Sympathomimetic
Mechanism of action:	Direct acting alpha and beta agonist α - 1: bronchial, skin, renal, and visceral arteriolar constriction β - 1: positive inotropic and chronotropic actions, increases automaticity β - 2: bronchial smooth muscle relaxation and dilation of skeletal vasculature
Indications and field use:	Cardiac arrest: VF, pulseless VT, asystole, PEA Symptomatic bradycardia: after atropine and transcutaneous pacing Acute bronchospasm: anaphylaxis, bronchiolitis, asthma, chronic obstructive pulmonary disease
Contraindications:	Pulmonary edema, hypothermia, hypertension Remember, however, there are no contraindications for the use of epinephrine in cardiac arrest.
Adverse reactions:	Ventricular arrhythmias, precipitation of angina or myocardial infarction, tachycardia, anxiety, hypertension, headache
Incompatibilities/drug interactions:	Potentiates other sympathomimetics Patients on monoamine oxidase inhibitors, antihistamines, and tricyclic antidepressants may have heightened effects.

TABLE 12-4	Continued

	These interactions, although important, should not prevent the use of epinephrine in cardiac arrest.
Adult dosage:	Cardiac arrest: First dose: 1 mg IV push (10 mL of a 1:10,000 solution); may repeat every 3-5 min Alternative regimens for second dose: Intermediate: 2-5 mg IV push, every 3-5 min Escalating: 1 mg, 3 mg, and 5 mg IV push, 3 min apart High: 0.1 mg/kg IV push, every 3-5 min Endotracheal: 2.0-2.5 mg diluted in 10 mL normal saline Profound bradycardia: 1-2 µg/min (add 1 mg to 500 mL normal saline or 5% dextrose in water to produce a concentration of 2 µg/mL Acute bronchospasm: 0.3-0.5 mg (0.3-0.5 mL of a 1:1000 solution). The dose may be repeated every 5-20 min to a total of three doses.

Pediatric dosage:	Bradycardia: IV/IO: 0.01 mg/kg (1:10,000, 0.1 mL/kg); ET: 0.1 mg/kg (1:1000, 0.1 mL/kg)
	Asystolic or pulseless arrest:
	    First dose: IV/IO: 0.01 mg/kg (1:10,000, 0.1 mL/kg); ET: 0.1 mg/kg (1:1000, 0.1 mL/kg) IV/IO doses as high as 0.2 mg/kg of 1:1000 may be effective.
	    Subsequent doses: IV/IO/ET: 0.1 mg/kg (1:1000, 0.1 mL/kg). Repeat every 3-5 min. IV/IO doses as high as 0.2 mg/kg (0.2 mL/kg of a 1:1000 solution) may be effective.
	Acute bronchospasm: give 0.01 mg/kg (0.01 mL/kg of a 1:1000 solution) subcutaneously (maximum of 0.35 mg/dose)

Routes of administration:	Cardiac: IV push, IV infusion, ET, IO Acute bronchospasm: subcutaneously, intramuscularly, IV, ET
Onset of action:	Immediate
Peak effects:	Minutes
Duration of action:	Several minutes
Dosage forms/packaging:	Prefilled: 0.1 mg/mL, 10-mL syringe, 1:10,000 solution Glass ampules: 1 mg/mL, 1:1000 solution Multidose 30-mL vial: 1 mg/mL
Generic name:	**Lidocaine hydrochloride**
Brand name:	Xylocaine
Class:	Antiarrhythmic
Mechanism of action:	Increases VF threshold, decreases phase-4 diastolic depolarization, suppresses premature ventricular ectopy
Indications and field use:	Cardiac arrest from VF/VT Stable VT, wide-complex tachycardias of uncertain type, wide-complex paroxysimal supraventricular tachycardia, and significant ectopy
Contraindications:	Prophylactic use in acute myocardial infarction patients not recommended. Reduce maintenance dose (not loading dose) in patients with impaired live function and left ventricular dysfunction.

TABLE 12-4	Continued	
Adverse reactions:	Drowsiness, confusion, fatigue, respiratory depression and arrest, cardiovascular collapse, tremors, twitching
Incompatibilities/drug interactions:	None known
Adult dosage:	Cardiac arrest from VF/VT: Initial dose: 1.0-1.5 mg/kg IV push for refractory VF may repeat at 1.0-1.5 mg/kg in 3-5 min; maximum total of 3 mg/kg (an additional countershock should be administered between these doses). A single dose of 1 mg/kg in cardiac arrest is acceptable. ET: use 2-2.5 times the IV dose to obtain equivalent blood levels compared with IV administration. Nonarrested patient: Stable VT and wide-complex tachycardia of uncertain type, significant ventricular ectopy: 1.0-1.5 mg/kg IV push. Repeat at 0.5-0.75 mg/kg IV every 5-10 min, maximum total 3 mg/kg. Maintenance infusion: On return of spontaneous circulation, start a continuous infusion at 2-4 mg/min. When given in the nonarrest setting to a responsive patient, lidocaine should be infused at no more than 1-4 mg/min.
Pediatric dosage:	1 mg/kg Maintenance infusion: 20-50 μg/kg/min. The infusion should contain 120 mg lidocaine in 100 mL 5% dextrose in water administered at a rate of 20-50 μg/kg/min (1-2.5 mL/kg/h)
Routes of administration:	IV bolus, followed by IV infusion May be given ET
Onset of action:	1-5 min
Peak effects:	5-10 min
Duration of action:	Bolus only, 20 min
Dosage forms/packaging:	Prefilled syringes, 5 mg/mL, 10 mg/mL, 15 mg/mL, 20 mg/mL Vials: 40 mg/mL, 100 mg/mL, 200 mg/mL
Generic name:	**Naloxone**
Brand name:	Narcan
Class:	Narcotic antagonist
Mechanism of action:	Competitive inhibition at narcotic receptor sites Reverses respiratory depression secondary to depressant drugs
Indications and field use:	Antidote for: Narcotics, Lomotil, Talwin, Darvon Given for acutely depressed levels of responsiveness (differentiates drug-induced coma from other causes).
Contraindications:	None
Adverse reactions:	Withdrawal symptoms, especially in neonates (nausea, vomiting, diaphoresis, increased heart rate, falling blood pressure, tremors) Be prepared for combative patient after administration
Incompatibilities/drug interactions:	None significant
Adult dosage:	Initial dose of 2 mg IV If necessary, dose may be repeated in 2 to 3 min intervals to a maximum of 10 mg

TABLE 12-4   Continued

	For ET administration, dilute medication with normal saline to a volume of 3-5 mL and follow with several positive-pressure ventilations
Pediatric dosage:	If less than or equal to 5 years of age or less than or equal to 20 kg: 0.1 mg/kg If greater than 5 years of age or greater than 20 kg: 2.0 mg
Routes of administration:	IV, ET
Onset of action:	IV, within 2 min
Peak effects:	Variable
Duration of action:	Approximately 45 min
Dosage forms/packaging:	Vials: 0.4 mg/mL (1 mL, 10 mL) 1 mg/mL (2mL)
Generic name:	**Nitroglycerin**
Brand name:	Nitrostat, Tridil
Class:	Vasodilator
Mechanism of action:	Coronary artery vasodilation Reduces workload on the heart by causing blood pooling and peripheral vasodilation Smooth muscle relaxant acting on vascular, uterine, bronchial and intestinal smooth muscle
Indications and field use:	Angina pectoris, congestive heart failure
Contraindications:	Hypovolemia, increased intracranial pressure, severe hepatic or renal disease
Adverse reactions:	Hypotension, bradycardia, headache
Incompatibilities/drug interactions:	IV: all other drugs
Adult dosage:	Sublingually: Initial dose of 0.3-0.4 mg, may be repeated at 5-min intervals to a total dose of three tablets if discomfort is unrelieved IV: Bolus of 12.5-25 μg may be administered before the initiation of a continuous nitroglycerin infusion (200-400 μg/mL) at a rate of 10-20 μg/min. The infusion should be increased by 5 or 10 μg/min until the desired hemodynamic or clinical response is achieved.
Pediatric dosage:	Not used
Routes of administration:	IV, sublingual, topical/transdermal, aerosol
Onset of action:	Immediate
Peak effects:	5-10 min
Duration of action:	1-10 min
Dosage forms/packaging:	Tablets: 1/150 gr (0.4 mg) IV: 50-mg/10-mL ampules

AV—atrioventricular; ET—endotracheal; IO—intraosseous; IV—intravenous; PEA—pulseless electrical activity; VF—ventricular fibrillation; VT—ventricular tachycardia.

CASE HISTORY FOLLOW-UP

As EMT–I Maloney is administering the albuterol via inhalation and preparing the stair-chair stretcher for the patient, the school nurse collapses at her desk. EMT–I Maloney and her partner rush to the nurse to find her face flushed and diaphoretic. Her pulse is 130, and she is developing stridorous respirations.

EMT–I Maloney is puzzled for a moment, thinking the only other time she ever saw a patient "crash" like this before was an anaphylactic reaction after a bee sting.

EMT–I Maloney takes the oxygen from Rosy and immediately begins to assist ventilations on the school nurse. Her partner prepares to start an IV of normal saline, while EMT–I Maloney takes off her gloves and contacts medical direction for orders.

The medical direction physician asks EMT–I Maloney what she thinks is going on, and the only thing she can think to say is that it looks a lot like an anaphylactic reaction she saw once. "Is the patient allergic to anything?" the medical direction physician asks.

EMT–I Maloney goes across the hallway to the office and asks, "Is the school nurse allergic to anything?"

"Only latex," the secretary responds.

EMT–I Maloney runs back across the hall and checks the box of gloves in the nurse's office. They are hypoallergenic nonlatex gloves.

"Doctor, she's only allergic to latex as far as we can find out, but she doesn't have latex gloves in the office."

"Are one of you wearing latex?" he asks.

"Sure, we both had on latex gloves, but we didn't touch her," EMT–I Maloney answers.

"Did one of you take your gloves off?" he asks.

"Yeah, my partner did, to call you and set up the stretcher," she says.

"Administer 0.3 cc of epinephrine 1:1000 subcutaneously stat," he orders.

EMT–I Maloney states the order back to him and administers the injection. In a few minutes the nurse is regaining responsiveness and breathing on her own easily. Rosy is doing well also, and she stares wide-eyed at her nurse.

Then, EMT–I Maloney realizes that when she 'snapped' off her gloves, she created a mist of cornstarch powder, which carried small latex particles into the air.

SUMMARY

A drug is any substance that, when taken into the body, changes one or more of the body's functions. Drugs may have as many as four names, including the chemical, generic, official, and trade name. Drugs may have natural sources such as plants, minerals, and animals, or they may be synthesized in the laboratory.

Consumers in the United States are protected by several regulations regarding drugs. All drugs sold in the United States must meet and maintain high standards for therapeutic results, patient safety, and packaging safety. To meet these standards, drugs must go through strict and accurate testing, which may take several years to complete. The FDA is responsible for final approval of all drugs.

There are several references for drug information. The *Physicians' Desk Reference* is widely used as a reference for drugs in current use.

Liquid drugs administered into the body by subcutaneous, intramuscular, or intravenous routes are called *parenteral drugs*. Drugs administered through the parenteral route are packaged in several ways, including prefilled syringes, ampules, and vials. The routes used by the EMT–I to administer drugs include sublingual, intravenous, subcutaneous, inhalation, endotracheal, or transdermal.

Administering drugs carries with it a tremendous responsibility. The EMT–I must be knowledgeable in the actions, indications, dosages, administration procedures, and side effects of the various drugs he or she may be called on to deliver. If the wrong drug or the incorrect dosage is given, the results can be fatal. EMT–Is may administer certain emergency drugs via local protocol or standing orders, with or without contacting medical direction.

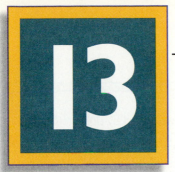

13

TRAUMA EMERGENCIES

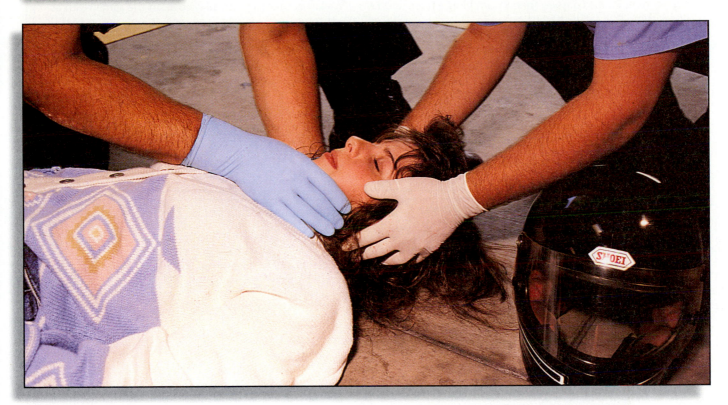

CASE HISTORY

It is 2:00 AM when EMT–Intermediates Walker and Fox are awakened by the alarm. "Unit 53...Respond to George's Corner Bar...Possible stabbing...Police are en route...Time out 02:03."

Within minutes, the EMT–Is are en route to the scene. EMT–I Walker's adrenaline is flowing.

EMT–I Walker knows the location of the bar well. In fact, he has been there a few times himself. It is not the nicest place, but it has always been a regular hangout for the "townies"—people like EMT–I Walker who grew up in the area. As the EMT–Is approach the scene, they see lots of

Case History, continued

emergency lights and several police cars in the parking lot. Two men in handcuffs are being questioned by police officers.

The EMT–Is grab their gear and make their way through the crowd of people surrounding the victim. The victim is positioned on his right side and is guarding his stomach through a blood-stained shirt. EMT–I Walker and his partner place the victim supine to begin their assessment. As EMT–I Walker rolls the patient onto his back, he realizes that he knows him. He was a good friend from high school, and EMT–I Walker occasionally still plays ball on the same team as the victim. This call is the first time EMT–I Walker has taken care of someone he knows. The patient looks up at EMT–I Walker and says with a frightened voice, "Man, I'm glad it's you. I've been stabbed."

EMT–I Fox applies high-concentration oxygen by nonrebreather mask and gets a baseline set of vitals while EMT–I Walker exposes his friend's abdomen. He sees a gaping 3-inch laceration just below the border of the patient's right rib cage. He finds a second, smaller wound just distal to the umbilicus. The abdominal wound is bleeding quite a bit, and EMT–I Walker knows the patient needs to get to the operating room. He prepares the pneumatic antishock garment on the long board, positions his friend, and loads him in the ambulance for transport.

LEARNING OBJECTIVES

Upon completion of this chapter, the EMT–Intermediate should be able to:

- LIST examples of blunt and penetrating trauma.
- LIST three signs associated with a skull fracture.
- DESCRIBE Cheyne-Stokes respirations.
- DESCRIBE the Cushing reflex.
- DESCRIBE decorticate and decerebrate posturing.
- DESCRIBE the mechanism of hypoperfusion.
- LIST four mechanisms of spinal injury.
- LIST three types of devices used to assist with spinal immobilization.
- IDENTIFY four instances in which rapid extrication techniques may be necessary.
- DESCRIBE a flail chest.
- LIST three signs or symptoms of a pneumothorax.
- LIST two early and two late signs or symptoms of a tension pneumothorax.
- STATE the importance of rapid transport to definitive care.
- LIST four signs or symptoms of abdominal trauma.
- DESCRIBE the position for a pregnant trauma patient that optimizes venous return to the heart.
- DESCRIBE the care of an amputated body part.
- LIST three types of burns.
- IDENTIFY one difference between open and closed bone injuries.
- LIST three signs or symptoms of a bone or joint injury.
- IDENTIFY three complications of musculoskeletal trauma.
- LIST three complications of splinting.

KEY TERMS

BATTLE'S SIGN

CHEYNE-STOKES RESPIRATIONS

CONTUSION

CUSHING REFLEX

DECEREBRATE POSTURING

DECORTICATE POSTURING

DEFINITIVE CARE

HEMATOMA

HEMIPLEGIA

HYPOPERFUSION

INTRACRANIAL PRESSURE

KINEMATICS

LEVEL OF RESPONSIVENESS

MULTISYSTEM TRAUMA

PARAPLEGIA

QUADRIPLEGIA

RACOON EYES

RAPID TRANSPORT

RULE OF NINES

SPINAL SHOCK

TRAUMA CENTER

INTRODUCTION

EMT–Is who read the newspaper usually come across many stories related to injuries caused by trauma. The man in the case history at the beginning of this chapter was injured by some type of traumatic event. How does this patient differ from someone who is lightheaded or who is having chest pain? According to statistics, trauma:

- Accounts for 60% of childhood deaths.
- Accounts for 80% of teenage deaths.
- Annually kills three times more Americans than died in Vietnam.
- Temporarily disables 11 million people each year.
- Permanently disables 450,000 people each year.
- Is a disease whose management accounts for 40% of all the healthcare costs in the United States ($100 billion) each year.
- Results in 5.1 million years in lost productivity from disabilities, at a cost of $65 billion.
- Results in 5.3 million years in lost productivity from deaths, at a cost of over $50 billion.
- Is the leading cause of death in people from ages 1 through 44 years.

KINEMATICS OF TRAUMA

KINEMATICS   The process of predicting injury patterns that may result from the forces and motions of energy.

When dealing with trauma, there are several things the EMT–I must do before even touching a patient. First, he or she must look at the situation and get an idea as to what may have happened. The EMT–I must assess the **kinematics** of trauma.

By first performing an overall assessment of the scene, the EMT–I is able to gain more information as to what occurred when the patient was injured. In addition, safety can be determined for the patient and the rescuer(s). When responding to the scene of a fall, for example, the EMT–I should consider the following when assessing the kinematics of the situation:

- How many patients are involved?
- How far did the patient fall?
- On what type of surface did the patient land?
- Was the patient wearing any type of protective gear such as a helmet, knee pads, elbow pads, etc.?
- Was the patient secured by any type of rope, and was he or she injured by that rope somehow in the fall?
- What type of environment is present? Is the temperature cold or warm? Is it raining or sunny? Is it during the day or night?
- Are there any other things that may present a danger to the EMT–I? Are there dangling ropes or wires, animals, hysterical bystanders, etc.?
- Did any material such as rocks or stones fall on top of the patient?
- Does the patient also have some underlying medical problem?

When responding to the scene of a motor vehicle accident, the EMT–I should consider the following when assessing the kinematics of the situation:

- How many vehicles were involved? What type of vehicles (cars, trucks, motorcycles) were involved? How fast were they traveling?
- What type of damage is present to the outside of the vehicles? Was it a head-on collision or did the car flip over? Is there any damage to the inside of the vehicles such as a sprung seat, cracked windshield, deformed steering wheel, etc.?
- Are there any identifying marks at the scene such as skid marks, broken glass, etc.? If skid marks are present, approximately how long are they?
- Are there any hazards in the area such as gasoline, downed power lines, etc.?
- How many patients are involved? Are the patients still in the vehicles or was anyone thrown from a vehicle or over the handlebars of

a motorcycle? In what position was the patient found inside the vehicle?

- Are any patients entrapped and is there easy access for patient extrication?

- Were the occupants in the vehicle(s) restrained? Did the occupants use shoulder belts or lap belts? Were air bags deployed? If any young children are involved, was some type of car seat used? Was the car seat properly restrained in the vehicle?

To better comprehend kinematics, a brief review of physics is necessary. Newton's First Law of Motion states that "a body at rest will remain at rest and a body in motion will remain in motion until acted upon by an equal and opposite force." For example, if a climber falls down a hill, he or she could remain in motion until the opposite force—the ground—is encountered. In the case of a motor vehicle accident, the vehicle is at rest until the engine starts. Once traveling down the road, it stays in motion until it hits another vehicle or slams into a stationary device such as a telephone pole. Applying the brakes also stops the motion.

The second principle of physics is that energy cannot be created or destroyed. It can, however, change its form. The forms of energy are mechanical, thermal, electrical, and chemical. For example, when the car crashes into a telephone pole, the energy is spread out over the frame of the car, the fenders, and other parts of the vehicle (mechanical). The more energy that is present, the greater the changes or damage will be to the structure of the car as well as the patient. If skid marks are noted, some of the energy of the car was transferred into the rubber, which burned onto the road from the tires (thermal). Electrical energy is displaced throughout the body during a lightning strike. If a corrosive hazardous material is spilled onto the skin, the chemical energy can destroy skin, muscle, and bones, depending on its strength and the duration of contact.

Kinetic energy also is involved, which refers to the object's weight and speed. When referring to people, the terms *weight* and *mass* are considered to be the same. *Speed* also is known as *velocity*. Therefore, this relationship can be expressed in the formula:

$$\text{Kinetic energy (KE)} = \frac{\text{Mass} \times \text{Velocity}^2}{2}$$

Speed, or velocity, is the determining factor in predicting the type of damage that occurs. If a patient weighing 120 lbs is traveling in a car at 30 miles per hour (mph), this results in 54,000 units of energy.

$$\text{KE} = \frac{120 \times 30^2}{2}$$
$$= 60 \times 900$$
$$= 54,000 \text{ units of energy}$$

If that patient's older sister is also in the car and weighs 130 lbs, this increases the kinetic energy to 58,500 units.

$$\text{KE} = \frac{130 \times 30^2}{2}$$
$$= 65 \times 900$$
$$= 58,500 \text{ units of energy}$$

However, if the first patient is now traveling at 40 mph (only 10 mph faster), the kinetic energy increases significantly.

$$\text{KE} = \frac{120 \times 40^2}{2}$$
$$= 60 \times 1600$$
$$= 96,000 \text{ units of energy}$$

When increasing the mass from 120 to 130 lbs, the kinetic energy only increases from 54,000 to 58,500 units of energy. However, when the speed is increased by only 10 mph, the kinetic energy jumps from 54,000 to 96,000 units of energy. Based on these calculations, an increase in speed is more deadly than an increase in mass.

 List examples of blunt and penetrating trauma.

Trauma can be either blunt or penetrating. With blunt trauma, there may be no external signs of injury; internal organs may be significantly damaged while the skin remains intact. Penetrating trauma involves some type of invasive injury to the body in which an opening is created. At the time of impact, significant force may have been involved.

Blunt injury occurs from any type of impact resulting in two forces: change of speed (shear) and compression. During a change in speed, the body accelerates (increases) or decelerates (decreases), which may cause shearing or tearing injuries. An instance when the body is going in a forward motion can be used as an example. When the head hits a stationary object, the brain slams against the front of the skull, which causes a bruise or laceration in the front and tearing of vessels in the back (Fig. 13-1).

When compression injuries occur during blunt trauma, an organ is compressed between two rigid structures. For example, with blunt trauma to the chest, the heart is compressed between the sternum and the spine (Fig. 13-2). The myocardial muscle is injured as a result. Compression injuries also can occur in the abdomen and cause damage to the liver, spleen, kidneys, and/or pancreas.

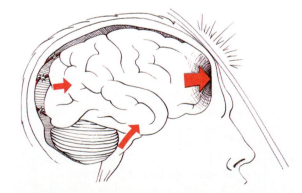

Fig. 13-1 Even after the forward motion of the skull has stopped, the brain continues to move forward inside the skull, causing injury.

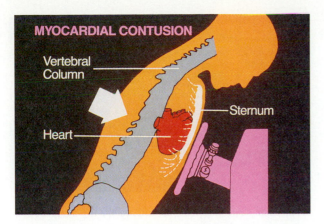

Fig. 13-2 The heart or myocardium is injured from blunt trauma to the chest.

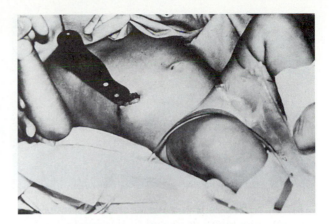

Fig. 13-3 A stab wound is an example of a low-energy injury.

With penetrating trauma, a temporary cavity is created (as happens with blunt trauma) as well as a permanent cavity when the skin is broken (eg, an opening in the chest wall from a gunshot wound). This injury is usually more evident, because bleeding from the opening may be apparent.

There are three levels to consider when discussing penetrating trauma: low energy, medium energy, and high energy.

Low energy

- Examples of weapons that have a low level of energy include those used by the attacker's hands, such as a knife, needle, or ice pick (Fig.13-3).

- These weapons produce low-velocity injuries and can be determined by examining the path of the weapon into the body. The potential for more injury exists, however, if the attacker moves the weapon around once it has entered the body.

Medium energy

- Handguns and some rifles are considered medium energies. Whenever possible, the EMT–I should attempt to identify the type and caliber of the gun or rifle as well as the approximate distance between the weapon and the patient (eg, close range versus approximately 10 feet away). This information will help to estimate the amount of damage produced. In general, tissue will be damaged along the track of the bullet as well as along the sides of the bullet's path (Fig. 13-4).

High energy

- Hunting rifles, assault weapons, and any other type of weapon that discharges high-velocity missiles are considered high energy. An increased amount of damage occurs to the sides of the path of the missile because of the increased energy. With any type of penetrating injury, the EMT–I must determine the number of wounds present. Any entrance and exit wounds should be

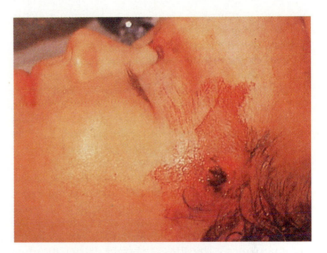

Fig. 13-4 Wounds produced by handguns are examples of medium-energy injuries.

noted. An entrance wound is usually round or oval and lies against the underlying tissue (Fig. 13-5). An exit wound is more explosive, looks like a starburst, and has no support from the underlying tissue (Fig. 13-6).

ASSESSMENT/MANAGEMENT OF THE TRAUMA PATIENT

The first step in managing the trauma patient is performing an accurate assessment of his or her injuries. Assessment is an essential prehospital care skill. All other care rendered is dependent on effective and efficient patient assessment.

Scene size-up

Patient assessment begins with the approach to the scene. The EMT–I should conduct a scene survey to assess the safety, scene, and situation. The scene must be safe for the rescuer(s) as well as the patient.

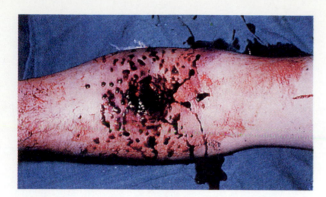

Fig. 13-5 This entrance wound demonstrates a high-energy injury produced by a powerful shotgun.

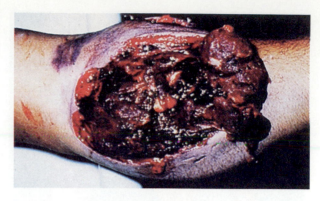

Fig. 13-6 An exit wound caused by a powerful shotgun fired at close range.

The EMT–I must be careful not to become a victim because he or she is too focused on gaining access to the patient. For example, if the call is for someone mauled by an animal, the EMT–I must make sure the animal who attacked the victim is not still loose or in the area. Another example is a domestic call in which the perpetrator with a weapon is still on the premises. The EMT–I should wait for law enforcement personnel before treating the patient. Also, the EMT–I should let fire or police personnel know if additional protective gear is required.

Next, the mechanism of injury or any other factors that may affect how the scene is managed should be determined. Is this an accident in a construction site requiring specialized extrication? Is the injured patient in a remote field that is not accessible by ambulance? The EMT–I should gather information from bystanders whenever possible.

The EMT–I should then work to gain more information about the situation. How many potential patients are on the scene? Is this a motor vehicle accident? How many motor vehicles are involved? Are these older individuals, children, young adults, etc.? Is additional help needed such as rescue equipment, additional ambulances, or hazardous materials teams? Did the patient have a seizure before falling off of the bicycle? Were any mind-altering substances involved (eg, drugs or alcohol)? When there are more patients than the unit can handle, the EMT–I must immediately call for additional help.

Once these factors have been determined and the scene is safe, the EMT–I can proceed to the actual hands-on patient assessment and treatment as described in the next section. To prevent unnecessary exposure to bloodborne pathogens, the EMT–I should always employ body substance isolation procedures while assessing and managing trauma patients.

Initial assessment

On examining the patient, a simultaneous, or global, assessment is what really takes place. First, the EMT–I should form a general impression of the patient's condition. Next, the EMT-I should determine if life threats exist, and the age, race, and sex of the patient. Then the EMT-I should assess the level of responsiveness, airway, breathing, and circulation. If the patient is speaking in complete, appropriate sentences, information can be immediately obtained about the patient's neurologic status as well as airway, breathing, and circulation. In this situation, the patient has an open airway, he or she is breathing, there is circulation, and the neurologic system is intact. If the patient is speaking, yet cannot complete a sentence because of shortness of breath, the EMT–I can immediately suspect a problem with breathing. By holding the patient's wrist, a radial pulse can be evaluated as well as the skin temperature and color and whether the skin is moist or dry.

The EMT–I can usually identify whether the patient is critical or not in about 15 to 30 seconds.

Level of responsiveness
The patient's level of responsiveness should be assessed. The EMT–I should avoid vague terms such as semicomatose, lethargic, etc., and use the following levels to maintain consistency:

    A = <u>A</u>lert
    V = Responds to <u>v</u>erbal stimulus
    P = Responds to <u>p</u>ainful stimulus
    U = <u>U</u>nresponsive

Airway with cervical spine control
The EMT–I should immediately provide manual in-line stabilization of the patient's head while assessing the airway. If necessary, the modified jaw-thrust should be used to open the airway:

- *If snoring is heard or patient is unresponsive:* The EMT–I should insert an oral airway (if no gag reflex is present) or nasopharyngeal airway (if a gag reflex is present), then should proceed to endotracheal intubation if necessary (after adequate basic life-saving ventilation/oxygenation).

- *If gurgling is heard or secretions, blood, or vomitus is present:* The EMT–I should suction the upper airway.

While opening the airway, the EMT–I should ask the patient, "Can you hear me? Are you OK? Where does it hurt?" The response gives the EMT–I a sense of the patient's mental status. Diminished mental status (disorientation, confusion, agitation, unresponsiveness) suggests possible head injury or cerebral hypoxia. With any sign of hypoxia or if the patient has sustained a serious mechanism of injury (eg, falling 8 feet from a scaffold onto a concrete sidewalk), oxygen therapy should be initiated at a 100% concentration via a non-rebreather face mask or bag-valve-mask device.

The EMT–I should tell the patient that he or she is there to help. While at the patient's head, the EMT–I should quickly inspect the neck for jugular vein distention and palpate for tracheal shift. The presence of either of these signs suggests conditions such as tension pneumothorax or cardiac tamponade.

Breathing (ventilation)

Next, the EMT–I should check for breathing by listening for air exchange and looking for adequacy of chest rise. Ventilatory rate and depth should be estimated and steps taken to ensure adequate ventilation of the patient.

If breathing is shallow, rapid (>30 breaths/min), or slow (<12 breaths/min), the EMT–I should assist ventilations with a bag-valve-mask device supplied with 15 L of oxygen and a reservoir. If breathing is 12 to 20 breaths per minute, supplemental high-concentration oxygen via a nonrebreather face mask should be considered. If breathing is between 20 and 30 breaths per minute (intermediate), the EMT–I should provide supplemental high-concentration oxygen via a nonrebreather face mask and monitor the patient closely.

If any potential respiratory problem exists, the chest should quickly be inspected for deformities, wounds, or bruising. The EMT–I should palpate the chest for equal expansion (symmetry), assess for pain, and then auscultate lung sounds. Any injury that may compromise breathing must be managed.

- *Open pneumothorax:* The EMT–I should cover the injury with occlusive dressing and tape three sides down.
- *Tension pneumothorax:* The EMT–I should lift one side of the occlusive dressing or perform emergency chest decompression.
- *Flail chest:* The EMT–I should immobilize the flail segment with bulky dressing or towels taped to chest.

Circulation

The EMT–I should check for a pulse. Is a pulse palpable? Is it fast or slow? Is it regular or irregular? The location of a palpable pulse also is important because it can be an estimate of the patient's systolic blood pressure.

- Radial indicates a pressure of at least 80 systolic, if present.
- Femoral indicates a pressure of at least 70 systolic, if present.
- Carotid indicates a pressure of at least 60 systolic, if present.

Next, the peripheral perfusion is assessed by checking skin color, temperature, and moisture. The EMT–I should look for and control major bleeding. If internal hemorrhage is suspected, the abdomen quickly should be exposed. The EMT–I should gently palpate the belly and look for signs of injury and also gently palpate the pelvis *without* rocking it.

Expose and protect from the environment

Removing the patient's clothes may help the EMT–I gain more information depending on the types of injuries suspected. The patient's body should be carefully examined for obvious signs of bleeding, unequal chest expansion, a distended abdomen, or other signs of possible life-threatening injuries. The EMT–I should logroll the patient to visually inspect the back. The EMT–I should take precautions to prevent hypothermia such as using a blanket after the clothes have been removed, exposing the patient in a warm environment when the weather is cold, and so forth. A more thorough examination will be done as part of the ongoing assessment.

Initial resuscitation

Oxygen therapy and ventilatory support should be initiated as soon as a problem is identified. The EMT–I should apply a rigid cervical spine immobilization device while maintaining manual in-line stabilization (after a quick examination of the neck). The device may be applied earlier in the process if it is readily available and the neck examination has been completed. Application of the pneumatic antishock garment (PASG) also may be necessary. The EMT–I should perform an ongoing examination of those body parts to be enclosed prior to applying the PASG. The patient is then secured to a long backboard (this step may occur during PASG application). If the patient is critical, immediate transport by air or ground should be provided. During transport, two large bore IVs (14-16 gauge) should be placed using macrodrip administration sets, normal saline or lactated Ringer's solution, and run at a wide open rate.

Focused trauma and detailed assessments

First, the EMT–I should reconsider the mechanism of injury. Then throughout the focused trauma and detailed assessments, the EMT–I should check to see if the patient's condition has changed (airway, breathing, circulation, and disability). The EMT–I should start by examining the head, including:

- Inspecting the mouth and nose
- Assessing the facial area

- Inspecting and palpating the scalp and ears
- Looking for any fluid from the ears or nose

When checking the patient's pupils, the EMT–I should remember the acronym PEARRL (pupils equal and round, reactive to light). Unequal pupils may suggest some type of neurologic abnormality.

If the cervical spine immobilization device is not yet in place, the EMT–I should examine the neck, checking the position of the trachea and jugular veins and palpating the posterior cervical spine. Any deformities should be noted by the EMT–I, and he or she should palpate for subcutaneous emphysema.

The chest is examined by inspecting for wounds, deformity, or bruising, palpating for symmetry, and auscultating lung sounds. Any areas of pain or guarding should be noted. The abdomen is then examined by inspecting and palpating all four quadrants. The EMT–I should palpate the pelvis, checking for instability.

During examination of the lower extremities, the EMT–I inspects and palpates the right and left legs. The motor, sensory, and distal circulation in each leg should be checked. The upper extremities are examined by inspecting and palpating the right and left arms. Motor, sensory, and distal circulation in each arm also should be checked.

Last, the EMT–I examines the posterior thorax/lumbar areas and buttocks by inspecting and palpating. The posterior examination may have been done earlier if the patient was rolled directly onto the backboard.

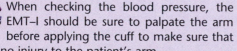

> **STREET WISE**
> When checking the blood pressure, the EMT–I should be sure to palpate the arm before applying the cuff to make sure that there is no injury to the patient's arm.

The EMT–I should perform baseline vital signs. If the patient's condition permits, the EMT–I may perform an extended neurologic examination, including the Glasgow coma scale (Table 13-1) and further evaluation of pupillary status.

Definitive field care

The EMT–I should identify and treat minor wounds and fractures appropriately if there are no life-threatening injuries. Otherwise, the patient should be immobilized to a long backboard. Transport should begin as soon as the patient is placed in the ambulance. Attempts at starting an intravenous line and a detailed ongoing assessment should be performed en route. Depending on local protocol, the EMT–I should communicate with the receiving facility as early as possible. In some areas of the country, the base hospital or medical direction will notify the receiving hospital. If the patient is critically injured, every effort should be made to transport the patient to a trauma center.

The EMT–I should continue to monitor the patient en route by checking to see if his or her condition has changed (airway, breathing, circulation, and level of responsiveness). Additional treatment should be provided as necessary. All examinations and treatments, including the scene survey and mechanism of injury, should be documented in writing whenever possible. The EMT–I should provide a verbal report to the receiving staff, which should include only details relevant to the care and treatment of the patient.

> **STREET WISE**
> With trauma patients, the EMT–I should be sure to:
> - Immediately establish and maintain spinal immobilization.
> - Check the level of responsiveness, then airway, then breathing, then circulation, while appropriately managing any life-threatening conditions along the way. The EMT–I can vary this order slightly by asking the patient if he or she can hear as the airway is opened, which gives a sense of the patient's mental status (disability).
> - Examine the back surface of the patient's body when logrolling him or her onto the long backboard or applying the PASG.
> - In critical situations, complete the ongoing assessment AFTER transport to the trauma center has been initiated. An intravenous line also can be started en route.
> - Initiate transport of the critical patient within 10 minutes as long as no extenuating circumstances are present (dangerous access, entrapment, prolonged extrication, etc.).
> - Continually reassess the patient. His or her condition may change during treatment and transport.

HEAD TRAUMA

Head injuries are the leading cause of death from trauma. These injuries may be particularly difficult to treat because the patient may be unresponsive and/or unable to provide a past medical history or details surrounding the incident.

Trauma to the head can result in several types of injuries including:

- Scalp injuries: closed soft-tissue injuries and open soft-tissue injuries (Fig. 13-7)
- Injuries to the face and neck
- Skull injuries: fracture (open, closed)
- Brain injuries: concussion, contusion, open injuries, hematoma, and hemorrhage

Head, face, and neck injuries are closely related. Trauma to one area is likely to involve injury to several areas. A force to the face also can injure the head and neck. Therefore, the EMT–I should assume that any

TABLE 13-1	Adult Glasgow Coma Scale*	
ACTION	**STIMULUS**	**POINTS**
Eye opening	Spontaneous	4
	To speech	3
	To pain	2
	None	1
Verbal response	Oriented x 4 (time, place, person, and situation)	5
	Confused	4
	Inappropriate words	3
	Incomprehensible sounds	2
	None	1
Motor response	Obeys (moves in response to command and pain)	6
	Localizes (changes location in response to pain)	5
	Withdraws (from pain)	4
	Abnormal flexion (decorticate)	3
	Abnormal extension (decerebrate)	2
	No movement	1
	Total score	

*A Glasgow coma scale of < 9 indicates severe neurologic injury.

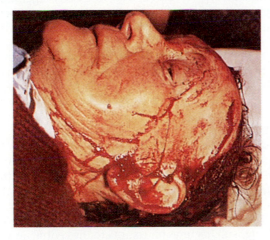

Fig. 13-7   Scalp lacerations can produce severe bleeding.

patient who suffers an injury to the upper torso has an injury to any of these areas until proven otherwise.

It is important to note the patient's level of responsiveness. If the patient experienced a period of unresponsiveness, the EMT–I should try to determine when it occurred and how long it lasted. He or she also should establish a baseline that can be used as a comparison if the patient's level of responsiveness improves or deteriorates while en route to the hospital. For example, if the patient is initially unresponsive yet is responding to verbal stimuli on arrival at the hospital, this change should be documented. Consequently, if the patient initially is alert and oriented and becomes responsive only to painful stimuli, this variation should be noted and documented.

Scalp injuries

The soft tissues of the head are vascular and contain many important structures. Closed and open injuries to the scalp can produce serious injuries.

A closed soft-tissue injury to the scalp occurs after a fall or following direct trauma such as an assault or motor vehicle accident. Closed injuries to the head should provoke a high index of suspicion that the brain or neck also may be injured. The EMT–I should assume a patient with a closed scalp injury has a cervical spine and brain injury until proven otherwise.

Open soft-tissue injuries to the scalp occur similarly to closed injuries. A knife, gunshot wound, or a sharp or blunt object can cause this type of injury. The EMT–I should look for items as described previously for closed soft-tissue injuries.

The scalp has a very rich blood supply, therefore the patient with an extensive open scalp injury may bleed significantly. The EMT–I should not use his or her fingers to stop the bleeding, because if the skull is fractured, this action may drive bone fragments into the brain. Instead, pressure should be applied over a broad area with the palm of a gloved hand (Fig. 13-8).

The EMT–I must control bleeding first. A bulky, bloody dressing should not be removed to examine the wound, because clots adhered to the dressing may be helping to control the bleeding. The dressing should be left in place, and reinforced as necessary.

The EMT–I should examine the wound when possible, but should not probe it with his or her fingers. If the scalp is avulsed, the skin flap should be replaced to its normal position. The EMT–I should wrap the avulsed tissue in dry or moistened sterile gauze, depending on local protocol, and transport it with the patient to the hospital.

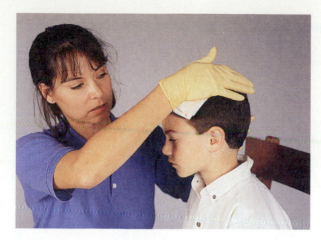

Fig. 13-8 Use an open-palmed hand when using pressure to control bleeding of the scalp.

> **HELPFUL HINT**
> The EMT–I should not delay transport while searching for an avulsed part. Someone from the scene should continue to search for the part and bring it to the hospital.

Skull fractures

A skull fracture is a break in the continuity of any of the bones of the skull. Generally, skull fractures cannot be definitely diagnosed without a radiograph. Uncomplicated skull fractures are often of minor significance. However, damage to underlying brain tissue or vascular structures of the meninges can be life threatening.

Skull fractures are classified as open or closed. An open skull fracture involves skin that has been disrupted, exposing the central nervous system. A closed skull fracture means the skin has not been broken.

Skull fractures also are described as depressed or nondepressed, depending on the location of fracture fragments in comparison with the uninjured bones. In nondepressed skull fractures, the pieces of fractured bone retain their normal alignment within the skull. In depressed skull fractures, the bony fragments have been forced inward toward the brain and may press on underlying structures (Fig. 13-9).

The EMT–I should suspect a skull fracture if the patient has:

- A history of trauma to the head with or without unresponsiveness
- An altered level of responsiveness
- Pupils sluggish to react or dilated
- Obvious penetrating or impalement injury
- Deformity of the skull
- Blood or cerebrospinal fluid draining from the nose or ears
- Raccoon eyes (may be a late sign)
- Battle's sign (may be a late sign)

 List three signs associated with a skull fracture.

Blood and cerebrospinal fluid drainage

Normally, the brain and spinal cord are contained within a closed system consisting of the meninges and cerebrospinal fluid (CSF). If the meninges are disrupted, cerebrospinal fluid may leak and drain into the nostrils or ear canal. CSF is normally clear and watery in appearance. Because bleeding can occur from a bone fracture, blood may mix with the CSF. Thus, drainage may appear watery or bloody. The EMT–I should consider any type of clear or bloody drainage from the nostrils or ears following head trauma an indication of a possible skull fracture.

> **RACCOON EYES:** Bilateral ecchymosis or bruising around the eye present with a basilar skull fracture; may be a late sign.

Raccoon eyes

Raccoon eyes are a black and blue discoloration that results from the collection of blood in the tissue around the eye sockets. Raccoon eyes suggest the presence of a basilar skull fracture and may not occur until 12 hours or more after the injury (Fig. 13-10).

> **BATTLE'S SIGN:** Ecchymosis or bruising behind the ears present with a basilar skull fracture; may be a late sign.

Battle's sign

Battle's sign is a discoloration of the skin at the mastoid region behind the ear. This sign is caused by an accumulation of blood after a basilar skull fracture, and may not occur until 12 hours or more after the injury (Fig. 13-11).

The EMT–I should evaluate patients suspected of having skull fractures for trauma to the central nervous system including the brain and spinal cord, and monitor them closely during transport so that any changes in their level of responsiveness can be rapidly identified. In addition, any related injuries such as facial and intracranial trauma, compromised airway, and spinal injuries should be anticipated by the EMT–I.

BRAIN INJURIES

Types of brain injuries include concussion, contusion, open injuries, hematoma, and hemorrhage. It is far more important that the EMT–I recognize the *presence* of a brain injury than it is that he or she determine its *precise nature*.

Signs and symptoms of brain injury can range from the brief loss of responsiveness seen with a concussion (usually 5 minutes or less) to the longer period of unresponsiveness (from 5 minutes to 1 hour) seen with a

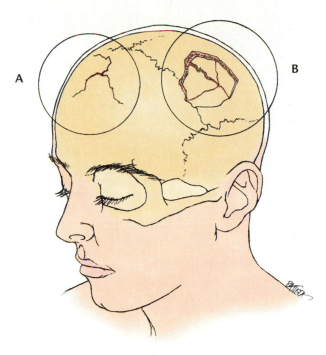

Fig. 13-9   A, A nondepressed skull fracture. B, A depressed skull fracture.

contusion. Brain tissue may be exposed if an open injury has occurred, and fractured bone fragments can lacerate or puncture the brain.

Bleeding within and around the brain can compress brain tissue, impair neurologic function, and lead to death. It is difficult to distinguish the different types of intracranial bleeding in the field. Therefore, the care for all sources of bleeding is the same: support the patient's oxygenation, ventilatory and circulatory functions while maintaining spinal precautions, and get the patient to definitive care, which can only be provided at the trauma center. It is important to document the patient's current level of responsiveness, any previous loss of responsiveness, ongoing neurologic status, and memory deficits at the scene and en route to the hospital.

Intracranial pressure

Continuous assessment of patients with potential or known brain injuries is important in order to detect signs of deterioration. The pressure within the intracranial compartment, the **intracranial pressure** (ICP), may increase. This increase can lead to further brain injury and death due to compression of vital brain structures. Several findings should suggest that the ICP is rising:

- A deterioration in the level of responsiveness (this is the most important sign to follow)

- Progressive neurologic deficits (especially paralysis)

- Vomiting (especially if projectile in nature)

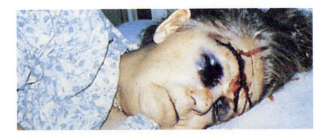

Fig. 13-10   "Raccoon eyes" may be seen with a basilar skull fracture.

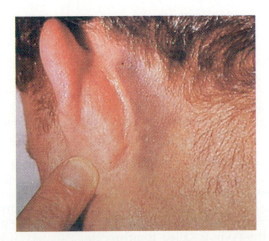

Fig. 13-11   "Battle's sign" may be present after a basilar skull fracture.

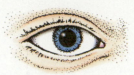
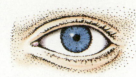

Fig. 13-12 Suspect injury to the brain whenever a patient's pupils are unequal in size.

- Unequal pupils (especially if one pupil is normal size and the other is markedly dilated (Fig. 13-12)

 Describe Cheyne-Stokes respirations.

- A repetitive pattern of slow, shallow breathing to rapid, deep ventilations back to slow, shallow breaths followed by a period of apnea (known as **Cheyne-Stokes respirations,** an early sign of increased ICP)

 Describe the Cushing reflex.

- Progressive increases in the blood pressure (especially the systolic reading), an increase in the respiratory rate, and a decreasing pulse rate (known as **Cushing reflex** or triad, a late sign of increased ICP)

Assessment of brain injury

The patient's **level of responsiveness** is extremely important in the evaluation of any brain injury. A change in the level of responsiveness is the *most significant sign* to follow when monitoring the patient with a brain injury. Patients who develop a sudden loss of responsiveness or decrease in their level of responsiveness should be transported immediately.

The patient with an altered level of responsiveness may be disoriented or confused or have garbled speech. The Glasgow coma scale (*see* Table 13-1) helps to evaluate and describe the patient's level of responsiveness.

Paralysis and abnormal posturing

> **HEMIPLEGIA:** A condition in which one side of the body is paralyzed.
> **PARAPLEGIA:** A condition in which the lower extremities become paralyzed.
> **QUADRIPLEGIA:** A condition in which all four extremities become paralyzed.

Patients with brain injury may have paralysis of any or all limbs. If the right side of the brain is injured, the patient's left side will be affected and vice versa. The injury may result in muscle weakness or paralysis of one or both sides of the body. Paralysis on one side of the body is called **hemiplegia.** Paralysis of the lower extremities is called **paraplegia.** Paralysis of all four extremities is **quadriplegia.**

The EMT–I must not allow a patient to attempt to move if a cervical spine injury is suspected. Movement without spinal immobilization may further aggravate the injury or cause an unstable fracture to sever the spinal cord. Once the spine has been immobilized appropriately, the EMT–I may proceed to check handgrips, foot motion, and sensation.

Other signs and symptoms

Certain findings suggest an injury to the brain. The patient may complain of a headache. The pupils may be unequal, dilated, or nonreactive. Occasionally an eye may be deviated to one side.

The EMT–I may note the presence of alcohol on the patient's breath or other evidence of drug intoxication. This finding is important because the presence of drugs and/or alcohol complicates the assessment and masks serious injuries. If the mechanism of injury suggests a brain injury, the EMT–I should initially attribute abnormal behavior to the injury and not to drugs or alcohol.

A patient with a brain injury may vomit, so the EMT–I should be prepared to suction as necessary. Blood or clear fluid (or a mixture) may be observed coming from the nose or ears, suggesting a CSF leak. Raccoon eyes or Battle's sign may be present, suggesting a coexisting fracture.

 Describe decorticate and decerebrate posturing.

Patients with brain injuries may assume abnormal body postures. The patient may be in this position during the assessment, or this posturing may follow the application of painful stimuli. **Decorticate posturing** is the position of a patient in which the upper extremities are flexed at the elbows and wrists. The legs also may be flexed. **Decerebrate posturing** is the position in which the arms are extended and internally rotated and the legs are extended with the feet in forced plantar flexion. It is a later sign of increasing ICP. The presence of either decorticate or decerebrate posturing suggests the presence of severe neurologic damage, and these patients should be transported quickly (Fig. 13-13).

Treatment

 Describe the mechanism of hypoperfusion.

> **HYPOPERFUSION:** Fluid passing through an organ or part of the body that does not have properly oxygenated blood.

The goal of treatment is to maintain cerebral oxygenation and perfusion while protecting the cervical spine. An oropharyngeal airway or endotracheal tube may be inserted if the patient is unresponsive and has no gag reflex. Insertion of a nasopharyngeal

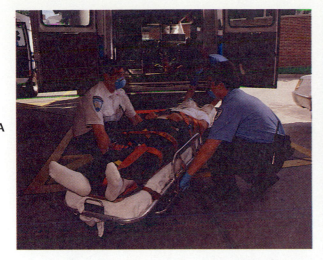

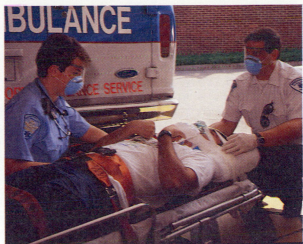

Fig. 13-13   A, A patient with decerebrate posturing. B, A patient with decorticate posturing.

airway and nasotracheal intubation are both contraindicated in basilar skull fractures.

Arterial carbon dioxide causes blood vessels to dilate, which takes up more intracranial space. Decreasing the carbon dioxide will cause the vessels to constrict and take less space, thus decreasing the ICP. With that theory in mind, the EMT–I should hyperventilate the patient with high-concentration oxygen (at least 24 to 30 breaths per minute in adults) to help decrease the ICP by "blowing off" excess carbon dioxide. The hyperventilation also will increase the oxygen available to brain cells with **hypoperfusion** (Fig. 13-14).

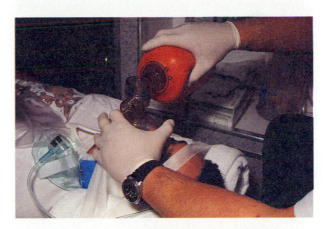

Fig. 13-14   Hyperventilation helps to increase cerebral oxygenation and perfusion in patients with suspected brain injury.

CLINICAL NOTES
Some current research raises questions about the use of hyperventilation in the management of acute head injury. Check you local protocols for direction.

As previously mentioned, the face and scalp are highly vascular and can produce a great deal of bleeding. Obvious bleeding should be controlled. Suction equipment should be readily available to manage vomiting. An IV of normal saline or Ringer's lactate also should be established at a keep vein open rate whenever possible. The rate can be adjusted if signs of hypovolemic shock are present.

If fluid or blood is coming from the nose or ears, the EMT–I should loosely cover the nostrils and/or ears with a clean dressing. The EMT–I should allow slight leaking to occur because this will prevent a complete tamponade of the fluid. If the fluid is not permitted to drain, the ICP may increase, thus increasing the amount of damage to the brain.

Serial vital sign determinations and frequent reassessments will help to detect signs of ICP as they occur. Any changes that suggest a progressive rise in ICP should be immediately reported to medical direc-

tion and/or the receiving hospital. In addition, this type of patient should be transported immediately.

Patients with head injuries should be immobilized based on the mechanism of injury. Forces significant enough to cause a brain injury also will traumatize the spinal cord. Cervical spine immobilization as well as the use of a long backboard are appropriate. Whenever possible, the long backboard should be raised so that the head is elevated. This positioning may help to decrease ICP.

SPINAL TRAUMA

Spinal injuries are physical trauma to the spinal cord, vertebral column, or surrounding connective tissues. Injury to any of these structures can affect the passage of nerve impulses to and from the spinal cord.

Injury to any section of the spinal cord can affect the communication between the brain and the rest of the body. The cord itself may be damaged directly, or injury can result from swelling around the cord or improper movement of the spine. If the cord is severed it cannot be repaired, because the central nervous system does not regenerate.

Anyone sustaining a head injury causing a loss of responsiveness, significant blunt trauma to the torso, significant injury above the clavicles, or a major fall must be considered also to have a spinal injury. A patient with spinal injury may be neurologically intact or may have deficits of movement and/or sensation. When nerve damage occurs, it may be partial or complete. With proper care, however, substantial recovery may be possible.

Although spinal injury can occur at any time, it is most common in patients between 16 and 35 years of age. It is during this age range when people are involved in the most violent types of activity. This trauma can leave the patient with devastating effects if not properly managed in the prehospital setting. EMT–Is must work to preserve as much function as possible for the patient.

Stable versus unstable spinal injuries

Nerve damage may or may not occur immediately following spinal injury. If deficits are present, the EMT–I's responsibility is to prevent further damage from taking place. If an injury exists but no nerve damage is present, the EMT–I must prevent such damage from occurring. It is impossible to determine in the field if any injury is stable or not, so the EMT–I must always care for the patient with any suspected spinal injury as though the injury was unstable.

Types of spinal injuries

Injury can occur to any part of the spinal column. Although isolated injuries can occur, most often trauma affects several different structures, such as vertebrae, ligaments, intervertebral disks, and the spinal cord.

Any portion of the spinal cord may be injured by direct or indirect trauma. Often the damage occurs from indirect trauma when a segment of vertebra presses against the cord (Fig. 13-15). In addition, the spinal cord can be contused or compressed when nearby injured tissues swell and constrict the cord. Injury also can be due to direct trauma, such as damage that occurs from a gunshot wound.

In all forms of spinal injury, the bottom line is whether the spinal cord is affected. If cord injury has occurred, the EMT–I must take steps to prevent additional damage. If the cord is not injured, the patient should be handled so that the risk of spinal cord damage is minimized. Because it usually is difficult to know if true spinal cord damage has occurred, the EMT–I should use every precaution for all suspected spinal injuries.

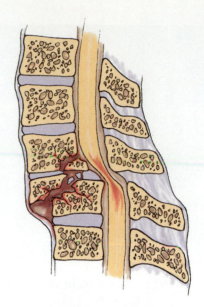

Fig. 13-15 An example of a spinal injury caused by a vertebra pressing against the spinal cord.

Mechanisms of spinal injury

Major causes of spine injury in adults include car accidents, shallow-water diving accidents, motorcycle accidents, and all other injuries and falls. In children, most injuries occur from falls from heights, falls from a tricycle or bicycle, and being struck by a motor vehicle. Remember that injury can occur to the cervical spine any time a significant force meets the head. This area of the spine is flexible and may not withstand the force of the impact. The cervical spine is, therefore, compressed directly, hyperextended, or hyperflexed. The forces that lead to spinal injury are flexion, rotation, extension, and compression. Many times, these forces occur in combination.

 List four mechanisms of spinal injury.

Flexion

Flexion injuries occur when the spinal structures are flexed violently forward such as when hitting one's head while diving. As a result, the supporting ligaments of the posterior spine are abnormally stretched, leading to tears or avulsions of the spinous processes of the vertebrae.

Mechanical pressure of one vertebra on another leads to "wedge" fractures of the body of the vertebra (Fig. 13-16). In the lumbar spine region, flexion forces, often after a fall, cause V-shaped compression fractures (Fig. 13-17).

Rotation

Rotation injuries of the cervical spine seldom occur as isolated events. Rather, a combination of flexion and rotation of the spine causes dislocation of the intervertebral joints. A pure rotational force applied

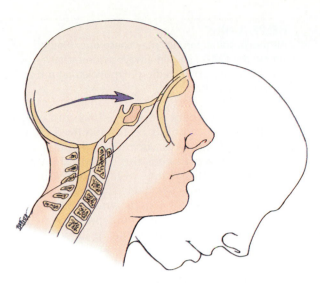

Fig. 13-16   Flexion injuries to the spinal column occur when the spinal structures are flexed forward violently.

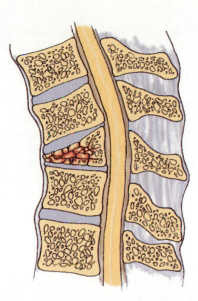

Fig. 13-17   Flexion forces can cause V-shaped compression fractures in the lumbar spine region.

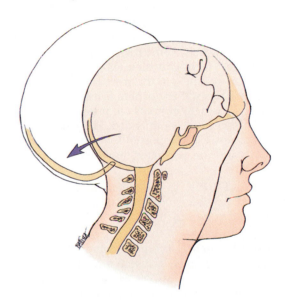

Fig. 13-18   Hyperextension injuries to the spinal column can occur when the spinal structures are forced back violently.

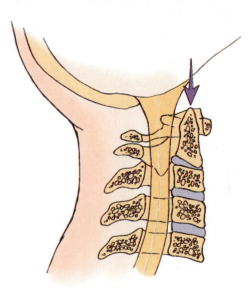

Fig. 13-19   A vertical compression injury occurs when force is exerted along the axis of the spine, compressing the vertebral disk into the body of the vertebra.

to the lumbar spine can result in an unstable fracture of the lumbar vertebrae.

Extension

Tears of the ligaments and vertebral instability occur with hyperextension (Fig. 13-18). Additionally, the skull may be forced down on the posterior aspects of the upper vertebrae, leading to fracture and patient death.

A combination of flexion and extension is responsible for many spinal injuries following motor vehicle accidents. One example is the classic "whiplash" injury. In this injury pattern, the head is "whipped" forward in a flexion motion and then back in an extension motion or vice versa. The spine, spinal cord, and adjacent structures are exposed to both types of forces.

Vertical compression

Vertical compression injuries occur when a force is directed along the axis of the spine. The invertebral disk is compressed into the body of the vertebra, leading to spinal cord damage. This type of injury occurs following a fall, especially when landing on the feet or if the head is hit by a heavy object (Fig. 13-19).

Lateral bending also can contribute to spinal injuries when the patient is hit from the side.

Examples include a side-impact motor vehicle accident or someone hit from the side while riding a bicycle or other riding toy. The chest and thoracic spine move sideways while the head stays in place until pulled along by the cervical attachments. Dislocations and bony fractures may occur.

Lastly, the spine may be pulled apart, causing the spinal cord to be stretched and torn. For example, this mechanism can occur to the cervical spine after a hanging, hence the term *hangman's fracture*. The force of the object around the neck as well as the weight of the body contribute to the injury.

Assessment of the patient with spinal injuries
Patient history
Assessment of the patient with spinal injuries must include a thorough review of the mechanism of injury. If there is any possibility that the patient may have a spinal injury, the spine must be immobilized. As the EMT–I moves the patient to complete the assessment, in-line spinal immobilization must be maintained. The following clues are indicative of possible spinal trauma:

- Mechanism of injury regardless of the absence of any other signs and symptoms
- Motor vehicle and motorcycle accidents
- Diving accidents
- Wounds of the face, head, neck, or shoulders
- Falls greater than 15 feet (for an adult)

> **HELPFUL HINT**
> The EMT–I should always assume that patients with severe injuries to the head or face also have injury to the spine.

- Pain, especially pain on movement
- Point tenderness
- Deformity
- Guarding of the spine area
- Paralysis, paresis, numbness, or tingling in the legs or arms at any time after injury
- Presence of gunshot wound to head, trunk, or back
- Unexplained shock
- Priapism (continuing erection of the penis) in male patients
- Loss of urine (incontinence)

> **HELPFUL HINT**
> The ability to walk after an accident does not exclude the existence of significant spinal trauma. Some patients with serious spinal injury initially are able to walk without difficulty.

> **HELPFUL HINT**
> Although spinal injuries may cause unexplained shock, the EMT–I should always assume that shock is caused by bleeding (hypovolemia) until proven otherwise.

If there is any doubt whether spinal cord injury exists, the patient should be immobilized. If the mechanism of injury is such that a spinal cord injury *may* have occurred, the patient should be immobilized. If other people were seriously injured or killed in the same accident, the EMT–I should immobilize the patient's spine. Immobilizing the patient does no harm and could preserve neurologic function or prevent further injury if spinal trauma is present.

Complications of spinal injury
Patients with spinal injury may develop several complications. If the cervical spinal cord is damaged, the patient may have difficulty breathing or respiratory arrest. The EMT–I should assume that patients with spinal injury will need respiratory support.

Injury to the spinal cord may lead to partial or complete paralysis. Some patients may have a "pins and needles" feeling in their extremities. Other may experience weakness in the arms and/or legs without specific paralysis. If the patient is responsive and any of these signs or symptoms are present, strong emotional support is recommended. The patient may be scared or upset at the possibility of present or future paralysis and the associated disability.

> **SPINAL SHOCK:** A complete transection of the spinal cord that causes the patient to lose sensation and voluntary movement below the injury.

Spinal shock is a form of neurogenic shock that results from complete transection of the spinal cord. There is complete loss of sensation and voluntary movement beyond the injury. The patient in spinal shock is hypotensive because of the loss of vascular control caused by the injury. As a rule, the patient will not have an elevated pulse rate. The patient's skin will be pink, warm, and dry and possibly even flushed due to vasodilation, especially below the level of the injury. Hypotension from spinal shock is difficult to treat.

The most common cause of shock and hypotension after trauma is hemorrhage. The EMT–I should assume that a trauma patient who is in shock has significant bleeding. The EMT–I should not attribute shock to spinal shock even if the patient appears to be paralyzed. These patients usually have life-threatening injuries and need immediate transport.

Emergency care
As with all other emergencies, the EMT–I should perform initial and ongoing assessments as previously described in this chapter. Life-threatening conditions

such as airway obstruction, respiratory arrest, cardiac arrest, or severe bleeding take precedence over spinal injuries. If spinal injury is suspected, movement of the spine should be limited whenever possible while treating critical injuries.

Patients with known or suspected spinal injuries present challenges for airway management. The EMT–I should not move or hyperextend the head of a patient with a possible spinal injury. To open the airway a jaw-thrust maneuver should be performed (Fig. 13-20).

The EMT–I should administer high-concentration oxygen and assist breathing as necessary. Suction may be necessary. Accompanying injuries should be treated and spinal immobilization maintained throughout treatment. One to two large-bore IV lines of normal saline or Ringer's lactate solution should be inserted once transport has been initiated.

Many people activate the EMS system for lower back pain even in the absence of trauma. Many conditions can cause back pain, and some of these, such as an abdominal aneurysm, can be life-threatening. If there is doubt about the severity of a patient's condition, the EMT–I should immobilize the spine.

Spinal immobilization

Anyone with the potential for spinal injury must be completely immobilized using the "joint above, joint below" theory. The joint above is the head, whereas the joint below is the pelvis. Essentially, the full body should be immobilized to prevent movement of the spine.

Spinal immobilization is a method of splinting the spine to prevent movement and additional injury to the vertebral column and spinal cord. The process has two steps: immobilization of the neck and immobilization of the body.

STREET WISE
The cardinal rule for spinal immobilization is identical to that for fractures: when in doubt, immobilize.

Neck immobilization

Immobilization of the cervical vertebrae is performed in two steps: manual stabilization and application of a rigid cervical spine immobilization device. The EMT–I should perform manual, in-line stabilization immediately when cervical spine injury is suspected. Manual stabilization:

- Helps establish and maintain the patient's airway.
- Places the head and neck into neutral alignment, which is the splinting position for the spine.
- Minimizes the risk of additional damage to the cervical spine.

Manual stabilization

The EMT–I should get into position at the top of the patient's head (if the patient is lying down) or

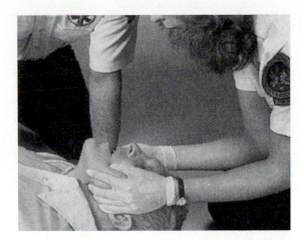

Fig. 13-20   Use a trauma jaw-thrust maneuver to open the airway on a patient with a suspected cervical spine injury.

behind the patient (if the patient is seated). The EMT–I should place his or her hands at the corner of the patient's jaw on both sides. The EMT–I should grasp the corner of the jaw and provide stabilization of the neck by wrapping his or her hands around the posterior portion of the neck. The patient's head should be placed in the neutral position in alignment of the spine. If the patient complains of pain, if the head is not easily moved into position, if muscle spasm occurs, or if the airway becomes compromised, **the EMT–I should not attempt this positioning.** A second EMT–I should apply a rigid cervical spine immobilization device. Constant manual inline stabilization should be maintained until the patient is properly secured to a backboard with the body and head immobilized.

HELPFUL HINT
Traction should not be applied to the head and neck. The EMT–I should simply stabilize the head and neck in a neutral, in-line position.

Cervical spine immobilization devices

While maintaining manual stabilization, the EMT–I should quickly inspect and palpate the neck area. A rigid cervical spine immobilization device should be applied, which reduces movement of the cervical spine and helps maintain neutral alignment of the head and neck. However, the device does not immobilize on its own, and movement of the head can still occur.

Soft cervical spine immobilization devices provide little, if any, stabilization of the injured spine. They are not strong enough to support the head nor do they prevent movement of the neck. The EMT–I should not use these soft devices.

List three types of devices used to assist with spinal immobilization.

There are many varieties of rigid cervical spine immobilization devices available for prehospital use. EMT–Is should consult their instructor and the manufacturer's written directions for the use of any particular device.

To apply a one-piece cervical spine immobilization device, the EMT–I must do the following:

1. Continue to provide manual stabilization during application of the device.

2. Properly measure the patient to determine the appropriate-sized device. Remove the patient's earrings, if present, and move the hair out of the way as much as possible. Place your fingers flat against the patient's neck under the corner of the mandible (jaw) to determine the height to the shoulder. Size the device to the same measurment as the patient's neck. The sizing depends on the type and the design of the type used.

3. Place the back portion of the device behind the patient's head (Fig. 13-21 A). Slide the front portion upward along the sternum until the device is around the neck.

4. Secure the device in place. Sometimes it is necessary to firmly mold the device around the neck while securing the Velcro to ensure a proper fit (Fig. 13-21 B).

5. Make sure the device is snug and the head is in neutral alignment.

To apply a two-piece cervical spine immobilization device, the EMT–I must do the following:

1. Continue to provide manual stabilization during application of the device.

2. Properly measure the patient to determine the appropriate-sized device. Remove the patient's earrings, if present, and move the hair out of the way as much as possible.

3. Place the anterior section under the patient's jaw and secure the Velcro around the back of the neck (Fig. 13-22 A).

4. Position the posterior piece behind the patient's neck, and connect it to the anterior piece using the Velcro straps (Fig. 13-22 B).

5. Make sure the device is snug and the head is in neutral alignment.

A rigid cervical spine immobilization device alone for spinal immobilization should never be used. It should always be combined with an appropriate body immobilization device, such as a long backboard, and some type of head immobilization to prevent lateral movement. The head immobilization device is used in conjunction with the rigid cervical spine immobilization device to immobilize the patient's head to the long backboard. Sandbags should not be used to help immobilize the head, because the weight of the sandbags can cause lateral pressure and movement of the patient's head if the board is tilted.

HELPFUL HINT

At times, patients will not fit into a standard rigid cervical spine immobilization device.
Should this happen, thick towels or blankets should be used to immobilize the neck.

Body immobilization

After manual neck stabilization and application of a rigid cervical spine immobilization device, the rest of

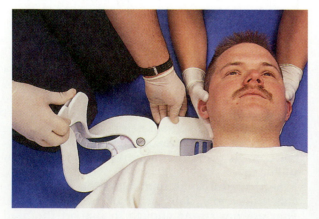
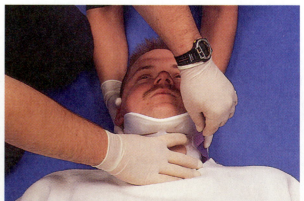

A
B

Fig. 13-21 Applying a one-piece cervical spine immobilization device. **A,** Carefully slide the back portion of the collar behind the patient's neck. **B,** Secure the collar with the Velcro straps to make a snug fit.

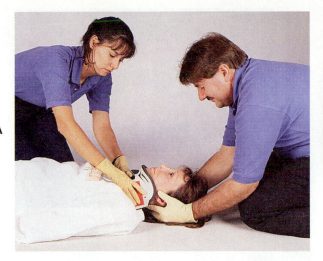 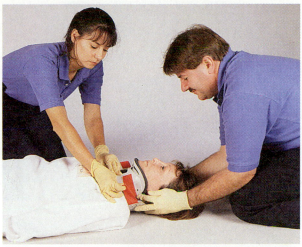

Fig. 13-22 Applying a two-piece cervical spine immobilization device. A, Place the anterior section under the patient's jaw and secure the Velcro around the back of the neck. B, Position the posterior piece behind the patient's neck, and connect it to the anterior piece using the Velcro straps.

the body and the spine should be immobilized. The patient's position will determine which immobilization device is best. Although techniques vary from device to device, some general guidelines apply, and the EMT–I should:

- Keep the patient's airway open.
- Maintain access to the patient to perform suctioning, oxygenation, ventilation, CPR, and bleeding control.
- Secure the patient firmly to any device used while keeping the spine in neutral alignment.
- Secure the head immobilization device to minimize lateral movement.
- Ensure that the patient will remain immobilized during transportation.
- Make the patient comfortable enough to cooperate as best as possible.

The techniques used to immobilize the spine depend on whether the patient is supine or seated. Outlined in the following sections are several methods to be used based on how the patient is found.

The seated patient
Some patients with a suspected spine injury may be in a seated position. Examples include patients who have sustained injury from motor vehicle accidents or falls and those patients who have moved after their injury.

During the scene assessment, the EMT–I should note if the patient is entrapped. If in doubt, he or she should call for assistance early. Patients found in the seated position must be immobilized in a short (half) spine board, vest-type, or similar device before being transferred to a full-body immobilization device *as long as their overall condition is stable.* Doing so will maintain neutral alignment and prevent movement of the patient's head and neck.

When employing a half spine board or vest-type device, several important rules must be followed. First, as soon as the EMT–I is at the patient's side, he or she immediately should provide manual stabilization. The head should be stabilized in a neutral, in-line position unless pain is encountered when moving the head to the neutral position. If the patient has too much pain, the head can be stabilized with towels or blankets in the position where movement is stopped. The EMT–I should apply a rigid cervical spine immobilization device if the head is in a neutral position. The EMT–I must avoid releasing manual stabilization before it is maintained with the immobilization device. **The patient's head should be secured to the immobilization device only after the device has been secured to the torso.** The apparatus used to secure the head must not obstruct the airway. During use of the device, the EMT–I should continually maintain neutral alignment. He or she should tightly secure the device while allowing for sufficient chest expansion. The EMT–I should avoid moving the patient excessively while applying the device, and should not pull on it to move the patient.

For our purposes, the Kendrick extrication device (KED) is demonstrated. Several models are available, so the EMT–I should review the equipment he or she has available to understand the general design and application sequence. To apply a vest-type device, the EMT–I should use the following procedure:

1. After ensuring scene safety, move to the patient and begin the initial assessment. Whenever possible, assume a position in front of the patient to minimize the patient's natural response to turn the head toward the EMT–I's voice. Throughout assessment and management of the patient, be sure to employ body substance isolation procedures.

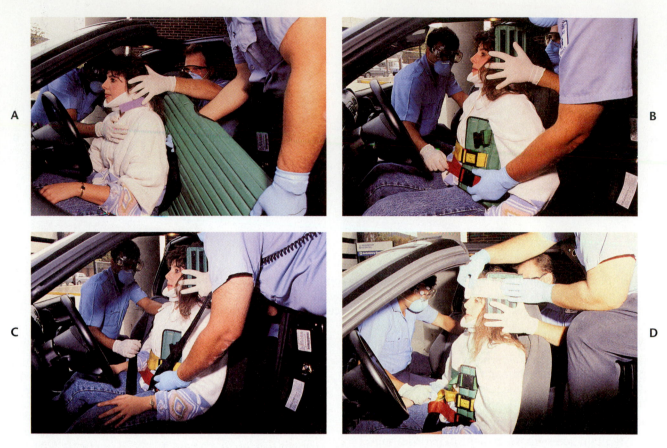

Fig. 13-23 Applying a vest-type cervical spine immobilization device. **A,** Move the patient forward and position the immobilization device. **B,** Position and fasten the color-coded torso straps. **C,** Apply the groin straps (if applicable), and reevaluate the position and tightness of the torso straps. **D,** While maintaining in-line immobilization, secure the patient's head to the device.

2. Move behind the patient. Place one hand on each side of the head, fingers spread wide, with the thumbs on the occipital area.

3. Place/maintain the patient's head in a neutral, in-line position. If the patient complains of extreme pain or if resistance is felt, do not move the head. Pad around it in that position.

4. Open the airway, if necessary, using the trauma jaw-thrust. Do not tilt the patient's head. Continue maintaining the head in a neutral position to ensure an open airway while preventing hyperextension. (If a partner or an EMT assistant has completed steps 2 through 4, assess the manual immobilization of the patient's head.)

5. If the patient is stable, assess motor, sensory, and distal circulation in all four of the patient's extremities.

6. Select a rigid cervical spine immobilization device of the appropriate size and apply it, without moving the patient. Remember to quickly inspect and palpate the neck before applying the device.

7. Carefully move the patient forward and position the immobilization device behind him or her (Fig. 13-23 A).

8. Bring the patient to the device. Stabilize the head while a partner slowly moves the patient backward.

9. Secure the immobilization device to the patient's torso so that it cannot move up or down, left or right. When using the KED, be sure that it is snug against the axillae (armpits).

10. Secure the device using the color-coded belts (Fig. 13-23 B). When pulling the straps tight, hold the buckles to prevent the device from rotating. Typically, the chest straps are applied first and then the groin straps. As the torso straps are tightened, be careful not to jerk or move the patient unnecessarily. Secure the leg straps so that the legs are not pulled upward (Fig. 13-23 C). In some EMS systems, use of the leg straps is optional. Check with the instructor or medical direction.

11. Reevaluate the position and tightness of the torso straps (torso fixation), adjusting as necessary. Check to ensure that chest expansion is not impaired by the tightness of the torso straps. On smaller patients, the chest section may interfere with respirations. In these cases, fold the chest section back to avoid interfering with breathing.

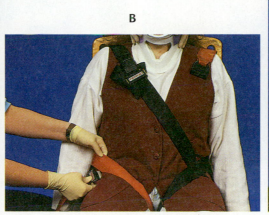
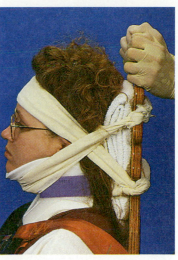

Fig. 13-24 Applying a short backboard cervical spine immobilization device. A, Slide the short backboard into place, with the top of the board even with the patient's head. B, Secure the patient's torso to the board. C, Secure the patient's head to the board.

12. Evaluate and pad behind the patient's head as necessary.

13. Secure the patient's head to the device being sure to maintain a neutral, in-line position (Fig. 13-23 D). Wrap the head piece around the patient. Pad any gaps between the patient and the device to ensure neutral alignment.

14. Secure the patient's head to the device using cravats, adhesive tape, or commercially prepared straps.

15. Reassess the patient before moving him or her to the long backboard; be certain that the patient is securely fastened to the device. Reassess motor, sensory, and distal circulation in all four extremities.

16. Move the patient to a long backboard.

17. Reassess motor, sensory, and distal circulation in all four extremeties.

    To apply the short (half) backboard, the EMT–I should use the following steps:

1. Complete steps 1 through 6 as described for the KED. Then, with the rigid cervical spine immobilization device already in place, continue to keep the patient in neutral alignment.

2. Slide the short backboard into position (Fig. 13-24 A). Ensure that the top of the board is even with the top of the patient's head.

3. Secure the patient's body to the board with 9-ft or larger straps (Fig. 13-24 B). Several techniques are acceptable.

4. Pad behind the head to ensure neutral alignment.

5. Secure the patient's head to the board with cravats or strong 2-inch or wider adhesive tape (Fig. 13-24 C).

6. Secure the wrists, knees, and ankles.

7. Reassess the patient prior to moving him or her to the long backboard; also be certain that the patient is securely fastened to the short backboard.

8. Transfer the patient to a long backboard. Be sure to lift the patient when transferring. Do not allow the bottom of the short backboard to strike the surface of the long backboard, because this will place additional pressure on the patient's head and neck. It may be necessary to loosen the leg straps to lower the patient's legs onto the long backboard.

9. If it is necessary to adjust the head portion of the short backboard, maintain manual stabilization.

Transferring to a backboard

To transfer a patient who has been immobilized with a rigid cervical spine immobilization device and short backboard (or vest-type device) to a long backboard, the EMT–I should follow these steps:

1. Make sure the short device is secure.

2. Move the ambulance cot with a long backboard on it next to the patient (in a motor vehicle accident, use the door opening of the vehicle).

3. Position the long backboard as close to the patient as possible. Place the end of the long backboard next to or under the patient's buttocks so that one end is securely supported on the car seat, chair, etc., and the other end on the ambulance cot. The backboard should be perpendicular to the cot.

4. Rotate the patient (with the device in place) and elevate his or her legs (Fig. 13-25 A).

5. Lower the patient to a supine position on the long backboard.

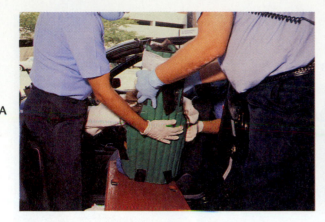
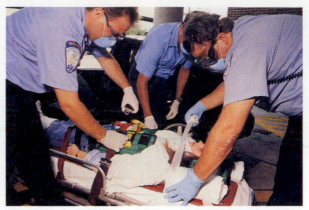

Fig. 13-25 Transferring an immobilized patient to a backboard. A, Rotate the patient in place and elevate the legs. B, Position the patient onto a long backboard and secure in place.

6. Lower the patient's legs onto backboard (in some patients it may be necessary to loosen the groin straps).

7. Slide the patient up until properly positioned on the long backboard. Avoid using the short backboard or vest-type device as a handle to move the patient. Keep the upper and lower body in line as much as possible.

8. Position the patient onto the long backboard (Fig. 13-25 B). If the patient is taller than the long backboard, let the feet extend beyond the device.

9. Secure the patient to the long backboard.

10. Position the long backboard onto the ambulance cot.

11. Securely fasten the device to the backboard.

12. Immobilize the patient's legs to the long backboard.

13. Secure the long backboard and the patient to the cot.

14. If the ambulance cot is not available, the long backboard can be held by others while the patient is lifted out of the seat and placed on the long backboard.

 HELPFUL HINT
If the patient is prone, stabilize the head while logrolling the patient into a supine position.

The supine patient

Many patients who are likely to have spinal injury are found lying down. Ideally, four people should be used to immobilize the spine of patients who are found in this position, but two to three people can accomplish the task. To perform this maneuver, the EMT–Is should follow these steps:

1. After ensuring scene safety, move to the patient and begin the initial assessment.

2. Employ body substance isolation procedures throughout assessment and management of the patient.

3. Approach the patient from the top of his or her head to limit the patient's motion before beginning cervical immobilization.

4. Place the hands alongside the patient's head.

5. Carefully move the patient's head into a neutral in-line position (Fig. 13-26 A). If the patient complains of extreme pain or resistance is felt, do not move the head. Continue to maintain the airway and manual stabilization of the head.

6. Open the airway, if necessary, using the trauma jaw-thrust. Do not tilt the patient's head.

7. If the patient is stable, evaluate motor, sensory, and distal circulation in all four of the patient's extremities.

8. Select an appropriately sized rigid cervical spine immobilization device and apply it without moving the patient. Use the largest device that does not cause hyperextension.

9. Position a long backboard alongside the patient.

10. Kneel next to the patient's midthorax.

11. The second partner should kneel next to the patient's knees. Each EMT–I should kneel within 1 inch of the patient, which allows the patient to be rolled and reduces excessive movement.

12. Straighten the patient's arms so that they are in a "palm-in" position next to the torso, and direct the second EMT–I to bring the legs together into neutral alignment. Do not raise the patient's arm to assist with the log roll, because this causes movement of the cervical and thoracic vertebrae.

13. Grasp the far side of the patient at his or her shoulder and wrist.

14. Direct the second EMT–I to grasp the patient's hip with his or her left hand just distal to the wrist and tightly grasp both pant cuffs at the

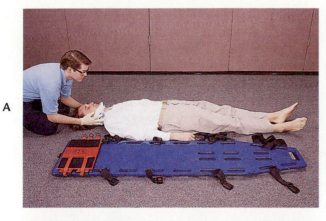
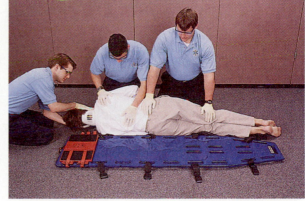
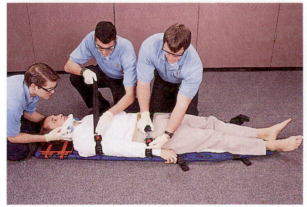
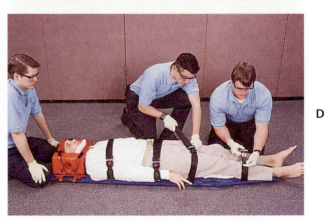

Fig. 13-26   Immobilizing a patient in the supine position. A, Move the patient's head into neutral alignment. Maintain an open airway and manual stabilization of the patient's head. B, Logroll the patient, and place the long backboard under the patient. C, Immobilize the patient's torso to the backboard. D, Immobilize the patient's head to the device in a neutral in-line position.

ankles with his or her right hand. (If the patient is wearing shorts or a skirt or no pants are available, a cravat tied around both ankles can be used instead.)

15. Usually the EMT–I at the head decides when the patient is logrolled. The other EMT–Is should follow the directions of the person at the patient's head.

16. With the patient's arms locked firmly at his or her sides, slowly roll the patient to the side (toward the EMT–Is) only until there is enough room to insert the long backboard (Fig. 13-26 B). Elevate the ankles as necessary to maintain lateral alignment. This must be done without compromising the integrity of the spine.

17. Slide the backboard close to the patient, and instruct the other EMT–Is as to when the patient will be rolled back down.

18. On command, roll patient back onto the board. This must be done without compromising the integrity of the spine.

19. Keeping the patient in neutral alignment, adjust the patient's position so that he or she is centered on the board and proper space

exists between the top of the board and the patient's head.

20. Ensure alignment by padding gaps or voids between the long backboard and the patient's body. Carefully place padding under the head to assist with alignment or to reduce patient discomfort.

21. Immobilize the patient's torso to the long backboard so that it cannot move up or down or laterally (Fig. 13-26 C). Place one strap over the nipple line and one strap over the iliac crests or use an X-strap technique.

22. Immobilize the patient's head to the device in a neutral, in-line position (Fig. 13-26 D) by placing pads or rolled blankets on each side of patient's head and fastening a strap tightly over the pads and patient's lower forehead. Place a second strap over the pads and rigid cervical spine immobilization device, and secure it to the long backboard.

23. Secure the patient's legs to the long backboard with one strap just above the knees and one strap midway between the ankles and knees.

24. If moving the patient over rough terrain or on steps, secure his or her feet to the board.

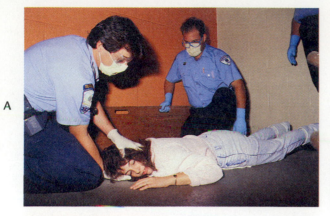

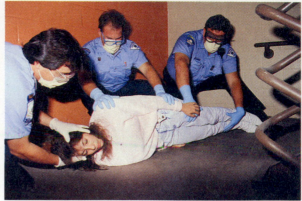

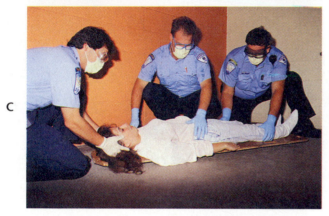

Fig. 13-27 Providing in-line stabilization for a patient found in the prone position. A, The EMT–I at the patient's head places his or her hands on the patient's head so that they will be in proper position after the logroll is complete. B, Roll the patient while carefully immobilizing head, neck, body, and spine. C, Roll the patient down onto a long backboard, and continue neutral alignment.

25. Place the patient's arms palm-in along his or her sides and secure them to long backboard.

26. Reassess motor, sensory, and distal circulation.

27. If the immobilized patient vomits, turn the entire board onto its side and suction as needed.

Patients found in a prone position require employment of a special technique to maintain the airway and provide in-line support as the patient is being logrolled (Figs. 13-27 A-C). The EMT–I stabilizing the head places one hand over the other, twisted about the patient's head. This puts the hands in the correct position after the roll. The prone patient is rolled into a supine position while carefully immobilizing the head, neck, and body. In extreme emergencies, when only two EMT–Is are available, the second EMT–I must control the entire body.

RAPID EXTRICATION TECHNIQUES

There are times when a patient with a spine injury must be rapidly removed from a vehicle without the benefit of full immobilization. **These techniques only are used when the patient's life is clearly at risk.** Rapid extrication techniques are used in two instances: an unsafe scene or patients with life-threatening injuries.

 Identify four instances in which rapid extrication techniques may be necessary.

During the scene assessment, the following conditions are examples that justify rapid extrication:

• Presence or threat of fire
• Rising water
• Danger of explosion
• Danger of structure collapse

Patients with life-threatening injuries also may require rapid removal. Some examples include:

• Patients in cardiac or respiratory arrest
• Patients whose airways cannot be maintained while in a sitting position
• Patients in whom bleeding cannot be controlled
• Patients who exhibit signs and symptoms of severe shock
• Patients whose mechanism of injury indicates the potential for rapid decompensation

 STREET WISE
The decision to employ rapid extrication techniques is not easy to make. The best guideline is, "Must this be done to save a life?"

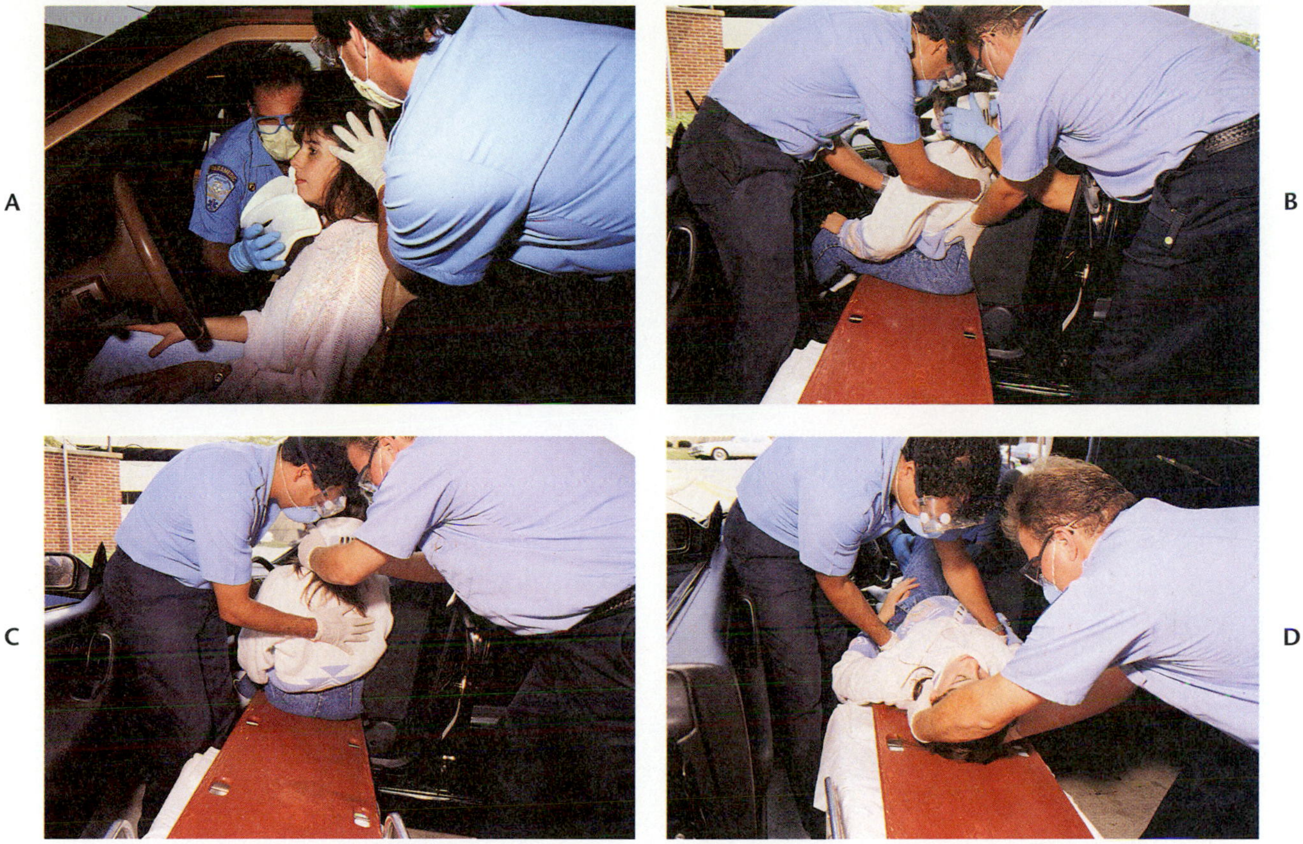

Fig. 13-28 **Steps involved in rapid patient extrication. A, Apply a rigid cervical collar. B, Begin rotating the patient toward the long backboard. C, Continue to rotate the patient onto the long backboard, maintaining neutral alignment. D, Slide the patient onto the long backboard.**

Rapid extrication requires a combination of three EMT–Is. A bystander can substitute for one EMT–I if necessary.

1. The first EMT–I stabilizes the patient's head.
2. The second EMT–I ensures that necessary equipment is gathered.
3. The third EMT–I applies a rigid cervical spine immobilization device (Fig. 13-28 A).
4. The second EMT–I places the long backboard on the stretcher and positions the stretcher at the door of the vehicle.
5. The first EMT–I directs the other EMT–Is to begin turning the patient toward the long backboard (Fig. 13-28 B, C). The EMT–Is must maintain neutral alignment and avoid sudden or jerking movements.
6. The third EMT–I takes control of the head, while the first and second EMT–Is slide the patient onto the long backboard (Fig. 13-28 D).
7. Move the patient to a safe area where additional care is provided.

MOTORCYCLE, FOOTBALL, AND OTHER HELMETS

For the EMT–I to properly manage the airway and cervical spine, access to the head is essential. If additional equipment *(eg,* shoulder pads or other protective equipment) is in place, the EMT–I must be careful to keep the head in neutral alignment (Figs. 13-29 A-C).

The EMT–I should remove helmets unless:

- The patient is obviously dead.
- The helmet is entangled into the patient's head.
- An impaled object penetrates the helmet and head.

Many experts disagree over whether protective helmets should be removed in the field. The EMT–I should review the types of protective equipment that are worn for various sports in addition to a helmet and work with medical direction and the athletic trainers in the area *before* an emergency occurs to establish the best policy and procedure for helmet removal.

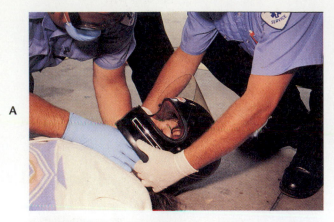

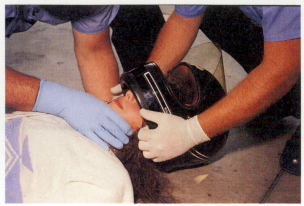

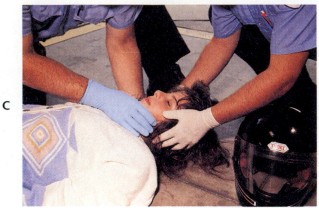

Fig. 13-29 Removing a motorcycle helmet from a suspected spinal trauma patient. A, Perform manual immobilization of the head and neck. B, The EMT-I above the patient's head pulls the sides of the helmet apart, while pulling the helmet off of the patient. C, The other EMT-I maintains immobilization of the patient's cervical-spine.

THORACIC TRAUMA

Chest injuries are the second leading cause of trauma deaths. These injuries can be caused by blunt mechanisms such as falls, motor vehicle accidents, or sporting accidents. Penetrating mechanisms such as gunshot or stab wounds also can produce thoracic or chest trauma.

Injuries that interfere with ventilation

It is vital for the EMT–I to initially recognize a chest injury and maintain ventilation and oxygenation before the patient suffers any lack of oxygen to the tissues. Several examples of thoracic injuries are described below:

Rib fracture

A rib can be broken depending on the amount of force exerted on the thoracic cavity. A simple fracture usually is not a threat to life. It becomes more serious when underlying tissue, blood vessels, and/or organs are damaged from the force of the injury or the broken end of a bone.

Signs and symptoms usually include pain when moving, decreased chest expansion due to discomfort, and local tenderness. High-concentration oxygen should be provided, especially because the patient may be hesitant to take a deep breath due to pain. The chest should be splinted using a sling and swathe around the patient's arm on the affected side. The EMT–I should make sure the patient can continue to take a deep breath and maintain an adequate tidal volume. The chest should not be restricted with tape or any other type of binding because this can lead to further pulmonary insult.

Flail chest

A flail chest occurs when two or more ribs are broken in two or more places. At least one section of the chest wall will move in a direction opposite that of the remainder of the chest, which is called *paradoxical motion*. It hinders the patient's breathing and produces hypoxia and hypercarbia (Fig. 13-30).

 Describe a flail chest.

The major symptoms are pain with movement and local tenderness. This type of injury may produce a great deal of pain. The patient may splint the area with his or her arm and avoid moving much air in and out of the lungs.

More importantly, there may be a serious injury (pulmonary contusion) to the lung under the area of the broken ribs, which further will lead to decreased oxygenation. Treatment consists of providing high-concentration oxygen and splinting the chest as described previously for a rib fracture. Some protocols may call for assisting the patient's breathing

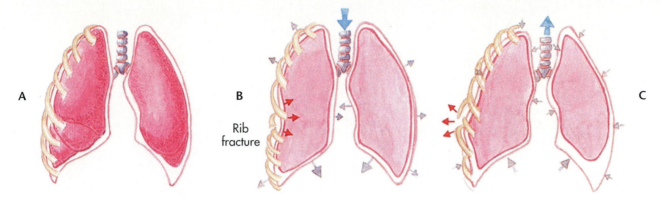

Fig. 13-30 A flail chest involves two or more ribs broken in two or more places. A portion of the rib cage then moves independently from the remainder of the chest. A, Normal lungs. B, Flail chest during inspiration. C, Flail chest during expiration.

with a ventilatory device supplied with a high-concentration of oxygen. Also, endotracheal intubation may be considered.

Pulmonary contusion

A pulmonary contusion usually occurs as a result of blunt trauma and is seen frequently under a flail chest. Bleeding occurs in the interstitial and alveolar areas of the lung. It also can be caused by penetrating trauma in the area around the initial injury. Treatment again consists of providing high-concentration oxygen and splinting as necessary to minimize pain.

Pneumothorax

When air is present in the pleural space, a simple pneumothorax exists. Air enters through an opening in the chest wall, an opening in the lung, or both. The lung begins to collapse as the pressure in the pleural space increases (Fig. 13-31).

 List three signs or symptoms of a pneumothorax.

Signs and symptoms include decreased or absent breath sounds on the affected side, pain, and dyspnea. The EMT–I should provide high-concentration oxygen and frequently reassess the patient. It is critical to monitor these patients for the development of a tension pneumothorax.

Open pneumothorax (sucking chest wound)

This open injury to the chest is caused by penetrating trauma. It creates an opening between the intrathoracic cavity and the outside of the body. The wound allows air to freely enter and exit the pleural cavity (Fig. 13-32).

Depending on the mechanism of injury, some wounds may seal independently (such as a small stab wound). Others, such as those caused by a shotgun blast, will create an opening. Air enters through the wound, producing a "sucking" sound.

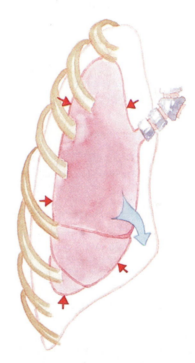

Fig. 13-31 A pneumothorax is created when air enters the pleural space.

The patient will have dyspnea and pain at the site of injury. There also may be a sucking or bubbling sound as air moves into the chest cavity.

The EMT–I should immediately cover the open area with a gloved hand, provide high-concentration oxygen, cover the open area with an occlusive dressing, and tape three sides of the dressing. This method creates a one-way valve, allowing the escape of air through the fourth, untaped side. It does not allow air back into the wound.

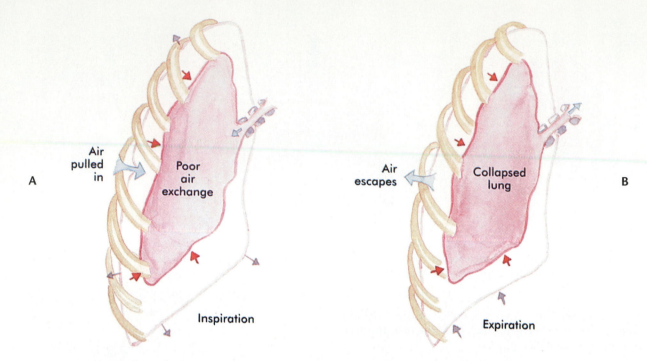

Fig. 13-32 Open pneumothorax. A, Air enters the pleural cavity during inspiration. B, Air exits the pleural cavity during expiration.

 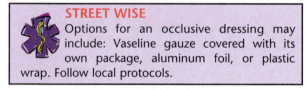

List two early and two late signs or symptoms of a tension pneumothorax.

Tension pneumothorax

When air enters the pleural space but does not exit, pressure builds inside the chest. This condition is a tension pneumothorax and is considered to be life threatening (Fig. 13-33). Because of the tension created, the lung on the side of the injury collapses, the mediastinum shifts away from the injury, and the heart becomes compressed, resulting in a decrease of blood flow back to the heart. Breathing becomes increasingly labored, and the blood pressure drops as cardiac output decreases.

Signs and symptoms of a tension pneumo-thorax can be divided into early, progressive, and late. Some of these signs and symptoms may be difficult to assess in the field.

Early signs

Decreased or absent breath sounds, dyspnea, and tachypnea despite any treatment.

Progressive signs

Increasing tachypnea and dyspnea, tympany (a low-pitched sound heard on percussion), and tachycardia.

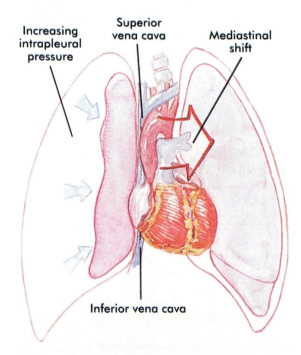

Fig. 13-33 Pressure builds inside the chest and causes a tension pneumothorax.

Late signs

Tracheal deviation (away from the injured side), jugular vein distention (may be absent if the patient is hypovolemic), signs of acute hypoxia, tympany, and narrowing pulse pressure.

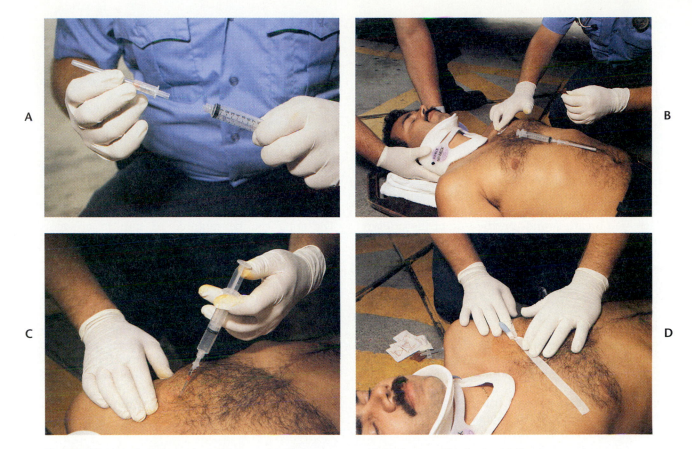

Fig. 13-34   Performing a needle decompression. **A,** Assemble the needle. **B,** Carefully cleanse the area over the second or third intercostal spaces. **C,** Insert the needle, and slide it over the rib. **D,** Attach a one-way valve to the catheter, and secure it in place.

When a tension pneumothorax is present, the patient can deteriorate quickly unless intervention is immediate. High-concentration oxygen should be provided to maximize whatever oxygen exchange is still occurring. To relieve the tension pneumothorax, the EMT–I should perform a needle thoracentesis. This skill should be performed under the auspices of proper medical direction.

Needle decompression or thoracentesis

To perform this technique, the EMT–I should do the following:

1. Assemble and prepare the necessary equipment (Fig. 13-34 A).
   - Needle (10 to 14 gauge)
   - Roll of 1/2-inch adhesive tape
   - Several alcohol or Betadine swabs
   - One-way valve or equivalent
   - Syringe (10cc)
2. Locate the second or third intercostal space on the midclavicular line. Cleanse this area with an alcohol or Betadine swab (Fig. 13-34 B).
3. Insert the needle and gently slide it over the rib (Fig. 13-34 C). In this manner, interference with

the blood vessels and nerves that run along the underside of the rib will not occur. A rush of air may be felt or heard.

4. Remove the needle from the catheter while being careful not to kink the catheter.
5. Attach the one-way valve to the catheter, and secure the entire device to the anterior chest (Fig. 13-34 D).
6. Auscultate breath sounds.

Tracheal/bronchial rupture

When blunt or penetrating trauma occurs, any part of the trachea or bronchial tree can be injured. Rupture of these structures may produce a hemothorax, pneumothorax, and/or subcutaneous emphysema. Most patients will have severe dyspnea and cough up bright red blood. The EMT–I should maintain patency of the airway and provide high-concentration oxygen. Transport to **definitive care** should be initiated as quickly as possible.

 State the importance of rapid transport to definitive care.

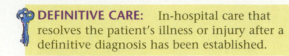

Injuries that interfere with circulation

Hemothorax

A hemothorax occurs when blood collects within the pleural space. Causes include bleeding from the lung or from blood vessels within the chest. The most critical symptoms are the loss of blood and associated hypotension.

Signs and symptoms primarily are related to the loss of blood. Confusion, anxiety, tachypnea, decreased breath sounds on the side of the injury, and other clinical signs of shock may occur. This injury is not routinely treated in the prehospital setting. The EMT–I should provide high-concentration oxygen and get the patient to definitive care at the hospital.

Hemopneumothorax

A hemopneumothorax is present when air and blood accumulate in the pleural cavity. It most often occurs with penetrating trauma. Signs and symptoms are the same as pneumothorax and hemothorax combined. Again, management is best accomplished in the hospital, so the EMT–I should apply high-concentration oxygen and initiate transport.

Myocardial contusion

Whenever blunt trauma occurs to the chest, the heart is at risk for injury. It can be compressed between the sternum and the spinal column, as seen when the patient strikes the steering wheel in a frontal motor vehicle accident. Injuries can involve a disturbance to the cardiac electrical system, bruising of the cardiac wall, or a complete rupture of the myocardium. This injury must be suspected in any patient suffering blunt chest trauma.

Some patients will exhibit no signs or symptoms of myocardial contusion. Others will complain of palpitations while displaying some dysrhythmia on the cardiac monitor. Oxygen, intravenous access, and antidysrhythmic drugs should be started. The EMT–I should continually reassess the patient's respiratory and cardiac status en route.

It is important to document the mechanism of injury, especially if no signs and symptoms are demonstrated. A broken steering wheel or bruising of the chest should be reported to medical direction and personnel at the receiving facility.

Pericardial tamponade

The pericardium is a membranous inelastic sac that encloses the heart. There is a potential space, the pericardial space, between the heart and the pericardium. This space can fill with blood, yet not expand with an increase in volume. As the space fills, the heart is compressed and cannot adequately expand to receive blood from the body. Cardiac output is decreased, leading to hypotension. This situation occurs despite the fact that the patient may have an adequate circulating blood volume (normovolemia).

Signs and symptoms are related to shock. As the pressure inside the pericardium increases, blood pressure drops and jugular vein distention may appear. The pulse pressure will narrow. The patient continues to worsen as the tamponade progresses. The EMT–I should provide high-concentration oxygen and initiate rapid transport to a trauma center for proper care.

Aortic rupture

The aorta can be ruptured or torn in accidents involving high energy. Shear forces will tear the heart and aortic arch away from the descending aorta, which is fixed to the thoracic vertebrae. Most of these patients bleed to death within the first hour after the injury. Specific diagnosis only can be made by an aortogram or specialized radiograph done at the hospital, and surgical repair is the only definitive care that will prevent most deaths. If the patient has unexplained shock and the mechanism indicates blunt trauma to the chest, aortic rupture should be suspected. The EMT–I should start high-concentration oxygen and rapidly transport the patient to a trauma center.

ABDOMINAL TRAUMA

Injuries to this area of the body also may be caused by blunt or penetrating mechanisms. Penetrating trauma usually is obvious, and blunt trauma can be particularly challenging to the EMT–I. It is important to assess the mechanism of injury and suspect abdominal trauma when there is unexplained shock.

 List four signs or symptoms of abdominal trauma.

Signs and symptoms may include abdominal pain, rigidity, tenderness, distention, bruising, guarding, pelvic instability, evisceration, and/or bleeding. The EMT–I should not waste time trying to document bowel sounds because this finding is not useful in the prehospital setting.

Evisceration

With this type of injury organ(s) protrude through the wound. The EMT–I should not attempt to replace the exposed organ(s). He or she should cover the exposed organs and the wound with wet, sterile dressings (use sterile water or saline), secure the dressings in place, and transport the patient.

Abdominal trauma in pregnancy

If the patient has sustained abdominal trauma and also is pregnant, priority should be given to treating

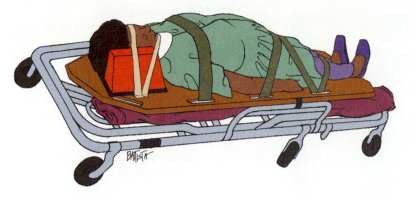

Fig. 13-35 Once a pregnant patient is fully immobilized, tilt the backboard approximately 10° to 15° to the left.

the mother. Signs and symptoms of shock may be present, and the patient should be transported as quickly as possible in an effort to save the mother and the fetus. High-concentration oxygen should be applied immediately. Some systems will authorize inflation of the legs of the PASG with proper medical direction.

 Describe the position for a pregnant trauma patient that optimizes venous return to the heart.

Once the pregnant patient has been immobilized to the long backboard, the board should be tilted to the left approximately 10° to 15°. This positioning will take pressure off the inferior vena cava and assist with blood return to the heart (Fig. 13-35).

SOFT-TISSUE TRAUMA

Soft-tissue trauma involves injury to the skin and surrounding structures. Injury can occur to the outer layer (epidermis) or the inner layer (dermis). Nerves, blood vessels, subcutaneous tissue, muscles, ligaments, and so forth can be affected depending on the mechanism of injury.

It is important for the EMT–I to focus his or her skills on identifying and treating life-threatening injuries. Blood loss is the most serious complication of soft-tissue injury and can represent a direct threat to life. Adequate steps should be taken to control bleeding to combat the onset of hypovolemic shock and its associated hypoxemia. Without the presence of major bleeding, most soft-tissue injuries do not require immediate treatment. The EMT–I should not become distracted and waste precious time treating a soft-tissue injury if the patient has any multisystem trauma.

The following are categories of soft-tissue injuries:

Closed wounds

 CONTUSION: Bruising below the dermis caused by blunt trauma.
HEMATOMA: Swelling caused by leaking blood vessels below the dermis; caused by blunt trauma.

Contusions and hematomas
Contusions and hematomas are caused by blunt trauma. With these injuries the blood vessels are torn beneath the dermis. Bruising or a contusion may result. The blood also may leak into deeper tissues and lead to swelling or a hematoma. A hematoma also may cause pain. Treatment includes applying cold to the area to encourage vasoconstriction, compressing the area to decrease bleeding, elevating the injured part whenever possible, and immobilizing when applicable to prevent motion.

Crush injuries
Crushing injuries are caused by a crushing force applied to the body. They usually involve the extremities, torso, or pelvis (Fig. 13-36). Crushing injuries can result in blood vessel injury and internal organ rupture. Symptoms include pain, paresis, or weakness (late finding), paresthesia, pallor, and pulselessness in the extremity (late finding). Treatment for a patient who has a crushing injury includes airway and breathing management, high-concentration oxygen, fluid replacement as needed (en route unless the patient is entrapped), immobilization, and rapid transport to a trauma center.

Compartment syndrome
Compartment syndrome is considered a surgical emergency. It is caused by blunt trauma or compressive forces to areas with a minimal ability to stretch. It develops as bleeding and swelling increase pressure in a closed area, which compromises circulation and leads to ischemia of the tissues. Ischemia causes

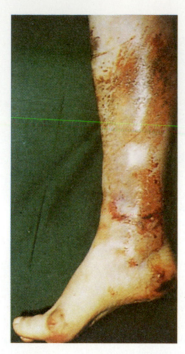

Fig. 13-36 **The appearance of a crush injury to the leg.**

tissue, muscle, and nerve damage. Signs and symptoms include extreme pain, swelling, tenderness, weakness of involved muscle groups, pain on passive stretching, and signs of ischemia at the site. Treatment is the same as for a crush injury; definitive care is necessary to restore circulation and correct metabolic abnormalities.

Crush syndrome
Crush syndrome is a life-threatening condition caused by prolonged compression or immobilization (beyond 4 to 6 hours). This condition is rare and the exact mechanism is unknown. Signs and symptoms appear after the patient is released from the crushing mechanism or immobilization. Shock and possible metabolic acidosis occur due to release of toxins and end-products of anaerobic metabolism. Treatment includes airway and ventilatory support, high-concentration oxygen, maintenance of body temperature, rehydration, some pharmacologic agents or arterial tourniquets (controversial), and surgical amputation (by a physician) if extrication is not possible.

Open wounds
Abrasions
An abrasion occurs when the outermost layer of skin is rubbed away by friction with a hard object or surface. Signs and symptoms include pain and minimal bleeding. Abrasions may involve loss of body fluids and/or blood depending on the size, depth, and location of the injury. Treatment includes cleaning the surface and removing any contaminants.

Lacerations
A laceration is caused by a tear, split, or incision into the skin. It can be caused by blunt or penetrating forces. Signs and symptoms include pain and bleeding. The amount of bleeding may be minimal or major depending on the site and mechanism. Treatment is directed at controlling hemorrhage and monitoring for signs and symptoms of hemorrhagic shock.

Punctures
Puncture wounds are caused by contact with sharp, pointed objects. Because of their nature, they may involve underlying tissues, and internal bleeding may be severe. Signs and symptoms include pain and bleeding (the amount will depend on the mechanism). Treatment for puncture wounds includes controlling hemorrhage and monitoring for signs and symptoms of hemorrhagic shock. If an object is impaled, the EMT–I SHOULD NOT REMOVE IT. He or she should control bleeding and stabilize the object. The object should only be removed if there is interference with airway management, ventilation, or chest compressions if needed.

Avulsion
An avulsion is the loss of full thickness of skin and usually is not repaired. Most commonly this injury involves fingertips, ear lobes, and nose tips. Signs and symptoms include pain and bleeding. If the tissue is still attached, the EMT–I should cleanse the area, return the skin to its normal position as much as possible, control bleeding, and apply a bulky dressing. If the tissue is separated, it should be treated as an amputation.

Amputation
An amputation involves partial or complete loss of a limb due to some type of mechanical force. Major bleeding is the most serious side effect and can be fatal. Signs and symptoms include pain, bleeding, and associated injuries dependent on the mechanism. The EMT–I should control the bleeding and save the amputated part.

 Describe the care of an amputated body part.

Care of an amputated body part begins with retrieving the part and placing it in a sterile dressing. The dressing may be dry or moistened with lactated Ringer's solution or normal saline depending on local protocol. Next, the part and dressing should be placed inside a plastic bag. The plastic bag is then placed on ice. The amputated part should be transported to the hospital with the patient whenever possible. However, transport of a critically injured patient should not be delayed to look for the amputated part. Someone else at the scene can look for the part, retrieve it, and meet the EMT–Is at the hospital. If fire or police personnel are left at the scene, they should be provided with the proper equipment and directions for saving the amputated part.

TREATMENT OF BLEEDING, WOUNDS, AND SHOCK

To manage an injury that is bleeding and progressively causing shock, the EMT–I should do the following:

1. Employ body substance isolation procedures.
2. Apply direct pressure to the wound with a gloved hand.
3. Elevate the wound (if it is on an extremity).
4. Apply a clean pressure dressing to the wound.
5. Bandage the wound.
6. Apply additional dressings if the wound continues to bleed. DO NOT remove blood-soaked bandages before applying additional dressings.
7. Locate and apply pressure to the appropriate arterial pressure point if the wound continues to bleed.
8. If the mechanism of injury or signs/symptoms indicate the victim is in compensatory shock:
   - Apply high-concentration oxygen via a nonrebreather face mask.
   - Properly position the patient (supine with the legs elevated).
   - Prevent heat loss (cover the patient as appropriate).
9. If the mechanism of injury or signs/symptoms indicate the victim is in profound shock:
   - Remove clothing or check for sharp objects.
   - Quickly perform an assessment of the areas of the body that will be covered by the PASG.
   - Position the PASG with the top of the abdominal section at or below the lowest ribs.
   - Secure the PASG around the patient.
   - Attach the hoses, open the stopcocks, and inflate the legs and the abdominal compartment of the PASG until:
     - the patient's systolic blood pressure returns to above 100 mm Hg *or*
     - the Velcro begins to crackle *or*
     - air leaks through the relief valves.
   - If an abdominal evisceration is present, DO NOT inflate the abdominal compartment of the PASG.
   - Check the patient's blood pressure and vital signs.
10. Close off the stopcocks as the device is inflated to maintain the air pressure in the garment.
11. Reassess the patient's vital signs and respiratory status.

The EMT–I should be aware that there is significant controversy regarding the use of the PASG. Some studies advocate the use of fluids over use of the PASG. Pulmonary edema has long been accepted as an absolute contraindication to use of the PASG. Major vascular injuries to the chest with uncontrolled bleeding is another contraindication because of the chance of increasing the hypovolemia and hypotension with the increased pressure. In addition, inflation of the abdominal section may be a relative contraindication in patients who are in the later stages of pregnancy. The EMT–I should check with medical direction regarding the policy or guidelines for use of the PASG when treating patients in shock.

> **STREET WISE**
> The EMT–I should remember to start body substance isolation precautions before beginning treatment. High-concentration oxygen should be administered via a nonrebreather face mask. If the bleeding continues, a tourniquet should be applied *only* after exhausting all other methods of bleeding control.

The EMT–I should consult with medical direction regarding the use of the PASG. If used, the garment should be positioned below the level of the lowest rib to prevent it from causing respiratory difficulty. The EMT–I should secure the garment so that it fits snugly around the patient's extremities and abdomen. All valves and hoses should face outward as the garment is applied.

Vital signs and lung sounds should be reassessed after inflation of the PASG, and appropriate spinal immobilization should be maintained if indicated. The EMT–I may start one or two large bore (14 to 16 gauge) IV lines using normal saline or lactated Ringer's and macrodrip administration sets en route to the hospital.

BURNS (THERMAL TRAUMA)

Burn injuries can be very distracting to the EMT–I and result in long-term disabilities for the patient. The EMT–I should focus on the treatment of life-threatening injuries if they are present even though the burn may consume his or her attention. The burn should be treated only when the EMT–I is sure there is no threat to the patient's airway, breathing, circulation, or neurologic status.

 List three types of burns.

Burns are classified according to depth.

Superficial
A burn is considered superficial when it involves only the epidermis (Fig. 13-37 A). The skin is usually reddened, and the patient complains of pain. The term previously used for this type of injury was a first-degree burn. No specific emergency treatment is recommended.

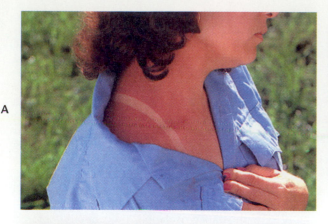

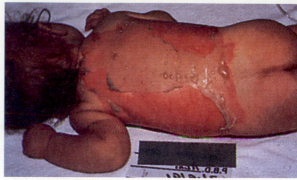

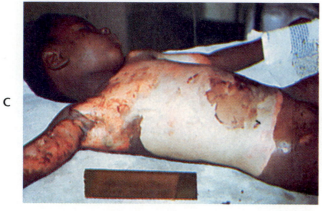

Fig. 13-37 Classifications of burns. A, A superficial burn involves only the epidermis. B, A partial-thickness burn involves the epidermis and dermis. No damage occurs to the underlying skin tissues. C, A full-thickness burn involves all layers of the dermis, and may involve bones, muscle, or underlying organs.

Partial thickness

A partial-thickness burn involves the epidermis and dermis but no underlying tissue (Fig. 13-37 B). This burn formerly was called a second-degree burn. There is intense pain, and the skin may appear white or red, moist, and mottled. Blisters usually are present. High-concentration oxygen and an intravenous line for fluid replacement should be initiated, using an area that has not been burned. Due to the intense pain, the EMT–I should consider pain relief for the patient whenever possible. The patient should be transported directly to a burn center when available.

Full thickness

A full-thickness, or third-degree, burn extends through all of the dermal layers. Subcutaneous tissue, muscle, bone, and/or organs also may be involved (Fig. 13-37 C). There is no pain associated with this burn, because nerves have been burnt away. However, there may be extreme pain in some areas due to partial-thickness burns surrounding the full-thickness burns. The skin may look very dry and leathery or appear white, dark brown, or charred. The EMT–I should start high-concentration oxygen and an intravenous line for fluid replacement, consider pain relief if pain is present, and initiate direct transport to a burn center when available.

Wound care for partial-thickness and full-thickness burns consists of first removing the burning process by cutting away clothes or removing the chemical in the case of a chemical burn. If blisters are present, the EMT–I should not break them open. The burn area should be covered with a clean, dry dressing. Some controversy exists regarding the use of wet versus dry dressings. It generally is recommended that wet dressings be used on up to 10% of the body surface area burned. The EMT–I should check with medical direction for specific treatment guidelines.

Severity of burns

When assessing a burn, it is important to consider the severity. This will provide information needed to make a decision on the patient's final destination (emergency department, burn center, etc.).

Elements that are used to categorize the severity of a burn include:

- The depth or degree of the burn
- The percentage of body surface affected
- Locations on the body that affect function, such as the face and upper airway, hands, feet, and genitalia
- Preexisting medical conditions

Also, patients who are under 5 or older than 55 years of age immediately should be evaluated at a burn or trauma center if they have serious burns. Medical direction should be consulted to make this referral.

⚷ RULE OF NINES: A system used to estimate the percentage of body surface involved in a burn injury.

Use the "rule of nines" to estimate the severity of the burn. The three levels of burn severity are minor, moderate, and major (Fig. 13-38).

Minor burns
Minor burns involve 15% or less of the body surface, and there is no involvement of the face, hands, feet, or perineum. Additionally, with minor burns there are no electrical burns, inhalation injuries, severe preexisting medical problems, or complications.

Moderate burns
With moderate burns, 15% to 25% of the body surface is involved, and there are no complications or involvement of hands, face, feet, or perineum. Additionally, there is no electrical injury, inhalation injury, associated injury, or severe preexisting medical problem.

Major burns
With major burns, 25% or greater of the body surface is involved, and there is functionally significant involvement of hands, face, feet, or perineum. Additionally, any one of the following will increase the severity of the burn to a major burn: electrical or inhalation injury, an associated injury, or preexisting medical problems.

MUSCULOSKELETAL TRAUMA

Musculoskeletal trauma involves injury to muscles and bones and can occur by a variety of mechanisms. Violence, sports and other recreational activities, as well as daily routines can cause damage to muscles, bones, and the related tissues.

The EMT–I frequently will see patients with these types of injuries. They are seldom life threatening unless circumstances such as uncontrolled bleeding are present. A fractured femur is one such injury that may produce severe internal bleeding. Fractures may be "limb threatening" if significant nerve damage is present or circulation is compromised to the injured extremity.

The goals of treating patients with musculoskeletal trauma are to:

- Control bleeding
- Prevent further injury
- Minimize permanent damage
- Reduce pain

 Identify one difference between open and closed bone injuries.

There are two types of bone injuries. An open injury occurs when there is a break in the continuity

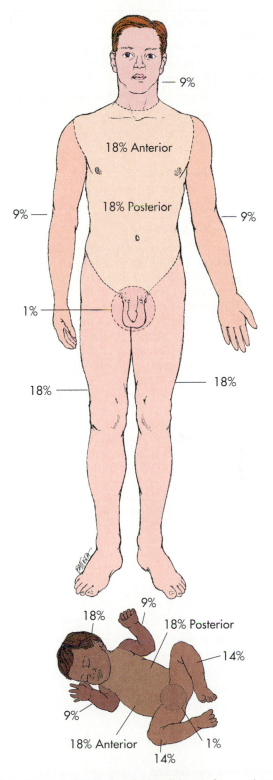

Fig. 13-38 The "rule of nines" is used to estimate the percentage of body area burned.

of the skin. A closed injury is present when there is no break in the continuity of the skin.

 List three signs or symptoms of a bone or joint injury.

Signs and symptoms of a bone or joint injury include the following:

- Deformity or abnormal position of an extremity
- Pain and tenderness
- Grating
- Swelling
- Bruising or discoloration
- Guarding
- Exposed bone ends
- Joint locked into position

When a patient presents with any of the previous chief complaints, a thorough examination should still be completed. The EMT–I should rule out any life-threatening or limb-threatening injuries first. After protecting against any body substances, the EMT–I should control bleeding. The limb should be returned to its anatomic position to restore sensory function unless severe pain or further damage results. If no immediate threats are found, the extremity should be splinted and prepared for transport. Application of cold items such as ice or cold packs may provide some assistance in reducing swelling and providing pain relief.

Splinting can be a very useful tool in controlling the injury until further evaluation is possible at a healthcare facility. It is important to prevent motion of any bony fragments, the bone ends, or abnormally positioned joints that may be present.

 Identify three complications of musculoskeletal trauma.

The following complications can occur from musculoskeletal trauma:

- Damage to muscles, nerves, or blood vessels caused by broken bones
- Conversion of a closed fracture to an open fracture
- Restriction of blood flow as a result of bone ends compressing blood vessels
- Excessive bleeding due to tissue damage caused by bone ends
- Increased pain associated with movement of bone ends
- Paralysis of extremities due to damage to the spine

Treatment for injured extremities includes controlling bleeding, splinting fractures, and preventing further injury. Various splinting techniques are discussed below. Oxygen administration and IV fluid therapy may be indicated, depending on the severity of the patient's condition.

Femur injuries

The femur is the largest bone in the body, and fractures of the femur can result in life-threatening bleeding. Several types of traction splints are available, including the Hare traction splint and Sagar traction splint.

Traction splinting (using the Hare traction splint)

To apply a Hare traction splint, the EMT–I should do the following:

1. Employ body substance isolation precautions. If the patient is wearing pants, cut the trouser leg to expose the injury site, and remove the shoe and sock.
2. Direct another EMT–I to manually stabilize the injured leg so that no motion occurs at the site of pain and/or swelling (Fig. 13-39 A).
3. Assess motor, sensory, and distal circulation in the injured extremity.
4. Direct the other EMT–I to pull on the distal leg to apply manual traction (Fig. 13-39 B). This may provide some pain relief.
5. Measure the splint against the uninjured leg (typically the pad is at the ischial tuberosity, and the end of the splint extends approximately 8 to 12 inches beyond the foot), and lock it in place.
6. Move the splint into position at the injured leg.
7. Open and adjust the four Velcro support straps (midthigh, above the knee, below the knee, and above the ankle).
8. While the other EMT–I lifts the injured leg, apply the splint by sliding it under the patient's injured limb so that the ischial pad is seated well against the ischial tuberosity (Fig. 13-39 C). Gently lower the leg.
9. Apply the proximal ischial strap (Fig. 13-39 D).
10. Apply the ankle hitch.
11. With the other EMT–I maintaining gentle manual traction on the patient's injured extremity, connect the "S" hook of the ratchet mechanism (of the splint) to the loops of the ankle hitch.
12. Wind the mechanism, which applies mechanical traction (Fig. 13-39 E). Without releasing manual traction, continue until the patient's pain is relieved.
13. Secure the splint support straps around the leg, and release manual traction once mechanical traction is adequate (Fig. 13-39 F).
14. Reevaluate proximal/distal securing devices.
15. Reassess motor, sensory, and distal circulation, and vital signs.
16. Secure the patient to a long backboard.
    - Logroll the patient onto the board.
    - Secure the patient's torso to a long backboard to immobilize the hip.

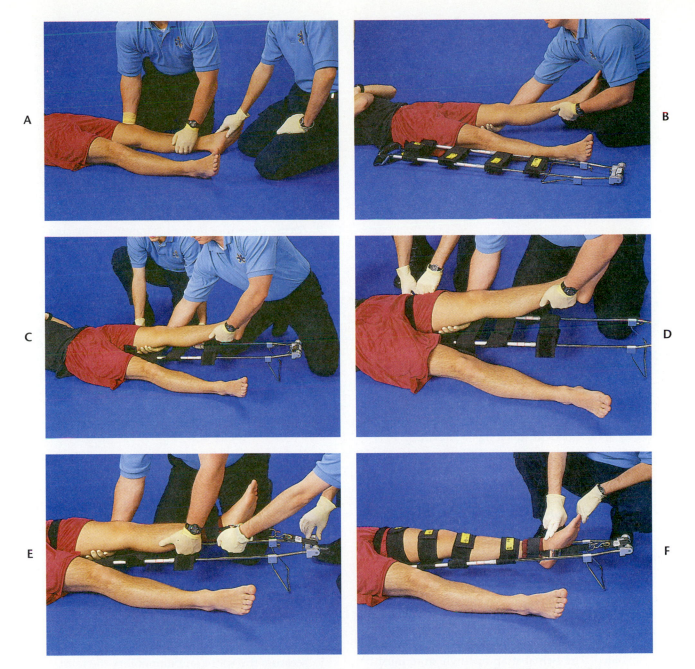

Fig. 13-39 Applying a traction splint. **A,** Provide manual stabilization to the injured leg. **B,** Applying manual traction to the injured leg may relieve some of the patient's pain. **C,** Slide the splint under the patient's leg. **D,** Apply ischial strap around the patient. **E,** Attach the distal securing device, and wind the ankle hitch for manual traction. **F,** Secure the support straps, and release manual traction.

- Secure the splint to the long backboard to prevent movement of the splint.
17. Pay careful attention to the injured leg in the ambulance, because it may extend past the end of the stretcher.

Traction splinting (using the Sager splint)
To apply a Sager splint, the EMT–I should do the following:

1. Employ body substance isolation precautions, cut the trouser leg to expose the injury site, and remove the shoe and sock.

2. Direct another EMT–I to manually stabilize the injured leg so that no motion occurs at the fracture site.

3. Assess motor, sensory, and distal circulation in the injured extremity.

4. Place splint medially between the legs.

5. Seat the perineal cushion against the groin and ischial tuberosity.

6. Apply the thigh strap snugly around the thigh of the injured leg.

7. Extend the inner shaft of the splint until the pulley wheel or cross bars are even with the patient's heel.

8. Apply the ankle harness(es) firmly around the ankle(s) above the medial and lateral malleoli.

9. Pull the control tabs on the ankle harness to shorten the ankle sling, pulling it up against the sole of the foot.

10. Pull out the inner shaft of the splint.

11. Extend the splint shaft to achieve the desired traction while observing the amount registered on the traction scale.

12. Check the thigh strap. Retighten to keep a snug fit.

13. Open and secure the three Velcro support straps (midthigh, below the knee, and above the ankle) around both legs.

14. Strap ankles and feet together.

15. Reevaluate proximal/distal securing devices.

16. Reassess motor, sensory, and distal circulation.

17. Secure the patient to a long backboard.

STREET WISE

A rough estimate for the initial amount of traction is 10% of the body weight per injured femur usually to a maximum of 15 lbs. For example, a patient weighing 100 lbs who has a single femur injury would require 10 lbs of traction. The same 100-lb patient with bilateral femur injuries would require 20 lbs of traction.

When immobilizing a patient with a suspected femur injury, the EMT–I must first remember that traction must be kept in place at all times once it has been applied. Rotating or extending the foot should be avoided. The ischial strap or thigh strap must be applied before instituting mechanical traction. The EMT–I should avoid applying supporting straps over the knee or injury site or applying the supporting straps too tightly. He or she also should avoid pulling too hard on the leg when applying mechanical traction. Motor, sensory, and distal circulation should be reassessed after splinting.

Long bone fractures

To immobilize various injuries and dislocations of the long bones, the EMT–I should do the following:

Lower extremity immobilization

1. Employ body substance isolation precautions, cut the trouser leg to expose the injury site, and remove the shoe and sock.

2. Direct another EMT–I to apply manual stabilization to the injured lower extremity (Fig. 13-40 A).

3. Assess motor, sensory, and distal circulation in the injured extremity.

4. Measure the splint(s) to the end of the leg (Fig. 13-40 B).

5. Place one padded board splint medially and one laterally (Fig. 13-40 C).

6. Pad the voids.

7. Immobilize the joint above and below the injury (Fig. 13-40 D).

8. Immobilize the foot in the position of function.

9. Secure the entire injured extremity by placing the patient onto a long backboard.

10. Reassess motor, sensory, and distal circulation in the injured extremity.

The EMT–I should handle the injured extremity carefully and not allow gross movement. Adjacent joints should be immobilized. Motor, sensory, and distal circulation should be checked before and after splinting. The splint should not be applied too tightly or too loosely.

Upper extremity immobilization

To immobilize the upper extremities, the EMT–I should do the following:

1. Employ body substance isolation precautions.

2. Direct another EMT–I to apply manual stabilization to the injured upper extremity (Fig. 13-41 A).

3. Assess motor, sensory, and distal circulation in the injured extremity.

4. Move the patient's hand into the position in which one most comfortably holds a baseball. This is called a *position of function.* To accomplish this, the wrist should be dorsiflexed approximately 20° to 30° with all fingers flexed slightly. Place a soft roller bandage into the palm of the patient's hand for immobilization (Fig. 13-41 B).

5. Measure the splint and immobilize the joint below the fracture by applying the splint to the palmar side of the hand and wrist. Secure it with a soft roller bandage throughout the length of the splint, making sure areas above and below the fracture are immobilized.

6. Secure the entire injured extremity by applying a sling and swathe (Fig. 13-41 C). A pillow may be placed between the arm and chest for patient comfort.

7. Reassess motor, sensory, and distal circulation in the injured extremity.

The EMT–I should handle the injured extremity carefully and not allow gross movement. Joints should be immobilized above and below the injury. Motor, sensory, and distal circulation of the injured

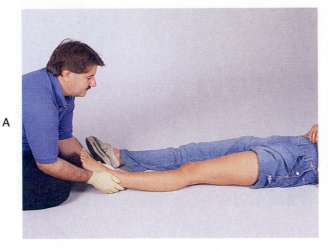
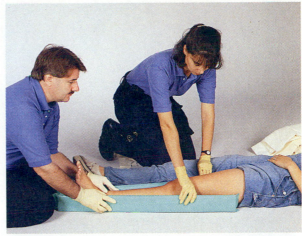
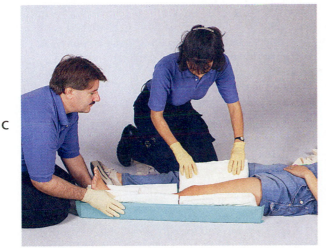
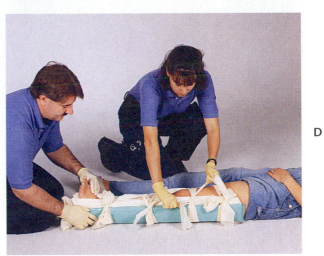

Fig. 13-40   Immobilizing a lower extremity. A, Apply manual stabilization to the injured lower extremity. B, Measure for the appropriate size splint. C, Place one splint medially and one laterally for complete stabilization and place padding between any voids. D, Immobilize the joint above and below the injury.

extremity should be checked before and after splinting. The splint should not be applied too tightly or too loosely.

Immobilization of a shoulder injury

To immobilize a shoulder injury, the EMT–I should do the following:

1. Employ body substance isolation precautions.

2. Direct another EMT–I to apply manual stabilization to the injured shoulder. If this is not possible, have the patient apply stabilization with the other hand.

3. Assess motor, sensory, and distal circulation of the arm on the same side as the injured shoulder.

4. Select proper splinting materials:
   - A sling, swathe, and pillow are effective for immobilizing an injury in which the patient presents with the upper arm positioned at

his or her side and is supporting the lower arm at a 90° angle across the chest with the uninjured arm.

5. Immobilize site of injury:
   - Position the sling over the top of the patient's chest with one point of the triangle extending behind the elbow on the injured side, one point over the shoulder, and one point lying across the patient's lap (Fig. 13-42 A).
   - Bring the bottom point of the triangle up over the patient's arm, taking the end up over the top of the patient's injured shoulder (Fig. 13-42 B).
   - Draw up on the ends of the sling so that the patient's hand is approximately 4 inches above the elbow.
   - Tie the two ends of the sling together, making sure that the knot does not press against the back of the patient's neck (Fig. 13-42 C).

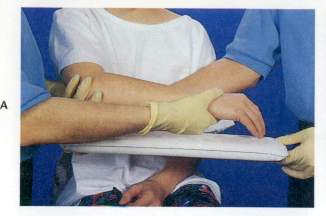

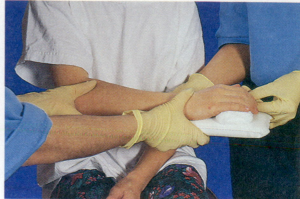

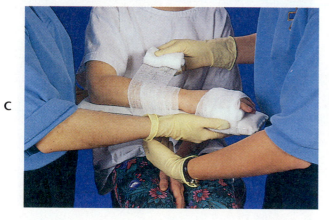

Fig. 13-41 Immobilizing an upper extremity. **A,** While performing manual stabilization of the extremity, measure the splint. **B,** Pad any voids to limit movement of the extremity. **C,** Secure the extremity to the board using gauze or cravats.

- Take hold of the point of material at the patient's elbow and fold it forward, pinning it to the front of the sling. If a pin is not available, twist the excess material and tie a knot in the point.

6. Place a pillow between the patient's arm and chest to make it more comfortable for the patient.

7. Secure the arm in place by tying a swathe around the chest and injured arm over the sling (Fig. 13-42 D).

8. Reassess motor, sensory, and distal circulation in the immobilized arm.

The bones should be immobilized above and below the injured joint. The joint should be supported so that it does not bear distal weight. Motor, sensory, and distal circulation should be assessed after splinting. The swathe should not be placed over the patient's arm on the uninjured side. The area where the knot is tied (against the back of the patient's neck) can be padded with bulky dressings if undue pressure is being applied. The patient's fingertips should be left exposed to detect any color or skin temperature changes that indicate a lack of circulation.

🍎 **List three complications of splinting.**

It is important to be careful when splinting an extremity. If the splint is too tight, complications can occur, including compression of nerves, tissues, and blood vessels. Distal circulation can be compromised, or the bone or joint injury can become worse because of improper treatment. Surrounding tissue, nerves, blood vessels, or muscles can be damaged from excessive movement.

If the patient complains of numbness or tingling of the extremity or if the feet or fingers become cool and/or mottled, the splint should be loosened. The EMT–I should reapply the splint and reassess the extremity.

Water rescue

Some situations may necessitate removal of a patient from water. The patient may have had a medical emergency (such as a seizure or syncope) or a traumatic emergency (such as that which occurs when diving into shallow water). Many victims of water-related emergencies suffer cervical spine trauma and are further injured during the removal process.

The EMT–I must get into the water to properly assess and treat the patient unless there are potential hazards to the EMT–I's safety such as downed electrical wires or fast-moving water. To ensure the safety of the EMT–I, he or she should put on a personal flotation device (PFD) (when indicated) before

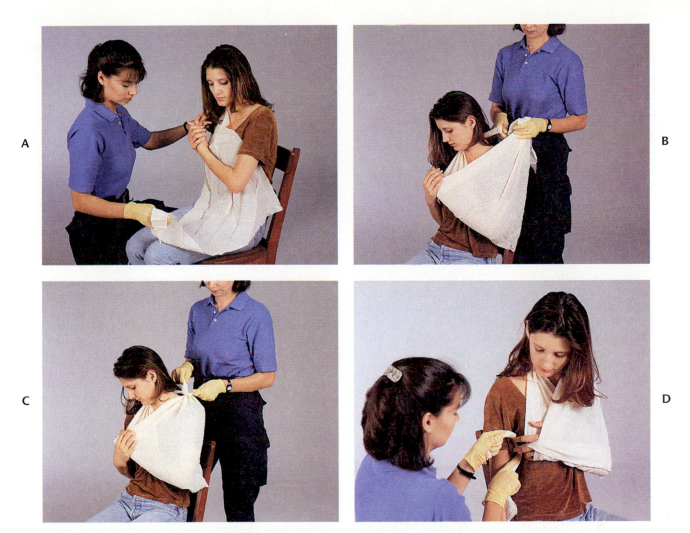

Fig. 13-42 Immobilizing a shoulder injury. A, Position the sling over the patient's chest. One point should be behind the elbow, one point over the shoulder, and the third point lying across the patient's lap. B, Bring the bottom point over the patient's arm over the injured shoulder. C, Tie the two ends of the sling together. D, Secure the arm in place using a swathe.

entering the water. Treatment includes attention to airway, breathing, and circulation. If the patient is not breathing, the EMT–I should begin rescue breathing. If there is no pulse, the patient should be rapidly removed from the water so that proper cardiac compressions can be started on a firm surface. If uncontrolled bleeding is present, the patient also should be removed from the water as quickly as possible, with minimal movement of the spine.

If spinal trauma is suspected in the absence of cardiac arrest, the EMT–I should maintain the patient in a neutral in-line position in the water while providing manual cervical spine stabilization. Depending on the size of the patient, several rescuers may need to be in the water. The EMT–I should gently position the patient onto a long backboard and remove the patient and board from the water. Further assessment and treatment should be performed once the patient is out of the water, and

the patient should be secured to the board. If the water is cool or the weather is cold, warm blankets and warm IV fluids should be used to increase the patient's body temperature. The EMT–I should remember the safety of the rescuers and help them get warm as soon as possible.

MULTISYSTEM TRAUMA

During the initial assessment, some patients may have injuries critical enough to be known as **multisystem trauma**.

MULTISYSTEM TRAUMA: Serious injury occurs to two or more major systems of the body; a rapid, accurate initial assessment is needed to recognize and treat hypoxia and shock.

Examples of patients fitting the classification of multisystem trauma are those with any:

- Decreased level of responsiveness
- Any period of unresponsiveness
- Dyspnea
- Significant bleeding
- Shock (compensated or decompensated)
- Incontinence
- Significant injury of the head, face, neck, thorax, abdomen, or pelvis
- History of major unstable medical problem
- Mechanism of injury that commonly produces significant internal injuries
- Unexplained systemic findings

Special consideration should be given to children, pregnant patients, and the elderly. The injuries of these patients may be more serious than they initially appear. In addition, injuries may have a more profound systemic impact or have a greater potential for rapidly decompensating.

The goal is to prevent death from ventilatory failure, circulatory failure (cardiac or fluid), or neurologic dysfunction whenever possible. This goal is accomplished through rapid treatment for hypoxia and hypoperfusion. Vital functions should be restored, and it is entirely appropriate to focus on this restoration above all else.

Patients with multisystem trauma must be considered unstable until they have been properly diagnosed in a hospital setting. At that time, definitive care can take place.

Treatment for patients with multisystem trauma

To approach the patient with multisystem trauma in a logical, rapid, and systematic way, the EMT–I should do the following:

1. Evaluate safety, scene, and situation.
2. Rapidly assess the patient: A = Airway (with cervical spine precautions), B = Breathing, C = Circulation to focus on ventilation, shock, and hemorrhage control.
3. Provide interventions for any life-threatening problems discovered in steps 1 and 2.
4. Reassess vital functions to evaluate effectiveness of the interventions.
5. Reassess the head, chest, and abdomen to locate potentially life-threatening conditions; rapidly provide meaningful interventions for any that are found.
6. Immobilize the patient and expedite transport to the closest appropriate facility.
7. Perform a rapid survey on the remainder of the patient and provide additional management while en route to the hospital.

Rapid transport and trauma centers

Patients with multisystem trauma require **rapid transport** to an appropriate facility. Rapid transport means that no more than 10 minutes (or less whenever possible) should be spent in the field with these patients unless the situation warrants a longer scene time (*eg,* entrapment, dangerous or hazardous environment, multiple patient scenario).

 RAPID TRANSPORT: Delivering the patient with multisystem trauma to definitive care without unnecessary delay; the EMT–I should spend no longer than 10 minutes in the field unless extenuating circumstances occur (entrapment, dangerous or hazardous environment).

If the patient does not have multisystem trauma or life-threatening injuries, more time can be spent treating individual injuries before transport. However, it is still important to initiate transport as soon as possible in case a hidden injury is present or a minor injury becomes worse.

Definitive care for trauma patients is control of hemorrhage. This care only can be accomplished in a facility that has immediate access to an operating room and the personnel associated with providing that level of care. Therefore, patients with multisystem trauma should be taken to a **trauma center** that has a well-rehearsed in-house team who can get the patient to definitive care within 10 to 15 minutes from arrival. At some trauma centers, the patient is taken directly to the operating room on arrival, which can save precious moments.

 TRAUMA CENTER: Hospital providing emergency and specialized intensive care to critically ill and injured patients; has a well-rehearsed in-house team that can place the trauma patient suffering with hemorrhage in the operating room within 10 to 15 minutes after arrival.

CASE HISTORY FOLLOW-UP

Before leaving the scene, EMT–I Fox had talked with police officers to get a description of the knife and the assailant. She knew this information would be important in predicting the patient's internal injuries. The assailant was a man and the knife had a 4-inch blade. The EMT–Is learned in EMT training that most men direct the knife upward when inflicting a stab wound. Based on the mechanism of injury, knowledge of anatomy, and the length of the blade, EMT–I Walker suspects possible lacerations to his friend's liver, pancreas, lungs, bladder, and intestines.

Per protocol, en route, EMT–I Walker establishes two IVs of lactated Ringer's solution, reassesses vital signs, and contacts medical direction. During the radio report, the patient tells EMT–I Walker that he feels faint and sick to his stomach. EMT–I Walker tells him to breathe slowly, but he starts to wretch and his intestines begin to eviscerate through the open wound in his abdomen. EMT–I Walker covers the protruding organs with wet, sterile dressings and secures the dressings in place. He prepares the suction and airway equipment and reassesses his friend's vital signs. His blood pressure is dropping. He is now tachycardic and barely responsive. EMT–I Walker inflates the leg compartments of the PASG and elevates the foot of the backboard. EMT–I Walker gives the trauma center an update and an estimated time of arrival of 5 minutes. They tell him they are waiting for their arrival and that the operating room staff is ready.

The EMT–Is deliver the injured patient to the emergency department. Before EMT–I Walker has had time to calm down from the call, his friend is on his way to surgery. On the way back to base, the EMT–Is discuss the role of EMS in managing life-and-death situations as well as routine interhospital transfers. They agree they are both important aspects of providing quality prehospital care. And yes, the EMT–Is both feel the job is worth it.

SUMMARY

Care for trauma patients begins with careful airway management with close attention given to protecting the cervical spine. The next step is to provide ventilatory support and administer high-concentration oxygen. Bleeding is controlled by broad manual pressure, and open wounds are dressed. Impaled objects should be left in place. Unresponsive patients should be transported in a supine position immobilized on a long backboard. One or two large bore (14 to 16 gauge) IV lines using normal saline or lactated Ringer's solution and macroadministration sets may be started en route.

Injuries to the head may be open or closed. The brain and surrounding structures may be injured by closed trauma. The EMT–I should assume that any injury sufficient to fracture the skull also has damaged the central nervous system. Signs of skull fractures include Battle's sign, raccoon eyes, and cerebrospinal fluid leak.

Spinal injuries are trauma to the spinal cord, vertebral column, or surrounding tissues. The spinal cord itself may or may not be damaged. Stable spinal injuries have a low likelihood of further nerve damage. Unstable spine injuries are high risk. Improper patient movement or handling can lead to further neurologic damage. It is impossible to distinguish stable from unstable spinal injuries in the field. Consequently, all patients with suspected spinal trauma are handled as though there is an unstable injury.

Patients with multisystem trauma require rapid transport to an appropriate facility. Rapid transport means that no more than 10 minutes (or less whenever possible) should be spent in the field with these patients. By performing a skilled assessment, the EMT–I can identify trauma situations and their proper management.

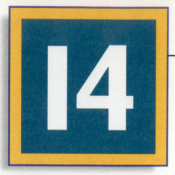

14

CARDIAC EMERGENCIES

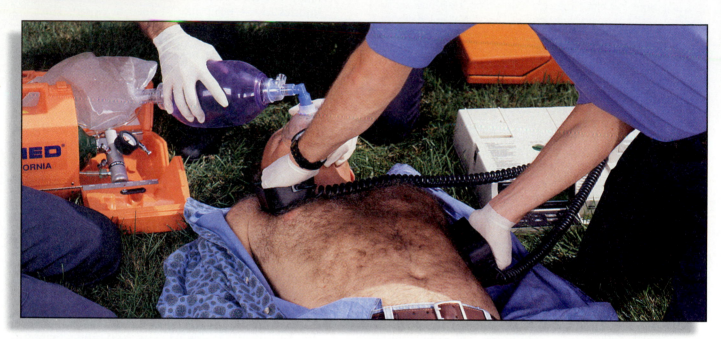

CASE HISTORY

At 2:21 PM EMT-Intermediates Adams and Graham are dispatched to 832-A Margaret Street, for a "patient with chest pain." The EMT-Is previously had taken care of Mr. Molino, aged 73 years, at that address several times. Three months ago he had a myocardial infarction, and he has had several episodes of congestive heart failure since that time.

The EMT-Is arrive at the patient's house 9 minutes later and find him sitting in his living room chair. "Hi, Mr. Molino, remember us? We're the crew that came here before for you." EMT-I Adams says.

He looks up at the EMT-Is and nods his head with recognition, but holds his fist over his chest and says, "I can't catch my breath."

"How long have you had the pain this time?" EMT-I Adams asks.

"About a half hour. I took two nitro pills. They aren't working." he responds.

EMT-I Adams places the patient on oxygen and attaches the electrocardiogram leads while EMT-I Graham takes the patient's blood pressure. EMT-I Adams prepares to start an IV of normal saline, while his partner takes the patient's vital signs.

LEARNING OBJECTIVES

Upon completion of this chapter, the EMT-Intermediate should be able to:

- IDENTIFY six risk factors for cardiac disease.
- DESCRIBE the proper mode of administration for sublingual tablet and sublingual spray nitroglycerin, and list the potential side effects and contraindications.
- LIST and differentiate between the symptoms of *angina* and *myocardial infarction* (heart attack).
- LIST three complications of myocardial infarction.
- DESCRIBE common features of cardiogenic shock.
- LIST five symptoms and signs of congestive heart failure.
- COMPARE the signs and symptoms of right-sided and left-sided congestive heart failure.
- DESCRIBE the signs and symptoms of dissecting thoracic aortic aneurysm, leaking abdominal aortic aneurysm, and ruptured abdominal aortic aneurysm.
- OUTLINE three risk factors for acute pulmonary embolism and describe the most common clinical signs and symptoms.
- LIST five causes of hypertensive crisis.
- IDENTIFY six symptoms of hypertensive crisis.
- LIST five causes of syncope.
- DISCUSS four main items to assess in patients who suffer syncope.
- DESCRIBE the cardiac conduction system.
- IDENTIFY the following components on a normal electrocardiogram tracing and describe the events of the cardiac cycle that they represent: P wave, PR segment, QRS complex, ST segment, and T wave.
- IDENTIFY each of the following cardiac rhythms on an oscilloscope monitor: normal sinus rhythm, sinus bradycardia, sinus tachycardia, premature ventricular contractions, ventricular tachycardia, ventricular fibrillation, and asystole.
- LIST the rationale for early defibrillation and describe the most common electrical disturbance resulting in cardiac arrest.
- LIST the indications for automated external defibrillation.
- DESCRIBE the proper steps for patient evaluation, placement, and use of an automated external defibrillator.
- LIST the contraindications for automated external defibrillation.
- DESCRIBE the proper steps for patient evaluation and administration of manual defibrillation.
- SUMMARIZE the general uses for each of the following agents in acute cardiac care: epinephrine, lidocaine, and atropine.

KEY TERMS

ACUTE PULMONARY EDEMA	DYSRHYTHMIA
ADRENALINE	ELECTROCARDIOGRAM (ECG)
ANEURYSM	EPINEPHRINE
ANGINA	HYPERTENSIVE CRISIS
APNEIC	ISCHEMIA
ASYSTOLE	LIDOCAINE
ATRIOVENTRICULAR NODE (AV NODE)	MYOCARDIAL INFARCTION (MI)
ATROPINE	NITROGLYCERIN
AUTOMATED EXTERNAL DEFIBRILLATOR (AED)	PALPITATION
BUNDLE OF HIS	PULMONARY EDEMA
CARDIOGENIC SHOCK	PULMONARY EMBOLISM
CONGESTIVE HEART FAILURE (CHF)	PULSELESS ELECTRICAL ACTIVITY (PEA)
DEFIBRILLATION	SINOATRIAL NODE (SA NODE)
DIAPHORESIS	SYNCOPE
DYSPNEA	THROMBOLYTICS

INTRODUCTION

Cardiovascular disease is a common cause of medical problems. Patients may present with symptoms ranging from chest pain to sudden collapse. The EMT–I should be familiar with the most important causes of cardiovascular emergencies: angina, heart attack (myocardial infarction), congestive heart failure, pulmonary embolism, aortic aneurysm, hypertensive crisis, palpitations, and syncope.

In the absence of any obvious trauma, the EMT–I should assume that a patient with chest pain has a myocardial infarction until proven otherwise.

GENERAL APPROACH TO A CARDIAC PATIENT

Cardiac signs and symptoms

The most common symptom of cardiac problems is chest pain. Cardiac chest pain typically is described as a squeezing, dull pressure often radiating (moving) down the arms or to the jaw. Other signs and symptoms may accompany cardiac chest pain, or by themselves may indicate possible cardiac disease:

- Sweating (diaphoresis)—The sudden onset of profuse sweating without preceding heavy activity can indicate a cardiac problem.

- Breathing difficulty (dyspnea)—An underlying heart or respiratory condition should be suspected in any person with shortness of breath.

- Anxiety and irritability—Patients who are uncomfortable for any reason, and especially those who are hypoxic, will feel anxious. By itself, the presence of anxiety or irritability does not necessarily indicate a cardiac condition, but it often is found in combination with other signs and symptoms noted in this section.

- Feeling of impending doom—The EMT–I should pay close attention to any patient who feels like he or she is about to die, because it is quite common for persons to have this sensation prior to cardiac arrest.

- Abnormal pulse rate—If the pulse is irregular, either too fast or too slow, the presence of a potential cardiac condition should always be suspected. However, numerous other problems (such as pain, bleeding, and neurologic problems) also can result in an abnormal pulse.

- Abnormal blood pressure—Many persons have high or low blood pressure for many different reasons. These findings by themselves do not necessarily indicate cardiac disease. However, in combination with other cardiac signs and symptoms, abnormally high or low blood pressure should suggest the possibility of a cardiac problem.

- Atypical cardiac pain—Pain is not always felt in the chest. Quite commonly, persons with angina or myocardial infarction (*see* below) have discomfort in the epigastrium (pit of the stomach), jaw, or arm. They may actually complain of indigestion as the first symptom of a heart attack. Any person with pain in the anterior portion of the body from the umbilicus (navel) to the jaw should be assumed to have cardiac problems until proven otherwise.

- Nausea and vomiting—Although these conditions are unlikely to be the sole manifestation of a cardiac problem, nausea quite commonly accompanies myocardial infarction. Vomiting is less frequent.

Initial Patient Assessment

NITROGLYCERIN: A tablet or spray commonly prescribed to cardiac patients; acts to dilate blood vessels to increase oxygen flow to the myocardium.

During the initial patient assessment, the presence or absence of respirations and pulse should be determined. A medical patient who is apneic and pulseless should immediately receive cardiopulmonary resuscitation. If the patient is over 12 years of age, the EMT–I should place the automated external defibrillator (AED) and use it according to the procedure detailed later in this chapter. In persons younger than 12 years of age or weighing less than 90 lbs, the EMT–I should perform CPR, call for paramedic assistance, and begin transport.

If the patient is responsive, and has a known cardiac history, the initial assessment and focused medical history and physical examination should be performed. The patient should be placed in a position of comfort. If the patient complains of chest pain or discomfort, the EMT–I should apply high-flow oxygen, if not applied already, and obtain baseline vital signs, including pulse oximetry.

The acronym "OPQRST" should be used to ask questions concerning:

- O = Onset—What was the patient doing when the pain started? Was the patient sitting, sleeping, exercising? Was there a period of emotional distress (such as a fight or the receipt of bad news)?

- P = Provocation—What makes the pain better or worse? What effect does breathing or movement have on the pain?

- Q = Quality—What does the pain feel like? Is it dull, aching, sharp, pressing, constricting? Is the patient able to describe the pain using a common metaphor, such as pressure "like an elephant is standing on my chest" or like a "hot knife is going through me."

- R = Radiation /relief—Does the pain go any-where? Does it radiate to the neck, jaw, teeth, back, arms, or legs? Does anything make the pain better (*eg*, nitroglycerin, rest)?

- S = Severity—How bad is the pain? On a scale of 0 to 10 (0 = no pain, 10 = the worst pain possible), how does the patient rate the discomfort?

- T = Time—How long has the pain been present? Has it been continuous, or does it come and go? What is the pain like now compared with when it started?

If the EMT–I suspects that a patient is suffering from cardiac pain and he or she has been prescribed **nitroglycerin** (NTG), he or she may assist the patient in administering the patient's own medication, if allowed by local protocols. If the patient has nitroglycerin and a blood pressure greater than 100 mm Hg systolic, the EMT–I may give one tablet or spray, as per local protocol. This dose may be repeated in 5 minutes if there is no relief and if authorized by medical direction, up to a maximum of three doses. Vital signs and chest pain should be reassessed after each dose.

If the patient's systolic blood pressure is less than 100 m Hg systolic, or if he or she does not have prescribed NTG, the EMT–I should apply high-concentration oxygen, continue with the focused assessment, and transport the patient to the hospital. The EMT–I should place the patient on a cardiac monitor and start an intravenous (IV) lifeline of normal saline as per local protocols.

Administration of Nitroglycerin

Nitroglycerin often is sold under the trade name Nitrostat (™). By dilating the blood vessels, NTG increases the oxygen supply to ischemic heart muscle (myocardium) and decreases the workload of the heart. To aid the patient in administration of NTG, the following criteria MUST be met:

- The patient must exhibit signs and symptoms of chest pain likely to be cardiac.

- The patient must have physician-prescribed sublingual NTG tablets or sublingual spray in his or her possession. Some EMS systems allow EMT–Is to carry NTG tablets or spray. The EMT–I should follow his or her local protocols.

- The EMT–I must have specific authorization by medical direction.

General contraindications to the administration of NTG include the following:

- Systolic blood pressure below 100 mm Hg. The EMT–I should follow local protocols. Some EMS systems require that the baseline blood pressure be higher than 100 mm Hg.

- Head injury

- Infants and children

- The patient has already taken three doses prior to the arrival of the EMT–I. Depending on circumstances and transport time, medical direction may allow the EMT–I to deviate from this recommendation if there is reason to suspect that the patient's NTG was inactive. The EMT–I should follow local protocols.

Nitroglycerin comes in several forms, the most common of which is the sublingual tablet. A sublingual spray is also available. Typically, protocols allow the EMT–I to assist the patient with administration of either form of this drug; each EMT–I should follow his or her local guidelines. The EMT–I should give one dose of NTG, repeated every 5 minutes if there is no relief of pain (and the blood pressure remains greater than 100 mm Hg) up to a maximum of three doses, with appropriate medical direction. NTG also is available in sustained-release tablets, a paste form, and in patches (Fig. 14-1). As a rule, the EMT–I should NOT aid a patient in taking any form of NTG except sublingual tablets or spray.

> ### CLINICAL NOTES
> Some patients take NTG as part of their regular medication regimen using a skin patch that slowly releases the drug into the body. If the EMT–I encounters such a patch, he or she should consult medical direction prior to either removing it or administering additional NTG orally or via spray. The same guidelines should be followed for encountering NTG paste, which usually is placed on the skin and covered by a transparent plastic wrap.

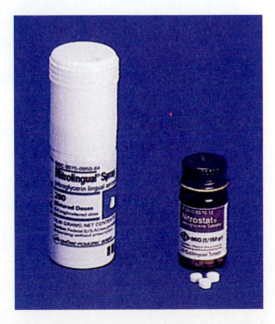

Fig. 14-1 Nitroglycerin can be found in several forms, including sublingual tablets and spray.

To administer nitroglycerin, the EMT–I should do the following:

- Obtain the appropriate order from medical direction (Fig. 14-2 A)

- Reconfirm that the systolic blood pressure is above 100 mm Hg.

- Check the expiration date of the nitroglycerin on the bottle. DO NOT give the medication if it is expired.

- Ask the patient to lift his or her tongue and place one tablet or spray one dose of medication under the tongue (Figs. 14-2 B, C). If actually placing the pill or spray, be certain to wear gloves. Without gloves some of the medication may be absorbed via the skin. DO NOT shake nitroglycerin spray prior to administration, because this will result in an incorrect dose being given to the patient.

HELPFUL HINT
The EMT–I should NOT shake NTG spray prior to administration.

- Recheck the blood pressure within 2 minutes following NTG administration (Fig. 14-2 D).

- Reassess the patient in terms of symptoms, especially the presence or absence of chest pain.

- If pain persists, seek medical direction prior to readministering either NTG tablets or spray.

Nitroglycerin commonly results in a headache following administration. By itself, the headache is not a contraindication for use or continuation of NTG. If the headache is very severe, further medication should not be administered without consulting medical direction. Typically, headaches from NTG are short-lived and subside within 5 to 10 minutes. NTG also may result in hypotension. Generally, this condition responds to elevation of the legs or a fluid challenge. The EMT–I should give a fluid challenge with caution, if at all, when the patient is in severe congestive heart failure.

STREET WISE
The EMT–I should not handle NTG tablets without gloves. If his or her hands are moist, the drug could be absorbed through the skin and cause the EMT–I to faint.

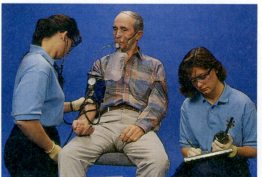
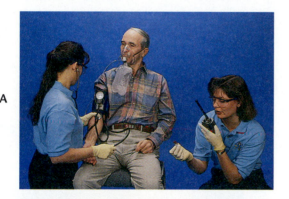
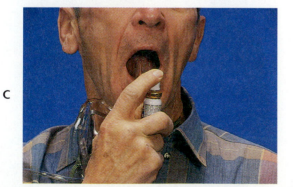
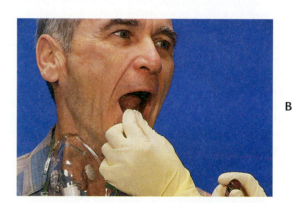

A

B

C

D

Fig. 14-2 Administration of nitroglycerin. A, Contact medical direction. B, Place the tablet underneath the patient's tongue, or C, Spray one dose of medication under the tongue. D, Reasses the patient's blood pressure.

ANGINA

ANGINA: Pain associated with decreased blood flow to the heart muscle.
ISCHEMIA: A lack of oxygen to the myocardium.
UNSTABLE ANGINA: A change in the pattern of stable angina, which may signify an impending myocardial infarction.

Introduction

Angina, also known as *angina pectoris,* is an intermittent attack of chest pain and related symptoms due to a reduction in blood flow to the heart muscle. Angina is brought on by exertion, emotional stress, or cold weather. The pain usually is relieved by rest or by administration of a medicine that dilates the coronary arteries. NTG is the most commonly used drug to treat angina.

Heart muscle suffers from lack of oxygen **(ischemia)** when the coronary arteries have been narrowed by atherosclerotic plaque (Fig. 14-3). Plaques consist of calcium, cholesterol, and connective tissue. The plaque reduces flow in the involved portion of the artery.

Angina results when the heart needs more oxygen than can be provided through the partially occluded coronary arteries. The heart muscle senses this lack of oxygen and develops anginal pain. The pain goes away when the stress is decreased and necessary oxygen supplies again flow to the myocardium.

Many cases of angina follow the above pattern: they come on with stress or exertion and are relieved by rest, nitroglycerin, or oxygen. This pattern of angina may persist for years in some patients and is called *stable angina.* Unstable angina, on the other hand, is angina that is either new in onset or differs from a patient's typical stable angina pattern. For example, a patient may have been awakened during the night with pain, which has never happened previously. Or, he or she may have pain that now occurs while the patient is at rest. Either way, a change in previously stable angina is often a warning sign of an impending myocardial infarction (heart attack).

Assessment

Chest pain is the most common symptom of angina. The pain is usually substernal (beneath the breastbone) and may radiate across the entire front of the chest. At times, the pain is felt primarily in the epigastric region. It may radiate down one or both arms, to the jaw, teeth, or neck. Often patients will describe the pain of angina as "squeezing," "pressure," "tightness," or "aching." Patients often have a desire to belch and may describe a feeling of indigestion.

Anginal pain usually does not vary with breathing or position changes. The patient may hold a clenched fist over the sternum while describing the pain. In addition, the patient may have shortness of breath, diaphoresis (sweating), weakness, and nausea.

As a rule, anginal attacks last less than 10 or 15 minutes. The symptoms are promptly relieved with rest or administration of NTG or oxygen.

Emergency care

To care for a patient with angina, the EMT–I should do the following:

- Request paramedic response if available, based on local protocols.
- Monitor the cardiac rhythm, if permitted by local protocols.

CLINICAL NOTES
Although most EMT–Is currently are not required to interpret cardiac rhythms, this skill is being taught in some programs. Basic rhythm interpretation is also an integral part of the National EMS Blueprint for the EMT–I level, meaning that all EMT–Is eventually will be required to have this skill. For these reasons, this topic has been included in the text. The EMT–I should follow his or her local protocols.

- Maintain a patent airway and administer high-concentration oxygen via a nonrebreather mask at 10 to 15 L/m.

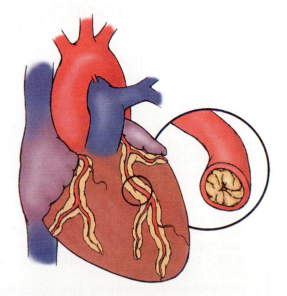

Fig. 14-3 The narrowing of coronary arteries leads to decreased blood flow to the heart muscle.

- Start an IV lifeline of normal saline via a microdrip at a keep vein open rate.

- Take vital signs every 5 minutes; place a pulse oximeter to monitor oxygen saturation, if available.

- Minimize patient activity. Do not allow the patient to move, especially if he or she is still having pain.

- Loosen restrictive clothing.

- If local protocol permits, help the patient take his or her own NTG tablets or sublingual spray.

- Transport the patient in a comfortable position. Unless the patient's condition deteriorates, do not use "emergency mode" (lights and siren) during transport, because the noise may increase anxiety.

- Watch for cardiac arrest. If the patient actually is having a heart attack, he or she is at a high risk for cardiac dysrhythmia. Have a defibrillator and airway management equipment ready.

Note: It is difficult to differentiate the symptoms of angina from those of a myocardial infarction (heart attack). The EMT–I should assume that a patient with chest pain is having a heart attack even if the pain stops and the patient feels fine. Patients with chest pain, especially if it is new in onset, should be transported to the hospital for evaluation.

> **STREET WISE**
> It may be impossible for the EMT–I to distinguish angina from a heart attack in the prehospital setting. The EMT–I should always assume the worst, *ie,* that the patient with chest pain may be having a myocardial infarction.

HEART ATTACK (MYOCARDIAL INFARCTION)

MYOCARDIAL INFARCTION: The death of heart muscle caused by a lack of oxygen.

Introduction

Heart attack, also called acute myocardial infarction, is death of an area of heart muscle due to complete blockage of blood flow in a coronary artery. The area of myocardium supplied by that artery receives little or no oxygen and dies.

Heart attack is the leading cause of death in America. Every year, more than 1.5 million Americans suffer a heart attack. Many heart attack victims die before reaching a hospital. Typically, victims die from cardiac dysrhythmia, a disturbance of the heart's normal rhythm.

The initial processes in angina and myocardial infarction (MI) are similar—partial blockage of a coronary artery due to atherosclerotic plaque. MI

occurs when the remaining open area (lumen) of the artery becomes occluded, usually due to a blood clot (**thrombus**) (Fig. 14-4). A small number of patients develop occlusion due to spasm in the muscles of the arterial walls (Fig. 14-5).

When the coronary artery becomes completely occluded, blood flow to the area of the heart that the artery supplies is markedly reduced. The heart muscle suffers chemical changes that result in symptoms, as well as damage to the myocardium. Eventually, a portion of the involved myocardium dies and is replaced with scar tissue.

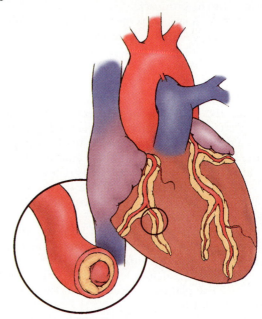

Fig. 14-4 Myocardial infarction occurs when an artery supplying oxygen to the heart is blocked.

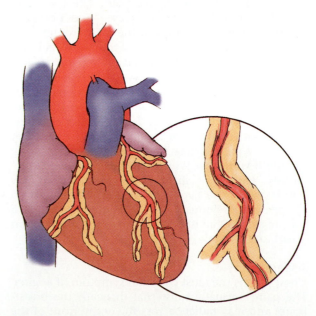

Fig. 14-5 Rarely, spasms in the muscles of arterial walls cause blockage of the artery.

CLINICAL NOTES
The fact that most patients with MI have occlusion of the artery by a blood clot forms the basis for treatment with chemical agents that break up the clot and restore flow. These agents are called *thrombolytic drugs*. They have their greatest benefit when administered within 4 hours of the onset of pain. Transport of these patients to the hospital should not be unnecessarily delayed.

Risk factors for heart attacks

 Identify six risk factors for cardiac disease.

Research has shown that certain factors increase the chances of a person experiencing a heart attack. The presence of any of these factors in a patient with chest pain should increase the EMT–I's suspicion of a heart attack:

- Cigarette smoking—Cigarettes double the risk for heart attack.
- Family history of heart attack or sudden death.
- Male sex—Men have a greater risk for heart attack than women. Women who take birth control pills or who are postmenopausal are at a higher risk than other women.
- Diabetes mellitus
- Hypertension
- Elevated blood cholesterol levels (hypercholesterolemia)
- Obesity
- Sedentary life style, failure to get sufficient aerobic exercise
- Stress

Assessment

 List and differentiate between the symptoms of angina and myocardial infarction (heart attack).

Patients with heart attacks have symptoms similar to angina. In fact, many patients have a history of anginal attacks. It may be difficult to differentiate the pain of angina from that of MI. Typically, however, there are differences. In MI:

- The pain lasts longer than 15 minutes.
- Respiratory distress may be more severe than with angina.
- The skin is often cold and clammy.
- The patient's pulse may be rapid or slow. Irregular heartbeats may be present.
- Hypotension and signs of shock may be present.

- The patient may deny the symptoms. Denial is common among heart attack victims; one-half of acute heart attack victims delay 2 or more hours before seeking medical attention.
- Cardiac arrest may occur.

Note: Elderly patients with heart attacks may not complain of chest pain. Their chief complaint is often only the sudden onset of weakness or shortness of breath. Sometimes, this event is referred to as a silent heart attack.

STREET WISE
Epigastric pain is common in acute MI. The patient may complain of indigestion rather than pain. Patients with epigastric discomfort should be assumed to have MI until proven otherwise. The EMT–I should consider the possibility of MI in patients who complain of left elbow pain, especially if no injury is obvious.

Complications of heart attacks

 List three complications of myocardial infarction.

Many patients with acute MI do quite well, whereas others may develop life-threatening complications. Problems that may develop during the prehospital phase of care include:

- Cardiac arrest—The most common time for cardiac arrest to occur is within the first hour of onset of symptoms. Arrest results from cardiac dysrhythmias that arise in ischemic heart muscle.
- Congestive heart failure—Mild heart failure occurs far more frequently than severe heart failure or pulmonary edema.
- Cardiogenic shock—Patients with MI who present in cardiogenic shock usually have suffered a massive heart attack.

Emergency care

To care for a patient with suspected acute MI, the EMT–I should do the following:

- If available and appropriate, request paramedic assistance.
- Maintain a patent airway and give oxygen at 15 L/m by nonrebreather mask. If the patient's condition deteriorates or he or she develops significant respiratory distress, intubate according to local protocols.
- Start an IV lifeline, normal saline via a microdrip at a KVO rate.
- Regularly monitor the vital signs and apply pulse oximetry if available.
- Monitor the cardiac rhythm, if permitted by local protocols.

- Minimize patient motion; do not allow the patient to move around, especially if he or she is still having pain.

- Loosen restrictive clothing.

- If local protocol permits, help the patient take his or her nitroglycerin tablets.

- If permitted by local protocol, administer chewable aspirin.

CLINICAL NOTES

The recommended dose of aspirin in patients with suspected MI varies from 80 to 325 mg. The American Heart Association recommends giving between 150 to 325 mg. Some of the research literature suggests that 80 mg are sufficient. In most localities, aspirin is only available in 80 and 325 mg tablets. Many EMS systems have their providers give two chewable 80-mg tablets (total dose of 160 mg). The EMT–I should follow his or her local protocols.

Early administration of aspirin decreases the chances of additional blood clot formation within the affected coronary artery.

- Transport the patient in a comfortable position. Unless the patient's condition rapidly deteriorates, DO NOT use "emergency mode" transport (lights and siren), because the noise may further aggravate anxiety.

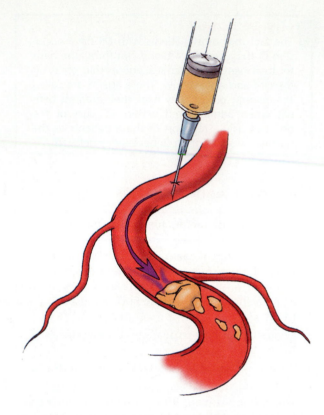

Fig. 14-6 Thrombolytic drugs act to dissolve blood clots.

Newer medical treatments for myocardial infarction

Because most patients with a heart attack have a thrombus occluding the coronary artery, doctors may try one of several techniques to eliminate the clot:

- **Thrombolysis**—"Clot busting" drugs, which chemically dissolve the clot (Fig. 14-6). These agents are referred to as thrombolytics and include streptokinase, urokinase, and tPA (tissue plasminogen activator). In some EMS systems, paramedic providers may administer these drugs in the field. EMT–Paramedics also may obtain a 12-lead electrocardiogram (ECG) to help in the rapid identification of patients who will need thrombolysis upon arrival at the hospital.

- **Balloon angioplasty**—Involves inserting a catheter into the coronary artery. A small balloon on the tip of the catheter is then inflated, which breaks apart the clot and parts of the atherosclerotic plaque, restoring arterial blood flow.

- **Coronary atherectomy**—A small catheter containing a blade (similar to that used by a plumber to clean out a sewer) is passed into the occluded

artery. The blade cuts away the clot and plaque, reopening the artery.

- **Laser angioplasty**—A small laser beam is used to burn away the clot and debris from within the artery.

- **Coronary artery stints**—Semirigid metal or plastic devices that are fitted inside a coronary artery. These serve to hold the vessel open.

Pharmacologic thrombolysis and balloon angioplasty have been used to treat MI for several years. Coronary atherectomy, laser angioplasty, and stints are still considered experimental techniques.

Circulation to the heart also can be restored by **coronary bypass surgery**, in which a vein taken from another area of the body is used to redirect blood around the blocked artery. Sometimes this surgery is abbreviated "CABG" and thus referred to as "cabbage."

- Watch for cardiac arrest and perform CPR and automated external defibrillation as indicated.

STREET WISE
The EMT–I should care for any adult with chest pain as though he or she is having a heart attack.

Some of the newer treatments for acute MI must be started as soon as possible following the onset of pain. Therefore, the EMT–I should make every effort to calmly but rapidly get the patient to the nearest appropriate emergency department.

CARDIOGENIC SHOCK

 CARDIOGENIC SHOCK: Cardiac failure whereby the heart cannot sufficiently pump blood to the rest of the circulatory system.

Describe common features of cardiogenic shock.

Introduction
Cardiogenic shock is caused by profound failure of the cardiac muscle, primarily the left ventricle. When greater than 40% of the left ventricle is nonfunctional, the heart loses its ability to efficiently pump blood into the systemic circulation. The mortality rate for cardiogenic shock is 50% to 80%. Cardiogenic shock can be caused by several factors including:

- Severe MI
- Severe heart failure.
- Cardiac valve muscle (papillary muscle) rupture.
- Trauma causing excessive pressure on the heart (*eg*, cardiac tamponade or tension pneumothorax)

Assessment
Along with the general signs and symptoms of shock, patients in cardiogenic shock may experience severe respiratory distress due to backup of fluid from the right side of the heart into the lungs. Patients also may have chest pain, if there has been an associated MI.
Signs and symptoms of cardiogenic shock include:

- Abnormal mental status due to decreased flow of blood and oxygen to the brain
- Collapse of peripheral veins
- Cold, clammy skin
- Rapid, shallow respirations
- Rapid, thready pulse
- Lowered oxygen saturation on pulse oximetry

The blood pressure may be high, normal, or low. Patients with preexisting hypertension (high blood pressure) may have a near-normal blood pressure even in moderately severe cardiogenic shock. EMT–Is should NOT rely on hypotension as a definitive indicator of shock.

 HELPFUL HINT
Hypotension is not a definitive indicator of shock.

Emergency care
To provide care for patients with suspected cardiogenic shock, the EMT–I should do the following:

- Call for more advanced cardiac response personnel, if available and appropriate.
- Secure and maintain a patent airway. Perform endotracheal intubation if necessary, according to local protocols.
- Administer high-concentration oxygen.
- Start an IV lifeline of normal saline at a KVO rate and give a 250 to 500-cc fluid challenge if called for by medical direction or local protocols.
- Monitor the vital signs and apply pulse oximetry frequently, at least every 5 minutes, if available.
- Monitor the cardiac rhythm, if permitted by local protocols.
- Transport the patient to the hospital.

CONGESTIVE HEART FAILURE AND PULMONARY EDEMA

 CONGESTIVE HEART FAILURE: An inability of the heart to pump blood caused by heart muscle damage.
PULMONARY EDEMA: An excessive backup of fluids in the lungs.

List five symptoms and signs of congestive heart failure.

Introduction
Congestive heart failure (CHF) is circulatory congestion due to inadequate flow of blood. It is caused by heart muscle damage that reduces the heart's ability to function as a pump. As a result of inadequate pumping, blood backs up in the tissues. CHF varies from mild to severe and may be chronic or acute in onset.

Causes of congestive heart failure
All forms of CHF result from the heart's inability to function as a pump. The most common cause is coronary artery disease, with or without acute MI. Other causes of CHF include:

- Cardiomyopathy, a disease of the heart muscle
- Drugs that adversely affect the ability of the heart to pump

- Hypertension
- Thyroid disease
- Heart valve disease

Right-sided versus left-sided congestive heart failure

 Compare the signs and symptoms of right-sided and left-sided congestive heart failure.

There are two types of CHF: right-sided and left-sided. To understand the differences, the EMT–I should think of the right and left sides of the heart as separate pumps with the lungs located between (Fig. 14-7).

With left-sided CHF, the pumping capability of the left ventricle is decreased. Fluid backs up into the lungs, causing pulmonary congestion. In its worst form, the lungs fill with large amounts of fluid, resulting in **pulmonary edema**. The signs and symptoms of left-sided CHF include:

- Shortness of breath—Dyspnea in patients with CHF is often worsened by lying down (orthopnea).
- Pink, frothy sputum
- Audible abnormal breath sounds (rales and wheezes)

In right-sided CHF, the pumping capacity of the right ventricle is impaired. Typically, this condition results from increased resistance to flow through the lungs caused by left-sided failure. Blood draining into the right heart backs up in the vascular system resulting in:

- Swelling (edema) of the extremities and lower back
- Abdominal swelling (ascites)
- Swelling of the liver and spleen
- Distention of the neck veins

Most patients with CHF have primarily left-sided symptoms, although in more severe cases, both left- and right-sided failure are present.

Assessment

The symptoms of CHF may be chronic, new in onset, or an acute worsening of a long-standing problem. Patients are usually short of breath. The patient may be in marked respiratory distress, especially if **acute pulmonary edema** is present. In addition, any of the following may be present:

- Diaphoresis
- Restlessness, anxiety—Patients in acute pulmonary edema feel as though they are, being "smothered."

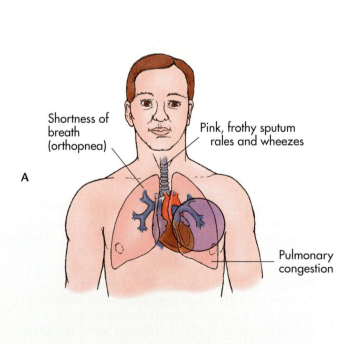
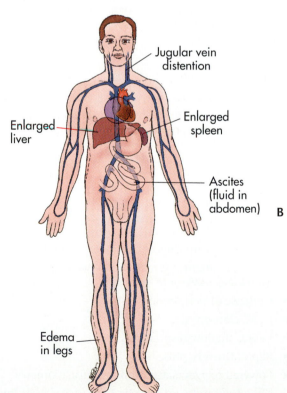

Fig. 14-7   CHF. A, Left-sided CHF results in a buildup of fluids in the lungs. B, Right-sided CHF results in a backup of blood in the vascular system.

- Shortness of breath—At night the patient may wake up unable to breathe; this symptom is called *paroxysmal nocturnal dyspnea*. Patients also may complain of orthopnea, or worsening of shortness of breath when lying down. The patient may state (if asked) that he or she sleeps sitting up or uses a number of pillows when sleeping to prevent shortness of breath at night.

- Distended neck veins

- Swollen, edematous legs

- Weakness, fatigue

- Tachycardia

- Chest pain—May be present if CHF occurs with acute MI.

- Cyanosis

- Increased systolic blood pressure—Most patients with acute CHF have elevated blood pressure. Patients with acute pulmonary edema and hypotension are "priority" patients who may rapidly deteriorate and develop respiratory or cardiac arrest.

Emergency care

To treat the patient with CHF, the EMT–I should do the following:

- Keep the patient in a sitting position, with the legs below the level of the heart if possible. Most patients naturally assume this posture (Fig. 14-8).

- Maintain a patent airway. If frothy secretions are present, suction as necessary.

- Use oxygen as required. The preferred route of administration is high-flow oxygen by mask if tolerated by the patient. Patients in acute pulmonary edema may not accept a face mask because it worsens the smothering sensation. In these cases, use a nasal cannula at 6 to 8 L/m.

- Be prepared to assist ventilation and possibly intubate if necessary, based on protocols.

- Start an IV lifeline of normal saline at a KVO drip rate.

- Monitor cardiac rhythm, if permitted by your local protocols. Dysrhythmias especially are likely in the face of acute pulmonary edema.

- Monitor the vital signs and apply pulse oximetry frequently, at least every 5 minutes, if available.

- If permitted by local protocols, assist the patient in taking his or her own NTG if the systolic blood pressure (BP) is greater than 100 mm Hg.

Patients with acute CHF may have an MI. Those patients in pulmonary edema need oxygen and drug therapy, and the EMT–I should request paramedic backup if available. It should be noted that the pneumatic antishock garment (PASG) is *absolutely* contraindicated in pulmonary edema.

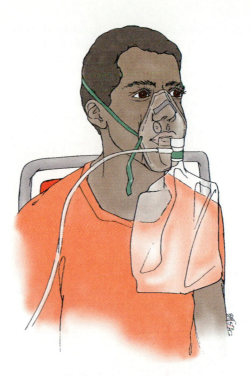

Fig. 14-8 Position the CHF patient in a sitting position and provide oxygen as required.

Drug treatment for acute pulmonary edema

Several drugs are used commonly in the treatment of acute pulmonary edema. The EMT–I may be required to assist an EMT-Paramedic in the preparation or administration of these medications. The EMT–I should NOT give any of these drugs unless trained and authorized to do so.

The major purpose of drug therapy in acute pulmonary edema is to reduce the workload on the heart. Common drugs used in the prehospital setting include:

- Nitroglycerin—Dilates both the veins and the arteries. Vasodilation decreases the amount of blood returned to the heart, thus decreasing the amount it must pump out with each stroke (preload). Arterial dilation decreases the workload against which the heart must pump (afterload). Generally, if the patient's systolic BP is greater than 100 mm HG, then sublingual or spray NTG is a first-line drug.

- Furosemide (Lasix ™)—Best known as a diuretic (causes urination) but has several effects in both CHF and acute pulmonary edema. Furosemide vasodilates, causing a decrease in the cardiac preload. In addition, it causes an exit of fluid from the lungs back into the circulatory system. Finally, the diuretic effect causes the kidneys to eliminate the excess fluid from the body. Furosemide usually is given intravenously in acute pulmonary edema.

- Morphine sulfate—A narcotic analgesic (painkiller) which also has significant effects on the central nervous system, causing dilation of both veins and arteries. As with nitroglycerin, both cardiac preload and afterload are reduced, allowing the heart to work more efficiently. Morphine usually is given intravenously in acute pulmonary edema.

AORTIC ANEURYSM

 ANEURYSM: A dilation of a portion of blood vessel that may cause a weakness or tear of the vessel wall.

Describe the signs and symptoms of dissecting thoracic aortic aneurysm, leaking abdominal aortic aneurysm, and ruptured abdominal aortic aneurysm.

Introduction

An **aneurysm** is an abnormal dilation of any portion of an artery. The EMT–I may encounter the following types of aneurysms of the aorta in the prehospital setting:

- Dissecting thoracic aortic aneurysm—Weakness and splitting of the connective tissue within the layers of the thoracic aorta, usually due to hypertension (high blood pressure).

- Ruptured or leaking abdominal aortic aneurysm— Weakness and abnormal dilation of the abdominal aorta; usually caused by atherosclerosis.

Dissecting thoracic aortic aneurysm

Dissecting thoracic aortic aneurysm most commonly is acquired and due to hypertension, although the weakness also can be congenital (at birth). It is more common in men than in women. Patients typically have a history of poorly controlled hypertension.

Blood enters a tear in the intimal lining of the vessel, causing a separation of weakened elastic and fibromuscular elements in the medial layer. The blood causes cystlike dilation of the media, resulting in a false passage for blood. Essentially, the walls of the aorta tear apart, much like layers of an onion, as the dissection proceeds (Fig. 14-9).

The most severe complications occur when the dissection involves various arteries that arise from the aorta. Blood is unable to flow properly into these arteries, resulting in impaired blood supply to the tissues that they supply. Life-threatening conditions, such as pericardial tamponade, myocardial infarction, and stroke may occur.

When dissection occurs, the patient suffers excruciating pain, usually starting in the anterior chest and moving downward and toward the back. Many

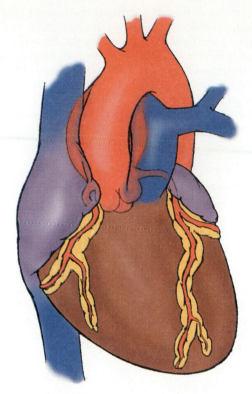

Fig. 14-9 Dissecting thoracic aortic aneurysms are the result of blood entering a tear in the intimal lining of the vessel.

patients complain of a "tearing" sensation when describing the onset of their pain. Some patients do not feel anterior chest pain; their symptoms are limited to severe pain between the shoulder blades. The pain may exactly mimic that of acute MI.

The physical examination findings vary greatly, depending on the severity and location of the dissection. If peripheral arteries are compromised, there often will be asymmetry of pulses between the right and left sides of the body. The EMT–I should be certain to check carotid, radial, and femoral pulses on BOTH sides in patients with suspected dissection. If the carotids are involved, the patient may have neurologic symptoms, similar to those of stroke. If the femoral arteries are affected, the femoral pulse will be decreased or absent on one side, and the leg, foot, or toes may be white or cyanotic, and are often cooler than the other side.

 HELPFUL HINT
The key to suspecting a dissecting thoracic aortic aneurysm is the presence of tearing chest pain, especially between the shoulder blades. The EMT–I should look for asymmetry of pulses, color, temperature, and neurologic signs. The presence of any asymmetry, in the face of typical pain, indicates a dissecting aneurysm until proven otherwise.

Persons with suspected dissection of the thoracic aorta are "priority" patients. They require gentle but rapid transport to an appropriate medical facility. The EMT–I should obtain paramedic backup, if available, but should NOT prolong transport time by waiting for help. While en route to the hospital, the EMT–I should provide the following care:

- Secure and maintain a patent airway.
- Administer high-concentration oxygen.
- Consider the use of PASG.

HELPFUL HINT
The use of PASG for suspected aortic dissection is highly controversial. Some experts believe that the increased blood pressure favors further dissection of the layers of the aorta. Local protocols or medical control directions should be followed.

- Initiate two large-bore IVs of normal saline, as long as the patient's blood pressure is greater than 90 mm Hg systolic. Keep the fluid rate KVO. DO NOT increase the IV rate without medical direction. Many EMS systems start IVs en route on these patients; follow your protocols.
- Monitor the cardiac rhythm, if permitted by local protocols.
- Monitor the vital signs, pulse oximetry, and peripheral pulses frequently, at least every 5 minutes.

Ruptured or leaking abdominal aortic aneurysm

An abdominal aortic aneurysm is a saclike widening in the abdominal portion of the aorta, usually caused by a combination of atherosclerosis and hypertension (Fig. 14-10). Most of these aneurysms are totally asymptomatic and are discovered on routine physical examination. Aneurysms that leak or rupture can lead to catastrophic circumstances. Patients have a 35% mortality rate if emergency surgery is required to attempt to repair the rupture. Abdominal aortic aneurysms are present in 2% to 4% of the adult population, the majority of which occur in elderly men.

Unless the aneurysm is leaking or actually has ruptured, the patient is likely to be asymptomatic. Symptoms include back pain, abdominal pain, nausea, vomiting, and signs of shock. With rupture, the symptoms come on quickly. The onset of severe abdominal pain is rapid, often radiating to the back and scrotum. Nausea and vomiting are common.

HELPFUL HINT
The EMT–I should strongly suspect ruptured abdominal aortic aneurysm in a middle-aged or elderly man with the sudden onset of abdominal or back pain and shock.

The patient appears quite ill and is very diaphoretic with signs of shock. A pulsating abdominal mass may

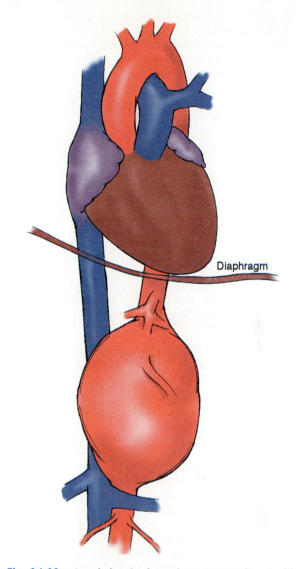

Diaphragm

Fig. 14-10 An abdominal aortic aneurysm is a saclike widening in the abdominal portion of the aorta.

be present. If the aorta already has ruptured, the most common finding is a markedly distended, tender abdomen and shock. Femoral pulses may be decreased. Occasionally, blood will dissect through the abdominal cavity into the groin, resulting in massive swelling of the scrotum with bluish discoloration, the so-called blue scrotum sign.

Patients with suspected rupture or leakage of an abdominal aortic aneurysm are priority patients. They require gentle but rapid transport to a medical facility. The EMT–I should obtain paramedic backup, if available, but should NOT prolong transport time by waiting for help. While en route to the hospital, the EMT–I should provide the following care:

- Secure and maintain a patent airway.
- Administer high-concentration oxygen.
- Consider the use of PASG.

- Initiate two large-bore IVs of normal saline, as long as the patient's blood pressure is greater than 90 mm Hg systolic. Keep the fluid rate KVO. DO NOT increase the IV rate without medical direction.
- Monitor the cardiac rhythm, if permitted by local protocols.
- Monitor the vital signs and peripheral pulses frequently, at least every 5 minutes.

PULMONARY EMBOLISM

PULMONARY EMBOLISM A blockage in a pulmonary artery; most often caused by a blood clot in the leg that breaks away, travels through the veins, and becomes lodged in the lungs.

Outline three risk factors for acute pulmonary embolism and enumerate the most common clinical signs and symptoms.

Introduction

Pulmonary embolism is the blockage of a pulmonary artery by foreign matter. In most cases, the obstruction is due to a piece of a blood clot that has broken away from a pelvic or deep leg vein and traveled to the lungs (Fig. 14-11). Other causes of obstruction include fat, amniotic fluid, air, or tumor tissue.

Pulmonary embolism is common, potentially lethal, and highly underdiagnosed. It is the third most common cause of death in the United States, with approximately 650,000 cases annually. Of these, 10% of patients die within 1 hour of the event. Among survivors, the diagnosis is missed in two out of three cases.

Risk factors for pulmonary embolism

Risks for pulmonary embolism include the following:

- Sedentary life style—Pulmonary embolism is common in hospitalized patients and in those who have completed long automobile or airplane trips.
- Obesity
- Thrombophlebitis—An inflammation of the veins.
- Use of oral contraceptives (birth control pills)

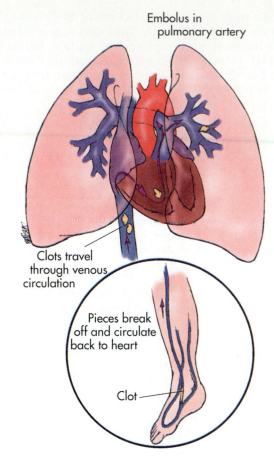

Fig. 14-11 Pulmonary embolism is the blockage of a pulmonary artery by foreign matter.

- Fracture of a long bone (femur, humerus)—The source of emboli is fat released from the bone marrow.
- Pregnancy—Amniotic fluid embolism may occur during delivery. It is often fatal.
- Surger—Patients may remain in the same position on the operating table for several hours, leading to blood clot formation in the veins of the pelvis and legs.
- Blood disease—Rare blood disorders can make a patient's blood more likely to clot (eg, polycythemia vera).

Pathophysiology of pulmonary embolism

The most common source of a pulmonary embolism is a blood clot that has formed in either the pelvic or deep leg veins. A piece can break off and travel through the venous system to the heart, then the lungs. As the clot passes through progressively smaller and smaller branches of the pulmonary circulation, it becomes lodged and blockage occurs.

The lung tissue supplied by the blocked artery becomes ischemic. If circulation to the lung is sufficiently compromised, the affected area dies. The process is similar whether the embolism consists of blood clot, fat, tissue, air, or other foreign matter.

Pulmonary emboli may be small or large. Large pulmonary emboli occlude major branches of the pulmonary arteries. When these occur, the heart is forced to pump blood against very high pressures, resulting in acute right-sided heart failure (acute cor pulmonale).

Assessment

Patients with massive pulmonary emboli often suffer cardiac arrest or a syncopal spell as the first symptom of the illness. Patients with smaller emboli may have the following signs and symptoms:

- Sudden, unexplained onset of chest pain that increases in intensity with a deep breath (pleuritic chest pain). The pain may be localized to the area of the chest overlying the involved lung tissue.
- Respiratory distress and shortness of breath. The patient's respiratory rate is almost always increased. The patient may hyperventilate.
- Wheezing or coughing up of blood (hemoptysis)
- Anxiety
- Shock
- Hypotension

 HELPFUL HINT
The signs and symptoms of pulmonary embolism are often similar to pneumonia, MI, or spontaneous pneumothorax.

Emergency care

To care for patients with suspected pulmonary embolism, the EMT–I should do the following:

- Maintain a patent airway, and intubate if necessary.
- Administer high-concentration oxygen.
- Monitor the cardiac rhythm, if permitted by local protocols.
- Place the patient in a comfortable position.
- Monitor the vital signs frequently, at least every 5 minutes.
- Start an IV lifeline of normal saline, at a KVO rate.
- Transport to the nearest appropriate medical facility.

HYPERTENSIVE CRISIS

 HYPERTENSIVE CRISIS: A sudden increase in blood pressure that leads to problems with the nervous system, the kidneys, or the heart.

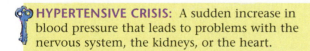
List five causes of hypertensive crisis.

Introduction

A hypertensive crisis is a sudden increase in the systolic blood pressure, the diastolic blood pressure, or both, which causes acute problems of the central nervous system, the heart, or the kidneys. Hypertensive crisis can be life-threatening. A delay in therapy can lead to stroke, MI, pulmonary edema, or death.

Causes of hypertensive crisis

The most common cause of a hypertensive crisis is an acute worsening of chronic hypertension. Many times patients have suddenly stopped taking their blood pressure medicines. Other causes of hypertensive crisis include:

- Drugs—Ingestion of cocaine is a common cause of hypertensive crisis.
- Amphetamines ("speed") and thyroid medicine toxicity cause a similar syndrome.
- Acute heart failure
- Pregnancy-associated hypertension (eclampsia or toxemia of pregnancy)
- Acute kidney infection or abnormal kidney function
- Dissecting thoracic aortic aneurysm
- Intracranial event—Stroke, head trauma, and brain hemorrhage. Almost all acute intracranial events are associated with a period of severe hypertension.

Pathophysiology of hypertensive crisis

Normally, the flow of blood within the brain is kept within a narrow range, regardless of the patient's blood pressure. This property is known as cerebral autoregulation. When a hypertensive crisis occurs, the brain's ability to maintain cerebral autoregulation is lost. As the blood pressure rises, so does the blood flow in the brain. As cerebral blood flow rises, the intracranial pressure increases, leading to symptoms of headache, drowsiness, vomiting, and visual disturbance.

The elevated blood pressure also places a stress on the heart and kidneys. As the blood pressure rises, so does the resistance against which the heart must pump blood. This increase in blood pressure places a strain on the myocardium, which may result in angina or MI. Similarly, increased vascular resistance interferes with blood flow through the kidneys, resulting in possible kidney failure.

 Identify six symptoms of hypertensive crisis.

Assessment

Patients with hypertensive crisis have markedly elevated blood pressure. Generally, the systolic pressure is greater than 250 mm Hg and the diastolic pressure greater than 120 mm Hg. However, these are not rigid criteria. Patients may have significant symptoms at lower readings. Local protocols should be followed. The following signs and symptoms may be present in hypertensive crisis:

- Severe headache or dizziness.

- Decreased level of responsiveness; the likelihood that an unresponsive patient with a significantly elevated blood pressure has an intracranial hemorrhage is quite high.

- Visual disturbances, such as blurred or double vision—The pupils may be unequal. Slowly reactive, pinpoint pupils in a hypertensive patient with an altered level of responsiveness indicate an intracranial hemorrhage.

- Nausea or vomiting.

- Chest pain, shortness of breath.

- Nosebleed (epistaxis)—Often results from elevated blood pressure whether or not a hypertensive crisis is present.

HELPFUL HINT

Spontaneous nosebleeds (epistaxis) in hypertensive patients may be difficult to stop. Bleeding tends to recur in these patients. These patients need evaluation in the hospital even if the bleeding has stopped by the time EMS providers arrive.

Emergency care

To provide emergency care for a patient with a suspected hypertensive crisis, the EMT–I should do the following:

- Maintain a patent airway and administer high-concentration oxygen.

- Start an IV lifeline of normal saline, at a KVO rate.

- Monitor the cardiac rhythm, if permitted by local protocols.

- Monitor the vital signs and pulse oximetry frequently, at least every 5 minutes.

PALPITATIONS AND SYNCOPE

Introduction

Palpitation is a sensation of pounding or racing of the heart. **Syncope** is a transient state of unresponsiveness due to inadequate perfusion of the brain from which the patient has recovered. These symptoms may occur together or individually.

 List five causes of syncope.

Causes of palpitations and syncope

Palpitations and syncope result from cardiac dysrhythmias, other types of heart disease, nervous system disorders, anxiety, and thyroid disease. The conditions also can be caused by a variety of drugs, such as caffeine, cocaine or amphetamines. The most common form of syncope is the simple fainting spell. Once the patient assumes the recumbent position, he or she rapidly regains responsiveness.

HELPFUL HINTS

The EMT–I should always consider the possibility of acute cocaine intoxication in a young patient with tachycardia, palpitations, diaphoresis, and chest pain. Cocaine also can cause acute MI.

Some people, particularly the elderly, experience fainting while straining on the toilet. This event is called *vasovagal syncope.* It results when increased abdominal pressure stimulates the vagus nerve, which travels near the stomach. Increasing the abdominal pressure while the breath is held is called the *Valsalva maneuver.*

 Discuss four main items to assess in patients who suffer syncope.

Assessment

To assess the patient who may have suffered a loss of responsiveness or feels dizzy, the EMT–I should assess the following:

- How long was the patient unresponsive? Patients who have had a simple fainting spell recover almost immediately after "hitting the ground."

- In what position was the patient when the syncopal episode occurred? Patients who have syncope while in the supine or recumbent position may have a cardiac dysrhythmia.

- Does the patient feel light-headed when going from lying down to sitting or sitting to standing? If so, the patient may have orthostatic hypotension.

- Is the patient pregnant? Women in the second and third trimesters of pregnancy may have syncope if they lie flat, allowing the uterus to compress the inferior vena cava. This compression decreases venous return to the heart, and syncope may result. This is called *supine hypotension syndrome of pregnancy.*

- Did the patient appear to have a seizure? Following even a simple fainting spell, the blood supply to the brain is transiently decreased. This decrease may result in one or two jerking movements. These movements are not actually a true seizure, however, a nonmedically trained person observing the event may report that the patient "fainted and had a seizure."

- Are the patient's vital signs normal? The vital signs may be normal, especially if the patient has recovered. The pulse may be normal, rapid, slow, or irregular.

HELPFUL HINT
Although a patient has recovered from a syncopal episode, he or she should be transported to the hospital for evaluation.

Emergency care

To provide care for patients with palpitations or syncope, the EMT–I should do the following:

- Administer high-concentration oxygen. Assist ventilations or intubate as necessary, according to local protocols.

- Monitor the cardiac rhythm, if permitted by local protocols. Cardiac dysrhythmias are a common cause of syncope.

- Start an IV lifeline of normal saline, at a KVO rate.

- Monitor the patient's vital signs and pulse oximetry. Transport the patient to the hospital for evaluation.

BASIC ELECTROCARDIOGRAM INTERPRETATION

 Describe the cardiac conduction system.

The cardiac conduction system

The heart muscle (myocardium) has the ability to generate and conduct electrical impulses. Normally, electrical signals begin in the right atrium and via specialized tissue, (the cardiac conduction system), travel throughout the heart (Fig. 14-12). As the electrical signal reaches various portions of the myocardium, it causes them to contract.

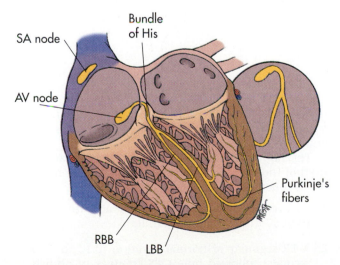

Fig. 14-12   The cardiac conduction system enables the heart to conduct electrical activity.

Normally, the cardiac impulse begins in the **sinoatrial node (SA node)** located high in the right atrium. From here, the current passes throughout both atria to the **atrioventricular node (AV node)**, located at the junction of the atria and the ventricles. The flow of electricity slows at the AV node to allow the atria to contract. Once the atria have contracted, the impulse continues from the AV node to the **bundle of His**. This structure rapidly divides into the left and right bundle branches. The bundle branches traverse the left and right ventricles, respectively, eventually dividing into very small Purkinje's fibers. These fibers are the smallest division of the conduction system and pass to all of the ventricular myocardial cells.

 Identify the following components on a normal electrocardiogram tracing, and describe the events of the cardiac cycle that they represent: P wave, PR segment, QRS complex, ST segment, and T wave.

Components of the normal adult electrocardiogram

The **electrocardiogram (ECG)** is a record of the electrical activity within the heart. Electrodes placed on the patient's skin detect the activity. These impulses, which appear as a series of waves or "blips," are then transferred to the ECG machine and displayed via a screen (oscilloscope) or printed onto moving graph paper.

The printed paper shows heavy vertical lines and smaller vertical lines. These lines divide the tracing into big and small "boxes," respectively (Fig. 14-13). The distance between the lines, or boxes, represents time. The time between two large lines is 0.2 second. Four smaller lines divide the large 0.2 second-box into five smaller 0.04-second boxes. The EMT–I can use these standardized distances to determine the length of any portion of an ECG complex.

The machine records positive electrical impulses as upward deflections and negative impulses as downward deflections. A flat or isoelectric line is produced if no electrical impulse is present. This series of waves and complexes is commonly known as the P wave, QRS complex, and T wave, and represents the normal cardiac conduction pattern (Fig. 14-14).

As the electrical impulse passes through the heart cells, it causes chemical changes within the cell. These changes are called *depolarization*. As the cell depolarizes, muscle fibers are stimulated to contract. Following depolarization and contraction, the chemical balance within the cell returns to the way it was prior to depolarization, or to the resting state (baseline). This process is called *repolarization*. The cardiac muscle relaxes during repolarization.

The P wave occurs first and represents movement of the electrical impulse (depolarization) through the atria, resulting in atrial contraction. Following this

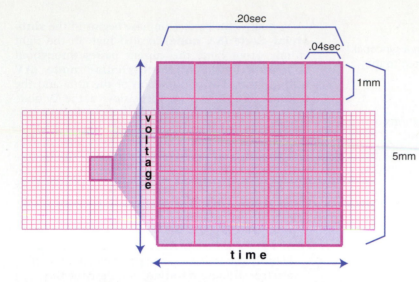

Fig. 14-13 ECG paper is a grid composed of standardized line distances and markings.

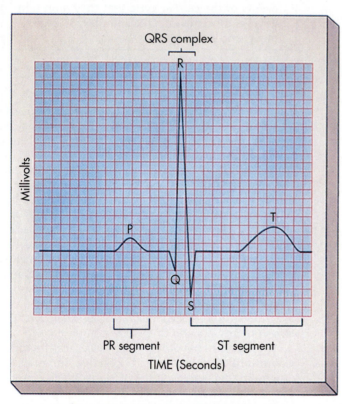

Fig. 14-14 An ECG is composed of P waves, QRS complexes, and T waves.

wave is a flat line, or electrical pause, called the PR segment, which represents the time delay that occurs as the impulse passes through the AV node.

Next is a larger wave, the QRS complex, which represents movement of the electrical impulse (depolarization) through the ventricles. This wave corresponds to ventricular contraction, or systole. The Q wave is the first downward deflection, the R wave is the first upward deflection after the P wave, and the S wave is the first negative deflection after the R wave. Another pause then occurs, known as the ST segment. During this period, repolarization of the ventricles is beginning. The T wave follows,

representing completion of repolarization. Atrial repolarization occurs during the QRS complex and is not visible on the regular ECG.

The normal ECG, representing a normal cardiac rhythm (normal sinus rhythm) (Fig. 14-15), consists of the following:

1. P waves occurring at regular intervals with a rate from 60 to100 beats per minute

2. A PR segment of normal duration (0.12 to 0.20 seconds) followed by a QRS complex of normal upright contour, duration (less than 0.12 second), and configuration.

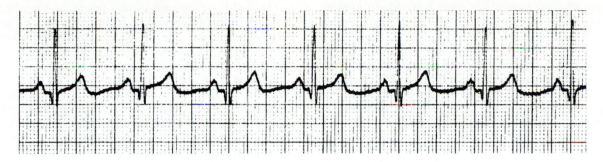

Fig. 14-15   An ECG representative of normal sinus rhythm.

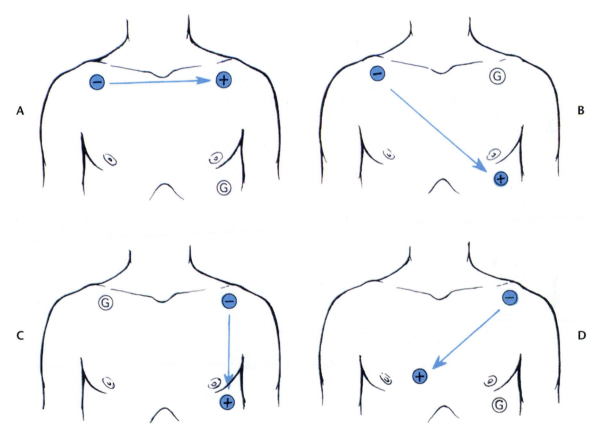

Fig. 14-16   A, Lead I placement. B, Lead II placement. C, Lead III placement. D, Lead MCL₁ placement.

3. A flat ST segment followed by a T wave of normal contour and configuration.

In a typical prehospital situation, the ECG tracing is monitored in one of four leads. Three electrodes are placed on the patient: positive, negative, and ground. Depending on the lead position, either lead I, lead II, lead III, or lead MCL₁ may be monitored (Fig. 14-16).

Routinely, lead II most commonly is used for continuous patient monitoring in the prehospital setting. This single lead shows the rate and regularity of the heartbeat—it does NOT give information about the pumping capability of the heart or the presence/location of MI. The MCL1 lead also is used in some jurisdictions, and local protocols should be followed.

Electrocardiogram analysis

 Identify each of the following cardiac rhythms on an oscilloscope monitor: normal sinus rhythm, sinus bradycardia, sinus tachycardia, premature ventricular contractions, ventricular tachycardia, ventricular fibrillation, and asystole.

There are two commonly used methods to analyze ECG tracings. One method is to observe the rhythm directly on the monitor screen or oscilloscope. In this manner the basic rhythm usually can be identified, but it may be difficult to ascertain details such as PR segment measurement or QRS complex duration. The other method is to print out a rhythm strip on paper. In this way the specific ECG components can be measured and plotted.

Dysrhythmias

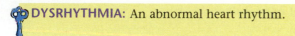 **DYSRHYTHMIA:** An abnormal heart rhythm.

The EMT–I MUST be able to recognize sinus rhythm, PVCs, and life-threatening dysrhythmias (VT, VF, asystole, and PEA). There are many other dysrhythmias that are beyond the scope of this text. As an introduction, a summary is presented of the major points to consider when evaluating an ECG rhythm.

The EMT–I should approach each ECG rhythm in a logical and systematic manner using the steps listed below every time he or she interprets an ECG rhythm. If a dysrhythmia is present, this finding should be compared with the EMT–I's assessment of the patient. This will determine the significance of the dysrhythmia and assist in any decision regarding patient treatment.

Step 1: Evaluate the rate
Several methods are available to calculate the heart rate. The following are most practical for use in the prehospital setting.

Method 1: Identify a 6-second interval on the ECG paper by identifying two 3-second marks at the top of the ECG paper. Count the number of QRS complexes and multiply by 10. This number will be the estimated heart rate per minute (Fig. 14-17).

Method 2: Locate an R wave on the dark line of a large box on the ECG paper. Give numbers to the next six dark lines to the right in the following order: 300, 150, 100, 75, 60, and 50. The line (and corresponding number) closest to the next R wave is an approximation of the heart rate per minute (Fig. 14-18).

Note: This method is accurate only if the rhythm is regular.

Step 2: Evaluate the rhythm
Measure the R-R interval (ventricular rate), and determine if it is regular. Is there an occasional irregular beat or is there a pattern of irregular beats? Is it "irregularly irregular" in which there is no relationship between the R-R intervals? Also measure the P-P interval (atrial rate). Determine if it is regular and constant.

Step 3: Evaluate the P waves
First and foremost, are P waves present? Are they regular, and is one present before every QRS complex? Are they upright or inverted as compared with the QRS complex? Do they all look the same? A normal, rounded P wave indicates that the impulse has originated in the SA node and denotes a "sinus" rhythm.

Step 4: Evaluate the PR interval
Measure the PR interval. Is it within the range of 0.12 and 0.20 seconds? Is the interval constant?

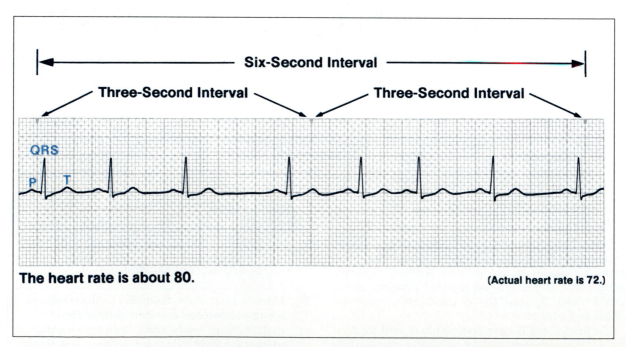

Fig. 14-17 The patient's heart rate can be estimated by counting the number of QRS complexes in a 3 or 6 second period and then multiplying by 20 or 10, respectively.

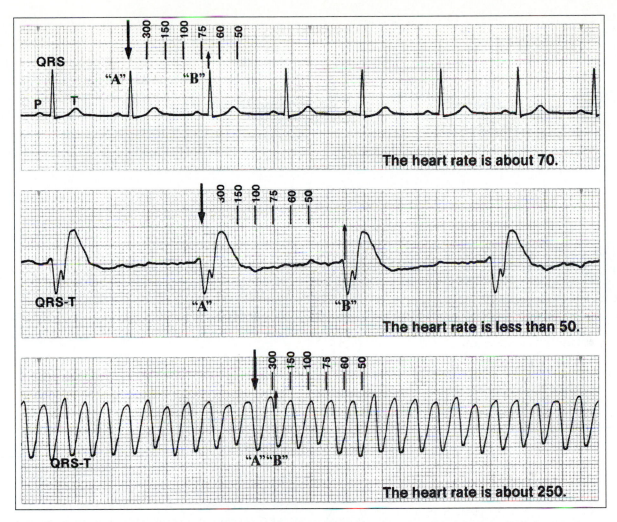

Fig. 14-18   The patient's heart rate can also be estimated by locating an R wave on a dark line and assigning the proceeding dark lines 300, 150, 100, 75, 60, and 50 until a second R wave is located.

Step 5: Evaluate the QRS complex

Are all complexes alike? Measure the QRS complex. Is it less than 0.12 seconds in duration?

Note: The rhythm is only considered "normal" sinus when these above standards are met.

Sometimes other markings are present on the ECG tracing that are not related to the heart's electrical activity. These are known as artifacts and can be caused by patient movement, shivering, muscle tremors, or 60-cycle current interference. In addition, the electrodes may be loose or improperly placed, the machine may not be functioning properly, or electrical interference may be present. Before finalizing the ECG interpretation, the EMT–I should reassess the patient and inspect the ECG machine. This step is especially important before treating potentially lethal dysrhythmias (Fig. 14-19).

Normal sinus rhythm

Normal sinus rhythm (NSR) (Fig. 14-20) is a heart rate of 60 to 100 beats per minute (BPM) in an adult. Each P wave is followed by a normal QRS complex, which is then followed by a normal T wave. Rates less than 60 BPM are bradycardias, and those greater than 100 BPM are tachycardias. If a P wave is followed by a normal QRS and T wave, as in normal sinus rhythm, a rate less than 60 BPM is called sinus bradycardia (Fig. 14-21), and a rate greater than 100 is called sinus tachycardia (Fig. 14-22).

Under most conditions, patients should be in normal sinus rhythm. Following exercise or with pain, fear, or excitement, persons often develop a slight sinus tachycardia (110 to 120 BPM). Rates over 120 BPM in an adult may indicate some type of underlying illness, such as blood loss or a heart or lung problem.

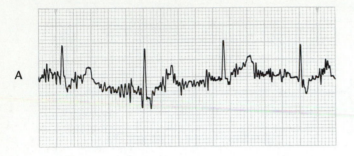

A

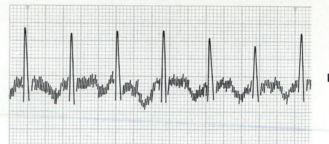

B

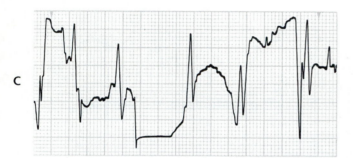

C

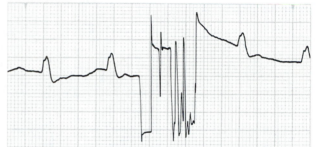

D

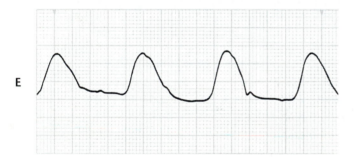

E

Fig. 14-19 A, ECG reading as a result of a muscle tremor. B, ECG reading as a result of AC interference. C, ECG reading as a result of loose electrodes. D, ECG reading as a result of biotelemetry-related interference. E, ECG reading as a result of external chest compressions.

Treatment of patients experiencing sinus tachycardia is directed toward correcting the underlying cause. Similarly, persons who are aerobically conditioned often have slower than usual heart rates (40 to 50 BPM). However, if a patient is symptomatic (eg, short of breath, chest pain, dizziness), the EMT–I should consider the presence of sinus bradycardia to be abnormal and potentially significant. Patients experiencing symptomatic bradycardia (chest pain, hypotension, etc.) should receive high-concentration oxygen, an IV lifeline of normal saline administered at KVO rate, and prompt treatment. Some EMT-Is may be permitted to administer atropine (a drug used to speed the heart rate) at a dose of 0.5 to 1.0 mg, IV push.

Premature ventricular complexes
Premature ventricular complexes (PVCs) (Fig. 14-23) are extra beats originating from the ventricle, which interrupt the normal rhythm. On the monitor, a wide, usually bizarre-looking QRS complex is seen, which is NOT preceded by a P wave. It appears earlier in the cycle than the normal set of complexes would be expected to occur. Following each PVC is a pause, sometimes called a compensatory pause.

Sometimes, PVCs all originate from one place in the ventricle. These beats look the same and are referred to as uniform (unifocal) PVCs. Other times, PVCs arise in several areas of the ventricles. These

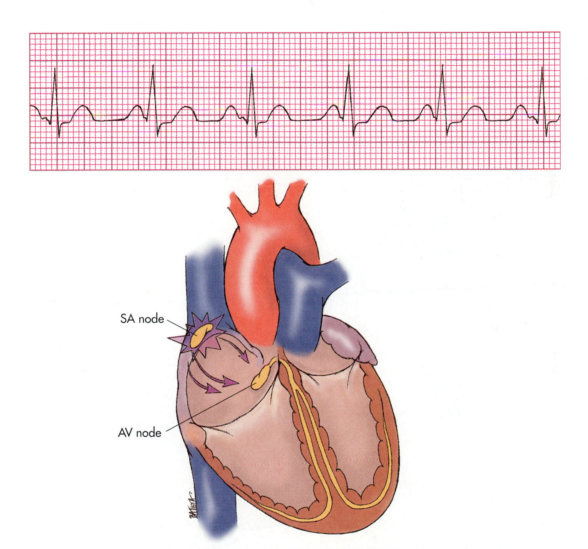

Fig. 14-20   A normal sinus rhythm is composed of a heart rate of 60-100 BPM, a P wave, a normal QRS complex, and a normal T wave.

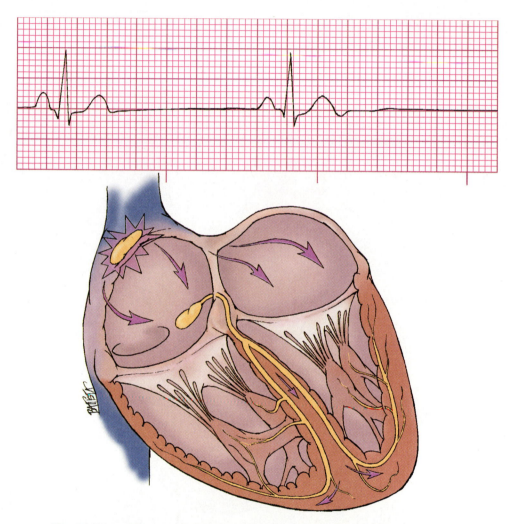

Fig. 14-21 Sinus bradycardia is composed of a heart rate less than 60 BPM, a P wave, a normal QRS complex, and a normal T wave.

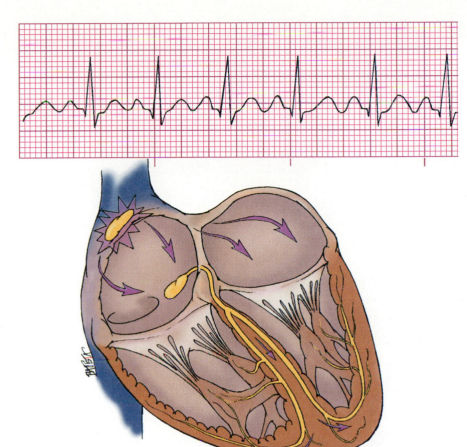

Fig. 14-22   Sinus tachycardia is composed of a heart rate greater than 100 BPM, a P wave, a normal QRS complex, and a normal T wave.

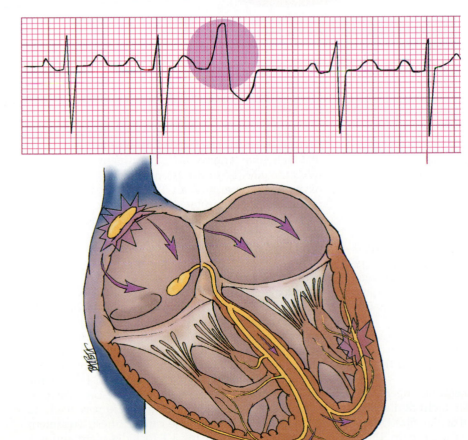

Fig. 14-23   Premature ventricular complexes lack P waves and have wide QRS complexes followed by a pause.

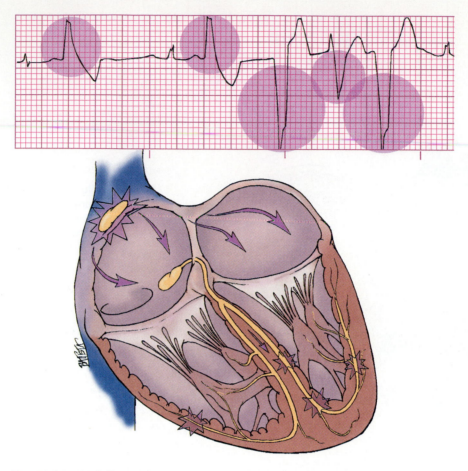

Fig. 14-24 Multiformed PVCs appear differently because they arise from several areas of the ventricle.

beats tend to appear different from each other and are called multiformed (multifocal) PVCs (Fig. 14-24).

PVCs may occur singly or more frequently. PVCs that are interspersed between normal beats are named depending on their frequency. Bigeminal PVCs are said to be present when every other beat is a PVC, regardless if unifocal or multifocal. If every third beat is a PVC, the condition is called trigeminal PVCs or ventricular trigeminy. Similarly, a PVC every fourth beat is ventricular quadrigeminy. Regular PVCs at greater intervals than every fourth beat have no special name and are simply referred to as frequent PVCs (Fig. 14-25).

PVCs may occur one after the other. Two PVCs in a row are a couplet or pair. Three or more PVCs in a row constitute an abnormal rhythm known as ventricular tachycardia (Fig. 14-26).

Frequent PVCs, especially if bigeminal, trigeminal, or couplets or runs of ventricular tachycardia may forecast the development of ventricular fibrillation. The EMT–I should pay special attention to these rhythm disturbances in persons with acute myocardial ischemia (angina, MI). Treatment of frequent PVCs includes administration of high-concentration oxygen, placement of an IV lifeline, and prompt transport. Some protocols may allow the EMT–I to administer lidocaine by IV push and continue maintenance infusion. (*See* First-Line Cardiac Drugs, this chapter.)

Ventricular tachycardia

Ventricular tachycardia (VT) (Fig. 14-27) is three or more PVCs in a row. It may come in bursts of 6 to 10 complexes or may persist (sustained VT). Typically, P waves are not discernable; the rhythm consists of frequent wide and bizarre QRS complexes at a rate of 150 to 220 BPM. T waves may or may not be present.

Clinically, VT is ALWAYS significant. Even if the rhythm results in a pulse, it should be considered as potentially UNSTABLE, *ie*, patients are very likely to develop worse rhythms and cardiac arrest. Treatment of a patient experiencing VT includes maintaining a

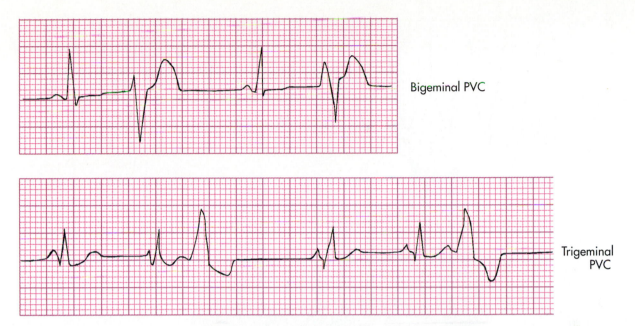

Fig. 14-25 PVCs present after every other beat are bigeminal PVCs. If every third beat is a PVC, the result is trigeminal PVC or ventricular trigeminy.

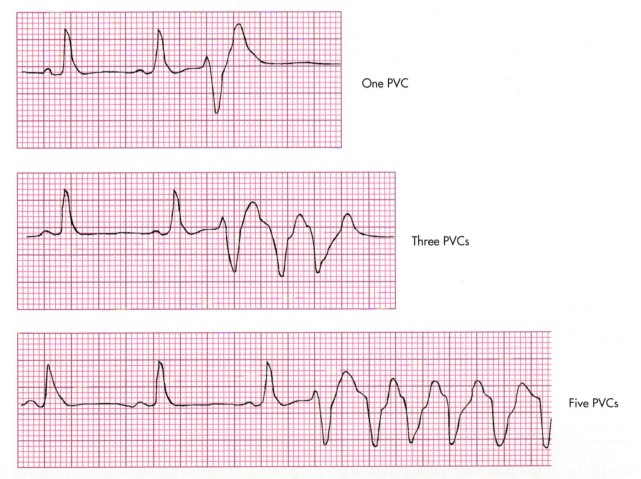

Fig. 14-26 PVCs can appear singularly, or many times. Three or more PVCs in a row are called ventricular tachycardia.

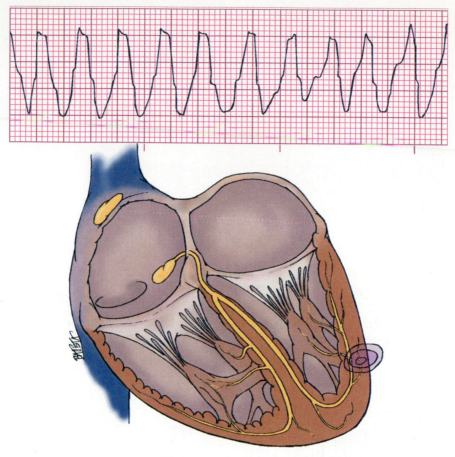

Fig. 14-27 Ventricular tachycardia may come in bursts of 6 to 10 PVC, or may persist.

patent airway, administering high-concentration oxygen, placing an IV lifeline, and prompt transport. Some protocols may allow the EMT–I to administer lidocaine at a dose of 1 to 1.5 mg/kg IV push. (*See* First- Line Cardiac Drugs, this chapter.) Patients with pulseless VT should be treated as though they are in ventricular fibrillation.

Ventricular fibrillation
Ventricular fibrillation (VF) (Fig. 14-28) is erratic firing of multiple sites in the ventricle. VF causes the heart muscle to wiggle, much like a handful of worms, rather than contracting efficiently. Within 10 seconds, the amount of blood pumped by the heart is essentially zero and unresponsiveness ensues. If the patient is not promptly treated (with defibrillation), death occurs. On the cardiac monitor, VF appears like a wavy line, undulating without logic. VF is the most common cause of prehospital cardiac arrest in adults.

Treatment includes prompt initiation of CPR and defibrillation, endotracheal intubation, placement of an IV of normal saline (in the antecubated fosse) and hemoport. Some protocols allow the EMT–I to pro-

vide advanced level care including administration of epinephrine (1.0 mg IV push every 3 to 5 minutes), repeat defibrillation administration of lidocaine (1.5 mg/kg IV push; repeat in 3 to 5 minutes to a total of 3 mg/kg) and repeat defibrillation.

 CLINICAL NOTES
The treatment of choice for pulseless ventricular tachycardia or ventricular fibrillation is prompt defibrillation.

Asystole

 ASYSTOLE: The absence of any electrical activity in the heart.

Asystole is the absence of any cardiac activity. Asystole appears as a flat (or nearly flat) line on the monitor screen. It is a terminal rhythm, and once a person has become asystolic, the chances of recovery are extremely low.

Many nonmedical conditions, such as misplacement of a lead or a loose wire, can mimic asystole (or VF) on the monitor screen. Before concluding that a

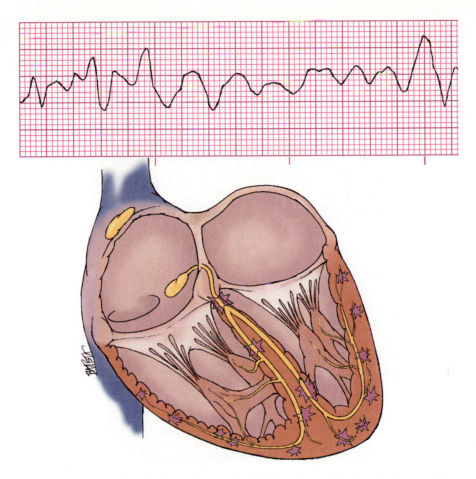

Fig. 14-28   Ventricular fibrillation is an erratic firing of multiple sites in the ventricles.

patient is actually in asystole, the EMT–I must assess for mechanical causes of this appearance on the monitor. If a patient is in cardiac arrest and appears to be in asystole, the EMT–I should check the following:

- Make sure all the leads are attached in the proper places to both the machine and the patient.

- Make sure the correct lead (eg I, II, III) is selected on the monitor.

- Check the rhythm in more than one lead.

- Make sure that the monitor batteries are functioning appropriately.

Treatment of asystole includes prompt initiation of CPR, endotracheal intubation, placement of an IV lifeline (in the antecubated fosse), and prompt transport. Some protocols may allow the EMT–I to administer epinephrine (1.0 mg, IV push, every 3 to 5 minutes) and atropine (1 mg, IV push, every 3 to 5 minutes to a total of 0.04 mg/kg).

Pulseless electrical activity (PEA) (Fig. 14-29) is a condition where there is a rhythm noted on the monitor that SHOULD result in adequate perfusion, but the patient is pulseless and apneic. In other words, there is electrical activity in the heart that is NOT appropriately converted to effective cardiac contraction.

This condition often is associated with severe underlying heart disease but the EMT–I should always consider the reversible causes of PEA:

- Hypovolemia (most common)

- Tension pneumothorax

- Hypoxia

- Pericardial tamponade

In consideration of these possibilities, many experts recommend a fluid bolus, in addition to high-concentration oxygen, CPR, and drugs (epinephrine and atropine), as part of the initial treatment for PEA. The EMT–I should follow his or her local protocols.

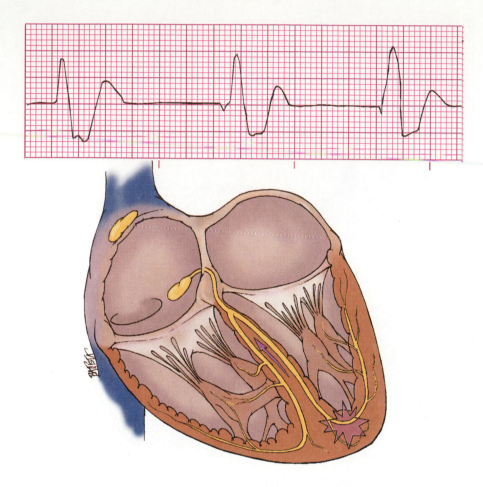

Fig. 14-29 An example of bradycardiac pulseless electrical activity.

GENERAL PRINCIPLES OF DEFIBRILLATION

 DEFIBRILLATION: An electrical shock delivered to the heart in order to restore an effective rhythm.

 List the rationale for early defibrillation and describe the most common electrical disturbance resulting in cardiac arrest.

Defibrillation is the delivery of an electrical shock to the heart in an attempt to terminate life-threatening rhythm disturbances such as ventricular fibrillation and pulseless ventricular tachycardia. By depolarizing a certain mass ("critical mass") of myocardium, it may restore an effective rhythm. Defibrillation also is referred to as unsynchronized countershock or asynchronous cardioversion.

Successful defibrillation depends on a number of factors including duration of time from onset of fibrillation, transthoracic resistance, energy output, and paddle placement. The paddles must make good contact with the skin, and adequate conductive gel, paste, or pads must be present. The operator should apply approximately 25 lbs of firm arm pressure to the paddles to optimize defibrillation.

The earlier that defibrillation is applied following the onset of VF, the more likely it is to be successful. In cases of witnessed VF (or VT without a pulse) in which a defibrillator is immediately available, the EMT–I should defibrillate prior to initiating CPR.

Resistance to passage of the countershock caused by the tissues of the chest is referred to as *transthoracic resistance*. The greater the transthoracic resistance, the less energy delivered to the heart. Factors that influence transthoracic resistance include delivered energy, electrode size, interface between the chest wall and the electrodes, the number and time interval between previous shocks, pressure applied to the electrodes, the phase of the patient's ventilation, and the distance between electrodes.

AUTOMATED EXTERNAL DEFIBRILLATION

Introduction

Because the early treatment of VF is crucial, several manufacturers have developed **automated external defibrillators (AEDs)**. The EMT–I does NOT need to be able to interpret cardiac rhythms to use an AED. Once properly attached to the patient, these devices automatically analyze the heart rhythm and electronically determine if VF is present If so, they will either automatically defibrillate the patient or advise the EMT–I to push a button, causing the machine to defibrillate the patient.

Types of automated external defibrillators

There are two types of AEDs (Fig. 14-30):

- Fully automatic defibrillators—These devices analyze the patient's cardiac rhythm, decide whether or not defibrillation is warranted, and automatically (after warning the operator) deliver a shock when appropriate.

- Semiautomatic defibrillators (also called shock advisory defibrillators)—These analyze the patient's rhythm and decide if a shock is warranted. If so, they advise the EMT–I of this fact. The EMT–I must actually push a button before the device will deliver a defibrillatory shock to the patient.

Each model operates differently. The EMT–I should follow the manufacturer's instructions for the use of each device.

Protocol for automated external defibrillation

The guidelines given here are generic in nature because each device operates differently. The EMT–I MUST be familiar with the operating features of his or her particular AED.

To use any AED, the EMT–I should perform the following basic steps:

- Recognize that the patient is in cardiac arrest.
- Prepare and attach the defibrillator pads or electrodes.
- Turn on the AED.
- Push the "analyze" button on the AED.
- Deliver the shock if indicated. The device will either automatically deliver a shock or instruct the operator (via audible and visible signals) to "Shock."

 List the indications for automated external defibrillation.

Many patients with cardiac arrest in the prehospital setting will have VF. If paramedic-level care is not immediately available, the MOST important thing

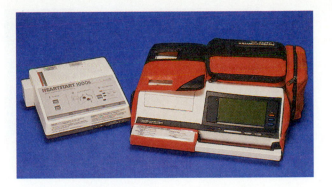

Fig. 14-30 Automated external defibrillators can be either fully automatic (left) or semiautomatic (right).

the EMT–I can do is to attach the AED and analyze the rhythm. If two or more EMT–Is are present, one should apply and operate the AED. The second EMT–I should perform CPR. If only one EMT–I is present, he or she should first verify cardiac arrest, then immediately apply the AED. Defibrillation should NOT be delayed to set up oxygen, IV lines, mechanical CPR devices, or other forms of care. Ideally, these preparations should proceed at the same time if sufficient personnel are available.

 Describe the proper steps for patient evaluation, placement, and use of an automated external defibrillator.

The EMT–I's first goal when providing care for a patient with cardiac arrest is to use the AED to quickly analyze for the presence of a dysrhythmia that is treatable by an electrical shock. After determining that a patient is in cardiac arrest (Fig. 14-31 A), the EMT–I should perform the following:

1. Place the AED close to the patient's left ear. If possible, perform all defibrillation protocols from the patient's left side. Some EMS systems have adopted different operator and device positions with equal success. Follow local protocols.

2. Turn on the power by either pressing the "power switch" or lifting up the monitor screen. At this point, the recording device is automatically activated (Fig. 14-31 B).

3. Open the adhesive defibrillation pads, attach them first to the cables, then to the patient's chest. Place one pad (right, or sternal) to the right of the sternum with the top edge at the bottom of the clavicle. Place the other (left, or apex) pad in the lower left chest, in the anterior axillary line (Fig. 14-31 C).

4. As soon as the pads are attached, stop CPR.

5. Push the "analyze" button. Most devices take between 5 and 15 seconds to interpret the rhythm. DO NOT touch or move the patient during the analysis phase (Fig. 14-31 D).

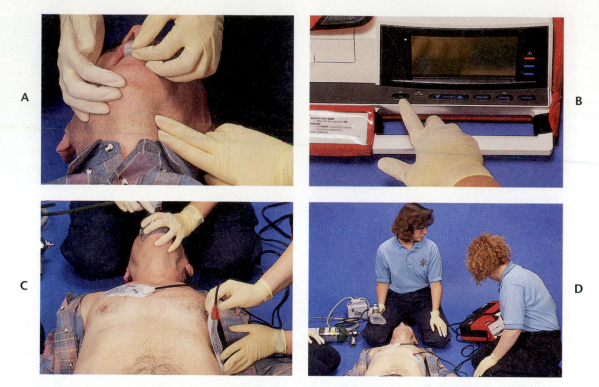

Fig. 14-31   Operating an AED. A, Perform an initial assessment to confirm cardiac arrest. B, Activate the device. C, Attach the electrodes and pads to the patient with the white electrode just below the clavicle and to the right of the sternum. The red electrode pad should be placed on the lower in the anterior axillary line. D, If the AED advises to shock, state loudly "clear" and push the "shock" button. Deliver the number of shocks indicated, up to three.

6. If VF or pulseless VT is present, the device will note that a shock is indicated. Depending on the model, this notification may consist of a written message on the display screen, an audible alarm, a voice-synthesized statement, or a combination of these. At this point, immediately state loudly, "Clear," so that no one is in contact with the patient when the shock is delivered.

7. If no shock is indicated, the patient does not have an electrically treatable rhythm. Check the pulse, and if the patient remains pulseless, continue CPR and transport to the hospital.

8. Automated devices will charge the capacitors and deliver a shock shortly after they have analyzed the rhythm to be VF or pulseless VT. A semiautomatic model will advise to push the "Shock" button to deliver a shock. The shock produces a sudden contraction of the patient's muscles.

9. DO NOT restart CPR or check for a pulse after the first shock is delivered. Instead, immediately press the "analyze" control. If the patient remains in a shockable rhythm, the device will again indicate that a shock is indicated. If indicated, proceed with delivery of a second shock.

10. If no shock is indicated, the patient does not have an electrically treatable rhythm. Check the pulse; if the patient remains pulseless, continue CPR, provide advanced life support according to local protocol (eg, IV, endotracheal intubation, first-line cardic drugs) and transport to the hospital.

11. Following the second shock, DO NOT resume CPR or check for a pulse. Instead, immediately press the "analyze" control If the patient remains in a shockable rhythm, the device will again indicate that a shock is indicated. If indicated, proceed with delivery of a third shock.

12. If no shock is indicated, the patient does not have an electrically treatable rhythm. Check the pulse; if the patient remains pulseless, continue CPR, provide advanced life support according to local protocol (eg, IV, endotracheal intubation, first-line cardic drugs) and transport to the hospital.

13. Use 200 joules (J) for the first shock, 200 to 300 J for the second shock, and up to 360 J for the third shock. Most currently available units will automatically set the required energy level.

14. Following the third shock, immediately perform CPR for 1 minute. After 1 minute of CPR, check for a pulse. If a pulse is present, monitor the patient, provide care as indicated, and transport to the hospital as soon as possible.

15. If the patient does not have a pulse following the third shock, provide advanced life support according to local protocol (eg, IV, endotracheal intubation, first-line cardic drugs) after 1 minute of CPR, immediately press the "analyze" button. Repeat sets of up to three "stacked" shocks, followed by 1 minute of CPR, as indicated. Follow the same guidelines as previously listed for the first series of shocks.

16. If a patient who initially develops a perfusing rhythm following defibrillation then re-arrests, start the analysis sequence again from the top of the algorithm.

To summarize, in the absence of paramedic-level care, if the EMT–I has an AED and is trained to use it, he or she should do the following:

1. Immediately apply the device to the patient in apparent cardiac arrest.

2. Always shock in sets of not more than three, as advised by the AED. If the first or second shock is successful, it is NOT necessary to give all three shocks.

3. The only time the EMT–I should touch the patient's chest following the initial assessment is to perform CPR for 1 minute.

4. Continue to shock in sets of up to three, as advised, followed by 1 minute of CPR (and the provision of appropriate advanced life-support problems) until the device confirms that no shock is indicated.

 List the contraindications for automated external defibrillation

Precautions for automated external defibrillation
Defibrillators do not discriminate—both the patient AND the EMT–I can be shocked if these devices are used inappropriately. The EMT–I should be certain to clear the area prior to delivery of a shock.

Defibrillation is of much less significance in pediatric arrest, in which VF is unlikely. Currently available AEDs should not be used in pediatric cardiac arrest, because they cannot deliver the appropriate amount of energy. Most experts also recommend that AEDs not be used in patients (adult or child) weighing less than 90 lbs. The EMT–I should follow local protocols and/or medical direction.

MANUAL DEFIBRILLATION

 Describe the proper steps for patient evaluation and administration of manual defibrillation.

Performing manual defibrillation
Prior to defibrillation, the EMT–I should place defibrillation pads on the patient's chest or apply conductive gel to the paddles. Resistance is very high if the metal electrodes are bare. All surfaces of the paddles should be touching the patient's skin. The EMT–I should push down with 20 to 25 lbs. of firm arm pressure. Resistance is also lower when the patient's phase of ventilation is at full expiration.

For defibrillation of VF and pulseless VT, the EMT–I should use up to three successive shocks at 200, 200 to 300, and 360 J, respectively. The EMT–I should use 360 J for subsequent shocks, which also may be delivered in sets of three. These "stacked shocks" are thought to decrease transthoracic resistance. In children begin with an initial dose of 2 J/kg. If repeat shocks are necessary, set the defibrillator at 4 J/kg.

Two commonly used positions for paddle placement are the standard and anterior-posterior positions. **Standard placement** calls for one defibrillator paddle to be placed to the right of the upper sternum just below the right clavicle, the other just to the left of the nipple in the midaxillary line (Fig. 14-32). With **anterior-posterior placement**, one paddle is positioned anteriorly, just to the left of the sternal border, and the other positioned behind the heart.

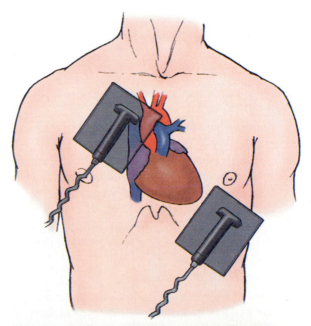

Fig. 14-32 Standard placement of defibrillator paddles calls for one paddle to be placed to the right of the upper sternum and the other to the left of the nipple in the midaxillary line.

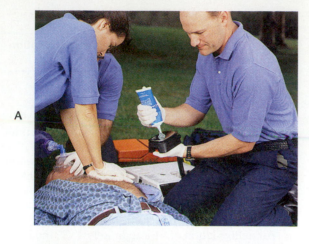
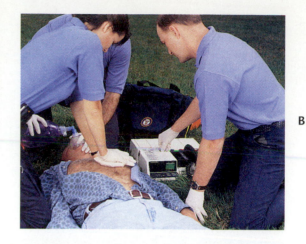
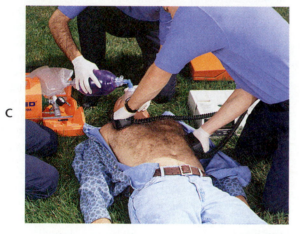
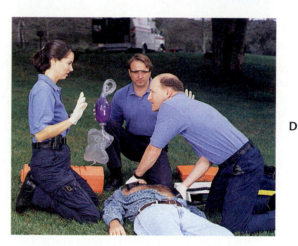

Fig. 14-33 A, Apply gel pads to the patient's chest or conductive gel to the defibrillator paddles. B, Select the appropriate energy level and charge the defibrillator. C, Apply the paddles to the correct locations on the chest with firm arm pressure. D, State "Stand clear" and verify that no one is touching the patient.

To defibrillate a patient, the EMT–I should do the following:

1. Prepare the equipment and bare the patient's chest.

2. Apply gel pads to the patient's chest or conductive gel to the defibrillator paddles (Fig. 14-33 A).

3. Select the appropriate energy level and charge the defibrillator (Fig. 14-33 B).

4. Apply the paddles to the correct locations on the chest with approximately 25 lbs of firm arm pressure (Fig. 14-33 C).

5. Reverify the dysrhythmia.

6. Instruct everyone to "stand clear," and make sure not to come in contact with the patient. Look in both directions to verify that no one is touching the patient or the stretcher (Fig. 14-33 D).

7. Depress the buttons on both paddles simultaneously to deliver the shock.

8. Observe the rhythm after the defibrillation.

9. If the rhythm changes, or following three sequential shocks, check the carotid pulse.

DO NOT stop to check the pulse between defibrillatory shocks if the monitor still shows VF.

If the patient has an automatic implantable cardioverter defibrillator or an implanted pacemaker, defibrillator paddles or self-adhesive electrodes should be placed at least 5 inches from the device. The EMT–I can identify the location of these devices by a visible scar on the chest or abdominal wall as well as by palpation.

If the patient has a NTG patch in place, it should be removed prior to defibrillation. The electrical current can cause the patch to explode and burn the patient.

 HELPFUL HINT

The EMT–I must remove NTG patches prior to performing defibrillation.

Safety and operational considerations

When defibrillating a patient, the EMT–I should keep the following additional precautions in mind:

- On an ongoing basis, check the batteries and defibrillator unit for proper operation.

- Make sure the electrode pads, if used, have not expired. Otherwise they may be dried out.

- Make sure that the paddles are clean from the last use.

- If using conductive gel or paste, make certain that the paddles are adequately coated.

- Make sure everyone is clear of the patient, including the operator, before delivering the countershock. Say "stand clear" loudly, and look around prior to discharging the defibrillator.

- Use extreme caution when defibrillating patients who are wet or in contact with metal. If unable to move them, be certain that no one else, including the operator, is in contact with the moisture or metal.

- Double-check the rhythm before delivering a countershock to ensure that the patient has not reverted to another rhythm.

- Make sure the synchronized mode is turned off when defibrillating VF.

- If the rhythm changes, or following three sequential shocks, check the carotid pulse.

FIRST-LINE CARDIAC DRUGS

 Summarize the general uses for each of the following agents in acute cardiac care: epinephrine, lidocaine, and atropine.

Introduction

An EMT–I may be called on to administer or to assist a paramedic-level provider in the administration of medications. The three drugs commonly used in acute cardiac emergencies are epinephrine, lidocaine, and atropine. The EMT–I should always follow local protocols when handling or assisting in the handling of any medication.

Epinephrine

Epinephrine, or **adrenaline,** is the most common drug used in treatment of cardiac arrest. It is indicated in all types of arrest (VF, pulseless VT, asystole, PEA) and in many life-threatening dysrhythmias. Administration of epinephrine raises the aortic diastolic pressure. The coronary artery perfusion pressure is the difference between the aortic diastolic pressure and the central venous pressure. Thus, epinephrine increases coronary perfusion pressure and increases a patient's chances of resuscitation from a cardiac arrest.

During a cardiac arrest, epinephrine usually is given intravenously, although it also may be administered via an endotracheal tube. In an adult, the initial IV dose is 1 mg. Repeat doses are given every 3 to 5 minutes, depending on the patient's response. Current American Heart Association guidelines allow for much flexibility in the amount of epinephrine given in repeat doses, so the EMT–I should follow local protocols.

Lidocaine

Lidocaine is an antidysrhythmic drug, which is administered to treat ventricular dysrhythmias (frequent PVCs, VT, VF). It stabilizes the cardiac membrane and decreases the frequency of rhythm problems. In cardiac arrest, the FIRST treatment of cardiac rhythm problems is defibrillation. Next is the placement of an endotracheal tube, IV line, and administration of epinephrine. Lidocaine is then only used when electrical shock fails or following successful defibrillation, to prevent recurrence. In a cardiac arrest, administration of lidocaine may increase the chances of the heart responding to subsequent electrical shocks.

In cardiac arrest, the dose of lidocaine is 1 to 1.5 mg/kg IV push. This dose may be repeated every 3 to 5 minutes to a maximum of 3 mg/kg. In frequent PVCs and ventricular tachycardic with a pulse associated with myocardial infarction, lidocaine may be given at a dose of 1.5 mg/kg and repeated in 0.5 to 0.75 mg/kg boluses every 5 to 10 minutes to a maxium of 3 mg/kg. A maintenance infusion of lidocaine at a dose of 2 to 4 mg per minute should be delivered following successful conversion of VF or pulseless VT. This maintenance infusion may also be used to maintain therapeutic levels of lidocaine when given in the treatment of PVCs and VT with a pulse.

Atropine

Atropine blocks discharge from the parasympathetic nervous system, leading to an increase in the heart rate. Indications include:
- Hemodynamically significant bradycardias
- Asystole

The initial dose of atropine is 0.5 to 1.0 mg IV push, unless the patient is in cardiac arrest, then the initial dose is 1.0 mg IV. Doses of atropine may be repeated every 3 to 5 minutes to a maximum dose of 0.04 mg/kg (approximately 3 mg in the average 70-kg person). Atropine may also be administered endotracheally at 2 to 2.5 mg.

CASE HISTORY FOLLOW-UP

After starting the IV and completing the history and physical examination, EMT–I Adams contacts medical direction for orders:

Continued

"MedCom, this is Metro 24, we have a 73-year-old male with chest pain and shortness of breath. The onset was approximately 30 minutes prior to our arrival, and the patient had taken two nitro [nitroglycerin] tabs SL [sublingually] without relief. The pain is squeezing, in the left anterior retrosternal region, and radiates to his left arm.

"His past medical history includes an acute MI 2 months ago, and several recent episodes of CHF, which required emergency transportation and ICU hospitalizations. He also has a past medical history of emphysema and uses a bronchodilator.

"He is responsive, alert, and oriented and in moderate distress. His vital signs are pulse 86 and irregular, respirations 26 and labored, with posterior-inferior bilateral crackles; BP is 156/96. He had central cyanosis on arrival; however, his color has improved with high-flow oxygen administration via nonrebreather mask.

"His ECG rhythm is normal sinus rhythm with approximately nine PVCs per minute and pulse deficits. His pulse oxygen reading is 88%.

"We started an IV of normal saline and are running it at a KVO rate. Do you have any further orders?"

Medical direction responds:

"Metro 24: Check the date of expiration of his nitro, and you can go ahead and give him one of yours. Contact us if his condition changes; we'll be waiting for you."

The oxygen, nitroglycerin, and reassuring care the EMT–Is provide for Mr. Molino give him some symptomatic relief.

SUMMARY

Cardiovascular disease is a common cause of medical problems. The most common symptom of cardiac disease is chest pain. During the initial patient assessment, the EMT–Is should immediately determine if the patient has a pulse. If the patient is in cardiac arrest, CPR should be started. In patients more than 12 years of age and weighing more than 90 lbs, the AED also should be applied.

If the patient is responsive, the EMT–I should take an appropriate history. If he or she complains of cardiac pain and has previously prescribed nitroglycerin, you may assist in the administration of this drug. Follow your local protocols and obtain permission from medical control prior to giving any drug.

Angina is an attack of chest pain and related symptoms due to lack of oxygen in the heart muscle. Various stresses may produce ischemia to the myocardium such as exercise, cold, or emotion. The underlying lesion in angina, as well as in MI, is an atherosclerotic plaque that narrows the lumen of the coronary artery.

Patients with angina complain of substernal chest pain. The discomfort may radiate to the epigastrium, arms, jaw, teeth, or neck. Other symptoms such as diaphoresis, shortness of breath, and nausea may be present. Anginal pain goes away with rest or with the administration of NTG.

A heart attack (or acute MI) occurs when the blood flow through a coronary artery is completely blocked. A thrombus occludes an artery whose lumen has already been narrowed by an atherosclerotic plaque. Cigarette smoking is the major risk factor for development of MI.

The pain of MI typically lasts more than 15 minutes. Patients often look pale and ill. It is common for heart attack victims to deny the severity of their illness. Elderly patients may not complain of chest pain; they are more likely to simply have weakness or shortness of breath. Complications of acute MI include cardiac arrest, CHF, and cardiogenic shock.

Cardiogenic shock occurs when greater than 40% of the myocardium is unable to effectively pump blood. The most common cause is acute MI, although other conditions, such as a ruptured valve, also may lead to shock. The blood pressure may be high, low, or normal. The EMT–I should NOT rely on the presence of hypotension to make a diagnosis of cardiogenic shock.

The EMT–I should care for patients suspected of experiencing MI with high-concentration oxygen, placement of a IV, monitoring the ECG rhythm, and transport in as calm and quiet a manner as possible. "Emergency mode" transport should not be used unless the patient's condition deteriorates. If the patient is in cardiogenic shock, an IV fluid bolus should be administered if mandated by local protocols.

Congestive heart failure is circulatory congestion due to inadequate flow of blood. CHF is caused by heart muscle damage. The most severe form is acute pulmonary edema. The most common cause of CHF is coronary artery disease. Both right-sided and left-sided CHF may occur.

Patients with CHF have shortness of breath, which is worse on lying down (orthopnea) and may awaken the patient at night (paroxysmal nocturnal dyspnea). Diaphoresis, cyanosis, and edema also may be present. Distention of the neck veins and hypertension are common. Hypotension in a patient with acute pulmonary edema is a serious sign, and these patients tend to deteriorate rapidly.

Aneurysm of the aorta commonly occurs in the abdomen (abdominal aortic aneurysm) and in the thoracic aorta (dissecting thoracic aortic aneurysm). Both types of aneurysms result in pain and may cause decreased peripheral pulses and shock. The PASG should only be used in these patients if local protocol allows.

A pulmonary embolism is the blockage of a pulmonary artery by foreign matter, usually by a blood clot that has broken loose in the veins of the pelvis and legs. This potentially lethal condition is relatively common and is often underdiagnosed. Patients may present with sudden cardiovascular collapse, pleuritic chest pain, anxiety, or shortness of breath. The EMT–I should administer high-concentration oxygen, start an IV lifeline, place the patient on a cardiac monitor, and transport to the hospital in a prompt fashion.

A hypertensive crisis is a sudden increase in the blood pressure, which results in functional disturbances of the central nervous system, heart, or kidneys. Without proper care, life-threatening complications can occur. The most common cause is an acute exacerbation of chronic hypertension. The EMT–I should consider ingestion of cocaine as a cause for hypertensive crisis in a young patient.

Patients with hypertensive crisis have markedly elevated blood pressure. Dizziness and headache may be present. If there is an alteration in the patient's level of responsiveness and pupillary abnormalities are present, the EMT–I should assume that the patient has an intracranial hemorrhage.

Palpitation is a sensation of pounding or racing of the heart. Syncope is a transient state of unresponsiveness from which the patient has recovered. Both conditions may be caused by heart disease, metabolic problems, or drugs. All patients with these symptoms should be transported to the hospital for evaluation.

The ECG is a graphic representation of the electrical activity of the heart and consists of a P wave (atrial depolarization), PR segment (delay of the electrical impulse at the AV node so blood may pass from the atria to the ventricles), QRS complex (ventricular depolarization), ST segment, and T wave (ventricular repolarization). Lead II is the most commonly used monitoring lead in the prehospital setting.

Cardiac dysrhythmias that commonly occur during cardiac arrest include VF, VT, and PEA. VF and pulseless VT are treated by administration of an electrical shock defibrillation. The EMT–I may administer this shock manually or via an AED. In either case, follow local protocols regarding indications for defibrillator use. The EMT–I should always adhere to recommended safety precautions. Defibrillators do not discriminate—they can shock the EMT–I as well as the patient.

An EMT–I may be called on to administer or to assist in the administration of cardiac drugs, especially during a cardiac arrest. Epinephrine is the most commonly used cardiac drug—it is indicated in all forms of cardiac arrest and works by improving the coronary artery perfusion. Lidocaine is an antidysrhythmic agent used in the treatment of significant ventricular dysrhythmias as a result of acute MI or myocardial ischemia. Atropine is given in an attempt to reverse excess parasympathetic nervous system tone that may perpetuate bradycardia or asystole.

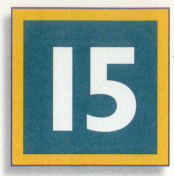

15

MEDICAL EMERGENCIES

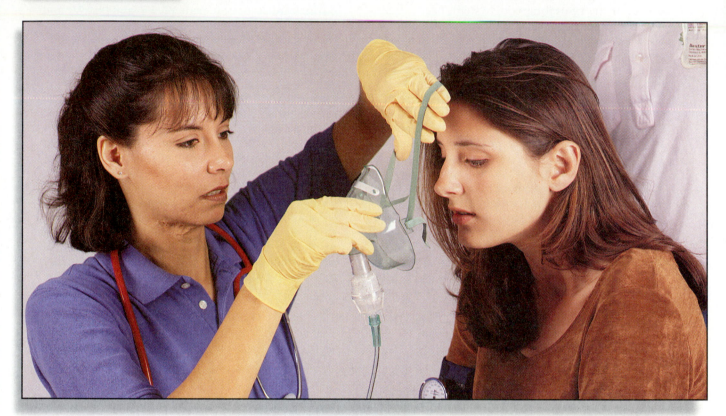

CASE HISTORY

EMT–Intermediates Stevens and Perez have been dispatched to a "man down" at a nearby park. En route, the EMT–Is are advised that a passerby witnessed a possible heart attack and called 9-1-1 via her cell phone. An Emergency Medical Dispatcher is on-line with the caller and is instructing her on how to position the patient, open his airway, and assess his breathing and circulation. The EMT–Is advise medical direction of the call and their 4-minute ETA to the scene.

On arrival, the EMT–Is find a large group of onlookers being contained by park security personnel. One of the security officers, a trained First Responder, is kneeling next to the patient and maintaining his open airway. He advises the EMT–Is that the patient is unresponsive and has shallow respirations and a rapid pulse. Another officer tells the EMT–Is that the man is a "regular" at the park. The patient is presumably homeless and often has to be removed from the park by law enforcement personnel.

Case History, continued

The middle-aged patient is pale and extremely diaphoretic. Per protocol, EMT–I Perez administers high-concentration oxygen and assists the patient's respirations while EMT–I Stevens begins the initial assessment. The physical examination is unremarkable, and the patient's vital signs are stable. The patient's ECG reveals a borderline sinus tachycardia. EMT–I Stevens makes radio contact with on-line medical direction and gives the hospital an initial patient report. Based on his general impression of the patient, EMT–I Perez requests an order for naloxone (Narcan) to rule out or reverse a possible narcotic depression.

The emergency department physician denies EMT–I Perez's request. Based on information provided in the radio report and the lack of available patient history, the physician instructs EMT–I Stevens to measure the patient's blood sugar to rule out hypoglycemia. Using a glucometer, the patient's serum glucose is measured dangerously low at 58 mg/dL. An IV is initiated, and 1 amp of 50% dextrose is administered. Immediately, the patient's respiratory status improves, and he begins to respond appropriately to verbal stimuli. The patient is packaged and made ready for transport to the emergency department.

The EMT–Is deliver the patient to the hospital and give a brief report to the emergency department nurse who will be assuming his care. The EMT–Is complete the necessary paperwork and replenish their supplies. Before leaving the hospital to return to service, the emergency department physician advises the EMT–Is that this call should be reviewed during a critique session as part of continuing education.

LEARNING OBJECTIVES

Upon completion of this chapter, the EMT–Intermediate should be able to:

- DESCRIBE the pathophysiology of anaphylactic shock.
- LIST the common signs and symptoms of anaphylactic shock.
- DESCRIBE the treatment of anaphylaxis.
- DESCRIBE the pathophysiology of asthma.
- DESCRIBE the signs and symptoms of asthma and list those that indicate a very serious condition.
- IDENTIFY the treatment for a patient experiencing an acute asthma attack.
- DEFINE the term *status asthmaticus.*
- LIST three priorities of care for COPD.
- IDENTIFY five conditions that may cause hyperventilation.
- DESCRIBE the care given to patients who hyperventilate.
- RECALL three patients who are at risk for pulmonary embolism.
- IDENTIFY four signs and symptoms of pulmonary embolism.
- DESCRIBE the mechanism of spontaneous pneumothorax.
- LIST five signs and symptoms of stroke.
- DESCRIBE the importance of airway management in the stroke patient.
- IDENTIFY five intracranial causes of coma.
- IDENTIFY five causes of coma that originate outside the nervous system.
- DESCRIBE the patient care priorities for coma.
- LIST four types of seizures.
- DESCRIBE the patient care priorities for seizure.
- LIST four causes of headache.
- DESCRIBE the patient care priorities for abdominal pain.
- LIST four causes of gastrointestinal bleeding.
- DESCRIBE the patient care priorities for gastrointestinal bleeding.
- DESCRIBE five signs and symptoms of hypoglycemia.
- DESCRIBE the care given to patients with hypoglycemia.
- LIST five signs and symptoms of diabetic ketoacidosis.

Continued

KEY TERMS

AEIOU-TIPS	DIABETES MELLITUS	HYPERVENTILATION
ANAPHYLACTIC SHOCK	DIABETIC KETOACIDOSIS	HYPOGLYCEMIA
ANAPHYLAXIS	EMPHYSEMA	MAST CELL
ANTIBODY	FACTS	POSTICTAL STATE
ANTIGEN	FROSTBITE	PULMONARY EMBOLISM
ASTHMA	GASTROINTESTINAL BLEEDING	SEIZURE
AURA	GRAND MAL SEIZURE	SPONTANEOUS PNEUMOTHORAX
BRONCHOSPASM	HEAT CRAMPS	STATUS ASTHMATICUS
CEREBROVASCULAR ACCIDENT	HEAT EXHAUSTION	STATUS EPILEPTICUS
CHRONIC OBSTRUCTIVE PULMONARY DISEASE(COPD)	HEAT STROKE	STROKE
	HISTAMINE	TRANSIENT ISCHEMIC ATTACK
COMA	HYPERGLYCEMIA	

INTRODUCTION

The EMT–I often will be called on to treat patients who are experiencing medical emergencies. Medical emergencies involve a broad range of conditions and signs and symptoms.

ALLERGIC REACTION AND ANAPHYLACTIC SHOCK

ANAPHYLAXIS: A severe allergic reaction; may cause breathing difficulty, circulatory problems, and ultimately, shock.

The terms *allergic reaction* and **anaphylaxis** often are used interchangeably. The differences in these terms are not absolute. Allergic reactions result from insect stings or exposure to substances to which an individual is sensitive. The symptoms and signs may include rashes, itchiness, a burning sensation of the skin, difficulty breathing, or hypotension. Anaphylaxis is an extremely severe allergic reaction; it includes airway edema, difficulty breathing, and vascular collapse leading to shock. This response can occur quickly and may lead to serious illness or death if not cared for immediately.

Pathophysiology

ANTIGEN: A foreign substance.
ANTIBODY: A substance in the body that functions to destroy foreign substances.
MAST CELL: A specialized white blood cell that releases histamine into the body.
HISTAMINE: Released into the body during anaphylactic shock; may cause airway compromise and vasodilation.

 Describe the pathophysiology of anaphylactic shock.

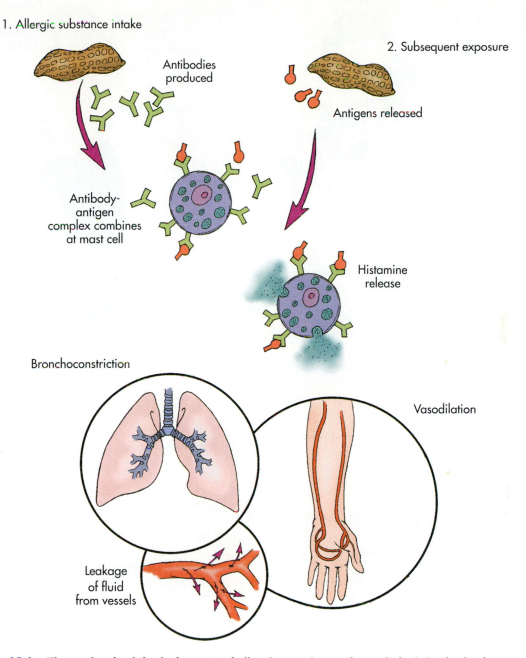

1. Allergic substance intake

Antibodies produced

2. Subsequent exposure

Antigens released

Antibody-antigen complex combines at mast cell

Histamine release

Bronchoconstriction

Vasodilation

Leakage of fluid from vessels

Fig. 15-1   **The pathophysiological events of allergic reaction and anaphylaxis in the body.**

When an **antigen** to which one is sensitive enters the body, it is attacked by a substance known as an **antibody.** Antibodies function to destroy foreign substances. In the event of anaphylaxis, however, the antibody does not destroy the antigen. Instead, the reaction between the antigen and the antibody triggers a series of events in the patient's body that lead to shock.

Shock occurs due to the release of chemicals from a specialized type of white blood cell known as a **mast cell.** The release is triggered by the antibody after it has reacted with the foreign antigen. Several types of substances are released from mast cells during anaphylactic shock. The most important of these substances is **histamine.**

The release of histamine causes the following responses:

- Sudden, severe bronchoconstriction/spasm, which can cause airway compromise

- Intense vasodilation

- Leaking of fluid from vessels due to a change in permeability

- Responses can range from mild to extreme, sometimes causing death (Fig. 15-1).

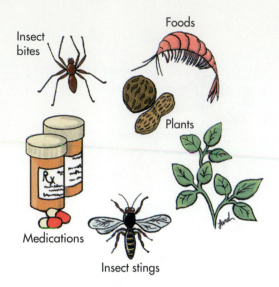

Fig. 15-2 Common allergens to the human body.

Mechanisms of anaphylactic shock

Antigens may enter the body through numerous channels (Fig. 15-2):

- Skin contact—irritants such as poison ivy, skin creams, cosmetics, and detergents
- Injection—medications such as penicillin, insect bites, and stings
- Inhalation—irritants such as molds, pollen, and perfumes
- Ingestion—foods or other substances such as chocolate, shellfish, and peanuts

Signs and symptoms of anaphylactic shock

 List the common signs and symptoms of anaphylactic shock.

The signs and symptoms of **anaphylactic shock** differ somewhat from other forms of shock and may develop rapidly or gradually. Anaphylactic shock presents a special challenge because profound airway compromise can develop quickly. Signs and symptoms include (Fig. 15-3):

- A sense of uneasiness or agitation, which is often the first symptom noticed by the patient
- Swelling of the soft tissues such as the hands, tongue, and pharynx

Patients may feel as if their tongue is swelling and their throat closing up.

 HELPFUL HINT
Listen for stridor in the upper airway and look for associated signs of respiratory distress. Observe for pharyngeal edema. The uvula and soft palate may be swollen. In some cases, the tongue may become so edematous that the airway is completely occluded.

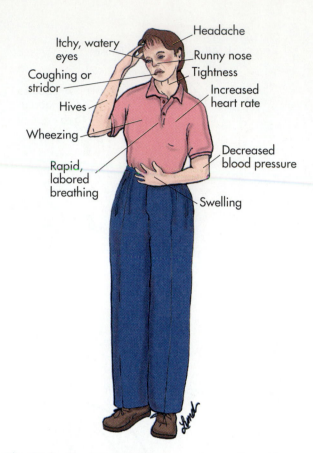

Fig. 15-3 Typical signs and symptoms of anaphylactic shock.

- Skin flushing and hives

 HELPFUL HINT
The typical rash consists of raised lesions called urticaria or "hives." The lesions may be widely disseminated or only noted in some localized areas. They may come and go fairly rapidly.

- Coughing, sneezing
- Wheezing due to spasms of the upper and lower airway, rales, rhonchi, or absent breath sounds

 HELPFUL HINT
Wheezing may be either grossly audible or only detectable by auscultation.

- Tingling, burning, or itching skin
- Abdominal pain
- Tachycardia
- Weak, thready pulse
- Profound hypotension (late sign)
- Confusion
- Decreased level of responsiveness
- Weakness
- Profuse diaphoresis

HELPFUL HINT
Patients in respiratory distress are usually sitting upright and forward and do not tolerate lying down

- Retraction of intercostal spaces and accessory muscle use
- Deep or shallow, labored respirations
- Cyanosis
- Anxiety
- Peripheral edema in the extremities

Unless there is a recent obvious insect sting, many cases of allergic reaction or anaphylaxis will not have any apparent cause. The EMT–I should ask the patient about:

- Recent insect sting or bite
- History of food or drug allergy
- Foods recently ingested
- Medications taken (name, dosage, when taken prior to reaction)
- New cosmetics, soaps, clothing, etc.

The EMT–I should also determine if there is a history of other significant medical conditions:

- Identify current medications
- Get a list of medications to bring to the hospital
- Perform a head-to-toe examination

Care for allergic reaction and anaphylactic shock

 Describe the treatment of anaphylaxis.

Care of an allergic reaction is generally supportive in nature. Benadryl administration, 25 mg, slow IV push or intramuscular, is appropriate if local protocols permit and:

- Vital signs are normal
- There are no respiratory symptoms
- The only manifestations of the reaction are itching, rash, and/or swelling on the outside of the body

Care of anaphylactic shock is similar to other types of shock:

- Aggressive airway management
- Ventilatory support
- Oxygen therapy
- Circulatory support

Administer epinephrine (1:1000) 0.1 to 0.5 cc subcutaneously if:

- Wheezing or stridor is present

- Edema of the pharynx, soft palate, or tongue is observed
- Manifestations of vascular compromise are noted (such as hypotension; confusion; weak, thready pulse; or tachycardia)

CLINICAL NOTES
The definitive treatment for anaphylaxis is epinephrine. Epinephrine vasoconstricts, has a positive inotropic action (the heart beats harder), bronchodilates, and directly counteracts released mediators. If the EMT–I is trained to administer subcutaneous epinephrine, he or she should do so (Fig. 15-4). Some patients may have their own physician-prescribed epinephrine for use in anaphylaxis. Even if the EMT–I is not allowed to give drugs, he or she can help a patient administer the drug to himself or herself. Anaphylactic shock can be a life-threatening emergency during which minutes can make the difference between life and death.

Care for anaphylactic shock includes the following:

- Provide continual reassurance to the patient.
- Ensure an adequate airway. Perform endotracheal intubation and administer high-concentration oxygen if:
  - The patient is unable to maintain an airway.
  - Ventilatory assistance is needed.
  - Respiratory distress is severe.
  - Cyanosis is present.
  - Significant hypotension (blood pressure [BP] < 70 mm Hg systolic) is present.
- If the patient is experiencing an allergic reaction but breathing adequately, administer high-concentration oxygen, 10 to 15 L/min (85% to 100%) by nonrebreather mask.
  - A nasal cannula delivering a 44% concentration of oxygen (flow rate of 6 L/min) may be used if the patient is afraid of or agitated by the oxygen mask.
- Establish an IV lifeline, using a large-bore cannula.
  - Use normal saline or Ringer's lactate with a macrodrip administration set.
  - Draw blood if time permits.
  - If BP is less than 90 systolic, run the IV wide open, reassessing vital signs after each 300 cc.
  - If BP is greater than 90 systolic, run the IV TKO.
- Administer epinephrine, 1:1000, 0.1 to 0.5 cc of 1:1000 solution subcutaneously; repeat, if necessary, two or more times at 10- to 20-minute intervals. If the patient has his or her own autoinjector (Epi-Pen), the EMT–I may assist in giving the injection. Repeat every 5 to 10 minutes if the patient's response to treatment is inadequate.

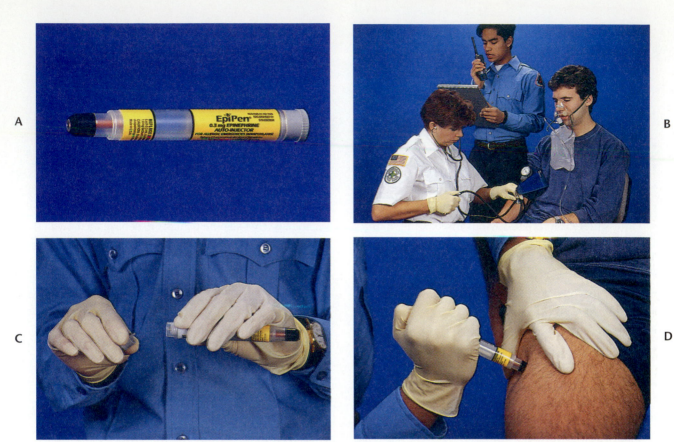

Fig. 15-4   Administering epinephrine to a patient experiencing an allergic reaction or anaphylactic shock. A, An epinephrine autoinjector. B, Consult with medical direction before assisting with Epi-Pen administration. C, Remove the cap from the injector. D, Insert the injector at a 90° angle laterally to the patient's thigh, between the waist and the knee. Hold the injector in place until the medication is injected.

- If wheezing or stridor is present, administer a nebulized bronchodilator treatment with medications such as albuterol (Proventil, Ventolin) or isoetharine (Bronkosol) by nebulizer if permitted by local protocols.
    - With albuterol, add the solution to 2.5 mL of normal saline (when dilutor is required), place in the nebulizer device, and deliver with a flow rate of 4 to 6 L/min.
    - With Bronkosol, place the solution (2.0 mL prefilled container of 0.25%) in the nebulizer device and deliver it with a flow rate of 4 to 6 L/min. (In some areas, these drugs come in prepackaged ampules and do not need to be mixed in saline; follow local protocols.)
    - Place the patient in a position of comfort.
- Identify priority patients and make the transport/backup decision. Rapidly transport the patient to the nearest appropriate medical facility.
- Move the patient to the ambulance on a stair chair or cot. Do not walk the patient to the

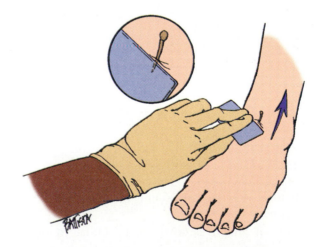

Fig. 15-5   Proper removal of a stinger.

vehicle. Place the patient in a position of comfort based on his or her physiologic needs.

- Continue to reassess the patient's vital signs and response to treatment.

- Apply electrocardiogram (ECG) electrodes and provide continuous monitoring if protocols permit.
- In the case of a bee sting, examine the sting site. If the stinger is still present, do not grasp it between your fingers or with a hemostat, tweezers, or any kind of grasping device. Take a flat object, such as a tongue depressor, and scrape it flat along the skin to remove the venom sac with or without the stinger (Fig. 15-5).

RESPIRATORY EMERGENCIES

Respiratory emergencies are extremely common. They are divided into two categories: acute and chronic. Both chronic and acute respiratory problems can present as life-threatening situations. Patients with chronic respiratory problems, such as chronic obstructive pulmonary disease (COPD) usually present with an acute worsening of their condition. In this sense, nearly all persons with respiratory problems who come to the attention of the EMT–I will have an acute condition. Many persons, however, are completely healthy prior to developing the problem in these situations; it is truly a new and acute respiratory emergency.

Acute asthma

ASTHMA: A common respiratory disease that causes sufferers to experience acute airflow obstruction in the lower portion of the airway.

Acute asthma is a recurring condition of reversible acute airflow obstruction in the lower airway. Approximately 8.9 million people in the United States suffer from asthma, with thousands dying each year. It is the most common chronic disease of childhood.

 Describe the pathophysiology of asthma.

Pathophysiology
Asthma is a chronic disease that involves the lower airway, beyond the level of the trachea and mainstem bronchi. It occurs when the bronchial airways narrow and make breathing difficult. It is not contagious and cannot be cured, but it can be controlled. Acute episodes of worsening, usually referred to as attacks, are the most likely reason these persons will seek emergency medical assistance.

People with asthma have extra sensitive bronchial airways, which are easily irritated. When the air tubes become irritated, four things happen:

1. **Bronchospasm**—The tiny muscle layers surrounding the bronchioles spasm and narrow the lumen of the airways. Bronchospasm is similar to pinching a drinking straw; it limits the movement of air. The result is wheezing, as air is forced through the narrowed airways. Shortness of breath follows because not enough air reaches the alveoli.

2. Increased mucus production—As a result of the irritation, the bronchial airways produce an abnormal amount of mucus. This secreted mucus is particularly thick, making it difficult to remove with coughing. Because mucus is no longer being removed through normal processes, it clogs the smaller bronchioles, further decreasing airway diameter and making breathing even more difficult.

3. Swelling and edema—Fluid collects in the lining of the irritated airways, causing them to swell, which further blocks the flow of air.

4. Inflammatory cell proliferation—White blood cells accumulate in the airway. These cells secrete substances that worsen the muscle spasm and increase mucus production.

The patient develops shortness of breath, wheezing, and cough. With proper care, many of these changes are reversible. A severe asthma patient may have ongoing inflammation in the lungs despite appearing clinically normal. The patient also may depend on daily medication to prevent attacks.

It is not known exactly why some people have asthma and others do not. It is known, however, that heredity plays a role. That is, if one member of a family has asthma, hay fever, or an allergic skin condition called eczema, another family member is more likely to develop asthma than someone who has no such family history.

Asthma can begin at any age, but it is most common in children and young adults. Approximately one third of the people who have asthma develop the condition before age 5 years. The good news is that approximately one third of the children who have asthma outgrow it before they reach adulthood. Conversely, adult asthma is usually persistent. One fourth of all asthma cases begin after age 50 years.

There are two kinds of asthma:

1. Extrinsic asthma—With this type of asthma some specific outside substance such as pollen causes the air tubes to narrow. The onset of extrinsic asthma is more common in childhood.

2. Intrinsic asthma—With this type of asthma no specific substance can be identified as causing the air tubes to narrow. The onset of intrinsic asthma is more common in adulthood.

Causes
The cause of an asthma attack is not always easy to identify. Asthma patients can be affected by chemicals, odors, smoke, and/or physical activity, any of which can irritate the bronchial airways. These causes are called *triggers* because they cause

bronchospasm, mucus production, and swelling during an asthma attack. Eight groups of common asthma triggers are:

1. Respiratory infections—Respiratory infections are the most common asthma triggers. They include colds, influenza, sinus infections, and so forth. These illnesses trigger asthma attacks because they temporarily inflame and damage the lining of the air tubes, causing bronchospasm, increased mucus production, and swelling. Asthma attacks that occur with a respiratory infection are usually worse than those that occur at other times.

2. Allergens—Allergens can trigger an allergic reaction, which irritates the bronchial airways. Children are more likely to have allergies that trigger attacks than are adults who develop asthma later in life. The most common allergens are pollen, dust, animal dander, lint, insecticides, food, mold, and drugs (eg, aspirin, penicillin, local anesthetics, and antiinflammatory drugs such as ibuprofen). Contrary to popular belief, food allergies are very rare. Nuts and seafood are the most common causes of food allergies that trigger asthma attacks.

3. Street drugs—Cocaine may cause acute asthmatic attacks in sensitive individuals.

4. Irritants—Irritant triggers can irritate the bronchi of nonasthmatic persons, but in persons who have asthma, they can trigger an attack. Examples of irritants include odors, cigarette smoke, air pollution, and fumes. Workplace irritants are particularly common among people who work in factories where a lot of dust or fumes are present.

5. Exercise—Exercise or fast breathing, especially during cold weather, irritates the bronchial airways, causing them to be more sensitive and produce more mucus, which can lead to an asthma attack. Exercise is a common trigger among children. It is natural for children to run and exercise outdoors, especially in the spring and fall when pollen fills the air.

6. Emotions—Any strong, subjective feeling or reaction may cause an asthma attack. Although there has been less research conducted in this area than with other asthma triggers, crying, yelling, or even laughing might trigger an attack. Stress from personal or work-related worries is a particularly powerful trigger.

7. Chemicals—Many people have severe asthma reactions to specific chemicals. Common examples include red and yellow dye (not only in food, but also in colored pills), sulfur dioxide in red wine, aspirin (as well as other antiinflammatory drugs), and sulfites, which are often used to preserve fruits and vegetables.

8. Changes in environmental conditions—A few people suffer from asthma attacks only once or twice a year. However, most people with asthma have some discomfort on a regular basis, and most experience at least some increased discomfort in the fall and spring when pollen levels are highest. Cold, wind, and humidity are examples of environmental triggers. Occasionally, hormonal variations during pregnancy or menstruation may make asthma either better or worse.

Assessment

 Describe the signs and symptoms of asthma and list those that indicate a very serious condition.

Many asthma patients keep medications at home to care for their asthma attacks. Usually, they try these remedies before calling EMS. Victims will many times report a recent upper respiratory infection, often with a cough. Given that many patients die from asthma, prompt, careful assessment and intervention in the field are essential. Often the patient is found sitting upright, leaning forward with the hands on the knees (tripod position), using accessory muscles to breathe and in obvious respiratory distress (Fig. 15-6). Respiratory distress is obvious with rapid, loud breathing and audible wheezing. Other common signs and symptoms of asthma include:

- Shortness of breath
- Extreme difficulty moving air in and out of the lungs
- Audible abnormal breath sounds (wheezing is the most common)
- Hyperinflated chest

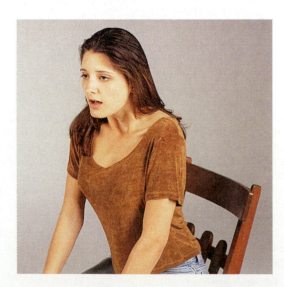

Fig. 15-6 **A patient experiencing an asthma attack.**

- Coughing, which may or may not be productive of sputum
- Tachycardia
- Hypertension
- Tachypnea
- Mild cyanosis
- Decreased oxygen saturation on pulse oximetry
- Anxiety, agitation, anxiousness
- Diaphoresis and pallor

The patient also may be unable to complete a phrase or sentence without having to stop to breathe. If the asthma attack is so severe that the patient cannot speak, arterial oxygen tension (PaO_2) is probably less than 40 torr (normal range at sea level is 80 to 100 torr).

The patient often will relate a history of acute or gradual onset of shortness of breath and wheezing from a previously healthy state. In many cases the patient will have taken his or her medication without relief. As the condition progresses, the patient must work harder to move sufficient air. Sometimes, patients overuse their medication when their breathing worsens, which may actually aggravate the attack.

The EMT–I must keep in mind that wheezes do not always indicate asthma. Wheezes also may be present with other diseases that cause dyspnea, such as heart failure, pulmonary embolism, pneumothorax, toxic inhalation, foreign body aspiration, or other pathologic states. The EMT–I should always consider the possibility of a foreign body in the airway, especially in young children with wheezing and no history of asthma. A complete history and thorough patient examination are necessary for appropriate emergency care decisions.

Certain signs indicate that a patient with an asthma attack is in very serious condition. EMT–Is should recognize these signs and manage these individuals as "priority" patients.

Signs and symptoms of a serious asthma attack include:

- Altered level of responsiveness such as sluggishness, exhaustion, agitation, and confusion. This sign indicates that insufficient oxygen is getting to the brain and carbon dioxide is building up in the blood. The victim may be agitated or drowsy.
- A "silent chest." An absence of breath sounds when auscultating the chest of the asthma patient means that there is severe narrowing of the bronchial passageways. These patients are said to be "too tight to wheeze." Air flow through the respiratory passageways is severely limited. *The partial or complete absence of lung sounds is a sign of danger.*
- Marked diaphoresis.
- Cyanosis.
- If the patient states that he or she is "too tired to breathe anymore."

Emergency care

 Identify the treatment for a patient experiencing an acute asthma attack.

Asthma patients are true medical emergencies. Treatment should be aggressive, and observation for deterioration that can be unexpected, rapid, and fatal must be vigilant. Initial patient management in the prehospital setting should include the following:

- Perform endotracheal intubation and ventilate using high-concentration oxygen if:
  - Unable to maintain an airway
  - Ventilatory assistance is needed
  - Respiratory distress is severe
  - Cyanosis is present
  - Significant hypotension (BP <70 mm Hg systolic) is present
- Calm and reassure the patient.
- If the patient is likely experiencing respiratory distress but breathing adequately, provide a high concentration of humidified supplemental oxygen (Fig. 15-7):
  - 10 to 15 L/min using a nonrebreather mask (85% to 100%) if the patient can tolerate the mask.
  - A nasal cannula delivering a 44% concentration of oxygen (flow rate of 6 L/min) may be used if the patient is afraid of or agitated by the oxygen mask.

 STREET WISE
Oxygen without humidification may not be as beneficial, but is better than none at all.

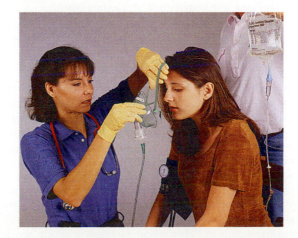

Fig. 15-7   Administer an aerosolized bronchodilator to asthmatic patients who are breathing adequately.

- Place the patient in a position of comfort. Typically this position is sitting upright, if the patient is having trouble breathing.
- Provide timely transport with treatment en route.
- Monitor vital signs, including pulse oximetry, frequently.
- Treat the bronchospasm:
  - Administer an aerosolized bronchodilator such as albuterol (Proventil), isoetharine (Bronkosol), or metaproterenol (Alupent)
  - Administer epinephrine (Adrenalin), at a dose of 0.1 to 0.5 cc of a 1:1000 solution, subcutaneously; and/or
  - Administer terbutaline (Brethine), 0.25 cc subcutaneously.
- Place an IV lifeline of normal saline or Ringer's lactate or 5% dextrose in water. DO NOT give epinephrine or terbutaline in the IV.
- Monitor the ECG for cardiac rhythm disturbances.
- Identify priority patients and make transport/backup decision.

 Define the term *status asthmaticus*.

Status asthmaticus is a severe prolonged asthma attack that does not respond to standard medications. Its onset may be sudden or insidious and is frequently precipitated by a viral respiratory infection. It is a true emergency that requires immediate transport because the patient is in imminent danger of respiratory failure. Prehospital treatment is the same as for acute asthma; however, rapid transport is more important. Patients should be closely monitored, and the EMT-I should anticipate the need for intubation and aggressive ventilatory support.

Chronic obstructive pulmonary disease (chronic bronchitis/emphysema)

 CHRONIC OBSTRUCTIVE PULMONARY DISEASE: A respiratory disease that causes decreased inspiratory and expiratory function.

Chronic obstructive pulmonary disease (COPD) is a progressive and irreversible disease of the airway marked by decreased inspiratory and expiratory capacity of the lungs. COPD may result from chronic bronchitis (excess mucus production) or **emphysema** (lung tissue damage with loss of elastic recoil of the lungs). Patients with COPD usually suffer from a combination of chronic bronchitis and emphysema.

Patients with COPD generally function at a certain baseline level until an event occurs that causes decompensation. This event is known as an acute COPD episode, and is usually when EMS is called for help.

Pathophysiology
Chronic bronchitis results from overgrowth of the airway mucus glands and excess secretion of mucus, which blocks the airway. These patients have a chronic productive cough.

Emphysema results from destruction of the walls of the alveoli. Normally, exhalation is a passive process resulting from elastic recoil of the lungs after they have expanded, similar to air coming out of a balloon after it has been blown up. The loss of normal alveolar structure leads to a decrease in elastic recoil, which creates resistance to expiratory airflow. Air is trapped within the lungs, resulting in poor air exchange.

Most patients with COPD have a combination of the features of both chronic bronchitis and emphysema. They have marked resistance within their airways to air movement. The work required to breathe is considerable.

After a period of time, the right side of the heart may develop failure due to the effort required to move blood through diseased lungs. This condition is known as chronic cor pulmonale and indicates severe COPD.

Causes
The major cause of COPD is cigarette smoking. Industrial inhalants (such as asbestos and coal dust), air pollution, and tuberculosis also contribute to the condition.

Assessment
The patient in an acute COPD episode will complain of shortness of breath with symptoms gradually increasing over a period of days. The patient may say he or she has "emphysema," "bronchitis," "COPD," or simply, "asthma."

 CLINICAL NOTES
Some patients with COPD refer to their disease as "asthma." This term is a misnomer, because patients with COPD never have totally normal airway function.

The patient's recent history prior to the acute COPD episode may include:
- A new cough or a change in the patient's previous pattern of cough and sputum production may appear.
- The patient may have stopped his or her medications (without the doctor's advice) because he or she was "feeling good."
- The patient may be on home oxygen.
- The patient may have a nebulizer at home with which to give himself or herself breathing treatments. This device may have failed to improve the patient's situation.

On assessment, the patient is usually seated upright, obviously short of breath. Other features include:

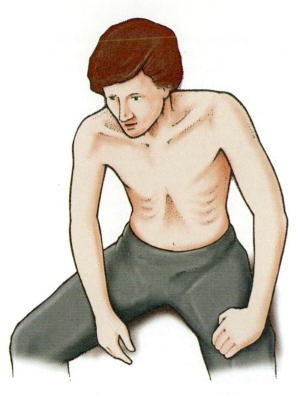

Fig. 15-8   A patient who is using accessory muscles to breathe is experiencing respiratory distress.

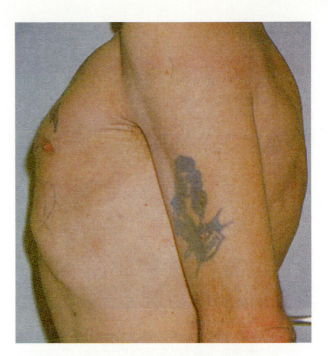

Fig. 15-9   A barrel-shaped chest is a sign that a patient is experiencing COPD.

- Tachypnea.
- Anxiety, because the patient may feel that he or she is suffocating.
- The patient may speak in short sentences because he or she is unable to get enough air to talk in longer phrases.
- Use of accessory breathing muscles (Fig. 15-8). Normally, most of the breathing effort is done by the diaphragm. A person in respiratory distress may use the supraclavicular and intercostal muscles of the rib cage. Use of accessory muscles causes the inward movement of these muscles during inspiration. This use is a sign of straining severely to breathe.
- Cyanosis.
- Cigarette stains on the fingertips, which suggests that the patient has been a heavy smoker for many years.
- The chest is often barrel-shaped (Fig. 15-9).
- Audible abnormal breath sounds such as wheezes, rales, and rhonchi may be noted. As with asthma, a silent chest, indicating that the patient is too tight to wheeze, is a serious sign (Fig. 15-10).

If the patient also has cor pulmonale, the following additional features are likely to be seen:

- Marked neck vein distention (although this finding may occur from COPD alone).

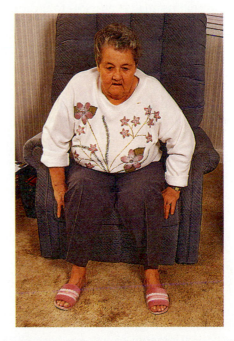

Fig. 15-10   A patient whose breathing is audibly abnormal or silent may be experiencing an acute COPD episode.

- Abdominal bloating (from fluid in the abdominal cavity).
- Leg edema.

 List three priorities of care for COPD.

Emergency care

To care for patients with an acute COPD episode, the EMT–I should:

- Transport the patient in a semisitting position.
- Give oxygen as per local protocol.
- Loosen restrictive clothing.
- Encourage the patient to cough up secretions. Do not force the patient to cough if it provokes non-stop spasms.
- Start an IV of normal saline at a TKO rate or an intermittent infusion device (heparin lock).
- Administer nebulized bronchodilator as per local protocol.

The use of oxygen in patients with COPD

There is disagreement in EMS about giving oxygen to patients with COPD. The basis for this argument is the fact that there are two separate respiratory drives:

- The carbon dioxide drive. When you hold your breath, CO_2 accumulates in the blood. After a period of time, the level of CO_2 gets high enough to stimulate breathing centers in the brain. The reflex response is to take a breath. The accumulation of carbon dioxide in our blood is the major stimulus that normally causes us to breathe.
- The hypoxic drive. A secondary mechanism that causes breathing is a lack of oxygen in the blood. If the level of oxygen in the blood drops very low, brain breathing centers are stimulated, leading to the reflex response of breathing.

A small number of patients with COPD do not effectively excrete carbon dioxide from their lungs. Carbon dioxide is always elevated in their bloodstream. These patients are called *carbon dioxide retainers*. These patients have lost their carbon dioxide drive to breathe. The only thing that stimulates breathing is the low level of oxygen in their blood (the hypoxic drive).

If a high level of oxygen is given to a CO_2 retainer, hypoxia, the only remaining stimulus for breathing, will be eliminated. The patient could develop hypoventilation and eventually respiratory arrest. Based on this logic, some EMS protocols limit the use of oxygen to low concentration. Others recommend the field use of Venturi masks to give precise oxygen concentrations.

Only a small number of patients with COPD are at risk for developing respiratory arrest from too high an oxygen concentration. Unfortunately, it is impossible to determine in the field who these patients are. A reasonable approach for the EMT–I to take is as follows:

- Unless the patient is in marked respiratory distress, give 1 to 3 L/min via nasal cannula. If the patient is on home oxygen, use the prescribed setting. This amount is not enough oxygen to harm the patient in the field even if the patient is a CO_2 retainer.

- If the patient is in severe distress and appears to require higher oxygen concentrations, use what you determine to be appropriate. Observe the patient carefully for changes in the respiratory rate and mental status. If the patient begins to deteriorate, the oxygen concentration may be decreased. Bear in mind that problems other than excessive oxygen can cause these patients to deteriorate. Assist their breathing as necessary.
- As a general rule, give the patient the amount of oxygen you consider necessary for his or her condition; do not withhold high-concentration oxygen, when required, just because the patient might be a CO_2 retainer in reality, because this is quite unusual.

HELPFUL HINT
Never withhold high-concentration oxygen from an ill or injured patient who requires it based on the unlikely possibility that he or she may be a carbon dioxide retainer.

Hyperventilation

Hyperventilation is a respiratory rate greater than that required for normal body function. It is the result of an increased frequency of breathing, an increased volume of air moved, or both. Hyperventilation causes an excessive elimination of carbon dioxide.

Pathophysiology

Excessive excretion (blowing off) of carbon dioxide results in low blood levels (hypocapnia), which disturbs the normal blood acid-base balance by increasing the pH. These pH changes can interfere with the normal function of other body systems.

Identify five conditions that may cause hyperventilation.

Causes

Many conditions can result in hyperventilation, including:

- Asthma attack
- COPD
- Myocardial infarction
- Pulmonary embolism
- Spontaneous pneumothorax
- Congestive heart failure
- Increased metabolism—Exercise, fever, hyperthyroidism, infection
- Central nervous system—Lesions, stroke, encephalitis, head injury, meningitis
- Hypoxia
- Accumulation of metabolic acids in the body, kidney failure, diabetic ketoacidosis, alcohol poisoning (methanol, ethanol)

- Drugs—Cocaine, amphetamines, aspirin, epinephrine
- Psychogenic factors—Acute anxiety, pain

STREET WISE
Many diseases cause patients to hyperventilate. Do not assume that the hyperventilating patient simply has anxiety.

Assessment
Signs and symptoms of hyperventilation include:

- Chest pain—The pain is usually in the center of the chest and often is described as sharp. The discomfort of hyperventilation may appear similar to myocardial ischemia.
- Dizziness, faintness—Although loss of responsiveness is possible, it is rare.
- Numbness and tingling of the face, fingers, and toes
- Tightness or a lump in the throat
- Spasm of the fingers and toes, known as carpopedal spasm
- Altered mental status
- Abnormal lung sounds
- Tachycardia—With this common sign, the patient may complain of palpitations.

Emergency care

 Describe the care given to patients who hyperventilate.

The major risk in caring for a patient with hyperventilation is to assume that anxiety is the cause of the symptoms. Many serious and life-threatening medical illnesses can cause hyperventilation. The patient's symptons can seem identical to those of someone with only a simple anxiety attack. A conservative approach demands that the EMT–I assumes the patient is seriously ill until the case is proven otherwise.

A discarded method of caring for hyperventilation is to have the patient breathe into a paper bag. The theory was that having the patient breathe his or her own CO_2 increases the level of that gas in the patient's bloodstream, allowing the normal respiratory control mechanisms to bring breathing down to a normal rate and depth. Plugging the portals of an oxygen mask also was done in the past for the same purpose.

CLINICAL NOTES
Rebreathing is no longer an acceptable practice. Many patients who appear to have simple hyperventilation actually have serious illness. Having the patient breathe into a paper bag causes a marked decrease in the available oxygen, and dangerous hypoxia can result.

To care for a patient with hyperventilation, the EMT–I should:

- Assume that there is an underlying medical cause of hyperventilation.
- Give oxygen generally 3 to 4 L/min by nasal cannula. Follow pulse oximetry. If the patient is hypoxic, deliver oxygen at 15 L/ min using a nonrebreather mask.
- If isolated anxiety hyperventilation is suspected, ask the patient to control his or her breathing. Suggest he or she breathe only when instructed, or have the patient count to five between breaths. Do not force the patient if he or she has an obvious respiratory difficulty.
- Do not have the patient breathe into a paper bag.
- Do not plug the portals of an oxygen mask in an attempt to have a patient rebreathe his or her carbon dioxide.
- If the patient has chest pain, place him or her on a cardiac monitor and start an IV lifeline.
- Transport the patient to the hospital as per local protocols.

STREET WISE
Do not use a paper bag or a blocked-off oxygen mask to care for hyperventilation. Give the patient the benefit of the doubt and administer oxygen.

Pulmonary embolism
Pulmonary embolism is the blockage of a pulmonary artery by foreign matter. In most cases, the obstruction is due to a piece of a blood clot that has broken away from a pelvic or deep leg vein. Other causes include fat, amniotic fluid, air, or tumor tissue. (*See* also Chapter 14, "Cardiac Emergencies.")

HELPFUL HINTS
Pulmonary embolism is common, potentially lethal, and highly underdiagnosed. It is the third most common cause of death in the United States. There are approximately 650,000 cases annually. Of these, ten percent of patients die within 1 hour of the event. Among survivors, the diagnosis is missed in two of three cases.

 Recall three patients who are at risk for pulmonary embolism.

Risk factors
Risks for pulmonary embolism include:

- Sedentary life style—Pulmonary embolism is common in hospitalized patients and in those who have completed long motor vehicle or airplane trips.

- Obesity.
- Thrombophlebitis, an inflammation of the veins.
- Oral contraceptives (birth control pills).
- Fracture of a long bone (femur, humerus)—The source of emboli is fat released from the bone marrow.
- Pregnancy—Amniotic fluid embolism may occur during delivery, and is often fatal.
- Surgery—Patients may remain in the same position on the operating table for several hours, leading to blood clot formation in the veins of the pelvis and legs.
- Blood diseases—Rare blood disorders can make a patient's blood more likely to clot.

Pathophysiology

The most common source of a pulmonary embolism is a blood clot that has formed in either the pelvic or deep leg veins. A piece can break off and travel through the venous system to the heart, then the lungs. As the clot passes through progressively smaller and smaller branches of the pulmonary circulation, it becomes lodged and blockage occurs.

The lung tissue supplied by the blocked artery becomes ischemic. If circulation to the lung is sufficiently compromised, the affected area dies. In addition to ischemia, the lung tissue releases various substances, including histamine, that causebronchoconstriction and wheezing. This release results in a worsening of blood oxygenation. The process is similar whether the embolism consists of blood clot, fat, tissue, air, or other foreign matter.

Pulmonary emboli may be small or large. Large pulmonary emboli occlude major branches of the pulmonary arteries. When these occlusions occur, the heart is forced to pump blood against very high pressures, resulting in acute right-sided heart failure (acute cor pulmonale).

 Identify four signs/symptoms of pulmonary embolism.

Assessment

Patients with massive pulmonary emboli often suffer cardiac arrest or a syncopal spell as the first symptom of the illness. Patients with smaller emboli may have the following signs and symptoms:

- Sudden, unexplained onset of chest pain which increases in intensity with a deep breath (pleuritic chest pain). The pain may be localized to the area of the chest overlying the involved lung tissue.
- Respiratory distress and shortness of breath. The patient's respiratory rate is almost always increased. The patient may hyperventilate.
- Wheezing or coughing up of blood
- Anxiety

- Shock
- Hypotension

 HELPFUL HINT
The signs and symptoms of pulmonary embolism are often similar to myocardial infarction or spontaneous pneumothorax. Pleuritic chest pain is sharp discomfort felt when taking a deep breath.

Emergency care

Emergency care for a patient with suspected pulmonary embolism includes the following:

- Maintain the patient's airway, ventilate with high-concentration oxygen, and assist breathing if necessary.
- Start an IV lifeline, watch for shock, and provide care as necessary.
- Place the patient on a cardiac monitor.
- Transport the patient in a position of comfort.

Spontaneous pneumothorax

 Describe the mechanism of spontaneous pneumothorax.

Spontaneous pneumothorax is a sudden accumulation of air in the pleural space. This condition is due to the rupture of a weak area on the lung surface. As the air enters the pleural space, the lung on the involved side collapses (Fig. 15-11). Spontaneous pneumothorax is a common cause of sudden-onset shortness of breath and chest pain in young individuals. It is more common in men than in women.

Causes

The most frequent cause of spontaneous pneumothorax is rupture of a congenital defect on the surface of the lung. A congenital bleb is an air-filled sac that has been present since birth. Young, tall, thin male smokers are most likely to develop pneumothorax from the rupture of a congenital bleb.

Other less common causes of spontaneous pneumothorax include:

- Menstruation—Spontaneous pneumothorax associated with menstruation is usually right-sided and occurs in women aged 20 to 30 years. It is thought to be secondary to the presence of endometrial tissue in the lung or pleura that ruptures after swelling during the menstrual cycle.
- Lung disease involving connective tissue of the lung.
- COPD—Spontaneous pneumothorax associated with COPD is usually secondary to rupture of defects that have formed from the destruction of normal lung tissue that results from COPD.

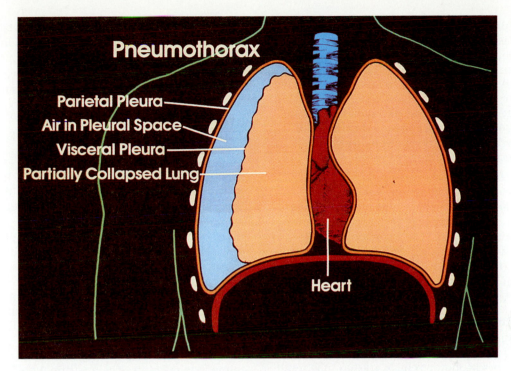

Fig. 15-11 A spontaneous pneumothorax is caused by a sudden accumulation of air in the pleural space of the lungs.

Assessment

Patients with spontaneous pneumothorax complain of the sudden onset of sharp chest pain accompanied by shortness of breath. The pain is often localized to the side of the lung involved. Decreased breath sounds are present on the involved side, and the patient's respiratory rate is increased. The patient may be coughing and be anxious or agitated.

Many times, the patient has only a simple spontaneous pneumothorax. The EMT–I should always, however, be on the watch for development of tension pneumothorax, the most dangerous complication of a spontaneous pneumothorax. The signs and symptoms of tension pneumothorax are:

- Increasing respiratory distress
- Weak pulse
- Cyanosis
- Hypotension
- Decreased breath sounds on the same side as the injury
- Distended neck veins
- Tracheal deviation away from the side of the injury (a late sign)
- Subcutaneous emphysema. Crepitus may be felt in the skin of the chest wall overlying the wound or injury.

Emergency care

Provide the following emergency care for a patient with suspected spontaneous pneumothorax:

- Maintain the patient's airway, give high-concentration oxygen, and assist breathing as necessary.
- Start an IV lifeline.
- Place the patient on a cardiac monitor.
- Transport the patient in the most comfortable position. Some EMS physicians believe that lying with the affected side down is more comfortable for the patient.
- If evidence of tension pneumothorax develops, immediately perform needle decompression, if authorized, as described in Chapter 13 "Trauma Emergencies."

Toxic inhalations
Categories of toxic gases

There are three categories of toxic gases the EMT–I may encounter:

- Inert gases—These gases generally cause no direct tissue toxicity. Inhalation displaces oxygen, and injury or death occurs as a result of asphyxiation. Common inert gas inhalations include carbon dioxide and the fuel gases (*eg*, methane, ethane, propane, acetylene). Inhalation of fuel gases in an attempt to get high ("gas huffing") also is popular in some areas. In this case, aberrant mental status, seizures, and cardiac dysrhythmias are more likely to occur than asphyxiation.
- Irritant gases—These gases cause direct irritation to tissues. They are inhaled into the lungs to a

variable degree, depending on their water solubility. Gases that are highly water soluble (eg, ammonia, chlorine) dissolve in the saliva and irritate mucous membranes of the mouth, nose, and pharynx. They tend to do less damage to the lungs. On the other hand, less water-soluble agents (eg, nitrous dioxide, phosgene) pass harmlessly through the upper airway, depositing in the bronchioles and alveoli. Here, they cause severe destruction of lung tissue.

- Systemic toxins—These gases poison the cells, leading to severe dysfunction. Agents such as carbon monoxide, cyanide, and hydrogen interfere with oxygen transport and delivery, resulting in immediate toxicity. The aromatic and halogenated hydrocarbons (eg, carbon tetrachloride, benzene, toluene) cause more chronic types of damage, especially to the liver and kidneys. They will not be discussed further here.

Sources of toxic gases
Accidents and fires are the most common sources of toxic gas. Tank-car rollovers, semitruck collisions, and other types of motor vehicle crashes may result in the release of toxic chemicals. Leaking chemical storage tanks also are a potential hazard. The byproducts of combustion from a fire are often poisonous because many common plastics give off cyanide when they burn. Carbon monoxide is universal in a fire, and home heaters and space heaters serve as sources of carbon monoxide when they fail to operate properly. Finally, the products of chemical reactions, such as in the production of silo gas, may result in toxic gas formation.

Pathophysiology
Several factors determine the effects of gas inhalation on the patient:

- Water solubility—If the gas is highly water soluble, it is absorbed into the saliva and remains in the upper airway; injury to the lungs and alveoli is uncommon. If the gas is not absorbed in the saliva, it travels further into the respiratory system, causing alveolar injury.
- Depth and rate of breathing—The amount of gas absorbed and the affected location may be affected by how fast and deep the patient is breathing. The effects of these parameters vary significantly from gas to gas.
- Smell—Some gases, such as hydrogen sulfide, rapidly cause olfactory fatigue, meaning that, over time, the patient is no longer able to smell and therefore avoid them. However, certain gases (eg, cyanide) have discernable odors, leading to rapid detection. Carbon monoxide has no odor, and it may go undetected in the atmosphere.
- Concentration of the gas
- Length of exposure

- Differences in host susceptibility—Certain individuals are more sensitive to toxic gas inhalation than others.
- Smoking habit—Cigarette smokers have lower resistance to toxic gas inhalation. This may be a result of a decrease in the lungs' ability to clear waste products.
- Underlying lung disease, such as COPD

Clinical presentation
Anoxia-causing gases typically result in sudden death without significant warning symptoms. Sometimes a headache will precede a sudden loss of responsiveness. Gases such as cyanide that cause metabolic problems typically act in one of two fashions. In large doses (eg, a gas chamber during a prison execution), sudden death results, and even immediate medical treatment could not reverse the effect. In cases in which the EMT–I may have a chance to provide care, the effects occur over several minutes to hours.

Irritant gases have three distinct periods of effects: immediate, delayed, and chronic. The immediate reaction occurs within 1 to 2 hours following inhalation. It consists of an irritant reaction resulting in laryngotracheobronchitis and bronchospasm. Persons who inhale carbon monoxide may suffer acute myocardial infarction or pulmonary embolus. The delayed reaction occurs 6 to 24 hours later. It consists of laryngeal edema, hoarseness, inspiratory stridor, and noncardiogenic pulmonary edema. Although complete recovery is usually the rule, chronic problems such as recurrent pneumonia and other severe lung disease can occur.

Field evaluation and care
The most important rule for the EMT–I in treating toxic inhalations is to protect himself or herself. If possible, the EMT–I should remove the victim from the area prior to providing emergency care. The EMT–I also must be certain to use necessary safety equipment to protect himself or herself. The following care should be provided to patients with toxic inhalation:

- High-concentration oxygen; intubate if necessary
- IV lifeline
- Nebulized bronchodilators as per medical direction
- Prompt transport to the nearest appropriate medical facility

Carbon monoxide poisoning
Carbon monoxide (CO) is a colorless, odorless, flavorless, and nonirritating gas that is a common source of poisoning. Carbon monoxide is a product of incomplete combustion of carbon-containing substances. Poisoning by carbon monoxide is the major cause of industrial deaths and deaths caused by fire. Sources of carbon monoxide gas around the home include barbecue grills, automobiles, and improperly ventilated heating systems. Gas heaters

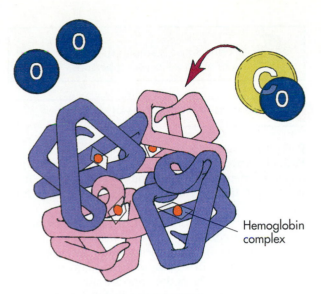

Hemoglobin complex

Fig. 15-12 Carbon monoxide has a stronger attraction to hemoglobin than oxygen. When carbon monoxide enters the body, it binds with hemoglobin, causing a decrease in the delivery of oxygen to tissue.

are among the most common source of domestic carbon monoxide exposure.

Pathophysiology

Carbon monoxide binds strongly with hemoglobin in red blood cells, producing a compound called *carboxyhemoglobin*. The strength of hemoglobin's bond with carbon monoxide is greater than that with oxygen (Fig. 15-12). As a result, the hemoglobin molecule is unable to carry oxygen. Perfusion may be severely impaired. Carboxyhemoglobin also directly affects the cellular energy transport system, leading to cell death.

Patient assessment

The EMT–I should suspect carbon monoxide poisoning in any patient exposed to fire or smoke or found in a closed space, particularly if several people in the same location have the same poisoning symptoms. The signs and symptoms of carbon monoxide poisoning include:

- Malaise, weakness, headache
- Confusion, dizziness
- Nausea, shortness of breath
- Drowsiness
- Unresponsiveness that may occur without warning
- Chest pain—Persons with carbon monoxide poisoning may develop acute myocardial infarction or pulmonary embolism.
- Cherry red skin and mucous membranes—This is a late sign and is actually rarely seen. The

absence of cherry red skin does not rule out carbon monoxide poisoning.
- Abnormal lung sounds (rales, rhonchi)
- Seizures
- Blisters on the skin

> **STREET WISE**
> Pulse oximetry may give inaccurate readings in cases of carbon monoxide poisoning. Oxygen saturation (SaO_2) readings may be falsely high.

> **HELPFUL HINT**
> Because carbon monoxide is odorless, colorless, and flavorless, protect yourself before entering a potentially hazardous environment.

Care of the patient with carbon monoxide poisoning

To care for a patient with carbon monoxide poisoning:

- Immediately remove the patient to fresh air. Be certain to use necessary safety equipment to protect yourself!
- Secure the airway, and ventilate as necessary.
- Provide high-concentration oxygen, and intubate if necessary.
- Initiate an IV lifeline.
- Care for life-threatening injuries.
- Make the patient comfortable and transport to the hospital as soon as possible.
- If the patient is unresponsive, combative, or hallucinating, consider transporting the patient to a specialty center with a hyperbaric chamber. Follow local protocols.

> **HELPFUL HINT**
> Hyperbaric oxygen is sometimes used to treat severe carbon monoxide poisoning. Extremely high concentrations of oxygen can be given in a pressurized vault in the hyperbaric chamber. At a pressure equal to three atmospheres, enough oxygen can be carried in the bloodstream to maintain perfusion without the need for hemoglobin. At these high pressures, the oxygen displaces carbon monoxide on the hemoglobin molecule, allowing the poisonous gas to be eliminated through the lungs.

NEUROLOGIC EMERGENCIES

Stroke

A stroke, or cerebrovascular accident (CVA), is a condition that results from a disruption of circulation to the brain, causing ischemia and damage to brain tissue. Neurologic symptoms persist longer than 24 hours. Recovery of function, to varying degrees, takes place over a period of weeks to months.

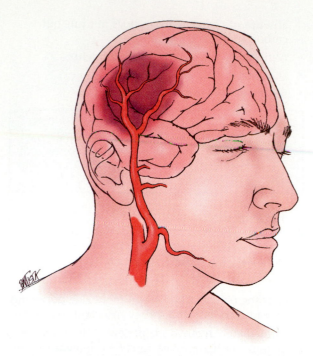

Fig. 15-13 A hemorrhagic stroke results from severe bleeding into the brain tissue as a result of the rupture of a weakened blood vessel.

Types of strokes

There are two types of strokes: occlusive and hemorrhagic. Approximately three out of four strokes are occlusive, caused by a blockage in a blood vessel due to either atherosclerotic plaque or an embolus. The most common source of emboli is the heart. Hemorrhagic strokes are caused by bleeding into the brain tissue due to rupture of a weakened blood vessel (Fig. 15-13).

Risk factors for stroke

Certain characteristics increase a person's chances of developing a stroke. The risk factors for stroke are similar to those for cardiovascular disease:

- Age (increases with age)
- Gender (more common among men)
- Race (more common among African-Americans)
- Hypertension
- Cigarette smoking
- Cardiac dysrhythmias (increases risk of embolus)
- Birth control pills (increases blood clotting)
- Alcohol consumption
- Elevated blood cholesterol levels
- Glue sniffing
- Cocaine use

Some factors, such as age, gender, and race cannot be modified. For those patients who have these factors, it is even more important to control those risks that *can* be modified.

 STREET WISE
Cocaine abuse is among the most common cause of stroke in young persons.

 List five signs and symptoms of stroke.

Patient assessment

Patients with a stroke may have gradual or rapid onset of neurologic symptoms. The patient may wake up in the morning with a deficit, or the symptoms may appear suddenly while awake.

The most common finding in stroke is paralysis. Usually, one complete side of the body is affected. This condition is called *hemiplegia*. Because nerve fibers cross sides in the brain stem, damage to one side of the brain affects the opposite side of the body.

The EMT–I also may notice facial droop on one side of the face, sagging muscles beneath the eye and cheek, and asymmetric movement of the mouth in stroke victims. The victim may have other neurologic deficits, such as impaired language or speech and decreased sensation.

The EMT–I should assume that the acute onset of slurred speech or hemiplegia is due to a stroke or cerebral hemorrhage.

Other signs and symptoms of stroke include:

- Seizures
- Dizziness
- Loss of responsiveness
- Stiff neck, headache
- Altered level of responsiveness
- Airway problems and hypoventilation
- Cardiac arrhythmias
- Nausea, vomiting
- Pupillary abnormalities (unequal, pinpoint)

Most stroke patients have an elevated blood pressure. A systolic blood pressure less than 100 mm Hg is unusual. If the patient is hypotensive, the EMT–I should suspect shock and provide care accordingly. Pinpoint pupils in a patient with an altered level of responsiveness suggest drug overdose or intracranial bleeding.

 HELPFUL HINT
If the unresponsive patient is hypotensive, consider drugs or shock as possible causes.

 STREET WISE
Pinpoint pupils are a common finding in certain drug overdoses. Determining the exact cause of pinpoint pupils is less important than supporting the airway, breathing, and circulation.

Describe the importance of airway management in the stroke patient.

Emergency care

To care for a patient with stroke, the EMT–I should:

- Establish and maintain the airway, and support ventilation as needed.

HELPFUL HINT

Airway problems are common in stroke; maintain the patency of the airway and provide oxygen.

- Give high-concentration oxygen by nonrebreather mask (15 L/min flow rate).
- Consider endotracheal intubation if the patient is unable to manage his or her own airway.
- Give nothing by mouth; be prepared for vomiting.
- Reassure the patient. Talk to the patient even if he or she is not able to respond. An unresponsive patient may still be able to hear.
- Start an IV lifeline.
- Place the patient on a cardiac monitor.
- If the patient is unresponsive, measure the blood sugar. Consider the use of dextrose (D50) IV and/or naloxone (*see* Coma, below), based on local protocols.

Transient ischemic attack

A **transient ischemic attack (TIA),** sometimes called a *ministroke*, is a stroke-like neurologic deficit that completely resolves within minutes to hours. People who have TIAs are at an increased risk for a stroke. In the field, it may be impossible to distinguish a TIA from a stroke. The patient care is identical. At times, a patient's symptoms and signs will have completely resolved by the time he or she is seen by EMS personnel, but it is still appropriate for the EMT–I to recommend evaluation at a hospital.

CLINICAL NOTES

Persons who have apparently had a TIA should be transported to the hospital for evaluation. These patients are at a high risk for stroke.

Coma

Coma is a state of unresponsiveness characterized by the absence of spontaneous eye movements and response to painful stimuli and vocalization. The comatose person cannot be aroused. Rather than simply referring to the patient as being "comatose," it is better for the EMT–I to describe the patient's status as "unresponsive to pain and verbal stimulus," or "responsive and alert."

HELPFUL HINT

Maintaining responsiveness requires the normal function and interaction of at least one of the two cerebral hemispheres and the ascending reticular activating system (ARAS). The ARAS consists of nervous tissue connections running from the brain stem to the thalamus. Dysfunction of the ARAS or the cerebral hemispheres can produce coma.

Identify five intracranial causes of coma.

Causes of coma

There are numerous causes of coma. Causes of coma originating from within the brain include:

- Intracranial bleeding
- Stroke
- Tumor
- Infection—meningitis, encephalitis
- Seizure

Identify five causes of coma that originate outside the nervous system.

Causes of coma arising outside of the nervous system include:

- Blood chemistry abnormalities—High sodium (hypernatremia), low sodium (hyponatremia), high calcium (hypercalcemia), low sugar (hypoglycemia), high sugar (hyperglycemia)
- Hypertensive crisis
- Kidney or liver failure
- Abnormalities of the endocrine gland—Underactive thyroid (hypothyroidism), underactive adrenal gland (Addison's disease), pituitary gland failure
- Vitamin deficiencies
- Drugs—Alcohol, narcotics, and depressant drugs ("downers," antidepressants, tranquilizers) are the most common cause of drug-induced coma.
- Psychiatric problems (catatonia)

STREET WISE

Use the **AEIOU-TIPS** mnemonic for causes of coma.

A = Acidosis, alcohol
E = Epilepsy
I = Infection
O = Overdose
U = Uremia (kidney failure)
T = Trauma
I = Insulin
P = Psychosis
S = Shock, stroke

Patient assessment

When assessing the comatose patient, the EMT–I should ask the following questions:

- When was the patient last well?
- How did the symptoms progress?
- Did any symptoms precede the onset of coma, such as seizures, confusion, or trauma?
- Are there any pill bottles, syringes, or strange odors present that may give a clue to drug intoxication? If medications, syringes, or other suspected drug paraphernalia are found, they should be brought to the hospital with the patient.

Patients who are in a coma are unresponsive and exhibit no response to stimuli. The EMT–I must pay attention to the following findings:

- Abnormal breathing—hypoventilation is common. Monitor the vital signs and pulse oximetry reading frequently.
- Evidence of trauma—suspect a spinal injury until proven otherwise.

> **HELPFUL HINT**
> Cervical spine injuries are common in unresponsive patients

- Abnormal pupil response
- Evidence of drug abuse, such as needle tracks
- Abnormal blood pressure—An elevated blood pressure suggests that some type of intracranial event may be responsible for the coma. Hypotension suggests drug intoxication or shock.

Emergency care

> **Describe the patient care priorities for coma.**

To care for a comatose patient, the EMT–I should:

- Establish and maintain the airway. Assist breathing, including endotracheal intubation, as necessary.
- Give high-concentration oxygen via non-rebreather mask or endotracheal tube, if necessary.
- Assume that the patient has a spinal injury and immobilize appropriately.
- Monitor the vital signs frequently.
- Transport the patient either supine or in the coma position.
- Be prepared for vomiting and airway problems.
- If local protocol allows and there is no evidence of eye injury, remove contact lenses.
- Remember that the comatose patient is totally dependent on the EMT–I. Avoid causing injury or aggravating preexisting problems.

- Start an IV lifeline of normal saline or Ringer's lactate TKO or heparin lock.
- Obtain a blood sugar determination (fingerstick), if possible.
- If permitted by local protocols, administer 1 ampule (25 gm) D50 IV if the measured blood sugar is less than 60 mg/dL. If unable to measure blood sugar in the field, follow your local protocols regarding the administration of IV D50.

CLINICAL NOTES

An ampule of dextrose (D50) contains 25 grams of dextrose dissolved in 50 cc of sterile water. This agent is indicated for persons with altered levels of responsiveness due to hypoglycemia. In many systems, a fingerstick blood sugar reading is done prior to administration of D50. In others, administration of this agent is routine in the treatment of unresponsive patients. Follow local protocols.

IV dextrose is highly acidic and very concentrated. Given improperly, it could result in severe tissue damage. Follow these guidelines:

1. Administer via a large-bore catheter in a large vein, if at all possible.
2. Double-check the patency of the IV prior to administration of D50.
3. Keep the injection site and the area above it as visible as possible.
4. Infuse into a fast-flowing IV line, instead of pinching the tubing above the injection port; depend on flow, not pressure, to administer D50.
5. Administer D50 slowly; 2 minutes is considered a minimum by many.

- Administer naloxone IV if no response to dextrose; use the dose recommended in the local protocols. The best route and dose of naloxone are not agreed upon. Many EMS systems start with 0.8 mg IV; others titrate the dose, based on the patient's respirations, whereas still others simply give 2.0 mg IV.

CLINICAL NOTES

The drug naloxone (trade name, Narcan) antagonizes the depressant actions of narcotics (*eg*, morphine, heroin, Demerol, Dilaudid, and codeine). It does this by affecting the place in the brain where these drugs bind. Narcotics are usually reversed within 5 to 10 minutes following administration of naloxone, somewhat slower if given intramuscularly. The effect lasts approximately 90 minutes. Patients respond differently to the administration of naloxone. Persons who have overdosed on Darvon (propoxyphene) may require large doses of naloxone to respond.

Many EMS systems recommend that EMT–Is only give enough naloxone to increase the respiratory rate to acceptable levels. If large doses of naloxone are given, the patient may suffer acute narcotic withdrawal. In addition to becoming violent, the patient may then refuse further treatment. Most narcotics remain in the body for at least 3 to 4 hours. Because naloxone wears off after 90 minutes, the patient could become symptomatic again after the EMT–I leaves. Some systems have changed their protocols, giving naloxone intramuscularly (2 mg IM) instead of intravenously. Large scientific studies are not yet available, but limited anecdotal experience suggests that the drug lasts longer when given via this route.

- Monitor cardiac rhythm.
- Realize that the apparently unresponsive patient may still be able to hear and understand. Even though he or she is unable to respond, continue to reassure the patient.

Seizure

SEIZURE: A sudden, intense episode of heightened electrical activity in the brain.

A **seizure** (convulsion) is a sudden episode of abnormal brain cell electrical activity resulting in a period of atypical muscular activity or abnormal behavior. Seizures spontaneously recurring over a span of years are termed *epilepsy*. Up to 6% of the population will experience at least one seizure at some stage of life. Three of four patients with epilepsy have their first seizure before 20 years of age.

Types of seizures

 List four types of seizures.

STATUS EPILEPTICUS: A series of seizures with no responsive intervals.

There are four types of seizures:
- Generalized major motor seizures—These seizures involve jerking movements, called *tonic-clonic seizure movements*, of the entire body as the muscles rapidly contract and relax. The victim may become incontinent of urine and feces. Generalized seizures, sometimes called **grand mal seizures,** usually last 2 to 5 minutes.
- Focal motor seizure—These seizures involve abnormal movements of a portion of the body, such as the arm and hand. The movements may spread to involve the entire body (generalized

seizure) or remain focal. Focal seizures generally last 1 to 2 minutes.
- Behavioral seizure—These involve brief "absence" spells or other abnormal behavior. The victim may make purposeless movements, such as smacking the lips and picking at his or her clothes. In children, these absence spells are called *petit mal seizures*. In adults, these events are usually due to temporal lobe epilepsy, named for the lobe of the brain in which they originate. These are often called *psychomotor seizures*.
- **Status epilepticus**—These are a series of seizures without an interval of wakefulness between them.

Causes of seizures
Seizures are not a disease, but a symptom of an underlying abnormality. Seizures may be idiopathic (no demonstrable cause) or secondary (due to a brain lesion or metabolic abnormality). Causes within the central nervous system (CNS) of secondary seizures include:
- Infection—Meningitis, brain abscess, encephalitis.
- Fever—Convulsions from fever (febrile convulsion) occur in children. Fever by itself is an uncommon cause of seizures in adults.
- Trauma—Immediately following head trauma, seizures can occur from damage to brain tissue. Late-onset seizures may be caused by the formation of scar tissue in the brain.
- Stroke
- Tumor—One of five patients over age 21 years with new onset seizures has a brain tumor as the cause.

Causes of seizures not directly involving the central nervous system include:
- Failure to take prescribed antiseizure medications—This is the most common cause of seizures in many patients.
- Metabolic abnormalities—Blood chemistry imbalance (low sodium, high calcium, low blood sugar), too much acid in the blood, hypoxia.
- Drug or alcohol withdrawal
- Overdose of drugs (especially tricyclic antidepressants or cocaine)
- Hypertensive crisis
- Liver or kidney failure

Patient assessment

POSTICTAL STATE: A period following a seizure lasting approximately 30 minutes, whereby the sufferer gradually returns to a normal state.

Many times, the amount of information available to the EMT–I at the scene is minimal. The patient often is of little help due to postseizure amnesia. Bystanders may not provide an accurate description of events. The mnemonic **FACTS** describes some of the historical information you should try to obtain about a seizure patient:

- F—Focus: Was there a single initiating movement, or was there simply generalized body involvement from the onset of the seizure?

- A—Activity: What movements took place during the event?

- C—Color: Did the patient become cyanotic during the seizure? C also stands for cocaine, a common cause of seizures in young individuals. Always ask the patient if he or she took drugs.

- T—Time: How long did the seizure last?

- S—Secondary information: What was the patient doing before the seizure? Was there an aura? Did incontinence occur? Did the patient bite his or her mouth or tongue? Is there a history of seizures? Is the patient on antiseizure medications?

Prior to a seizure, some patients will notice the presence of an **aura.** An aura is a warning sign that consists of seeing, hearing, or smelling something unusual before losing responsiveness. A few patients may tell the EMT–I that they "feel as though they are about to have a seizure." The EMT–I should observe these patients carefully and provide appropriate care should a seizure occur.

Most generalized seizures follow a typical pattern:

- An aura may occur.

- The patient develops a glassy-eyed stare and becomes unresponsive.

- Unresponsiveness rapidly develops.

- Alternating tonic-clonic muscle movements of the entire body occur.

- The patient may hold his or her breath and become cyanotic.

- The patient may drool or vomit.

- The patient may become incontinent of urine or feces.

- Generally, the seizure lasts less than 5 minutes.

Following a seizure, the patient is usually in a **postictal state.** This state is a period of decreased responsiveness after a generalized seizure. As the patient gradually wakes up, he or she may look at the EMT–I but not be able to respond.

Generally, the postictal period lasts less than 30 minutes. At times, patients may have a prolonged postictal period that mimics coma. When the patient is completely awake and lucid, he or she generally does not remember the seizure. If a patient develops another seizure before becoming lucid, he or she is in status epilepticus.

A patient's behavior during the postictal period may be unusual. Most patients are disoriented, and some become violent. The EMT–I should be alert for violent postictal behavior and be prepared to restrain the patient as necessary. Remember, patients with violent postictal behavior are not aware of what they are doing.

STREET WISE
Watch for violent postictal behavior.

HELPFUL HINT
A small percentage of patients will have a neurologic deficit following a seizure. This deficit is called Todd's postictal paralysis and lasts up to 2 hours. This condition may appear identical to a stroke. A small number of patients actually suffer injury to the head or spine during the seizure. If cervical spine tenderness or neurologic deficit is present, assume that spinal injury has occurred and immobilize the patient.

Some patients may have bitten their mouth or tongue during the seizure. The EMT–I should care for these wounds the same as for any other open wound.

Emergency care

Witnessing a seizure is extremely disturbing for bystanders, relatives, and healthcare providers. The EMT–I must maintain a calm, concerned, and professional attitude toward the patient. If the patient is a child, the family may be hysterical. The EMT–I should calm and reassure them but not compromise patient care.

 Describe the patient care priorities for seizure.

There is nothing an EMT–I can do to stop a seizure. The EMT–I should care for the seizure patient as follows:

- Maintain the airway as best as possible. Many patients with seizures develop transient airway obstruction during seizure. If the obstruction is due to muscle spasm, it will not respond to standard airway procedures.

- Do not insert airways, jaw screws, or bite bars between the teeth of a seizing patient. You will likely damage the patient's teeth as well as your fingers.

- Assist ventilation as required during the postictal state.

- Be prepared to suction the patient during the seizure. It is common for the mouth to become full of secretions and vomitus. Suction this material using a rigid tip device. Do not force the suction catheter between the patient's teeth.

- Give high-concentration oxygen by nonrebreather mask.

- Do not restrain the patient. The seizure cannot be stopped by restraining muscle movements. The best approach is to let the seizure take its course. Place a pillow, rolled blanket, or other padding material beneath the patient's head to help prevent injury.

- Start an IV lifeline. This may be difficult during the seizure; in this case, wait until the seizure movements have lessened.

- Place the patient on a cardiac monitor. Sometimes life-threatening dysrhythmias can cause seizures because of decreased blood flow to the brain.

- Keep alert for violent postictal behavior.

- Keep bystanders and nonessential EMS personnel back to avoid frightening or embarrassing the patient as he or she wakes up.

- Check oxygen saturation via pulse oximeter.

- Transport the patient in the coma position following a seizure.

 HELPFUL HINT
Many patients fail to take antiseizure medication regularly. Some are compliant with medication but need to have the dosage adjusted. Transport all patients who have had seizures to the hospital for evaluation.

Headache

 List four causes of headache.

Although most headaches result from minor ailments (such as fever, anxiety, or tension), some are due to potentially serious conditions:

- Brain tumors
- Intracranial bleeding
- Hypertensive crisis
- Meningitis
- Poisoning

Patient assessment

The location of head pain varies, depending on the cause. The onset of pain may be gradual or rapid. In addition to pain, other symptoms may be present:

- Visual disturbances, such as blurred vision
- Nausea, vomiting
- Vertigo (spinning of the room)
- Stiffness of the neck

 HELPFUL HINT
Consider the rapid onset of severe headache to be due to intracranial bleeding until proven otherwise. The patient often states that it is the worst headache of his or her life. If you suspect that the patient has an intracranial hemorrhage, transport immediately to the nearest appropriate hospital.

- Neurologic deficit, such as hemiplegia
- Elevated blood pressure
- Unequal or pinpoint pupils
- Eye pain with bright light (photophobia)

Emergency care

The EMT–I should assume that any patient with a headache severe enough to lead him or her to activate the EMS system has a dangerous condition. The EMT–I should provide the following care:

- Monitor the airway, breathing, and circulation carefully.
- Prepare for vomiting.
- Reduce bright lights.
- Place an ice pack to the head over the area of pain.
- Give oxygen via nasal cannular or nonrebreather mask.

GASTROINTESTINAL EMERGENCIES

Acute abdominal pain

The focus of this section is on acute abdominal pain not due to injury. See Chapter 13, "Trauma Emergencies," for information on abdominal injuries.

The EMT–I should approach the patient with acute nontraumatic abdominal pain as follows:

- Does this patient have a life-threatening condition, including severe pain or shock? If so, rapidly provide necessary care and transport the patient as "priority."

- If the patient does not have a life-threatening illness, care for the patient and transport him or her to the nearest appropriate hospital.

It is NOT necessary for the EMT–I to make a diagnosis in the field. The signs and symptoms of many abdominal conditions are similar. It may be impossible to determine in the field if the EMT–I is dealing with a potentially life-threatening situation or not. The EMT–I should always assume that a serious condition may be present until proven otherwise.

Anatomy review

The abdominal cavity extends from the diaphragm to the pelvic bones and contains the organs of digestion, the organs of the urinary and reproductive tracts, the vertebral column, and major blood vessels.

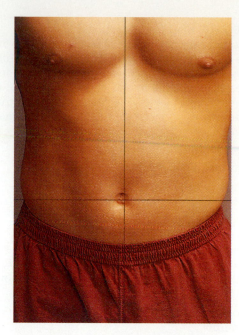

Fig. 15-14 **The four quadrants of the abdomen.**

For descriptive purposes, the abdomen is divided into four quadrants (Fig. 15-14).

Causes of acute abdominal pain

There are many diseases that may cause acute abdominal pain. Four diseases are immediately life-threatening:

- *Acute myocardial infarction*—The pain of acute myocardial infarction may occur anywhere from the umbilicus upward (*see* Chapter 14, "Cardiac Emergencies").

- *Ruptured abdominal aortic aneurysm*—This is an out-pouching of the abdominal portion of the aorta due to atherosclerosis. Aneurysm formation weakens the wall of the artery. If the aneurysm ruptures, severe abdominal and back pain, as well as shock, result. The patient may easily bleed to death.

- *Ruptured ectopic pregnancy*—This condition occurs when the fertilized egg implants outside the uterus. Internal structures may rupture, causing severe internal bleeding. The patient has abdominal pain, vaginal bleeding, and shock (*see* Chapter 17, "Obstetric and Gynecologic Emergencies").

- *Ruptured viscus*—Viscus is a general term for any hollow organ. The most common viscus to rupture is the duodenum, usually due to a peptic ulcer. The patient develops the sudden onset of sharp epigastric pain and shock, and the abdomen is rigid.

Other common causes of acute abdominal pain that are not usually life-threatening include:

- *Peptic ulcer disease*—Erosions in the lining of the gastrointestinal tract. Ulcers result from excess acid production by the stomach and are associated with stress, cigarette smoking, and the intake of certain drugs (steroids and antiinflammatory agents). Symptoms include gnawing upper abdominal pain and nausea, which is often relieved with food or antacids.

- *Gastritis*—Inflammation of the lining of the stomach resulting from drugs, alcohol, or infection. Gastritis is characterized by loss of appetite, nausea, vomiting, and epigastric discomfort after eating. The pain may be relieved with antacids.

- *Pneumonia*—Infection and inflammation of the tissues of the lungs; pneumonia of the lower lobes of the lungs can cause upper abdomen pain.

- *Pancreatitis*—Inflammation of the pancreas due to stones that block the ducts. The pain is epigastric and radiates straight through to the patient's back. Nausea and vomiting are common.

- *Kidney stones (nephrolithiasis)*—Kidney stones are the formation of small rocklike structures in the kidney. The passage of a stone down the urinary tract causes severe, intermittent pain. The discomfort starts in the flank and radiates to the abdomen and groin. Nausea and vomiting are common.

- *Pelvic inflammatory disease (PID)*—Inflammation of the female internal genitalia usually due to a sexually transmitted disease. The patient complains of lower abdominal pain; she may have vaginal discharge, fever, and chills.

- *Appendicitis (inflammation of the appendix)*—Results from obstruction of the lumen of the appendix. The patient initially has pain around the umbilicus, which then localizes to the right lower quadrant. Loss of appetite (anorexia) is common. Rupture of the appendix can result in peritonitis, an inflammation of the abdominal cavity.

- *Cholecystitis (gallbladder attack)*—Occlusion of the gallbladder duct, leading to inflammation and pain. The pain is usually intermittent, located in the right upper quadrant, and is accompanied by nausea. Pain may radiate to the posterior scapula or right shoulder. Attacks are often self-limited and may be brought on with the ingestion of fatty foods.

- *Pyelonephritis (kidney infection)*—The patient has flank pain, which may radiate to the abdomen; discomfort with urination; nausea; and vomiting.

- *Diverticulitis*—Diverticula are small, saclike outpouchings in the intestine. Infection of these leads to cramplike abdominal pain in the left lower quadrant. Diverticulitis may be accompanied by fever, diarrhea, or constipation.

- *Bowel obstruction*—A blockage of the intestinal tract. The symptoms include cramping pain, vomiting, abdominal tenderness, and distention of the abdomen.

- *Nonabdominal causes*—Sickle cell anemia crisis, black widow spider bite, diabetic ketoacidosis, anaphylactic shock.

 STREET WISE
Assume that any patient with right lower quadrant abdominal pain has appendicitis until proven otherwise.

Patient assessment

Patients with an acute abdominal condition complain of localized or diffuse pain. The abdominal organs have nerve receptors for pressure, but not for pain. Often, abdominal discomfort is vaguely located and referred to other parts of the body. Conditions that originate in the abdomen can cause pain in locations quite distant such as the neck, shoulder, or flank. Other signs and symptoms of an acute abdominal condition include:

- Nausea, vomiting
- Diarrhea
- Decreased appetite
- Chills, fever
- Painful urination
- Blood in the urine, stool, or vomitus
- Vaginal bleeding or discharge

 HELPFUL HINT
Vaginal bleeding in a woman of childbearing years is assumed to be due to an ectopic pregnancy until proven otherwise. Do not perform a vaginal examination in the prehospital setting.

- Cough (if pneumonia is present)
- Chest pains, shortness of breath (in myocardial infarction)

  On examination, evaluate for the following:

- General appearance—Patients with acute abdominal conditions may be lying extremely still (any movement worsens the pain) or writhing in pain (common with kidney stones and gallbladder attacks).
- Abdominal tenderness to palpation—The abdomen may be soft, rigid, or distended. There may be localized or diffuse tenderness to palpation.
- Signs of shock
- Fever
- Pulsating mass in the abdomen—This sign suggests an abdominal aortic aneurysm.
- Guarding—The patient may lie on the back or side with the knees drawn toward the chest.

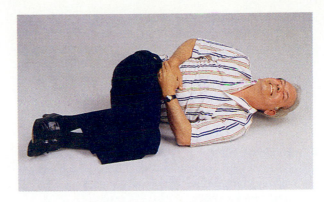

Fig. 15-15 Often, the most comfortable position for a patient experiencing acute abdominal pain is flat on the back with the knees drawn up to the chest.

Emergency care

 Describe the patient care priorities for abdominal pain.

To provide care for patients with acute abdominal pain, the EMT–I should:

- Maintain the airway. Give oxygen and assist breathing if necessary.
- If leaking or ruptured abdominal aortic aneurysm is suspected, transport the patient immediately. Perform other treatments en route.
- Allow the patient to lie in a comfortable position. Many times the best position is flat on the back with the knees drawn up (Fig. 15-15).
- Do not give anything by mouth.
- Start an IV lifeline; if the patient appears to be dehydrated or is hypotensive, give a fluid bolus as per local protocol. The usual dose is 500 to 1000 cc of normal saline or Ringer's lactate IV as rapidly as possible.
- Care for shock if present. Use the pneumatic anti-shock garment (PASG), if necessary, according to local protocols.
- Be prepared for vomiting. Have suction equipment available.
- Always consider the possibility of acute myocardial infarction in a patient with abdominal pain, especially if the location is epigastric.

Gastrointestinal bleeding

Gastrointestinal bleeding refers to hemorrhage anywhere in the gastrointestinal (GI) tract (from the mouth to anus) due to a lesion of the mucosa (lining). GI bleeding accounts for 1% to 2% of hospital admissions in the United States.

Approach to gastrointestinal bleeding

Gastrointestinal bleeding can rapidly result in life-threatening hypovolemic shock. The chances of determining the exact cause of GI bleeding in the field are slim. Rather than trying to determine the cause of the GI bleeding, the EMT–I should evaluate the following:

- Is the patient's airway open? Airway obstruction due to vomiting of blood is common.

> **HELPFUL HINT**
>
> Patients who vomit blood may have a high risk of airway compromise. The EMT–I should monitor and care for shock.

- Is the patient in shock?
- Is active bleeding present?

 List four causes of gastrointestinal bleeding.

Causes of gastrointestinal bleeding

Causes of GI bleeding are divided into upper and lower sources. Upper GI bleeding originates anywhere in the GI tract from the mouth to the duodenum. Most commonly, the patient vomits blood, but if the bleeding rate is sufficient, blood will be passed via the rectum as well. Because of the action of gastric fluids, vomited blood usually has the appearance of coffee grounds.

Lower GI bleeding results from bleeding due to a lesion of the GI tract below the level of the duodenum. Blood from these lesions always passes rectally and may appear as bright red blood passing from the rectum or red-streaked or tarry-looking stool.

> **STREET WISE**
>
> It is not important that the EMT–I figure out the exact cause of the bleeding. More importantly, the EMT–I should recognize that the patient has GI bleeding and provide care accordingly.

Common causes of upper GI bleeding include:
- Peptic ulcer disease
- Gastritis
- Esophageal varices—Dilation of veins of the esophagus due to liver disease. This is a common cause of upper GI bleeding in alcoholic patients.
- Esophagitis—Irritation of the esophagus, similar to that which occurs in gastritis.

Common causes of lower GI bleeding include:
- Diverticulosis—Diverticula may become inflamed (leading to diverticulitis), or may bleed.
- Tumors, hemorrhoids, polyps—These commonly result in lower GI bleeding, but usually the bleeding is not significant in the prehospital setting.

All patients with rectal bleeding are considered high-risk patients. The EMT–I should monitor them and care for shock.

Patient assessment

Patients may report use of aspirin, alcohol, or anti-inflammatory agents such as ibuprofen. The patient may vomit blood, which either is bright red or looks like coffee grounds. Blood passed by the rectum may be bright red or appear as dark, tarry stool. During assessment, the EMT–I should pay special attention to:

- Airway patency
- Signs and symptoms of shock
- Abdominal pain
- Fever

> **CLINICAL NOTES**
>
> Hematochezia is the presence of bright red blood in the stool. Melena is black, tarry stool caused by digested blood passing slowly through the GI tract.
>
> Hematemesis is the vomiting of blood. Coffee ground vomitus is the vomiting of liquid resembling coffee grounds. The appearance is due to digestion of the blood by stomach acid.
>
> More than 80% of patients with upper GI bleeding have fever. The reason for this is unclear.

Emergency care

 Describe the patient care priorities for gastrointestinal bleeding.

To care for a patient with gastrointestinal bleeding, the EMT–I should:

- Maintain control of the airway.
- Give high-concentration oxygen by nonrebreather mask. If the patient is nauseated or vomiting, use nasal cannula (4 to 6 L/min).
- Assist breathing as necessary.
- Care for shock, if present. Patients with GI bleeding are at a high risk for shock. Use the PASG as needed, as per your local protocols.
- Start an IV lifeline; if the patient appears dehydrated or is hypotensive, give a fluid bolus as per local protocol. The usual dose is 500 to 1000 cc of normal saline or Ringer's lactate IV as rapidly as possible; follow local protocols.
- Anticipate vomiting and be prepared to suction the patient.
- Give nothing by mouth.
- Assume that any patient with ongoing GI bleeding has a significant, potentially life-threatening lesion and provide care accordingly.

DIABETIC EMERGENCIES

 DIABETES MELLITUS: A disease whereby an insufficient amount of insulin is produced to regulate blood sugar levels in the body.

Diabetes mellitus is a disease of the endocrine system involving the hormone insulin. Insulin regulates the blood sugar level and moves sugar molecules from the blood into the cells, where they are metabolized. In addition, insulin prevents the breakdown of fat tissue in the body. Persons with diabetes do not produce enough insulin to regulate the blood sugar level. As a result, the blood sugar level may become too high (hyperglycemia) or too low (hypoglycemia). Either condition can result in potentially life-threatening problems.

> **CLINICAL NOTES**
> Measurement of the blood sugar level is usually done in a hospital laboratory. A useful but less precise measurement of blood sugar level involves chemically treated paper strips exposed to a drop of blood obtained by a fingerstick. Fingerstick measurements of the blood sugar level may be easily done in the field (usually by advanced life-support providers), home, emergency department, or hospital wards (Fig. 15-16).

If a known diabetic patient has an altered level of responsiveness or neurologic symptoms, the EMT–I should ASSUME that he or she has low blood sugar and care for the patient accordingly.

Hypoglycemia

Hypoglycemia is an abnormally low blood sugar level. This condition is sometimes called *insulin shock*. However, these patients are rarely in shock. Because circumstances other than insulin overdose lead to low blood sugar, the preferred term is hypoglycemia.

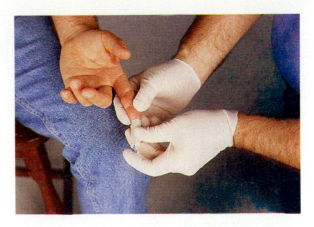

Fig. 15-16 A measurement of blood sugar using a fingerstick.

Causes of hypoglycemia

Causes of hypoglycemia include the following:

- Medications (insulin, oral diabetic medications)
- Excessive exercise (causes overly rapid absorption of insulin)
- Endocrine diseases
- Alcohol consumption
- Poor diet
- Hypothermia (severe cold exposure)
- Liver disease

Hypoglycemia in a diabetic patient most frequently occurs because the patient has taken his or her insulin, but not eaten enough food. Insulin forces sugar into the cells. Due to the inadequate dietary intake, too little sugar remains in the blood to maintain homeostasis. Low levels of blood sugar interfere with the function of the central nervous system.

Fingerstick blood sugar determination

To properly perform a fingerstick blood sugar determination:

1. Use either the patient's index or middle finger.
2. Clean the fingertip with an alcohol swab.
3. Gently squeeze the finger at the joint below the fingertip.
4. At the same time, use either a small needle or special fingerstick lancet to pierce the skin of the fingertip. The tip should not go in more than 1 to 2 mm. Do this in a rapid "in and out" fashion. Do not leave the lancet or needle in place or twist it around.
5. Immediately remove the lancet or needle.
6. Using a gloved hand, gently squeeze the fingertip to express a drop of blood from the wound.
7. Place the drop of blood on the chemical reagent strip; begin timing.
8. When the proper period of time has passed (this depends on the type of reagent strip), use a cotton ball and wipe the remaining blood from the strip.
9. Use either a measuring device (glucometer) or the color scale on the reagent container to determine the patient's blood sugar.

Patient assessment

 Describe five signs and symptoms of hypoglycemia.

Hypoglycemia generally develops rapidly, over a few minutes to a few hours. The signs and symptoms of hypoglycemia include:

- Shakiness, weakness

- Diaphoresis

- Rapid pulse and respiratory rate

- Altered level of responsiveness. The patient may appear intoxicated.

- Slurred speech

- Neurologic deficit (unusual)

- Seizures (unusual in adults; more common in children)

Severe hypoglycemia causes a marked alteration in the level of responsiveness. The patient often is unconscious. It may be impossible to differentiate hypoglycemia from a stroke, because hypoglycemia can cause paralysis and altered levels of responsiveness. Hypoglycemia by itself usually does not result in hypotension. The EMT–I should look for another cause of the patient's symptoms if hypotension is present.

 STREET WISE
Hypoglycemia by itself does not usually result in hypotension. Look for another cause of the patient's symptoms if hypotension is present.

The EMT–I should ALWAYS ask the diabetic patient, "Did you eat today? Did you take your insulin (or other diabetic medication) today?"

Emergency care

 Describe the care given to patients with hypoglycemia.

To care for a patient with known or suspected hypoglycemia, the EMT–I should:

- Control the airway and assist breathing as necessary. Patients with an altered level of responsiveness may have partial airway obstruction.

- Give oxygen by nasal cannula at a rate of 6 L/min.

- Monitor the electrocardiogram (ECG).

- If the patient is responsive, give orange juice with two packets of sugar dissolved in it. Alternatively, have the patient take a dose of oral glucose solution, corn syrup, or candy.

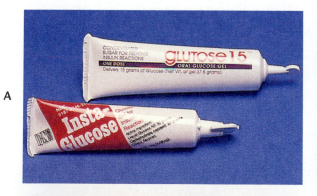

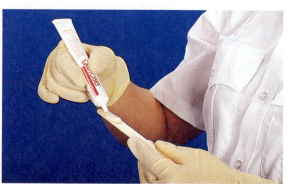

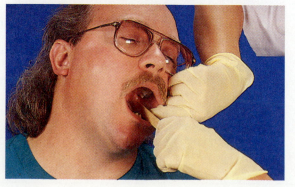

Fig. 15-17 Administering oral glucose to a patient experiencing hypoglycemia. **A,** Various types of oral glucose. **B,** Administer the full tube of glucose. **C,** Place the glucose between the patient's cheek and gums.

- Unless the symptoms are extremely mild, start an IV lifeline; draw blood PRIOR to giving any fluid or sugar (D50).

- If permitted by local protocols, administer 1 ampule of D50 (25 g of dextrose in 50 cc water) IV if the measured blood sugar is less than 60 mg/dl. If you are unable to measure blood sugar in the field, follow local protocols regarding the administration of IV D50.

- If unable to start an IV through which to give dextrose (D50), place liquid glucose or glucose paste into the patient's mouth (Fig. 15-17). Try to place it onto the inner cheeks. Oral glucose is contraindicated if the patient is unresponsive and has no gag reflex.

HELPFUL HINT

Follow local protocols regarding placing liquid glucose or glucose paste in the mouth of an unconscious patient.

- If you are in doubt as to whether the conscious patient has hypoglycemia or hyperglycemia (diabetic ketoacidosis), always assume the patient is hypoglycemic and give sugar. Never give a diabetic patient insulin in the field.

- Transport the patient to the hospital for further evaluation and treatment.

Hyperglycemia and diabetic ketoacidosis

Hyperglycemia is an elevation of the blood sugar level above normal. The most common cause of hyperglycemia is diabetes. **Diabetic ketoacidosis** (sometimes called *diabetic coma*) is a metabolic condition consisting of hyperglycemia, dehydration, and the accumulation of abnormal compounds, called *ketones* and *ketoacids*, in the body.

Causes of diabetic ketoacidosis

Diabetic ketoacidosis (DKA) occurs when a patient with diabetes has inadequate insulin circulating in the blood to properly control the blood sugar level. The patient's blood sugar rises significantly and the fatty tissue breaks down. The body forms compounds called *ketones* and *ketoacids* from the fat tissue. These substances change the acid-base balance in the body, harming the patient. The elevated blood sugar level makes the patient urinate more frequently than usual, leading to dehydration and loss of body chemicals (particularly potassium).

The most common reason a diabetic patient develops DKA is an infection. This stress results in an increased insulin requirement in the body.

Unless the diabetic patient recognizes the need to increase the daily dose of insulin when sick, metabolism and the regulation of blood sugar level become abnormal.

CLINICAL NOTES

The terms *diabetic coma* (for diabetic ketoacidosis) and *insulin shock* (for hypoglycemia) are misleading. Patients in DKA are not usually in a coma, and hypoglycemic patients are rarely in shock. Avoid the use of these confusing terms—use hypoglycemia, hyperglycemia, or diabetic ketoacidosis.

Patient assessment

 List five signs and symptoms of diabetic ketoacidosis.

Diabetic ketoacidosis has a relatively slow onset. Patients with DKA have symptoms that become worse over a matter of hours to days. The signs and symptoms are:

- Weakness

- Nausea and vomiting

- Abdominal pain

- Frequent urination

- Thirst

- Rapid, deep, sighing respirations (Kussmaul respirations)

- Alterations in the level of responsiveness

- A fruity, acetone-like odor to the breath

- Normal or mildly decreased blood pressure

- Rapid, weak pulse

The acetone-like odor described in DKA is not always present. Not all people are able to detect this odor. The EMT–I should not rely on the breath odor to suspect DKA.

Emergency care

To care for a patient with suspected hyperglycemia or diabetic ketoacidosis the EMT–I should:

- Maintain the airway, and assist breathing as necessary.

- Give high-concentration oxygen.

- Monitor the ECG rhythm.

- Start an IV lifeline. Because many of these patients are significantly dehydrated, give a fluid bolus as per local protocol. Many systems use 500 to 1000 cc of normal saline or Ringer's lactate as rapidly as possible.

- Watch carefully for shock and care for the patient accordingly.

- Give nothing by mouth. An exception to this rule is when the patient is responsive or when it is uncertain whether a patient has hypoglycemia or hyperglycemia. If unable to check the finger-stick blood sugar, always assume hypoglycemia is present and give sugar. Never give a diabetic patient insulin in the field!

- Transport the patient to the hospital as soon as possible.

>
> **STREET WISE**
> If a diabetic emergency is present and the patient has an altered level of responsiveness or neurologic symptoms and the EMT–I is unable to check the blood sugar, the EMT–I should ASSUME that the patient has low blood sugar and care for him or her accordingly.

Hyperglycemic hyperosmolar nonketotic coma

Hyperglycemic hyperosmolar nonketotic coma (HHNC) refers to a state in which the blood sugar is markedly elevated but no acidosis or accumulation of ketones is present. As a result, high levels of glucose in the cerebrospinal fluid leads to dehydration of the brain and decreased levels of responsiveness.

 Describe the most common presentation of hyperosmolar hyperglycemic nonketotic coma.

Persons with HHNC are typically over 60 years of age. Their underlying health is poor, and often these persons are in a nursing home or other assisted-living setting. HHNC is precipitated by infection, extreme cold, or dehydration. The typical history is that of gradual deterioration in mental status over 4 or 5 days. Other signs and symptoms include:

- Altered mental status; the patient may be unresponsive or may appear to have had a stroke.

- Evidence of dehydration—Poor skin turgor, furrowed tongue.

- Kussmaul respirations and fruity breath odor— Although these signs are present in diabetic ketoacidosis, they are conspicuously *absent* in HHNC.

The treatment for patients with HHNC is the same as that described previously for diabetic ketoacidosis.

General management of a diabetic emergency

 Describe the care given to patients with hyperglycemia.

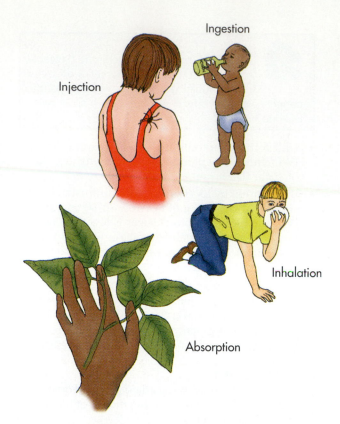

Fig. 15-18 The four mechanisms of poisoning: ingestion, inhalation, absorption, and injection.

As a reminder, the EMT–I should follow these general guidelines when dealing with any type of suspected diabetic emergency:

- Manage the airway with supplemental oxygen and assisted ventilation, including endotracheal intubation when necessary.

- As per local protocols, draw blood before giving any medication or IV fluid; take a fingerstick blood sugar reading if possible.

- Monitor vital signs and the ECG.

- Administer dextrose (D50) as per protocol.

POISONING EMERGENCIES

Poisoning is the ingestion, inhalation, absorption, or injection of any harmful substance. Nearly one half of all poisonings involve prescription drugs. Many poisonings are unintentional but preventable. Poisoning is most common among children under 10 years of age. In adults, most poisonings are suicide attempts or drug abuse.

 Identify four routes of exposure to poison.

Routes of poisoning

There are four routes by which poisons are introduced into the human body (Fig. 15-18):

- Ingestion—A poison may enter the body by the mouth and be absorbed in the gastrointestinal tract. Ingestion is the most common poisoning route.

- Inhalation—Toxic fumes or gases may be inhaled into the lungs. The material may damage the lungs or be absorbed into the blood, leading to systemic toxicity. Carbon monoxide poisoning is an example of inhalation exposure.

- Absorption—Substances may pass through the skin into the bloodstream. Many chemicals dissolve easily in the fat of the skin. These materials are the ones most likely to cause poisoning by absorption. Pesticides and agricultural chemicals are often absorbed this way.

- Injection—Toxic material may be injected by needles or insect stingers.

Patient assessment

 List four items of information needed when assessing a patient who ingested a poison.

When caring for a poisoning patient, the EMT–I should try to gather the following information about the event:

- What was taken.
- How much was ingested.
- When the poisoning occurred.
- What, if anything, has been done for the patient.

The patient may say that he or she took a poison. If the patient is a child, the parent may be able to tell or show the EMT–I the substance involved. The EMT–I should always bring any containers, pills, syringes, and pill bottles to the hospital with the patient. If the patient vomits, the EMT–I should try to collect the vomitus in a plastic bag and bring it to the hospital for analysis.

Signs and symptoms of poisoning vary, depending on the particular substance involved. They may include:

- Burning and tearing of the eyes
- Respiratory distress, wheezing, chest pain
- Cyanosis
- Nausea, vomiting, diarrhea
- Excessive sweating or salivation
- Weakness
- Headache, dizziness, seizures
- Altered level of responsiveness (ranging from hyperactivity to coma)
- Pain, burning, or itching of the skin
- Burns or stains around the mouth

 Identify five areas to assess with a poisoned patient.

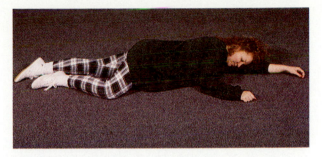

Fig. 15-19 The proper position for a poisoning patient.

Physical findings may help identify the poison involved.

- *Pulse*—Tachycardia suggests stimulant ingestion. Bradycardia may be caused by various heart medications, as well as by pesticide poisoning.

- *Respiratory rate*—Isolated increases in the respiratory rate, especially in children, suggest the possibility of aspirin toxicity (which causes hyperventilation). Depressed respirations occur from narcotics, sedatives, and carbon monoxide poisoning.

- *Temperature*—Can be elevated from aspirin and stimulants and lowered (hypothermia) with alcohol, sedatives, narcotics, and pesticides.

- *Blood pressure*—May be decreased if the patient took depressant or narcotic agents. The BP is often elevated if the patient has taken cocaine or amphetamines.

> **STREET WISE**
> It is NOT necessary to determine the exact substance taken by the patient. The main goal in managing a poisoning victim is maintenance of the airway, breathing, and circulation, and definitive treatment at an appropriate medical facility.

Poisoning may affect a number of body systems. Indications of poisoning may be apparent during the focused history and physical examination:

- Respiratory system—Many poisonings cause respiratory depression and partial airway obstruction. Inhaled toxins may cause respiratory distress and wheezing.

- Cardiovascular system—Some poisonings can cause irregular heart rhythm, chest pain, shock, and cardiac arrest.

- Neurologic system—Poisonings may result in changes in the pupil size. Narcotics usually cause constricted pupils, whereas stimulants result in pupillary dilation.

Care of the poisoned patient

Control of airway, breathing, and circulation is the first concern in poisoning management. For any type of poisoning, the EMT–I should provide the following care:

- Assess and maintain the airway, and monitor vital signs and pulse oximetry frequently.
- Place the patient on a cardiac monitor.
- Position the patient to prevent aspiration (left lateral recumbent position, head down) (Fig. 15-19).
- Give high-concentration oxygen by mask. If the patient is vomiting, use nasal cannula (6 L/min). If the patient is unresponsive, consider endotracheal intubation, per local protocol.
- Use the PASG as necessary, per local protocols.
- If the patient is uncooperative, violent, or suicidal, restrain according to local guidelines. Be sure to document the need for restraints in the run report. Do not be a hero—call for police assistance with violent patients.
- Notify the hospital of the suspected substances involved.

After providing life-maintaining care, the EMT–I should consult the local Poison Information Center or medical direction for specific advice. Depending on the patient's condition, this may be done en route to the hospital. The EMT–I should bring all suspect material and containers to the hospital.

Ingested Poisons

🍎 **Describe the proper use of syrup of ipecac.**

The EMT–I should care for poisoned patients as recommended by the Poison Information Center or medical direction. Some EMS systems advise giving syrup of ipecac to induce vomiting. Because syrup of ipecac is not universally accepted, the EMT–I should consult local protocols before giving ipecac. Vomiting should not be induced if the patient is having seizures or if the EMT–I suspects ingestion of acid, lye, or petroleum products. Vomiting also should not be induced if the patient has a decreased level of responsiveness or may lose responsiveness. Transport should not be delayed to wait for ipecac to take effect.

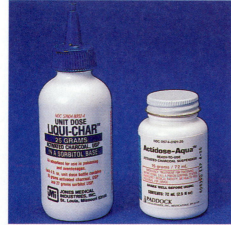
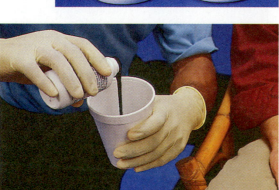
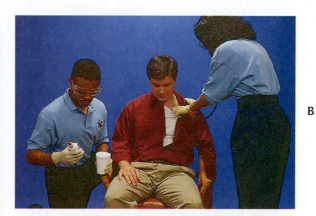
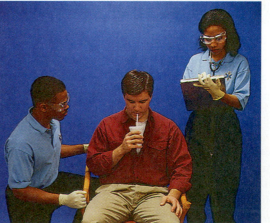

Fig. 15-20 Administering activated charcoal to a poisoned patient. A, Various types of activated charcoal. B, Shake the container to suspend the medication in the fluid. C, Pour the liquid into a container. D, Have the patient drink the full dose.

Some protocols advise the administration of activated charcoal to absorb the poison (Fig. 15-20). The EMT–I should not give charcoal until ipecac has caused vomiting. Otherwise, the charcoal will absorb the ipecac and vomiting will not occur.

> **CLINICAL NOTES**
>
> Syrup of ipecac is a drug that produces vomiting by irritating the lining of the stomach. It is used to empty the stomach in certain cases of poisoning. Some poison centers recommend that ipecac be limited to home use, when the patient does not require hospital evaluation.
>
> The dosage of syrup of ipecac is 30 mL for adults and 15 mL for children given by mouth, followed by several glasses of water. Do not give ipecac to children under 9 months of age.
>
> Do not induce vomiting if the patient is:
>
> - Is comatose or has an altered level of responsiveness
> - Is seizing or has a history of seizures
> - Is in the third trimester of pregnancy
> - Has a history of cardiac problems
>
> Do not induce vomiting if the patient has ingested:
>
> - Corrosives, such as strong acids or alkali
> - Petroleum products
> - Iodine, silver nitrate, or strychnine
>
> The preferred method of care in the hospital is activated charcoal and/or gastric lavage. Gastric lavage involves placing a tube into the stomach, through which fluids are given to dilute and rinse the stomach contents. The liquid is then removed through the gastric tube by suction.
>
> Activated charcoal, in addition to absorbing and neutralizing many poisons, serves as a marker to indicate when a poison has passed through the digestive tract. Cathartic drugs, such as magnesium citrate, also are sometimes given to speed passage of substances through the digestive system.

Inhaled Poisons

Inhaled poisons may be odorless and colorless. The EMT–I should not place himself or herself at risk when caring for a victim of inhalation poisoning. The EMT–I should survey the scene to make sure it is safe to approach the patient. It may be necessary to wait for respirators or other specialized equipment before caring for the patient.

Care begins by removing the patient from the source of exposure. The EMT–I should move the patient to an area outside or with freely circulating air.

🍎 **List the common signs and symptoms of carbon monoxide poisoning.**

Carbon monoxide poisoning should be suspected in all victims of fire. The EMT–I should assist breathing as necessary and provide high-concentration oxygen by nonrebreather mask. The EMT–I should keep the patient at rest and transport to the hospital as soon as possible.

Absorbed Poisons

Care for absorbed poisoning involves reducing the contact of the toxic material on the patient's skin:

- Brush off any visible chemical.
- Flush the affected area with large amounts of water.
- Remove contaminated clothing while flushing.
- Protect yourself from exposure to the poison.

HEAT EXPOSURE EMERGENCIES

Heat is generated by muscular activity and through metabolic reactions in the body. As the body temperature increases, changes occur in each organ system. If an individual gradually exposes himself or herself to a hot environment, the body acclimates, or becomes used to the heat. Heat is dissipated from the body by four mechanisms (Fig. 15-21):

- Radiation—Transmission of heat through space.
- Conduction—Transmission of heat from warmer to cooler objects in direct contact.
- Convection—Transfer of heat by circulation of heated particles.
- Evaporation—Loss of heat at the surface from vaporization of liquid.

In humans, conduction is not a major mechanism of heat loss unless the clothing is removed and the

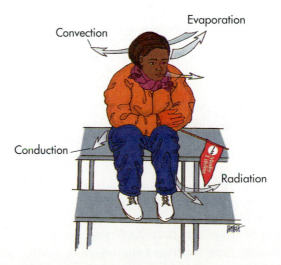

Fig. 15-21 The four mechanisms of heat dissipation: radiation, conduction, convection, and evaporation.

individual lies on a cool surface. Convection also is hindered by clothing. At room temperature, 75% of heat dissipation is by radiation and convection. Evaporation, the loss of moisture from the lungs and skin, accounts for approximately 25% of heat loss.

As the ambient temperature approaches body temperature, radiation is no longer effective to dissipate heat. The body may actually pick up heat by conduction and convection. At high temperatures, evaporation becomes the only effective method of heat dissipation. High humidity seriously impairs heat dissipation, because evaporation occurs slowly.

Most heat injury syndromes occur in individuals who are unacclimated. Three types of heat-related syndromes can develop: heat cramps, heat exhaustion, and heat stroke.

Heat cramps

Heat cramps are cramps or pains in the muscles, especially the muscles of the abdomen and lower extremities, which occur in a hot environment. Heat cramps are the most common of the heat injury syndromes.

The cause of heat cramps is excessive loss of salt and water in the sweat. Cramps usually occur in the young unacclimated individual who engages in exercise or heavy labor in hot climates and sweats profusely.

Patient assessment

Signs and symptoms of heat cramps include:

- Muscle twitching, followed by painful spasms, especially involving the lower extremities and abdomen
- Nausea and vomiting
- Weakness
- Diaphoresis
- Hypotension and tachycardia

 Describe care provided for patients with heat cramps, heat exhaustion, and heat stroke.

Care of the patient with heat cramps

To care for victims of heat cramps, the EMT–I should:

- Remove the patient to a cool environment.
- If the patient is completely responsive, give sips of cool water. Avoid liquids that are extremely cold, salty, or sweet, because they may cause nausea or vomiting.
- Start an IV lifeline. A fluid bolus of 500 to 1000 cc normal saline will often decrease pain—follow local protocols.
- DO NOT give the patient salt pills.
- Provide high-concentration oxygen by nonrebreather mask (15 L/min flow).
- Transport the patient to the hospital.

Heat exhaustion

Heat exhaustion is a more severe loss of fluid and salt than occurs in heat cramps, usually following exertion in a hot, humid environment.

There is a high incidence of heat exhaustion in young children, individuals on water pills (diuretics), and debilitated persons who are unable to maintain an adequate oral water intake or those having prolonged bouts of diarrhea.

Patient assessment

Signs and symptoms of heat exhaustion include:

- Lack of skin coloration (pallor)
- Profuse sweating
- Hypotension, especially with positional changes
- Headache, often with weakness and fatigue
- Thirst
- Normal or slightly elevated temperature

Care of the patient with heat exhaustion

To care for victims of heat exhaustion, the EMT–I should:

- Remove the patient to a cool environment.
- Give high-concentration oxygen by nonrebreather mask (15 L/min flow rate).
- Do not give anything by mouth.
- Initiate IV lifeline; give a fluid bolus as per your local protocols.
- Monitor the ECG.
- Transport the patient to the hospital as soon as possible.

Heat stroke

Heat stroke, or sun stroke, a failure of the body's temperature regulation mechanisms, is an extreme medical emergency. Heat stroke develops when the body is no longer able to get rid of heat. Unlike the heat exhaustion victim, the person in heat stroke sweats very little or not at all. Usually the skin is hot, red, and dry. As heat accumulates, body temperature can reach a dangerously high level.

Patient assessment

Some heat stroke patients may have 1 or 2 days of lethargy, fatigue, weakness, nausea, vomiting, and dizziness prior to developing full-blown heat stroke. Other cases develop rapidly. These victims become confused or irrational and lose responsiveness within a period of minutes.

The EMT–I should suspect heat stroke in any individual who loses responsiveness in a hot environment. Signs and symptoms of heat stroke include:

- Altered level of responsiveness
- Increased body temperature
- Minimal or no sweating

- Collapse
- Signs and symptoms of shock
- Nausea and vomiting
- Shortness of breath

Care for victims of heat stroke

Rapid cooling is vital for the victim of heat stroke. Time is extremely important. If the victim's body temperature is not quickly lowered, permanent brain damage may result.

To care for heat stroke victims, the EMT–I should:

- Place the patient in a cool environment, such as an air-conditioned ambulance, as soon as possible.
- Remove the patient's clothing.
- Cool the patient immediately by applying ice packs to the neck, axillae (armpits), wrists, and groin.
- Give high-concentration oxygen by nonre-breather mask.
- Start IV fluids (normal saline or Ringer's lactate) at 250 to 500 cc/h.
- Monitor the ECG.
- Wrap the patient with wet sheets if there is good ambient airflow present. Do not postpone transport in order to cool the patient in the field.
- Transport the patient to the hospital as soon as possible. Use the air conditioner in the ambulance as well as any available fans to cool the patient.

COLD EXPOSURE EMERGENCIES

Frostbite

Frostbite is the formation of ice crystals within the tissues. These crystals damage the blood vessels and other tissues. Eventually, frostbitten tissues may die.

The worst tissue damage occurs when an area freezes, thaws, and then refreezes.

Patient assessment

The signs and symptoms of frostbite depend on the stage at which the patient is seen:

- Initially the frostbitten extremity appears waxy, yellowish-white, or bluish-white (Fig. 15-22).
- Whether the skin of a frostbite victim feels soft or firm to frozen depends on the severity of injury. In severe frostbite, the area is hard, cold, and insensitive to pain.
- With rewarming, the extremity becomes flushed with a red to purple-burgundy color.
- Swelling appears within hours of thawing and may persist for days to weeks.
- Following thawing, fluid-filled blisters may form.
- After 9 to 15 days, a black, hard scar will form over the frostbitten area.
- If tissue death occurs, the area will appear moist and weeping with pus (Fig. 15-23).

Generally, there is an initial cold sensation in frostbite, which subsides, leading to numbness. The patient may say that the affected area feels "like a stump." This feeling is due to lack of oxygen.

Following thawing, there is severe, throbbing pain. This pain may last for several weeks. There also may be tingling and burning due to nerve damage that lasts for 3 to 4 weeks. Postthawing pain tends to be severe, requiring strong medications for relief.

Other symptoms may develop up to 4 years later. These symptons consist of cold feet, excess sweating, and numbness. The symptoms are worse in the winter. Patients who have had one bout of frostbite develop an exaggerated response to cold and are therefore more susceptible to another episode.

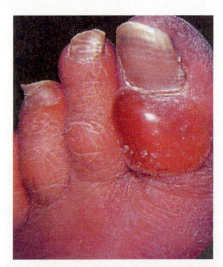

Fig. 15-22 A frostbite injury after thawing has occurred.

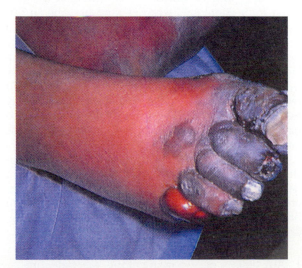

Fig. 15-23 A severe frostbite injury may be dark in color with swelling.

List the care for frostbite.

Care of the patient with frostbite
To care for a patient with frostbite, the EMT–I should:

- Rule out the presence of other significant injuries or illnesses such as total body hypothermia, fractures, or bleeding.
- If the patient has total body hypothermia, do not care for a frostbitten extremity until the body's core temperature is normal.
- Transport the patient to the hospital as soon as possible.
- Protect the involved site by covering it and handling it gently.
- Do not break any blisters. Cover them with dry, sterile dressings.
- Do not allow the patient to smoke. Smoking constricts blood vessels and aggravates hypoxemia to the involved area.
- Do not allow the patient to drink alcohol.
- Do not rewarm frostbite in the field. An exception is if a limb is frozen to an object that cannot be moved. In this case warm the area just enough to move the patient.
- Do not rub a frostbitten area, especially with ice or snow. This can cause severe tissue damage.

Hypothermia
Generalized hypothermia is a condition in which the core or internal body temperature is less than 95° F due to either decreased production of heat or increased heat loss from the body.

Causes and predisposing factors
The three primary causes of hypothermia are cold water immersion, cold weather exposure, and "urban hypothermia." Cold water immersion is the principal cause of death following boating accidents. With the exception of wool, wet clothing loses 90% of its insulating value. Thus, soaked individuals are essentially nude. Cold weather exposure runs a close second in terms of incidence. Finally, cold stress in the poorly heated homes of elderly, intoxicated, or debilitated patients (referred to as *urban hypothermia*) can cause fatal hypothermia.

Conditions that may contribute to hypothermia include the use of central nervous system depressants (such as downers or alcohol), infections, endocrine system diseases, brain dysfunction, and burns. Hypothermia also may occur while skiing, camping, or hiking.

People predisposed to hypothermia include:

- Any elderly person living alone, especially one with chronic disease or who has suffered a stroke.
- People who are intoxicated with alcohol.
- Children less than 1 year of age.
- Victims of submersion injury, especially in cold water.
- Patients suffering head trauma, especially if the accident occurred outdoors.
- Any patient with a history of trauma and subsequent blood loss with shock.
- Any person lost or immobilized in cold weather, especially if the individual is wet.

Victims of hypothermia stop shivering when the body temperature is below 90° F.

Patient assessment
The signs and symptoms present in a hypothermic patient depend on the stage of severity. Patients with mild hypothermia (90° F to 95° F) have the following signs and symptoms:

- Shivering and vasoconstriction—Victims stop shivering when the body temperature is below 90° F
- Loss of fine motor control, such as that required for starting a fire
- Increased blood pressure, heart rate, and respiratory rate
- Mild alterations in the level of responsiveness
- Lack of coordination

Patients with signs of moderate hypothermia (82° F to 90° F) have the following signs and symptoms:

- Muscular rigidity and stiff movements
- Progressive decrease in the respiratory and heart rate
- Glassy stare with marked depression in the level of responsiveness
- The BP may be difficult to detect, although the carotid pulse is usually still present

Patients with severe hypothermia (less than 82° F) have the following signs and symptoms:

- Deep coma
- Rigidity
- Patient appears pulseless and apneic
- Pupils are fixed and dilated

Severe hypothermia mimics clinical death. It may be impossible to distinguish a patient who is still alive, but profoundly hypothermic, from the victim of a cardiac arrest. Patients who have been pronounced dead from hypothermia have actually awakened in the morgue.

Care of the patient with hypothermia

 Describe the care for hypothermia.

To care for the patient with hypothermia, the EMT–I should:

- Handle these patients gently. Rough handling may precipitate cardiac dysrhythmias.

- Perform CPR as necessary. Check the pulse for 30 to 45 seconds before beginning chest compressions.

- Give high-concentration oxygen by nonrebreather mask (10 to 15 L/min).

- Give warm fluids if the patient is completely responsive. Observe the patient carefully to prevent aspiration. Do not give fluids before or during an aeromedical transport to reduce the chances of aspiration.

- Start an IV lifeline. Hypothermic persons tend to be dehydrated. Consider a fluid bolus of 500 to 1000 cc normal saline or Ringer's lactate as rapidly as possible, if allowed by local protocols. IV fluids are especially helpful if they are able to be warmed to approximately 104° F prior to administration.

- Care for other life-threatening injuries or conditions. Dress and protect frostbitten extremities.

- Remove wet clothing and maintain the patient in a warm, draft-free environment.

- Follow local protocol for rewarming. In some areas, rewarming is not attempted if the ETA to a hospital is less than 1 hour. Simply cover the patient with a blanket and transport him or her in a warm ambulance compartment to the hospital as soon as possible. Remove wet clothing prior to covering the patient.

- If local protocol includes rewarming or if the ETA is greater than 1 hour, begin controlled rewarming with hot packs placed over the carotids, head, lateral thorax, and groin.

- Do not try to rewarm the patient's extremities.

- Chemical hot packs can cause burns. Pad these with towels before placing them next to the skin.

CLINICAL NOTES
Do NOT attempt to rewarm the extremities alone. This causes vasodilation of the arms and legs, resulting in a bolus of cold blood flowing into the central circulation. The patient's core temperature may actually decrease, resulting in what is called the "afterdrop phenomenon." In addition, if the patient is somewhat dehydrated due to hypothermia ("cold diuresis"), then vasodilation will worsen intravascular volume status, leading to "rewarming shock."

CASE HISTORY FOLLOW-UP

En route back to base, the EMT–Is discuss how important it is to keep an open mind and to consider "all the possibilities" when assessing and managing an unresponsive patient. EMT–I Perez realizes that his assessment was tainted by the park officer's report that the patient was indigent. And he was hasty in concluding that a drug overdose was the most likely cause of the patient's condition. Although drug use was a possibility, it should not have been his initial assumption. He learned in school that in cases of coma of unknown origin, naloxone (Narcan) should only be considered after hypoglycemia is ruled out. Administering the narcotic antagonist would have delayed the delivery of the life-saving glucose. The medical direction physician is right—this will be a good call to critique in a continuing education class.

SUMMARY

Anaphylactic shock is a severe, life-threatening allergic reaction. It occurs in response to various antigens. These antigens react with antibodies, resulting in the release of histamines and other vasoactive substances from mast cells. The patient develops swelling, itching, shortness of breath, and signs of decreased cardiac output. Immediate treatment is essential and consists of airway, IV fluids, and epinephrine.

When dealing with breathing problems, the EMT–I must remember that the cause of the patient's distress may not be obvious to him or her. The EMT–I's job is to:

- Identify that a problem exists, rather than to make a specific diagnosis.

- Stabilize the patient, administer oxygen, and provide other care as necessary.

- Transport the patient to the hospital.

Acute asthma is a recurring episode of reversible airflow obstruction in the lower airway. Acute asthma occurs in response to a number of stimuli. Patients with an acute asthma attack are usually seated, in obvious respiratory distress. Signs of a severe attack include an altered level of responsiveness, a silent chest, marked diaphoresis, and cyanosis. Care consists of airway maintenance, humidified oxygen, administration of bronchodilators or epinephrine, and transportation to the hospital. It is important to reassure the patient.

Chronic obstructive pulmonary disease (COPD) is a progressive and irreversible disease of the airway. COPD is usually a combination of chronic bronchitis and emphysema. The major cause of COPD is cigarette smoking. Acute COPD episodes usually develop over several days. The patient has gradually increasing shortness of breath, and may have increased sputum production. Patients with severe long-standing COPD may have chronic cor pulmonale.

Care for patients with an acute COPD episode includes airway maintenance, placing the patient in a seated position, and giving the appropriate concentrations of oxygen. There is disagreement among EMS experts over the correct amount of oxygen to give COPD patients. Local protocols should be followed.

Hyperventilation is a respiratory rate greater than that required for the exchange of respiratory gases. As a result, excess quantities of carbon dioxide are blown off. Numerous conditions, many of them serious, are linked with hyperventilation. The EMT–I should always assume that patients with hyperventilation have a serious medical illness until proven otherwise. The EMT–I should give appropriate concentrations of oxygen and transport the patient to the hospital. The patient should not be asked to breathe into a paper bag. The EMT–I should not plug the portals of an oxygen mask in an attempt to have the patient rebreathe carbon dioxide, because this may result in dangerous hypoxia.

Pulmonary embolism is the blockage of a pulmonary artery by foreign matter, usually a blood clot, fat, amniotic fluid, air, or tumor tissue. There are many risk factors for pulmonary embolism, the most common of which is prolonged bedrest.

Massive pulmonary embolism can cause syncope or cardiac arrest. Smaller emboli are associated with sharp, pleuritic chest pains and shortness of breath. The symptoms may be similar to pneumonia, myocardial infarction, or spontaneous pneumothorax.

The EMT–I should give oxygen and transport the patient to the hospital.

Spontaneous pneumothorax is a sudden accumulation of air in the pleural space. Eventually, the lung on the affected side collapses. Rupture of a congenital defect in young men is the most common cause of this disease. Patients have a sudden onset of shortness of breath, anxiety, and pleuritic chest pain. Decreased breath sounds often are heard over the affected lung. Watch for development of tension pneumothorax. The EMT–I should give oxygen and transport the patient with the affected side down.

STREET WISE

Most illnesses that cause shortness of breath are potentially life-threatening. The EMT–I should relieve airway obstruction, maintain the airway, give oxygen, calm the patient, and transport to the hospital.

A stroke is a sudden disruption of circulation characterized by impairment of circulation to the brain tissues, resulting in ischemia and neurologic deficits that last more than 24 hours. Strokes may be either occlusive or hemorrhagic in nature. The risk factors for stroke are similar to those of heart disease.

Patients with stroke have neurologic deficits. The most common finding is hemiplegia, which is paralysis of one side of the body. Most patients have an elevated blood pressure as well. Pinpoint pupils in a patient with an altered level of responsiveness suggest intracranial bleeding. When caring for a patient with a stroke, the EMT–I should pay particular attention to the airway, because these patients tend to hypoventilate.

Coma is a state of profound unresponsiveness that may be due to one of many causes. A markedly elevated blood pressure suggests that an intracranial event may be responsible for the coma. The EMT–I should always assume that a comatose patient has a spinal injury until proven otherwise. The EMT–I should be prepared for vomiting and airway problems.

A seizure is a sudden period of exaggerated brain cell activity resulting in a period of atypical muscular activity or abnormal behavior. There are four types of seizures: focal, generalized, behavioral, and status epilepticus. The most common type of seizures seen in the field are generalized grand mal seizures. Many causes, within or outside of the central nervous system, may lead to seizures.

Often, the history in seizure patients is minimal. Following a seizure, the patient may be in a postictal state for up to 30 minutes. Postical behavior may be extremely violent, and patients do not usually remember the seizure. Status epilepticus is a series of seizures without a lucid period between them. Patients with epilepticus should be immediately transported to the hospital.

The EMT–I should maintain the airway of a seizing patient as best as possible. The EMT–I should never insert any object or his or her hands between the patient's teeth. Suctioning the mouth in front of the teeth with a rigid tip device may be helpful. The patient should not be restrained, but the EMT–I should protect the patient from injury.

A headache may occur for many reasons. Some causes of headache are serious. A patient who has a headache severe enough to call EMS has a potentially dangerous condition.

Acute nontraumatic abdominal pain may be caused by life-threatening diseases, such as ruptured abdominal aortic aneurysm, myocardial infarction, ruptured internal organs, or ruptured ectopic pregnancy. Many less harmful conditions can cause severe abdominal pain as well.

Patients with severe abdominal pain need to be evaluated at the emergency department. The EMT–I should allow the patient to lie in a comfortable position, not give anything by mouth, observe for shock, and provide care accordingly.

Gastrointestinal bleeding can originate from a lesion of the mucosa anywhere along the digestive tract. The patient can bleed severely enough to develop hypovolemic shock. Airway control is of primary importance, especially in upper GI bleeding with hematemesis. The EMT–I should care for shock and transport the patient to an appropriate hospital as soon as possible.

Diabetes is a disease of the endocrine system resulting from a lack of insulin. Insulin regulates the blood sugar level. Abnormal levels of insulin may result in either hypoglycemia or hyperglycemia. The EMT–I should always ask the diabetic patient if he or she ate and took his or her insulin (or other diabetic medication).

Hypoglycemia is low blood sugar. There are many causes of hypoglycemia. Most commonly, the diabetic patient takes his or her insulin and eats improperly. Symptoms develop rapidly and vary from shakiness to unresponsiveness. It may be impossible to distinguish hypoglycemia from alcohol intoxication or stroke.

To care for the responsive hypoglycemic patient, the EMT–I should give sugar in any of the following forms: orange juice with two added packets of sugar, glucose solution, candy, or corn syrup. The EMT–I should care for the unresponsive patient according to his or her local protocol. Some EMS systems allow EMT–Is to place sugar solution into the mouth of an unresponsive diabetic patient.

Hyperglycemia is an elevation of the blood sugar level. Diabetic ketoacidosis (DKA) is an abnormal metabolic condition resulting in hyperglycemia and the accumulation of ketones and ketoacids in the blood. The patient with DKA is severely ill and dehydrated. The EMT–I should provide care for shock if present and transport the patient to the nearest appropriate hospital as soon as possible.

Poisoning results from the ingestion, inhalation, absorption, or injection of a harmful substance. Most poisonings occur by oral ingestion. Evidence and information at the scene can help determine the poisoning agent. Poisoning may cause many different signs and symptoms.

The EMT–I should care for all poisoned patients by first opening and maintaining the airway. Syrup of ipecac or activated charcoal should be administered only if directed by the EMT–I's EMS system protocols. The regional Poison Information Center or medical direction base should be contacted before giving any care beyond life-saving measures. The EMT–I should not take risks when caring for the victim of an inhalation or exposure poisoning. Violent or suicidal patients should be restrained according to local protocols.

Heat exposure emergencies include heat cramps, heat exhaustion, and heat stroke. Of these emergencies, heat stroke is the most serious. Immediate cooling is critical to recovery from heat stroke.

Frostbite is the formation of ice crystals within the tissues. The signs and symptoms vary depending on the stage of frostbite. The EMT–I should care for the affected area carefully. The EMT–I should not rub the skin or attempt rewarming in the field.

Generalized hypothermia may be mild, moderate, or severe. Patients with severe hypothermia may appear to be in cardiac arrest. The EMT–I should perform CPR as necessary but should check the pulse for 30 to 45 seconds prior to beginning compressions. If local protocol permits, the EMT–I can begin rewarming in the field. Otherwise, the patient should be transported as soon as possible.

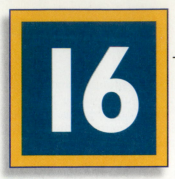

16

OBSTETRIC AND GYNECOLOGIC EMERGENCIES

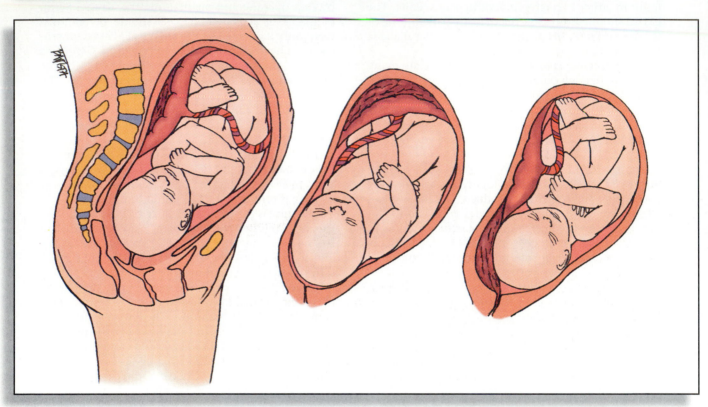

CASE HISTORY

EMT–Intermediate Bradley is dispatched at 3:25 AM to 42 Markingham Park, for a "woman in premature labor, contractions are 2 minutes apart, and she's bleeding." EMT–I Bradley arrives at the address in 4 minutes. He notices that the front lights are on and the door is open.

As EMT–I Bradley approaches the patient, her husband comes up to him and says, "She's 7½ months, and she's bleeding. Please get her to the hospital right away."

EMT–I Bradley looks at the patient and sees that she is crying and afraid. "We're going to take good care of you and your baby," he says, in the most confident and supportive voice he can manage.

Bradley takes the patient's vital signs as his partner places her on oxygen and applies the electrocardiogram electrodes. Her pulse is 124, respirations are 24 between contractions, and her blood pressure is 94/76. Her respirations are easy and

Case History, continued

quiet. EMT–I Bradley opens the obstetrics kit and places the sterile pads under the patient's buttocks and covers her belly. He sees that the baby is crowning.

His partner says that the patient is in sinus tachycardia and auscultates her breath sounds.

"We're going to have to deliver the baby right here," EMT–I Bradley tells her. "It's coming right now."

LEARNING OBJECTIVES

Upon completion of this chapter, the EMT–Intermediate should be able to:

- RECALL the physiologic changes in "normal" vital signs in pregnant patients.
- DESCRIBE supine hypotensive syndrome.
- IDENTIFY four signs of impending delivery.
- LIST the three stages of labor.
- DESCRIBE the priorities for newborn care.
- IDENTIFY and list management procedures for postdelivery bleeding.
- IDENTIFY four high-risk or "priority" situations involving prehospital childbirth.
- LIST two causes of abdominal pain in pregnant patients.
- IDENTIFY two causes of vaginal bleeding during the third trimester of pregnancy.

KEY TERMS

ABRUPTIO PLACENTA	PERINEUM
AMNIOTIC SAC	PLACENTA
BREECH PRESENTATION	PLACENTA PREVIA
CERVIX	PREECLAMPSIA
ECLAMPSIA	PROLAPSED CORD
ECTOPIC PREGNANCY	SPONTANEOUS ABORTION
FALLOPIAN TUBES	SUPINE HYPOTENSIVE SYNDROME
FETUS	UMBILICAL CORD
MENSTRUAL CYCLE	UTERINE RUPTURE
MISCARRIAGE	UTERUS
OVARIES	VAGINA

THE FEMALE REPRODUCTIVE SYSTEM

Anatomy

An EMT–I should be familiar with the structures of the female reproductive system (Fig. 16-1).

Ovaries—A walnut-sized pair of glands located on each side of the uterus in the upper pelvic cavity. The ovaries produce mature ova (eggs) and secrete primarily female sexual hormones (estrogen and progesterone).

Fallopian tubes—A pair of muscular tubes that extend from the uterus into the pelvic cavity. Each tube has a funnel-shaped open end, which is close to an ovary. The tubes provide a passageway for the transport of sperm to the ova and transport the ova back to the uterus by wavelike, muscular contractions.

Uterus—A hollow, muscular organ shaped like an inverted pear located in the pelvic cavity between the urinary bladder and the rectum. The uterus is divided into three parts: the fundus, the body, and the cervix. The inner lining of the uterus, the endometrium, serves as the site of implantation of the fertilized egg as well as the organ of menstruation. During pregnancy, the fetus develops within the uterus.

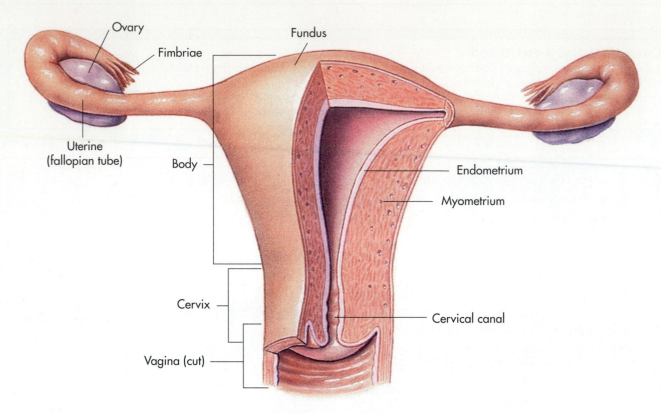

Fig. 16-1 **The female reproductive system.**

Cervix—The interior, narrow portion of the uterus that opens into the vagina. During labor, the cervix will thin out (efface) and dilate to allow the fetus and placenta to pass into the birth canal or vagina.

Vagina—The birth canal or passageway between the uterus and the external genitalia or perineum. The vagina is the female sex organ that receives the penis during intercourse. It also provides a passageway for menstrual flow and for the fetus and placenta during delivery.

Perineum—The external female genital region between the urinary opening (urethra) and the anus or rectal opening. This area includes the external female genitalia and the opening of the vagina. The labia are structures that protect the vaginal and urethral openings.

During pregnancy, certain organs or structures develop that are not present in the nonpregnant state (Fig. 16-2).

Placenta—A disk-shaped spongy organ that develops in the uterus during pregnancy. The placenta exchanges oxygen and nourishment from mother to baby and transfers waste products from the baby to the mother's bloodstream via blood vessels in the umbilical cord. It also manufactures hormones vital to the maintenance of the pregnancy. When the placenta passes from the vagina following delivery of the baby it is sometimes referred to as the *afterbirth*.

Umbilical cord—The attachment between the fetus and the placenta. The umbilical cord contains two arteries and one vein, providing continuous blood flow from mother to fetus and from fetus to mother. The blood, oxygen, and nourishment to the baby from the mother are carried via the umbilical vein. The arteries carry deoxygenated blood from the fetus back to the placenta.

Amniotic sac—Protective membranous sac that insulates and protects the fetus during pregnancy. The sac contains 500 to 1000 cc of amniotic fluid. The fluid is normally clear in color. Together, the sac and fluid protect the fetus while in the uterus.

Fetus—The unborn child.

Physiology

MENARCHE: The onset of menstruation in a female.
MENOPAUSE: The point at which a woman stops menstruating.

Each month the uterus is stimulated by hormones to develop a thickened inner lining or endometrium. If an egg is fertilized by sperm it is implanted in the uterus and nourished by this lining and pregnancy begins. If no egg is fertilized, the uterus sheds the lining, which is composed of cells and blood. This process is known as the **menstrual cycle** or menstrual period.

The onset of menstruation, or menarche, usually occurs in girls between the ages of 8 and 14. The average menstrual cycle lasts 28 days, but there is a

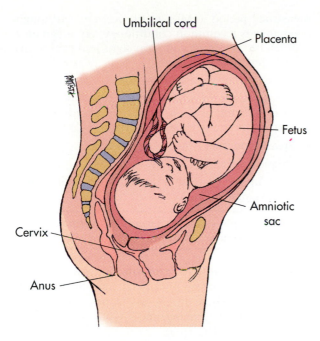

Fig. 16-2   The female anatomy during pregnancy.

great deal of individual variation. The onset of menstrual flow is counted as the first day of the cycle. Menstruation generally lasts for 3 to 7 days.

Under the influence of hormonal changes, an egg is released by an ovary on approximately the 14th day of the cycle. This process is known as ovulation. The egg then travels down the fallopian tube toward the uterus, where it will be implanted if it is fertilized. If not fertilized the egg will be shed with the menstrual flow.

Generally, between the ages of 35 and 60 years, the menstrual cycle and a woman's reproductive years come to an end. This process, known as **menopause,** may occur gradually or suddenly. When menopause occurs, the woman will no longer have a menstrual period.

GYNECOLOGIC AND OBSTETRIC HISTORY

Basic principles

Patient assessment always begins with scene size-up and initial assessment. The EMT–I should correct any life-threatening conditions before proceeding into the focused history and physical examination.

Female patients with a variety of complaints may have a dysfunction of the urinary tract, the gastrointestinal tract, or any of the reproductive organs. An accurate gynecologic and obstetric history is essential to the assessment of these patients. Whenever possible, another woman should be present during patient evaluations that involve the examination of the genitalia or sexual history taking.

HELPFUL HINT
Many patients feel uncomfortable speaking candidly about genital or urinary conditions. Adolescents may be particularly reluctant to discuss these conditions honestly while their parents are present. If the patient seems uncomfortable or embarrassed, the EMT–I should ask only those questions that are necessary for immediate care and make every effort to ask the questions in as private a setting as possible. As a healthcare provider, the EMT–I's professional demeanor will increase the patient's comfort level. A more complete history may be obtained at the hospital.

History of present illness

A directed history is an attempt to pinpoint the patient's problem. It is not necessary for the EMT–I to make a diagnosis in the prehospital setting, but important points to elicit include:

- Where is the pain/problem? Is there any referred pain?
- When did the symptom(s) start?
- What was the patient doing at the onset of signs and symptoms?
- How severe is the pain? Use a scale of 0 to 10 with 0 being pain-free and 10 being the worst pain the patient could ever imagine having.
- Has anything aggravated or alleviated the signs or symptoms (*eg*, movement, self-medication)?
- Are there any other symptoms, such as vaginal bleeding, vaginal discharge, fever, diarrhea, constipation, nausea, or vomiting?

Past medical history

The patient's past history is vital in determining the nature of her current problem. The EMT–I should try to elicit the following information:

- When was the patient's last menstrual period? Was it normal for this patient? Is there any possibility of pregnancy?
- Does the patient have any previous or current medical problems or conditions?
- Is the patient taking any prescription or over-the-counter medicines?
- Does the patient have any allergies?
- Does the patient have any past gynecologic problems including abnormal bleeding or discharge, infections, surgeries, cysts, or growths?

CLINICAL NOTES
The patient's last normal menstrual period is often abbreviated LNMP and is indicated by the date of onset of the flow of the most recent menses. For example, if a woman's last normal menses started on March 26th and ended on March 30th, the LNMP = 3/26.

Contraception and substance abuse history

Many substances may be harmful and alter the growth and development of the fetus during pregnancy. Commonly abused substances include cigarettes, alcohol, and drugs. In addition, it is important to ascertain whether or not the patient uses medications or condoms or other practices to prevent pregnancy. The EMT–I should consider assessing the use of the following:

- Use of oral contraceptives (birth control pills)
- Other types of birth control (intrauterine device, diaphragm, sponge, foams/jellies, surgical sterilization, hormone implant)
- Cigarette—Number of packs per day?
- Alcohol—Last use of alcohol? Frequency of use?
- Street drugs, including marijuana and cocaine

Obstetric history

Part of a routine gynecologic history is an obstetric history. This portion of the history is particularly important if the patient has a pregnancy-related problem. The EMT–I should ask the following questions:

- Has the patient had any previous pregnancies? How many? Were there any complications?
- Deliveries—were they full term? Premature?
- Has the patient had any previous Cesarean sections?
- Has the patient had any previous abortions or miscarriages?
- Is the patient pregnant now? Have there been any signs or symptoms of pregnancy such as a missed period, morning sickness, breast tenderness, or urinary frequency?
- If pregnant, has the patient had prenatal care? When is her due date (also known as estimated date of confinement)? Are there any known complications of this pregnancy such as multiple births or breech?

> **CLINICAL NOTES**
>
> Standard obstetric histories are abbreviated using the symbols G (gravida) to refer to the number of pregnancies including the current pregnancy, P (para) for the number of previous live births, and A (abortion) to indicate the number of miscarriages or elective abortions. For example, a woman who is currently pregnant with her fourth child, has delivered two previous live births, and had one miscarriage would be described as a G4P2A1.

PREGNANCY

Signs and symptoms

Pregnancy and childbirth are natural conditions. Full-term pregnancies last approximately 280 days (40 weeks) from the first day of the patient's last menstrual period (LMP) until delivery. Although pregnancy is a common condition, every pregnancy is different. The most common signs and symptoms of early pregnancy include:

- Missed or late menstrual period
- Nausea and vomiting (although typically referred to as morning sickness, nausea and vomiting may occur at any time of the day)
- Breast tenderness and enlargement
- Frequent urination

Later in the pregnancy abdominal swelling and fetal movements will occur.

> **Recall the physiologic changes in "normal" vital signs in pregnant patients.**

Physiologic changes during pregnancy

Pregnancy leads to significant changes in nearly all body systems. These alterations in physiology from the nonpregnant state become important in cases of illness or injury (Fig. 16-3).

Respiratory system

Pregnant women will develop an increased respiratory rate and depth. During the fourth to fifth month the fetus begins to take up increased space in the abdominal cavity and will compromise the ability of the diaphragm to flatten completely. The expectant mother will become tachypneic to compensate for this decreased volume of the thoracic cavity. As a result of the increased respiratory rate, a respiratory alkalosis develops.

Cardiovascular system

The cardiovascular system is significantly affected during pregnancy. An increase in the total blood volume of 40% to 50% occurs, which is referred to as *hypervolemia of pregnancy*. There is a proportionately greater increase in the amount of plasma than in red blood cells (RBCs), resulting in a dilution in the concentration of RBCs. This condition results in physiologic anemia. In addition, there is an increase in the number of white blood cells and in cardiac output during pregnancy. The expectant mother also is prone to develop blood clots in her legs.

Vital signs

The normal range for vital signs changes during pregnancy. The resting heart rate typically increases 10 to 20 beats per minute and the normal blood pressure (BP) drops 10 to 15 mm Hg from nonpregnant levels.

Gastrointestinal

There tends to be decreased motility of the gastrointestinal organs and upward displacement of the diaphragm during pregnancy, which results in a decrease in movement of foodstuffs through the gastrointestinal tract. For this reason, an increased risk of vomiting and aspiration occurs in the later stages of pregnancy and heartburn is common.

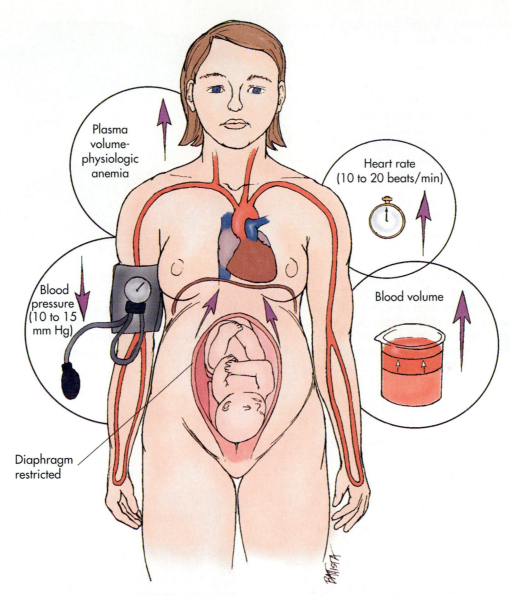

Fig. 16-3 Physiologic changes observed in the pregnant female.

Urinary

The bladder is displaced anteriorly and superiorly in pregnancy and is very vulnerable to penetrating or blunt trauma. Due to an increased cardiac output, the pregnant woman makes more urine, which leads to increased frequency of urination. The risk of urinary tract infections also increases during pregnancy.

Minor and common problems with pregnancy

Pregnancy is divided into three trimesters, each lasting approximately 13 weeks. During each trimester, the patient may suffer from any of a number of minor but common problems. Although bothersome, these complaints are not often dangerous to either mother or baby, and may include:

- First trimester:
    Frequent urination
    Nausea and vomiting
    Breast pain/tingling/tenderness
    Weakness and fatigue
- Second trimester:
    Constipation
    Heartburn
    Leg cramps
- Third trimester:
    Hemorrhoids
    Varicose veins
    Leg cramps

Braxton-Hicks contractions (painless irregular uterine contractions)

Pregnancy-associated illnesses

Various medical and surgical conditions may arise during pregnancy. Many of these are related to the physiologic changes noted previously.

 Describe supine hypotensive syndrome.

Supine hypotensive syndrome

> **SUPINE HYPOTENSIVE SYNDROME:** When in a supine position, a restriction of the flow of blood to the placenta due to the fetus compressing the inferior vena cava.

As the uterus enlarges, at approximately 20 weeks' gestation, the weight of the pregnant uterus may compress the inferior vena cava when the mother is in a supine position. This compression will result in hypotension and a restriction of blood flow to the placenta, which is called **supine hypotensive syndrome**. Although easily relieved, this situation can be fatal to the fetus if uncorrected. The easiest treatment is prevention—by keeping the pregnant woman positioned on her left side rather than in a supine position. In pregnant trauma victims, the EMT–I should apply immobilizing devices as he or she normally would, using caution to not compress the uterus with the straps. Once the patient is immobilized, the backboard should be tilted to place the patient with her left side down. A turnout coat, blankets, or other suitable objects can be placed under the board on the mother's right side to keep the board tilted to her left (Fig. 16-4).

> **HELPFUL HINT**
> Anatomically, the vena cava lies slightly to the right of the midline, so by tilting to the left the gravid uterus will shift off the vena cava. Whenever possible, pregnant patients should be transported on the left side to prevent supine hypotensive syndrome.

Appendicitis

Although appendicitis is common in patients of all ages and both sexes, it occurs in one out of every 1000 pregnancies. The appendix normally is located in the right lower quadrant of the abdomen. Pregnancy causes many organs, including the appendix, to be displaced superiorly. Appendicitis is more difficult to assess during pregnancy, especially in the last two trimesters, partially due to this anatomic change. The appendix is two to three times more likely to rupture in the pregnant patient. The EMT–I should care for the pregnant patient as he or she would any patient presenting with abdominal pain. The EMT–I should give her nothing by mouth, administer oxygen, consider

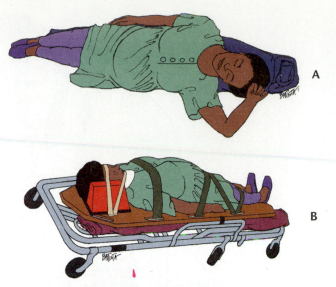

Fig. 16-4 A, Transport a pregnant patient on her left side to reduce pressure placed on her circulatory system by the baby. B, If a pregnant patient is immobilized on a long board, tilt the board on her left side.

an intravenous (IV) lifeline, and transport with her left side down as per local protocols.

Pregnancy-induced hypertension

> **PREGNANCY-INDUCED HYPERTENSION:** A rise in blood pressure in a pregnant female.

Pregnancy-induced hypertension will be a problem in approximately 5% of all pregnant women in the United States. Pregnancy-induced hypertension is defined as a rise in systolic BP of 30 mm Hg or a rise in diastolic BP of 15 mm Hg above the woman's normal baseline values. If the patient's baseline BP is not known, a blood pressure of 140/90 also is considered hypertensive during pregnancy. Pregnancy-induced hypertension alone is not considered life threatening.

Preeclampsia and eclampsia

> **PREECLAMPSIA:** During pregnancy, hypertension and excess fluid retention.
> **ECLAMPSIA:** A condition whereby a pregnant female experiences seizures in addition to preeclampsia; usually occurs during the third trimester of pregnancy.

Preeclampsia is an abnormal state during pregnancy characterized by hypertension and fluid retention. **Eclampsia** is defined as the occurrence of seizures in addition to the syndrome of preeclampsia. Eclampsia peaks during the third trimester and is life threatening to both the mother and fetus. Both preeclampsia and eclampsia may occur up to 1 week after delivery.

Women more likely to have pregnancy-induced hypertension or preeclampsia include:

- First-time pregnancy in a woman under 20 years or over 35 years of age
- Multiple gestation (twins)
- Preexisting hypertension
- Diabetes mellitus
- Family history of preeclampsia or eclampsia
- Previous preeclampsia or eclampsia

Signs and symptoms of preeclampsia/eclampsia include:

- Elevated blood pressure—In mild cases, the patient's BP is approximately 140/90 mm Hg; in severe cases, it may be as high as 160/110 mm Hg. The EMT–I should not rely solely on the presence of hypertension, however, because preeclampsia may exist without elevated blood pressure.
- Fluid signs—Signs include puffiness around the eyes, face, and fingers and legs swelling. The EMT–I should listen for rales in the lungs.
- Excessive weight gain—Most experts consider the following to be abnormal:
  - Greater than 3 pounds per month during the second trimester.
  - Greater than 1 pound per week during the third trimester.
  - A sudden weight gain of 4.0 to 4.5 pounds per week anytime during the pregnancy.
- Headache—A transient headache indicates a mild case, whereas a very severe headache may indicate severe preeclampsia.
- Visual disturbances (blurring/double vision)
- Irritability or change in mental status
- Epigastric abdominal pain
- Protein in the urine (tested at hospital or doctor's office)
- Decreased urine output

The onset of seizures or coma heralds eclampsia, which requires emergency treatment. Any patient with seizures during pregnancy or labor, or soon after delivery must be suspected of having eclampsia.

To care for the patient with preeclampsia or eclampsia, the EMT–I should do the following:

- Ensure that the airway, breathing, and circulation are secured.
- Administer oxygen by nonrebreather mask at 10 to 15 L/min.
- Start an IV lifeline per protocol.
- Place the patient on her left side and transport.
- Provide seizure care as needed.

- Protect the airway and the patient from injury.
- Use medications to stop the seizure and control the blood pressure as recommended by local protocol and medical direction.
  - Valium (diazepam), 5 to 10 mg IV
  - Magnesium sulfate, 2 to 4 g slow IV
  - Hydralize (Apresoline), 5 mg slowly IV, to lower blood pressure
- Avoid emergency lights or siren during transport as they may precipitate seizures.
- Notify the receiving hospital of your patient's status and your ETA.

Trauma during pregnancy

A call to care for a pregnant trauma patient creates fear and anxiety in many emergency care providers. Pregnancy can complicate the patient assessment and cause an alteration in vital signs. No matter how minimal trauma may appear, all pregnant patients who experience blunt or penetrating trauma should be evaluated by a physician.

Due to the physiologic changes previously noted, the pregnant woman has an increased heart rate and lower blood pressure. Therefore, changes in vital signs may be difficult to interpret. In addition, the increased blood volume of pregnancy may allow greater blood loss to occur before signs or symptoms develop. By the time the EMT–I even notices a change in vital signs the pregnant patient may have lost 35% of her circulating blood volume. Maternal hypovolemia will decrease blood flow to the uterus and reduce oxygen delivery to the fetus. The fetus will suffer harm before the EMT–I notices signs and symptoms of decreased perfusion in the mother.

To provide general prehospital care for the pregnant trauma patient, the EMT–I should do the following:

- Assess the airway, breathing, and circulation.
- Administer oxygen by nonrebreather mask at 10 to 15 L/min.
- Provide IV fluid resuscitation as per local protocols.
- Provide spinal immobilization—Immobilize a pregnant trauma patient as any other patient. Tilt the board and patient on the left side, as noted previously.
- Transport the pregnant trauma patient to the closest appropriate medical facility.
  - Keep in mind that this facility should have trauma, obstetrics, gynecologic, and newborn intensive care unit capabilities.
- Reassure the patient.
- Notify the receiving hospital of the patient's injuries and ETA.

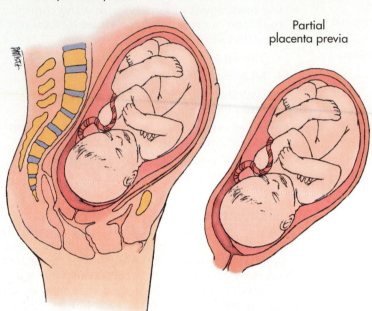

Total placenta previa

Partial
placenta previa

Fig. 16-5 Placenta previa is an abnormal positioning of the placenta low in the uterus.

Third trimester bleeding and abdominal pain

> **PLACENTA PREVIA:** An abnormal positioning of the placenta in the uterus.
> **ABRUPTIO PLACENTA:** The premature detachment of the placenta.

Vaginal bleeding in the third, or last, trimester indicates a serious and potentially life-threatening emergency for both the mother and fetus. The three common causes of third-trimester hemorrhage are noted below. (Prehospital care for these conditions is the same regardless of the suspected condition.)

Placenta previa

Placenta previa is the abnormal positioning of the placenta within the uterus. If the placenta implants low in the uterus it will be the presenting part (Fig. 16-5). At the onset of labor, with the dilation of the cervix, the placenta will begin to detach. Once the placenta delivers or begins to separate, the fetus will not receive oxygen or nutrients. Predisposing factors include multiple pregnancies, rapid succession of pregnancies, mothers over the age of 35 years, and previous history of placenta previa. Typically, the patient presents with profuse, painless bright red bleeding from the vagina. The uterus may be soft or may develop contractions.

Abruptio placenta

Abruptio placenta is the premature detachment of a normally situated placenta. This detachment may be complete or partial and can occur in any stage of pregnancy but is usually a third-trimester

complication (Fig. 16-6). Signs and symptoms of abruptio placenta include:

- Sudden onset of severe and constant lower abdominal pain
- Dark vaginal bleeding—However, bleeding may occur behind the placenta with no obvious external bleeding. Visible blood loss should NOT be used as a guide for internal blood loss in this condition
- Soft, tender, or contracting uterus
- Shock

Risk factors for developing either abruptio placenta or placenta previa include a history of preeclampsia (at least 25% of cases), chronic hypertension, multiple pregnancies, previous abruptio placenta, motor vehicle trauma, or cocaine use.

> **HELPFUL HINT**
> To differentiate placenta previa from abruptio placenta, the EMT–I should look for painless bleeding in placenta previa and uterine pain and tenderness with less obvious bleeding in abruptio placenta.

Uterine rupture

Uterine rupture occurs most commonly after the onset of labor. The patient will complain of severe abdominal pain, which may appear to be the onset of normal labor or a severe contraction. Contractions will then cease as the uterus ruptures. This condition has a high mortality rate for both mother and fetus. Risk factors for developing uterine rupture include a history of uterine surgery (including Cesarean section), trauma, prolonged or obstructed labor, and an abnormal fetal presentation.

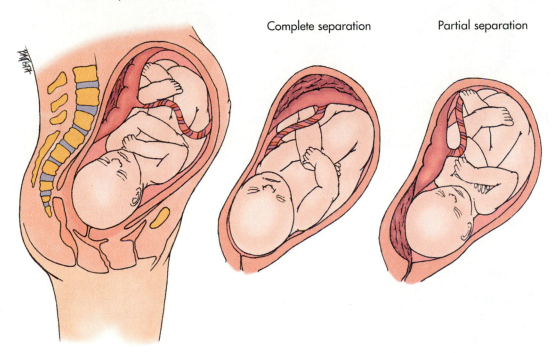

Partial separation

Complete separation   Partial separation

Fig. 16-6 **Abruptio placenta is a premature detachment of an otherwise normal placenta.**

Signs and symptoms of uterine rupture include:
- Continuous severe abdominal pain
- Minimal vaginal bleeding
- Tearing sensation in abdomen
- Nausea
- Shock
- Easily palpable fetus in abdomen

Care for the patient
It is often difficult to distinguish between the possible complications of late pregnancy. To provide care for any patient who is in her third trimester of pregnancy and complains of either abdominal pain or bleeding, the EMT–I should do the following:

- Administer oxygen by nonrebreather mask at 10 to 15 L/min.
- Continuously monitor the patient's vital signs.
- Place the patient on her left side.
- Provide resuscitation as per local protocol.
- Consider application of the pneumatic antishock garment (PASG), but inflate the legs only (as per protocol).
- Provide rapid, gentle transport to the closest *appropriate* hospital with obstetric and neonatal care.
- Notify receiving hospital to alert the obstetrics staff and of the ETA.
- Reassure the patient.

NORMAL LABOR AND DELIVERY

 Identify four signs of impending delivery.

Labor and delivery are natural events. In general, the EMT–I only assists the mother and the baby as necessary. In fact, prehospital childbirth most often will be "unexpected" rather than "emergency" childbirth.

 List the three stages of labor.

Labor
Labor occurs in three stages. The length of each stage of labor varies from patient to patient and from pregnancy to pregnancy. Most often, the second stage of labor will be approximately one half as long as the first stage.

The stages of labor include (Fig. 16-7):

- First stage—Beginning of regular contractions to complete dilation of the cervix (10 cm)
- Second stage—Complete cervical dilation to delivery of the baby
- Third stage—Delivery of baby to delivery of the placenta

Patients in labor may experience any or all of the following signs or symptoms:

- Contractions—Contracting of the uterus that occurs when the baby begins to move into the birth canal. These contractions are timed from the beginning of one contraction to the begin-

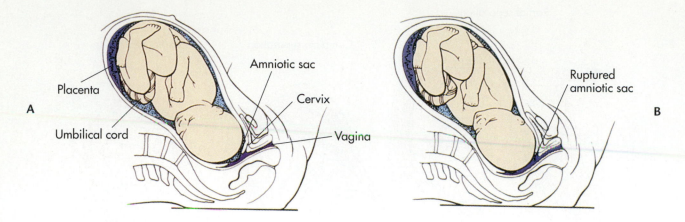

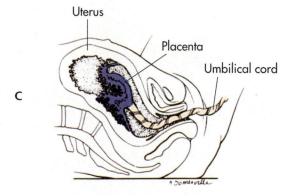

Fig. 16-7 **Stages of labor. A, The fetus moves into the birth canal. B, The cervix completes dilation. C, The placenta separates from the uterus.**

ning of the next. As labor progresses, the contractions usually become stronger and closer together, lasting 30 to 60 seconds and occurring every 2 to 3 minutes.

- Ruptured membranes (or breaking of the "bag of waters")—This usually occurs spontaneously and is characterized by a gush or slow leak of fluid. The amniotic fluid is usually clear but may be tinged with meconium. The patient may not be aware of this rupture. Occasionally, the patient's membranes may not rupture until the actual delivery.

- Bloody "show"—The passage of a mucus, blood-tinged discharge, often referred to as a *mucus plug*, usually occurs in early labor.

- Pain—Abdominal pain or back pain or both. Labor is very painful and is very hard work. Every patient's pain tolerance varies. Each stage of labor brings a greater awareness of stronger, longer contractions to the patient.

- Transition—Occurs close to delivery. The patient may panic and be "out of control" with overwhelming contractions. Expect a very irritable patient attempting rapid breathing exercises. Most patients cannot speak through contractions at this point of labor.

- Urge to push—Either to have a bowel movement or to simply push the baby out. Occurs close to delivery.

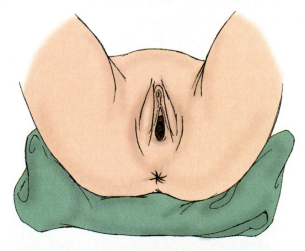

Fig. 16-8 **Crowning, when the fetus's head bulges at the perineum, marks the final stage of labor and imminent delivery.**

- Crowning—The appearance of the baby's head bulging at the perineum shortly before delivery. Marks the beginning of the final stage of labor (Fig. 16-8).

Delivery is often imminent when a woman with her first pregnancy has the urge to move her bowels, the "bag of waters" has broken, and crowning is present (Fig. 16-9).

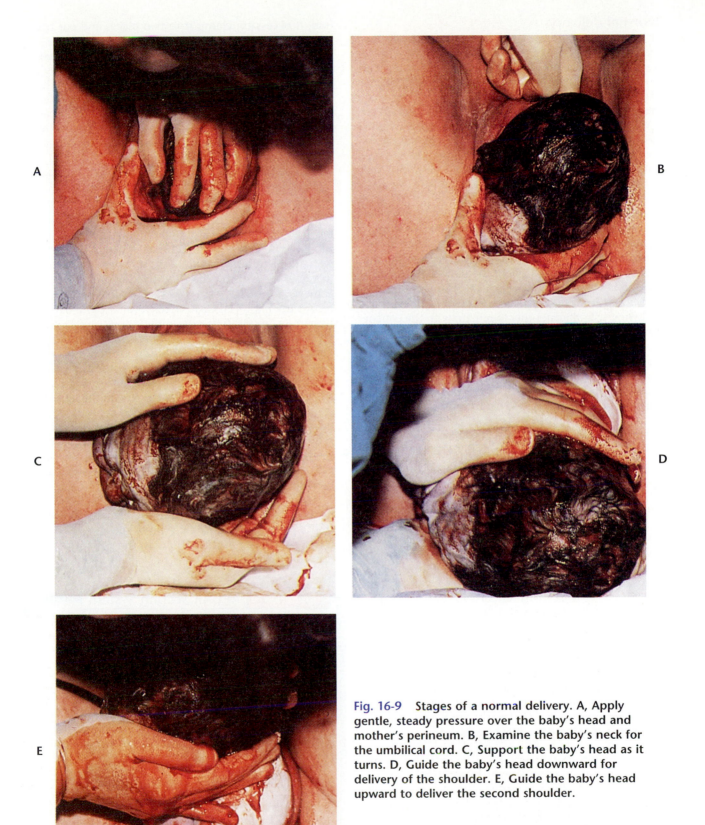

Fig. 16-9 Stages of a normal delivery. A, Apply gentle, steady pressure over the baby's head and mother's perineum. B, Examine the baby's neck for the umbilical cord. C, Support the baby's head as it turns. D, Guide the baby's head downward for delivery of the shoulder. E, Guide the baby's head upward to deliver the second shoulder.

Normal delivery

If labor is imminent, it will be obvious simply by examination of the external genitalia. The EMT–I should assess for the likelihood of delivery using the above guides. If the patient is at the pushing stage, she should be encouraged to push during the contractions and to relax in between contractions. The EMT–I should provide as much assistance and support to the mother as possible. If birth is not imminent, as noted by the absence of crowning or contractions not occurring every 2 to 3 minutes, the mother should be placed on her left side (if tolerated) and transported to the hospital.

If birth is imminent, the patient should be placed in a semireclining position on your stretcher or a firm, comfortable surface (Fig. 16-10). The stretcher is preferred because the patient can be moved rapidly. The EMT–I should be sure to help the patient protect her privacy and avoid embarrassment. Many times, the patient will have a spouse or "coach" with her. Allowing a significant other to remain with the patient can be very helpful.

It is important for the EMT–I to remember to prepare equipment, especially necessary in delivery are cord clamps or ties, a scalpel or scissors to cut the cord, warm towels, sheets or other linens (Fig. 16-11) and a bulb suction apparatus. Body substance isolation precautions must be taken when assisting in a delivery.

If the membranes have ruptured, the EMT–I should observe the color of the fluid. If the fluid is not clear, the EMT–I is dealing with a "meconium baby." Meconium is a fetal waste substance produced by the baby in distress. If the baby aspirates during delivery, the baby may suffer severe respiratory damage. Thick, dark meconium increases the potential severity of aspiration. The baby's airway must be suctioned PRIOR to its first breath to prevent meconium aspiration (Fig. 16-12). After deep suctioning of the baby, the mother should be encouraged to push and deliver the baby's shoulders. Excessive stimulation of the baby's nares should be avoided until thorough suctioning is complete.

HELPFUL HINT

The EMT–I may need to remove thick meconium from the airway prior to the baby's first breath. By performing direct laryngoscopy with a laryngoscope and suctioning below the vocal cords, serious complications may be avoided.

An explosive delivery can be prevented by applying gentle, steady pressure over the baby's head and the mother's perineum. A slow, controlled delivery will avoid or minimize injury to the infant and mother. Just before delivery, the baby's neck should be examined for the umbilical cord. If the cord is wrapped around the baby's neck, the EMT–I should slip the cord over the baby's head. If the cord will not slip easily over the head, the EMT–I should place his or her fingers between the baby's neck and the cord,

and, if necessary, clamp it in two places and cut the cord between the clamps (Fig. 16-13).

The time of birth should be noted and recorded. The EMT–I should continue suctioning the baby's mouth and nose with a bulb syringe to clear the baby's airway. The baby's mouth should be suctioned first, then the nose. Positioning the baby's head slightly lower than the rest of the body may allow retained fluids in the airway to drain into the airway to be suctioned (Fig. 16-14).

 Describe the priorities for newborn care.

After the baby is delivered, the EMT–I should begin to stimulate breathing by drying the baby and rubbing the spine (Fig. 16-15). Because the baby is wet and has a large surface area, it is very important to preserve warmth. The baby will begin to cry and achieve a normal skin color. The EMT–I should record the baby's APGAR scores (evaluate the baby's heart rate, respiratory rate, muscle tone, reflex irritability, and color) (Table 16-1) at 1 and 5 minutes after delivery. Until the umbilical cord is cut, the baby should remain level with the mother's vaginal area. This positioning prevents the mother and baby from becoming hypotensive. After the umbilical cord stops pulsating, usually 20 to 30 seconds after delivery, the cord should be clamped in two places. It is best to leave 6 to 9 inches of cord from the baby. Using a sterile knife or scissor (provided in commercial obstetric kits), the EMT–I should cut the cord between the clamps (Fig. 16-16).

The placenta usually will deliver within 20 minutes after delivery of the baby. If the placenta delivers in the presence of the EMT–I, he or she should place it in a plastic bag and bring it with the patient to the hospital (Fig. 16-17).

TABLE 16-1	APGAR Scoring System		
SIGN	0	1	2
Appearance (Skin Color)	Blue, pale	Body pink, blue extremities	Completely pink
Pulse Rate (Heart Rate)	Absent	<100/minute	>100/minute
Grimace (Irritability)	No response	Grimace	Cough, sneeze, cry
Activity (Muscle Tone)	Limp	Some flexion	Active motion
Respirations (Respiratory Effort)	Absent	Slow, irregular	Good, crying

From: Aehlert B: Pediatric Advanced Life Support Guide, 1994, St. Louis: Mosby–Year Book, Inc.

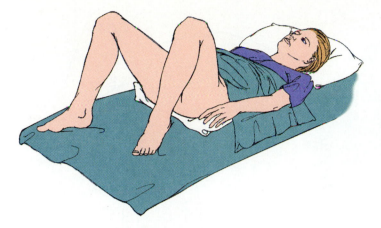

Fig. 16-10   If birth is imminent, position the patient in semi-reclining position.

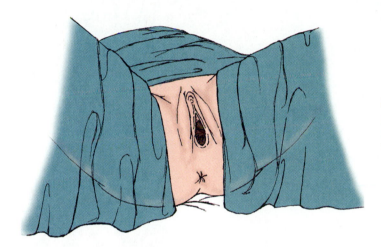

Fig. 16-11   Prepare necessary equipment prior to birth including warm towels, sheets, or other linens to create a sterile field for delivery.

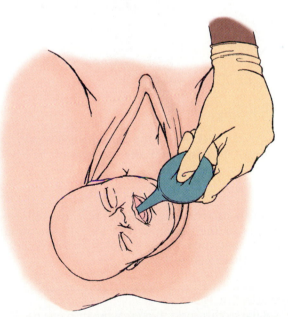

Fig. 16-12   Suction the baby's airway to open the passages and encourage breathing. This is especially important if meconium is present.

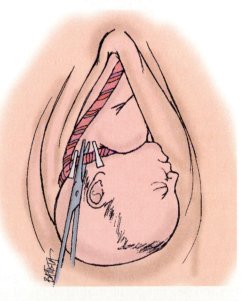

Fig. 16-13   If the cord cannot be removed from the baby's neck, clamp it in two places and cut between the clamps.

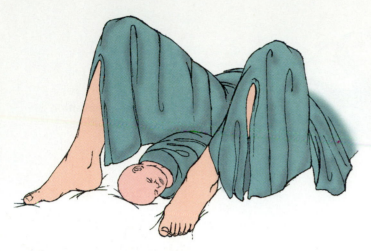

Fig. 16-14 Position the newborn baby's head at a lower level than the rest to permit any remaining fluids to drain for suctioning.

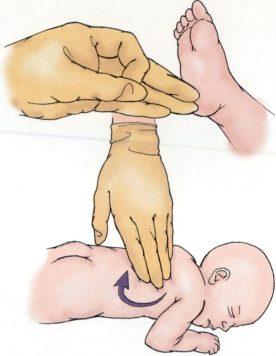

Fig. 16-15 If necessary, stimulate the baby by flicking the foot or rubbing the back.

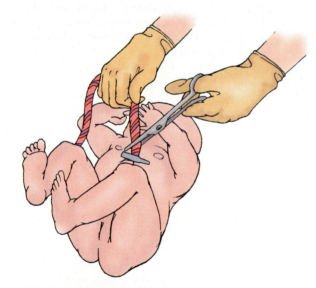

Fig. 16-16 Leaving approximately 6 to 9 inches of cord for the baby, clamp the cord in two places and cut between the clamps.

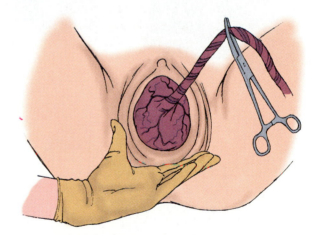

Fig. 16-17 Delivery of the placenta will usually occur within 20 minutes after delivery of the baby.

 Identify and list management procedures for post-delivery bleeding.

The mother will have a moderate amount of postpartum bleeding. To reduce bleeding, the EMT–I should place the dry, warm baby with the mother and encourage the mother to breastfeed the baby, which will reduce the bleeding by constricting the uterus. Massage the mother's lower abdomen (Fig. 16-18). This also will stimulate uterine contractions and reduce bleeding following delivery of the placenta. The EMT–I then should apply a maternity sanitary napkin and cold pack to the mother's perineal area.

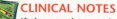 **CLINICAL NOTES**

If the mother soaks through more than one pad in 15 minutes or less, bleeding is excessive. Normal postpartum blood loss is less than 500 cc.

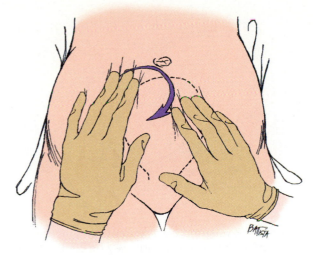

Fig. 16-18   If postpartum bleeding is excessive, manage the bleeding by massaging the mother's abdomen.

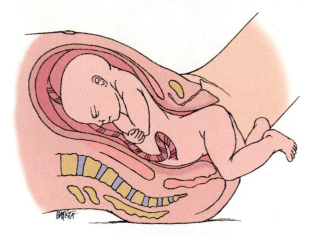

Fig. 16-19   Breech presentation is a delivery in which the baby's head is delivered last.

If the mother is experiencing excessive bleeding, the EMT–I should take the following actions:

- Administer oxygen by nonrebreather mask at 10 to 15 L/min.
- Continue to place sanitary pads over the vagina. Do not pack anything inside the vagina.
- Continue to massage the lower abdomen.
- Apply and inflate the PASG per local protocol.
- Establish IV access and administer IV fluids per protocol.

 Identify four high-risk or "priority" situations involving prehospital childbirth.

Abnormal presentations

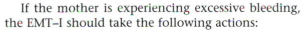
BREECH PRESENTATION: In childbirth, a delivery in which the baby's buttocks or feet present before the head.
PROLAPSED CORD: In childbirth, a delivery in which the umbilical cord presents during delivery.
LIMB PRESENTATION: In childbirth, a delivery in which the baby's arm or leg presents during delivery.

An abnormal presentation is when the first body part passing through the cervix is not the baby's head. Multiple births, although not technically abnormal in presentation, often are complicated by abnormal presentations such as breech.

Multiple Births
Multiple births are given special consideration by prehospital providers because the babies are generally smaller in size than single babies. In addition, multiple-birth babies are often premature and small because the uterus sometimes cannot expand to hold two or more full-sized infants. Lower birth weight babies have difficulty regulating body temperature. The baby will exhaust all efforts in keeping warm and probably will not succeed alone, and will depend on the EMT–I's efforts to survive.

To provide care for the woman with suspected multiple births, the EMT–I should do the following:

- Obtain an accurate history to determine if the mother is carrying more than one baby.
- If, after delivery of one baby, the abdomen remains unusually large, suspect multiple births.
- Follow normal delivery procedures for each birth.
- With multiple births, there may be a shared placenta or a placenta for each baby.
- Follow the same resuscitation procedures for newborns in distress with special attention to warming procedures.
- Be prepared to treat postpartum hemorrhage after multiple-birth deliveries.

Breech presentation
Breech presentation includes any delivery in which the buttocks or feet present first rather than the head of the baby (Fig. 16-19). Breech deliveries make up only 3% to 4% of all deliveries. Preterm deliveries, however, are breech 20% to 30% of the time. Babies in breech presentation have an increased risk for birth trauma. To provide care for the woman and baby in breech presentation, the EMT–I should do the following:

- Do not try to push the baby back in.
- Encourage the mother to push during the contractions.

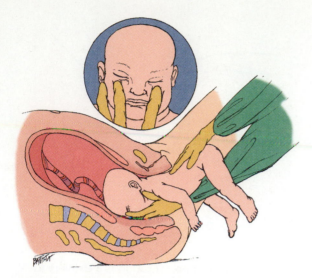

Fig. 16-20 Manage the breech presentation with a "V" shape around the nose and mouth.

- Do not attempt to pull the baby out.
- Allow the baby's legs and trunk to deliver. Support the trunk by wrapping a towel around the body and supporting it on your arm.
- If the baby does not deliver within 3 minutes or begins to breathe before the head is delivered, put a gloved hand in the vagina. Turn the baby to face the mother's back.
- Form a "V" with the fingers on either side of baby's nose and mouth; gently guide the baby's head out by lifting the body slightly anteriorly (Fig. 16-20).
- If the baby's head does not deliver within 3 minutes, transport the mother either with her buttocks elevated or in a knee-chest position while maintaining the "V."
- Administer oxygen by nonrebreather mask at 10 to 15 L/min.
- Start an IV lifeline in the mother.
- If delivery occurs, be prepared to resuscitate the baby.
- Notify the receiving hospital so they can prepare personnel and equipment.

Prolapsed cord

A **prolapsed cord** is a condition in which the umbilical cord is the presenting part during delivery. This condition is an emergency complication of delivery, because the cord will be compressed between the baby and the mother's pelvis, cutting off fetal circulation prior to delivery. Breech presentation, preterm deliveries, and multiple gestations increase the likelihood of a prolapsed umbilical cord (Fig. 16-21).

To care for the woman and the baby with a prolapsed cord, the EMT–I should do the following:

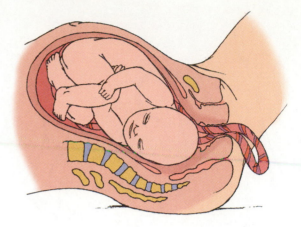

Fig. 16-21 Prolapsed cord presents an emergency to the infant because the cord may be compressed.

- Elevate the baby off the cord by inserting a gloved hand in the vagina and pushing up on the baby's head.
- Monitor for pulsations in the cord. A pulsating cord indicates a viable baby.
- Position the mother in a knee-to-chest or head-and-torso-down position (Fig. 16-22). If unable to do so, place her supine with the hips elevated.
- Transport rapidly but carefully.
- Do not push the cord back in under any circumstance.
- Cover the exposed cord with a warm, moist gauze or cloth pad.
- Administer oxygen to the mother by nonrebreather mask at 10 to 15 L/min.
- Establish IV access in the mother.

Limb presentation

Limb presentation occurs when an arm or a leg is the presenting part during delivery (Fig. 16-23). Again, this situation often is complicated by preterm delivery. There is little the EMT–I can do for this condition. To provide care for the woman and the baby in limb presentation, the EMT–I should do the following:

- Transport the patient to the hospital.
- Do not attempt delivery in the prehospital setting.
- Administer oxygen to the mother by nonrebreather mask at 10 to 15 L/min.
- Establish an IV lifeline in the mother.

Summary of high-risk deliveries

The following prehospital childbirth situations are "priority" conditions:

- Uncontrolled predelivery or postpartum bleeding from the mother

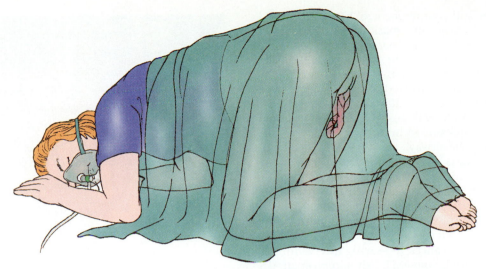

Fig. 16-22 If presented with a prolapsed cord, transport the mother in the head and torso down position.

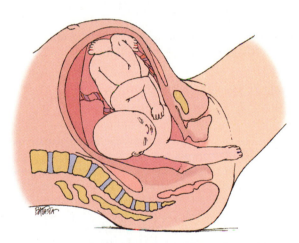

Fig. 16-23 Limb presentation is a condition in which an arm or leg is the presenting part.

- Breech presentation
- Prolapsed cord
- Limb presentation
- Severe abdominal pain with rigidity (other than labor)
- Any time more than drying and stimulation are needed to resuscitate an infant

CARE OF THE NEWBORN IN DISTRESS

Unfortunately, there are times when it becomes necessary to resuscitate a newborn baby. Complications can develop during the pregnancy, labor, or delivery. Assessment of the newborn actually begins prior to delivery, with an accurate history. A mother at risk may have had problems regarding the pregnancy, prenatal

care, and previous deliveries. Once the baby is delivered, assessment must begin immediately. Normal vital signs for the newborn are: heart rate 160; blood pressure 80; respirations 40.

 HELPFUL HINT
In most instances, basic life support, including warming and stimulation, is all that is necessary to successfully resuscitate the newborn.

The baby should be positioned on his or her back with the head slightly lower than the rest of the body. The EMT–I should suction the mouth first, then the nose, with a bulb syringe device for up to 15 seconds and then evaluate the baby. If the baby still does not cry, he or she should be stimulated by gently rubbing the soles of the feet or the back. There is no need to spank the baby.

The baby should be dried thoroughly, any wet towels discarded. The rubbing action taken to dry the baby provides stimulation. It also allows the baby to be kept warm until arrival at the hospital. Using a different towel, the EMT–I should wrap the baby to keep him or her as warm as possible. The head should be covered with a blanket, towel, or hat to prevent heat loss through the head.

The EMT–I should clamp the cord after it stops pulsating, and inspect it for blood loss. After cutting the cord as described previously, the EMT–I should place the baby against the mother's skin for warming.

If the baby does not respond within 30 seconds to these above techniques, the baby should be positioned with its head in a sniffing position. A rolled towel can be placed under the baby's shoulders to promote good positioning, but the EMT–I should avoid hyperextending the head, because this may cause airway collapse. Oxygen is administered by holding a mask near the baby's face until his or her condition improves (skin color goes from cyanotic to pink).

If the baby still is unresponsive, he or she should be ventilated by bag-valve mask with 100% oxygen at a rate of 40 to 60 breaths per minute. When using an oropharyngeal airway, the EMT–I should ensure that the correct size is used. During insertion, the airway should not be rotated at a 180° angle as is done for adults, because it may cause damage to the baby's mouth and tongue. Instead, the EMT–I should use a tongue depressor to hold the tongue in place while inserting the airway.

If the baby starts breathing on his or her own, the respiratory rate and depth and heart rate should be assessed. If the heart rate remains below 100 beats per minute, ventilations should be continued with 100% oxygen. If the baby's pulse is absent or below 60 BPM, initiate CPR.

At this point, advanced life-saving intervention is necessary. If possible, the EMT–I should meet an ALS unit while en route to the hospital. If ALS is unavailable or too far away, the EMT–I should transport the baby immediately. Notify the receiving emergency department to be ready for a newborn resuscitation.

> **HELPFUL HINT**
> Cardiac arrest in the most newborns is usually secondary to respiratory failure.

Guidelines for newborn resuscitation

After the baby has been dried and suctioned, if respirations are inadequate or the heart rate is below 100 BPM, the EMT–I should do the following (Fig. 16-24).

- Properly position the baby. Quickly provide blow-by oxygen near the baby's mouth and nose. Do not aim directly at the face or eyes.

- Begin bag-valve-mask resuscitation with 100% oxygen at a rate of 40 to 60 breaths per minute.

- If the pulse is absent or below 60 BPM, begin CPR. CPR should also be provided if the heart rate is between 60 and 80 but does not increase even with 30 seconds of positive-pressure ventilation and supplemental oxygen.

- Babies most often experience cardiopulmonary arrest due to hypoxia. For this reason, initial therapy consists of ventilation and oxygenation. However, when these measures do not resolve the problem, IV fluids and medications including atropine, epinephrine, lidocaine, and naloxone may be administered. Fluid therapy should consist of 10 mL/kg of saline or lactated Ringer's solution given by syringe over a 5 to 10 minute period.

- Transport in "priority" mode to the closest appropriate hospital. Notify them in advance that a newborn resuscitation will be arriving.

Note: It is imperative that the baby be kept warm during resuscitation and transportation. The EMT–I should make sure the baby is well wrapped and has a

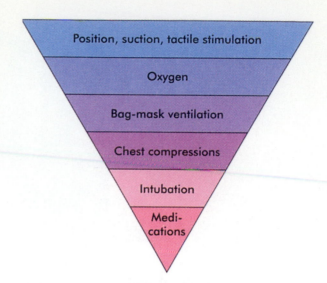

Fig. 16-24 Pyramid represents the relative frequencies of newborn resuscitative measures.

head cover. The ambulance should be warm enough to be uncomfortably hot for the EMT–Is.

NONTRAUMATIC FEMALE GYNECOLOGIC EMERGENCIES

Nontraumatic female gynecologic emergencies most often include complaints of abdominal pain, vaginal bleeding, or vaginal discharge. Proper assessment and good history taking are essential for proper care. Women often are embarrassed under these situations, so the EMT–I should respect the patient's feelings as much as possible. If a female companion or healthcare provider is available, ask her to assist with the evaluation.

The combination of abdominal pain and vaginal bleeding not associated with a normal menstrual cycle indicates infection or an obstetric emergency such as an abortion or ectopic pregnancy. The patient may not even be aware that she is pregnant, because some women have irregular menstrual cycles.

Ectopic pregnancy

> **ECTOPIC PREGNANCY:** The implantation of a fertilized egg outside of the uterus; usually occurs in the fallopian tube.

An **ectopic pregnancy** occurs when a fertilized egg implants itself anywhere outside the uterus, usually in the fallopian tube. This implantation can occur anywhere, including in an ovary, the cervix, or the abdominal cavity. The developing embryo cannot grow in the limited space available within the fallopian tube and will eventually stretch the tube to the point of rupture (Fig. 16-25).

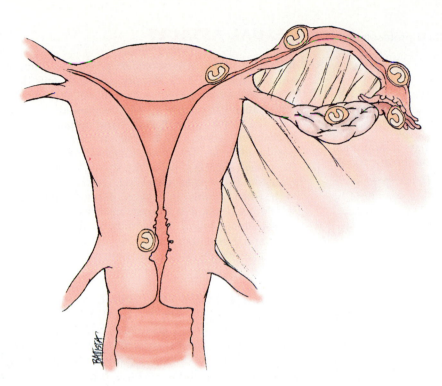

Fig. 16-25 A pregnancy is considered ectopic if the embryo implants itself outside the uterus. This situation can be life-threatening to the mother.

Some women are at higher risk for the development of ectopic pregnancy, including patients with a history of pelvic inflammatory disease (PID), prior ectopic pregnancies, users of the intrauterine device (IUD) for birth control, or a history of tubal ligation or tubal surgery.

Signs and symptoms of ectopic pregnancy may include:

- Weakness
- Dizziness or syncope
- Abdominal pain—Localized or generalized; in 25% of cases, the pain is referred to the shoulder.
- Late menstrual period or an abnormal last menstrual period (*eg*, lighter than usual flow)
- Nausea and vomiting
- Vaginal bleeding or spotting

Ectopic pregnancy is the leading cause of maternal death during the first trimester of pregnancy. Unrecognized shock is usually the main culprit. Time is critical, so the EMT–I should not wait for vital signs to change before suspecting ectopic pregnancy. Prehospital care includes oxygen by nonrebreather mask, IV lifeline and fluid resuscitation as needed, and use of the PASG as necessary and according to local protocol. The patient should be transported in the "priority" mode to the hospital.

Spontaneous abortion (miscarriage)

Spontaneous abortion or **miscarriage** is the sudden unexpected loss of pregnancy. It usually occurs in the first 3 months of pregnancy but can occur up until the twentieth week. After 20 weeks fetal loss is referred to as *intrauterine fetal demise* or *stillbirth*. A spontaneous abortion can be very distressing and emotionally traumatic for both the mother and the father. The EMT–I should be supportive and reassuring if this condition is suspected. Signs and symptoms of spontaneous abortion may include:

- Abdominal pain and/or cramps—The pain may feel like labor or severe menstrual cramps.
- Vaginal bleeding—Varies from spotting to profuse bleeding with clots. The passage of tissue like material also may be noted.
- Shock.

 List two causes of abdominal pain in pregnant patients.

Care for the female patient with abdominal pain

Many conditions that may cause abdominal pain are difficult to assess, even in the hospital. To provide appropriate prehospital care for any female patient of childbearing years who complains of abdominal pain, the EMT–I should do the following:

- Maintain airway, breathing, and circulation.
- Deliver oxygen at 10 to 15 L/min by nonrebreather mask, especially if signs of shock are present.
- Suspect shock and treat accordingly.

- Establish an IV lifeline as per local protocols.
- Consider use of the PASG if shock is present.
- Keep the patient warm.
- Let the patient assume a comfortable position.
- Reassess vital signs every 5 to 10 minutes, and consider pulse oximetry.

Patients with abdominal pain may be apprehensive and upset. It is sometimes comforting for the patient if a female EMT–I provides emergency care and support.

 Identify two causes of vaginal bleeding during the third trimester of pregnancy.

TRAUMATIC VAGINAL BLEEDING OR VAGINAL PAIN

Causes
Vaginal bleeding or pain can be caused by any of the following:

- Sports/recreational injuries such as horseback riding or bicycle seats
- Sexual assault or rape
- Childbirth
- Insertion of a foreign body into the vagina

Associated vaginal bleeding may occur with the injury, and lacerations to the perineal area may need suturing.

Prehospital care for vaginal bleeding
Regardless of the cause, to provide care for the patient with vaginal bleeding the EMT–I should do the following:

- Move the patient to a safe, private area such as the ambulance.
- Examine the affected area only if necessary (*eg*, to rule out crowning).
- Explain all procedures and steps before doing them (*eg*, "I am going to take your blood pressure now.")
- Respect and maintain the patient's privacy.
- Continue to provide emotional support.
- Perform necessary procedures. Vaginal or perineal injuries usually can be treated in the prehospital setting like other soft-tissue injuries. Apply an absorbent dressing and ice to the area for patient comfort.
- If bleeding is significant, administer oxygen, start an IV lifeline, and apply the PASG as needed.
- Reassess vital signs every 5 to 10 minutes, including pulse oximetry.

SEXUAL ASSAULT

In cases of alleged or possible sexual assault it is important for the EMT–I to identify and treat any head, chest, abdominal, or extremity trauma. If possible, a female friend or relative should be allowed to remain with the patient. Patient care is the number one priority, but an effort must be made to avoid destroying possible evidence. Therefore, if the EMT–I must remove the patient's clothes, he or she should carefully place each item in a separate paper bag. These articles should be handled as little as possible. Likewise, the victim should not be allowed to wash any affected areas. The EMT–I should follow local protocols regarding treatment and transportation of sexual assault victims, and should constantly reassure the patient.

CASE HISTORY FOLLOW-UP
EMT–I Bradley supports the baby's head as it presents in a downward orientation on the next contraction and immediately suctions the mouth and nose with a rubber bulb aspirator. He notes that there is no meconium staining or odor.

As the patient contracts again, EMT–I Bradley is able to support the baby's chest and right arm. His partner breaks a heat pack and wraps a blanket around it. The patient breathes with heavy puffing breaths and screams with each contraction, and the baby fully delivers.

It is a baby girl, purple and covered with white pasty fluid. EMT–I Bradley immediately dries the baby off with a clean towel, wraps her in the warm, dry blanket, and places her on her mother's belly. She is not moving yet.

EMT–I Bradley suctions the baby's mouth and nose again, and then rubs his fingertips gently on her spine to stimulate her. Finally, she begins to move.

SUMMARY
The major structures of the female reproductive tract include the ovaries, uterus, fallopian tubes, cervix, vagina, and perineum. During pregnancy, the placenta provides oxygen and nourishment to the growing fetus through the umbilical cord. The amniotic sac and fluid protect and cushion the fetus. Each month, the uterine lining is stimulated by hormones to prepare for possible pregnancy. If no pregnancy occurs, the lining is shed during menstruation.

An accurate history is essential in dealing with any obstetric or gynecologic emergency. Important components include the history of the present illness, past medical history, contraception and substance abuse history, and obstetric history.

Pregnancy and childbirth are usually normal, naturally occurring processes. Early symptoms of pregnancy include missed menstrual periods, nausea and vomiting, breast tenderness, and frequent urination. As the pregnancy progresses, abdominal swelling becomes prominent. During pregnancy, the woman's body undergoes many normal physiologic changes. These changes result in hyperventilation, hypervolemia, and physiologic anemia. In addition, there is a decrease in the movement of foodstuffs through the gastrointestinal tract and increased urinary frequency. As a result of these changes, the patient may suffer various predictable maladies during the three trimesters of pregnancy.

Sometimes more severe illnesses develop in conjunction with pregnancy. Supine hypotensive syndrome results from compression of the inferior vena cava when the mother is in a supine position, which causes decreased circulation to the baby. This problem can be prevented by keeping the pregnant patient positioned on her left side.

Appendicitis is more difficult to detect during pregnancy due to an upward displacement of the appendix. Rupture of the appendix is also more likely during pregnancy.

Pregnancy-induced hypertension, or elevated blood pressure, occurs during pregnancy in 5% of women. By itself, it may not be harmful, but if associated with excess weight gain and fluid retention, a condition of preeclampsia occurs. If the patient develops eclampsia, seizures will occur. Women with suspected preeclampsia and eclampsia should be treated as "priority" patients.

Trauma during pregnancy poses a risk to both the mother and the unborn baby. As part of the physiologic changes during pregnancy, the mother's blood volume increases and her normal blood pressure decreases. The EMT–I should NOT wait for signs of significant hypovolemia in the mother to develop, but should provide high-flow oxygen, and an IV lifeline and transport the patient promptly to an appropriate facility.

Third-trimester bleeding and abdominal pain may occur as a result of either placenta previa, an abnormal positioning of the placenta, or abruptio placenta, premature detachment of a normally situated placenta. Either condition is life threatening to both the mother and the baby. The EMT–I should administer oxygen, start an IV lifeline, and transport the patient to the nearest appropriate hospital as soon as possible. Uterine rupture may occur as a complication of labor, but also may occur prior to labor or with trauma.

Normal labor and delivery is a natural event. Labor occurs in three stages. During the first stage, contractions begin and the cervix dilates. In the second stage, the cervix finishes dilation and the baby is born. In the third stage, the placenta is delivered. Signs of imminent delivery include crowning, an urge to move the bowels, and breaking of the "bag of waters."

If labor is imminent, it will be obvious by examination of the patient's external genitalia alone. If the membranes have ruptured or if they rupture in the EMT–I's presence, he or she should note the color of the fluid. Normal amniotic fluid is clear. Dark or cloudy fluid may indicate the presence of meconium, a substance produced by a baby in distress. The EMT–I should be certain to suction the infant thoroughly PRIOR to the first breath, to avoid aspiration of this material.

An explosive delivery can be prevented by maintaining gentle pressure over the baby's head and the mother's perineum. The EMT–I should observe carefully for the presence of the umbilical cord wrapped around the baby's neck and should treat accordingly. Following delivery, the EMT–I should suction and dry and warm the baby, which should result in spontaneous breathing from the stimulation. The cord should be clamped and cut when it stops pulsating. The placenta usually will deliver within 20 minutes. To reduce maternal bleeding, the mother should be encouraged to breastfeed the baby following delivery. Massaging her lower abdomen may help control bleeding as well.

In abnormal presentation the first body part out of the cervix, the "presenting part," is not the baby's head. Abnormal presentation can be breech, prolapsed cord, and limb presentations. Multiple births also are considered as an abnormal or high-risk delivery. In a breech delivery, the baby's head should be delivered if it does not spontaneously deliver after delivery of the legs and the trunk. A prolapsed cord or limb presentation presents another emergency situation. The EMT–I should appropriately position the mother, administer oxygen, and transport to the nearest appropriate hospital as soon as possible.

If the newborn is in distress, necessary resuscitation should be provided. Oxygen and respiratory assistance are all that is required in most cases. If the baby's pulse rate is below 60 BPM, the EMT–I should call for ALS and begin CPR. If ALS is not available, the mother and baby should be transported to the hospital as soon as possible.

Nontraumatic gynecologic emergencies most often include complaints of abdominal pain, vaginal bleeding, or vaginal discharge. A good history is essential for proper care. The three most common problems are infection of the reproductive tract, an ectopic pregnancy, or spontaneous abortion or miscarriage. It is often difficult, if not impossible, to differentiate these conditions in the prehospital setting. The EMT–I should maintain airway, breathing, and circulation, and use an IV lifeline and PASG as per local protocols.

Trauma to the female genital area is painful and embarrassing for the patient. If possible, a female EMT–I should help provide care. It is important to respect the patient's privacy throughout the encounter.

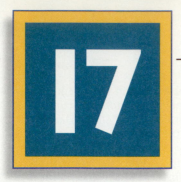

17

PEDIATRIC EMERGENCIES

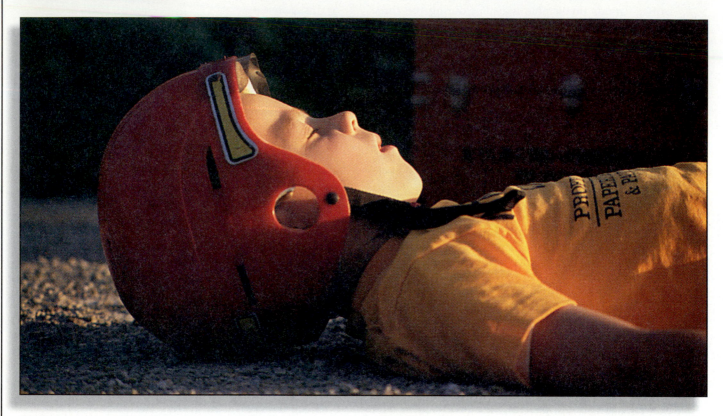

CASE HISTORY

Finally, after a series of busy 24-hour shifts at the fire department, EMT–Intermediate Ward is on a much-deserved "four day." The kids are in bed, and EMT–I Ward and her husband are enjoying a quiet evening at home watching an old movie on TV. On the way to the kitchen to get some popcorn, EMT–I Ward hears her youngest child call out to her. She goes to his room and finds him sitting upright in his bed, struggling to breathe. She sees that classic tripod position that he uses whenever it is a "bad" attack. He is wheezing, his color is not good, and he is telling his mom that he "can't catch his breath." EMT–I Ward attempts to calm him while her husband gets the inhaler. She tells her son to breathe slow and deep, but he is using "everything he's got" to move that air in and out.

EMT–I Ward administers one inhalation of his prescribed albuterol, but, as usual, there is little response. The inhalers just are not doing much good anymore. He is still using accessory muscles to

CASE HISTORY, continued
breathe, and his color is not improving. Quietly, she tells her husband to call the ambulance and let the emergency department know he is on his way. EMT–I Ward recalls his last attack and the trouble they had reversing his bronchospasm. Her son spent 2 days in the pediatric intensive care unit, and she was afraid that she might "lose him."

Within minutes, the Ward's quiet evening at home has become a busy EMS scene. An ambulance, a pumper, and two police cars are parked out front. EMT–I Ward's husband is asking the neighbors to stay with the other children while they are both at the hospital. EMT–I Ward tells her coworkers that this is her child's third asthma attack in several weeks and that the last one required hospitalization. She lets them know he has had one dose of albuterol and that his medication includes corticosteroids to help reduce his inflammatory response. She helps them apply an oxygen mask to her son, and she quickly carries him to the ambulance.

LEARNING OBJECTIVES

Upon completion of this chapter, the EMT–Intermediate should be able to:

- NAME the narrowest part of the child's upper airway.
- RECALL the characteristics of the various pediatric developmental stages and how the EMT–I should approach the patient at each stage.
- RECOGNIZE the signs and symptoms of increased respiratory effort in the infant or child.
- RECOGNIZE the normal vital sign values for the various pediatric age groups.
- IDENTIFY the type of endotracheal tube used in children less than 8 years of age.
- LIST at least three techniques for bag-valve-mask ventilation in the infant or child.
- RECOGNIZE two characteristics of the following: croup, epiglottitis, asthma (reactive airway disease), and bronchiolitis.
- IDENTIFY the signs and symptoms of the infant or child with dehydration.
- DESCRIBE the treatment of an infant or child in status epilepticus.
- IDENTIFY the signs and symptoms of the infant or child with meningitis.
- DEFINE drowning and near drowning.
- IDENTIFY common poisons ingested by children.
- LIST the causes of pediatric trauma in order of the most common to the least common.
- LIST the most important intervention for a child with head trauma.
- DESCRIBE the process for pediatric immobilization.
- LIST two signs of blunt trauma to the abdomen in the pediatric patient.
- DESCRIBE treatment for a child with hypothermia.
- LIST five indicators of child abuse or maltreatment.
- RECOGNIZE examples of cognitive and physical disabilities.
- DESCRIBE treatment of an obstructed tracheostomy in an infant or child.
- IDENTIFY family issues encountered when working with children that have special needs.

KEY TERMS

BRONCHIOLITIS

BROSELOW TAPE

CRICOID CARTILAGE

CROUP

DROWNING

EPIGLOTTITIS

FONTANELLES

INTRAOSSEOUS INFUSION

MENINGITIS

NEAR DROWNING

PNEUMONIA

THE PEDIATRIC PATIENT

Epidemiology

In rural and urban areas, approximately 10% of all EMS treatment is for children under 14 years of age. Children between 5 and 14 years of age are most commonly seen because of trauma. Medical illness is the most frequent reason given for children less than 5 years of age. In children less than 2 years of age, serious illness, including cardiopulmonary arrest is most common.

It is critical that the EMT–I be trained to deal with emergencies involving infants and young children. Once trained, the prehospital provider must maintain those skills, particularly in areas in which pediatric field experience is limited. In many instances, the majority of pediatric patients seen are not in severe distress. However, a critically ill pediatric patient can present at any time. Workshops, continuing education programs, and other clinical opportunities must be made available to EMS personnel to enhance the level of care rendered to pediatric patients.

Anatomic differences

Infants and children are anatomically different from adults. The term *infant* is used to refer to those individuals under the age of 1 year, whereas the term *child* is used to refer to those individuals from age 1 to 8 years. More specific classifications are listed below. Remember that these are only guidelines. The patient's weight is the key to providing treatment.

Airway

Occlusion of the upper airway is one of the major causes of death in the prehospital setting when not appropriately managed. Therefore, it is important for the EMT–I to be aware of the significant anatomic differences between adult and pediatric airways. First, the overall size of the pediatric airway is smaller. Therefore, the airway of an infant or child is more likely to become occluded by foreign bodies, blood, vomit, or loose teeth. Secondly, a child less than 8 years of age has a larger tongue in comparison with the size of the mouth, a large and floppy epiglottis, and an airway that is narrowest at the **cricoid cartilage**. Lastly, the tonsils and adenoids (found in the posterior aspect of the pharynx) also may affect the patency of the airway. The weak muscles of the neck also may lead to obstruction, due to their inability to hold the various anatomic structures clear of the airway.

> Name the narrowest part of the child's upper airway.

 CRICOID CARTILAGE: The narrowest part of the child's upper airway.

Pediatric Classifications	
Neonate:	Birth to 1 month
Young infant:	1 to 5 months
Infant:	6 to 12 months
Toddler:	1 to 3 years
Preschooler:	3 to 5 years
School age:	6 to 12 years
Adolescent:	12 to 15 years

The location of the vocal cords in a child is also different than in an adult. The cords of a child sit more superior and anterior on the cervical spine than an adult. In infants the cords are located at approximately the first (or second) cervical vertebra. As the child grows, the cords begin to move downward closer to the level of the third vertebra.

Internal organs

In infants and children, the internal organs are larger in proportion to body size. The skeletal structure is smaller; therefore, the internal organs are basically "packed" into a smaller space. Because of this relationship, there is a higher incidence of internal injuries to infants and children. The organ that is most often injured is the liver. This difference in size and structure explains why multisystem injuries occur more often in childhood than in adulthood.

Head, neck, and bones

Because the head of an infant is so large, many childhood accidents usually involve a head injury. Cervical injuries can occur more easily because the head is large and heavy, exerting more pressure on the cervical spine. In medical situations the child may complain of a sore, stiff, or swollen neck.

Infants also have **fontanelles**, or soft spots, on the tops of their heads. Fontanelles are spaces between the bones of the infant's cranium that are covered by a tough membrane. The diamond-shaped, anterior fontanelle can be palpated until approximately 18 to 24 months of age. The posterior or triangular-shaped fontanelle usually closes approximately 2 months after birth. These fontanelles will bulge with any increase in intracranial pressure and be depressed when dehydration is present. The EMT–I should gently palpate the fontanelles during the infant's assessment.

Children's bones are different as well. They are softer and have less calcium and fewer other minerals as compared with an adult. Therefore, an injury to the child's bone may be no more than a bending of the bone rather than an actual break. Similarly, a child's ribs are more pliable and can withstand more force. They are injured less frequently than are an adult's. The result is that the underlying lung can be injured very easily without an overlying rib fracture.

Nervous system

The child's control of the nervous system is also immature. Their nerves are not well insulated, and their reflexes are less developed. An infant or child really does not know how to flinch when an object suddenly comes at them.

Approaching the pediatric patient

 Recall the characteristics of the various pediatric developmental stages and how the EMT–I should approach the patient at each stage.

Children can present unique challenges to the EMT–I simply because of their age and level of understanding. This section reviews the stages that children go through as they grow and how the EMT–I should handle each stage. The EMT–I should incorporate this information into his or her assessment and treatment of pediatric patients.

The psychologic aspect of injury and illness in the pediatric patient should be considered. Most children do not have the ability to understand what is occurring around them. They may be aware that something is hurting them or is painful. They become fearful of voices with which they are not familiar or the tones of those voices. If the psychologic aspect is not taken into account in the prehospital setting, the pediatric patient may experience significant psychologic scarring in future years. The goal for all patients is care of the total person.

The parents of the injured child also must be considered as part of the child's psychologic environment. The parents must know what is happening. They often will require psychologic assistance in dealing with their injured or ill child. They may feel responsible for the child receiving the injuries or that there was something they did or did not do to cause the injury. In dealing with parents, many EMT-Is have found the following to be helpful.

First, the EMT–I must remember that they are the authorities at the scene, and patient care is their top priority. Parents can be their greatest allies or their greatest obstruction. If the parents are calm, the EMT–I should make eye contact and have them assist with the care of their child. However, if the parents are not able to control their emotions, others should be sought at the scene to assist with the parents. The EMT–I should always keep the parents informed.

Finally, the EMT–I should not forget to take into account his or her own personal psychologic well being. The stress of the job is tremendous, and being exposed to pediatric illness and/or injury can be devastating. Pediatric emergencies are ranked among the highest in creating stress for the healthcare provider. The EMT–I should be sure to seek assistance from peers or even professional help should he or she be confronted with a particularly stressful situation. The EMT–I is important as well.

Before interacting with the child, the EMT–I should ask the following questions:

- What is the child's chronologic age and/or approximate weight?
- What is the child's level of understanding? (Note: It may not always match the age.)
- Is someone present whom the child knows and/or trusts (*eg*, parents, older siblings, caregivers, teachers) who can be with the child to offer emotional support?
- Does anyone know the child's medical history or other information that may be helpful to the EMT–I (*eg*, details of the accident, type of seizure activity)?
- Are there any special circumstances present (*eg*, language barrier, physical or mental disabilities, special equipment)?

To adequately care for children, it is also essential to have equipment specific to the pediatric population. The EMT–I should work with personnel in his or her area to ensure access to the appropriate pediatric equipment.

GENERAL PEDIATRIC ASSESSMENT

Initial and ongoing examinations

The initial examination includes assessment of the airway, breathing, and circulation. The airway must be patent, and breathing and circulation must be of the appropriate rate and quality.

Responsiveness

A brief neurologic examination should permit the classification of the patient's mental status. The EMT–I should use the acronym AVPU to determine if the pediatric patient is alert, responsive to verbal stimuli, responsive to painful stimuli, or unresponsive. These results should be adjusted based on the child's age and baseline mental status, if known.

Respiratory status

Respiratory distress in a pediatric patient can be a life-threatening event by itself. For this reason, prompt assessment of the child's respiratory status should be accomplished immediately. According to the American Heart Association (AHA), approximately 90% of pediatric cardiopulmonary arrests start as respiratory problems. Early identification and intervention is the best way to *prevent* pediatric cardiac arrest and can significantly enhance the child's future quality of life. Once the pediatric patient arrests, the prognosis is poor.

 Recognize the signs and symptoms of increased respiratory effort in the infant or child.

The first sign of respiratory distress in an infant is usually tachypnea. Other signs of respiratory distress that may be present in infants or children are increased respiratory rate and/or effort, diminished breath sounds, decreased level of responsiveness or response to parents or pain, poor skeletal muscle tone, and/or cyanosis.

As the child's respiratory effort increases the following signs and symptoms may be present:

- Nasal flaring
- Intercostal, subcostal, and suprasternal inspiratory retractions
- Head bobbing
- Grunting
- Stridor
- Prolonged expiration

If an infant or child is acutely ill, a slow or irregular respiratory rate is a dismal sign. This sign usually indicates that the child's status is declining due to fatigue, central nervous system depression, or hypothermia. Many times the child will be tachypneic for a period of time, become fatigued from working so hard, and slow his or her rate of breathing. The EMT–I should not be fooled into thinking the child is improving because the respiratory rate drops. In reality, the child may progress to respiratory arrest and possibly cardiac arrest if not treated appropriately.

The EMT–I should assess the neck for trauma, jugular venous distention, and tracheal deviation. The chest should be checked for deformities, contusions, abrasions, penetrations, paradoxical motion, accessory muscle usage, and intercostal retraction. With a stethoscope, the EMT–I should listen anteriorly, posteriorly, and under the arms to do an adequate assessment. The child should have equal breath sounds bilaterally. These sounds can be transmitted easily across the thorax because the child's chest wall is so thin. Therefore, it may be difficult to identify areas of decreased function on one side because the EMT–I will be able to hear sounds from the lung on the other side.

Circulatory status

Many of the usual heart rates for infants and children show normal tachycardia. Sinus tachycardia also can occur as a result of stress due to hypovolemia, hypoxia, anxiety, fever, pain, increased carbon dioxide, or cardiac impairment.

Bradycardia usually occurs when the child can no longer maintain adequate tissue oxygenation. This condition is usually a precursor to cardiopulmonary arrest and should be treated quickly. Many times, proper oxygenation will cause the heart rate to rise, increasing the child's cardiac output.

Infants have short, chubby necks, which makes it extremely difficult to palpate the carotid artery. Therefore, the brachial artery should be palpated on the inside of the upper arm between the infant's elbow

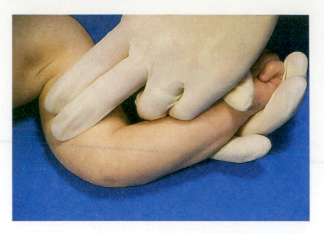

Fig. 17-1 In infants, palpate the brachial artery for a pulse.

and shoulder (Fig. 17-1). The carotid artery can be palpated for children older than 1 year of age (Fig. 17-2).

Skin color, temperature, and capillary refill also should be evaluated. The EMT–I should be aware that young children have poor collateral circulation, especially in a cold environment, so capillary refill may not provide an accurate assessment of perfusion.

The intent of the initial examination is to detect any life-threatening injuries and treat them. The purpose of the focused history and physical and detailed examination is to obtain a more detailed accounting of the patient's condition.

Focused history and physical and detailed examination

The focused history and physical and detailed examination is a reexamination of the patient. All the components of the initial assessment should be included. However, this survey may be performed slowly so that a greater understanding of the patient's condition can be reached.

This ongoing assessment should include vital signs: pulse, respirations, blood pressure, and pupillary reaction. If the child is less than 3 years of age, a blood pressure may not be necessary.

Continuation of the focused history and physical and detailed examination includes evaluation of the abdomen for rigidity or tenderness. The pelvis is checked for stability. The lower and upper extremities are evaluated for trauma and distal pulses as well as for sensation and motor function. Finally, the posterior aspect of the patient is assessed.

Vital signs
Normal values

Vital signs in infants and children vary with age. In addition, "normal" vital signs actually can vary from patient to patient.

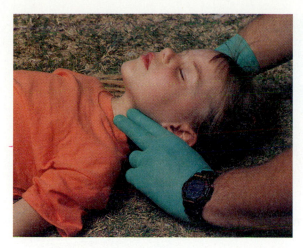

Fig. 17-2   In children, palpate the carotid artery for a pulse.

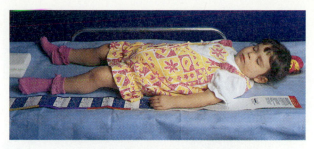

Fig. 17-3   A Broselow resuscitation tape can be used to identify the proper range of vital signs for a pediatric patient.

 Recognize the normal vital sign values for the various pediatric age groups.

It may be difficult for the EMT–I to remember all of this information. A more practical method is to keep some type of reference material in the ambulance. A resuscitation tape developed by Broselow and colleagues (the **Broselow tape**) is an example of a tool that can be used (Fig. 17-3).

Pulse oximetry

Pulse oximetry provides continuous monitoring of a child's arterial oxygen saturation. It evaluates oxygenation and not the effectiveness of ventilation (elimination of carbon dioxide). It is quite useful as an adjunct, but the EMT–I should not rely solely on this tool. If the child's clinical status is questionable (*eg*, tachypnea, cyanosis, decreased heart rate), yet the pulse oximeter reading is within normal limits, the EMT–I should rely on his or her assessment and treat the child for respiratory distress regardless of the number on the machine.

An infant sensor is used on the ear lobe and also can be applied to the nares, cheek at the corner of the mouth, or the tongue, if the child is unresponsive. Adult sensors can be used around the hand or foot of an infant. Regardless of what type of sensor is used, the EMT–I should be familiar with the particular device available to him or her.

PROCEDURES AND EQUIPMENT FOR MANAGEMENT OF AIRWAY, BREATHING, AND CIRCULATION

A child's airway must be managed in a specific manner to ensure its patency. Procedures with pediatric patients are relatively easy to perform, however, there must be attention to detail.

The appropriate method of opening the child's airway is to use the chin-lift or jaw-thrust maneuver. To perform this maneuver, the EMT–I places the fingers on the angle of the mandible and pulls gently anteriorly. This motion opens the airway, clears the tonsils and adenoids from obstructing the airway, and brings the tongue forward, allowing air to move more freely. Depending on the age and size of the child, a small blanket roll may be placed under the base of the neck or shoulders to assist in maintaining a "sniffing position." If after performing these procedures the airway is still obstructed, suction may be needed to help clear the airway.

The tongue is the primary cause of airway obstruction in the infant or child. Two other potential causes are foreign objects and swelling from infections. If the tongue is the culprit, the head must be repositioned. Airway obstruction from an object is managed by first visualizing the object. If something is seen in the airway, it must be removed with the EMT–I's fingers or Magill forceps. If forceps are used, the EMT–I should be careful to avoid the adenoids and tonsils, because they are very vascular and may complicate the situation with bleeding if injured. If nothing is seen in the airway, the EMT–I should not blindly sweep the mouth because this may result in the object moving deeper into the airway.

If there is a foreign body obstruction, the Heimlich maneuver may be performed on older children but should never be performed on infants. Infants may benefit from back blows or chest thrusts. It is essential that the EMT–I maintain proficiency in basic cardiac life support and pay particular attention to those aspects of managing the pediatric airway.

A suction device may be more helpful in removing fluids that may be causing the obstruction. If an infant requires suction, a bulb syringe may prove to be more effective. Another means of suctioning infants is to wrap a piece of gauze around the finger and gently clear the pharynx. In older children, powered suction devices may be used but should be set on the lowest setting possible.

It is *crucial* that basic life-support measures be initiated as soon as the need for airway management and/or ventilatory assistance is identified. Adequate

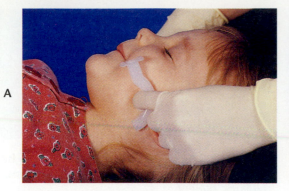
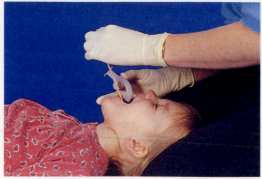

Fig. 17-4 Using an oropharyngeal airway in a pediatric patient. A, Measure the airway from the corner of the mouth to the angle of the jaw. B, Using a tongue depressor to move the tongue, insert the airway right side up.

Average vital signs by age			
Age	Pulse	Respirations	Blood pressure
Newborn	120-160	40-60	80/40
1 year	80-140	30-40	82/44
3 years	80-120	25-30	86/50
5 years	70-115	20-25	90/52
7 years	70-115	20-25	94/54
10 years	70-115	15-20	100/60
15 years	70-90	15-20	110/64
Adult	60-80	12-20	120/80

Source: Sanders, MJ: Mosby's Paramedic Textbook, Mosby–Year Book, St. Louis, 1994.

artificial ventilation can buy critical minutes and also may be just enough to deter further respiratory and/or circulatory compromise.

Airway adjuncts
Oropharyngeal airway
An oropharyngeal airway can be used in an unresponsive infant or child to maintain a clear, unobstructed airway when there is no gag reflex. It is very important to select the proper size airway so that no harm is done to the child. The airway is measured the same as for the adult. The airway should reach from the corner of the mouth to the angle of the jaw (Fig. 17-4 A).

Oropharyngeal airways come in many different sizes. The age of the child will assist in the determination of the size of the device. However, it is important to measure the airway to ensure a proper fit. If the EMT–I attempts to place an oropharyngeal airway that is too large in the mouth of an infant or child, vomiting or trauma to the soft tissues may occur. If an oropharyngeal airway that is too small is

placed into the airway, it may fail to adequately open the airway and may push the tongue back causing an obstruction.

The best method of airway insertion is to depress the tongue with a tongue blade and insert the airway device over the blade (Fig 17-4 B). If a tongue blade is not available, the AHA suggests inverting the airway and using the curved side as a substitute blade. The airway should be turned 180° as it reaches the back of the oropharynx. The EMT–I must be *extremely* careful not to lacerate or tear any of the anatomic structures. Correct positioning of the child's head must be maintained to ensure a patent airway once the device is in place.

Nasopharyngeal airway
Again, it is important that the nasopharyngeal airway is the proper size. The EMT–I should measure the length of this airway from the tip of the patient's nose to the tragus (small extension of the outside cartilage of the ear anterior to the external opening) of the ear. He or she then lubricates the airway with a water-soluble substance and gently inserts it into one of the child's nares. This device may need to be suctioned to maintain patency.

If the properly sized nasopharyngeal airway is not available, a 3-mm endotracheal tube should be used as a substitute. The EMT–I should use the same measurement (from the tip of the nose to the tragus) and shorten the endotracheal tube. The 15-mm attachment should be firmly reinserted so the tube does not go in past the nares (Fig. 17-5).

Suction equipment
If the child is crying, he or she swallows air and is prone to vomiting. Frequent suctioning may be necessary because of the presence of vomitus, saliva, mucus, blood, teeth, and so forth. A force greater than 120 mm Hg should not be used for an infant or child to avoid traumatizing the airway during the procedure.

Also, a flexible plastic catheter should be used whenever possible. A large-bore (tonsil-tip) catheter

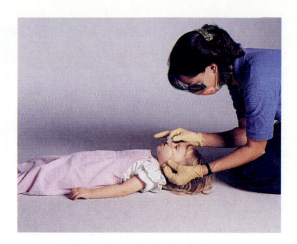

Fig. 17-5 **If necessary, a 3mm endotracheal tube can be used as a substitute for a nasal airway in a pediatric patient.**

may be used for larger amounts or thicker material, but the EMT–I must be cautious not to be too vigorous. The EMT–I must not cause soft-tissue damage to the oropharynx and increase the obstruction because of bleeding.

The heart rate should be monitored during suctioning. Irritation of the posterior pharynx, larynx, or trachea produces vagal stimulation, which in turn causes the heart rate to drop. If the heart rate decreases, the EMT–I should stop the procedure and hyperventilate the child with high-concentration oxygen.

Once basic life-support skills have been performed on the infant or child, consideration should be given to more advanced procedures. The EMT–I must continue to reassess the patient to determine if these skills should be attempted at the scene, en route to the hospital, or not at all.

Endotracheal intubation
Once the decision has been made to initiate an advanced airway procedure, intubation remains the method of choice. This method provides the most effective airway control and allows direct ventilation of the lungs.

Indications
Indications for intubation of the child include the following:

1. Inadequate central nervous system control of ventilation
2. Functional or anatomic airway obstruction
3. Excessive work of breathing leading to fatigue
4. Need for high peak inspiratory pressure or positive end-expiratory pressure to maintain effective alveolar gas exchange

Prior to intubating the infant or child, several considerations should be taken into account. First, the size of the endotracheal tube should be determined. The

easiest and quickest way to determine the appropriate size endotracheal tube is to use the external nostrils as a guide. Generally, but not always, the nares should accept the endotracheal tube size that is to be placed into the trachea. If the tube is too small, it will not secure the airway. On the other hand, if the tube is too large, damage to the vocal cords may occur.

Several other methods may be useful when determining endotracheal tube size for the pediatric patient. The EMT–I can look at the outside diameter of the patient's little finger or use the following formula for children older than 2 years of age:

$$\frac{\text{Endotracheal}}{\text{tube (in mm)}} = \frac{\text{Age in years}}{4} + 4$$

Using the length (height) of the infant or child is actually more accurate than using the age. Resuscitation tapes help with this method. The EMT–I should keep in mind that math is often a difficult task to perform when a child is seriously ill and use whatever method best meets his or her needs.

Once the endotracheal tube size has been selected, a handle and blade must be prepared. The laryngoscope handle for a pediatric patient has a smaller diameter and therefore uses smaller batteries, which allows for greater control of the handle and more importantly, the blade. Using a pediatric handle will actually make the intubation easier.

The blade selection for intubation also is measured, and it is important to select the proper size blade. For intubation of infants and toddlers, a straight blade (or Miller blade) is recommended because it provides better visualization. For older children, a curved blade (or Macintosh blade) may be more helpful.

As a general rule, the endotracheal tube sizes outlined in Table 17-1 should be used for pediatric intubation.

 Identify the type of endotracheal tube used in children less than 8 years of age.

Procedure
To perform endotracheal intubation in the pediatric patient, the EMT–I should do the following:

1. Begin artificial ventilations and provide high-concentration oxygen as soon as it is available. Suction the airway as necessary, and hyperventilate the child prior to the intubation attempt.

2. Assemble the laryngoscope and blade. Check the light to make sure it works *before* attempting intubation. Also, a straight blade is easier to use in the child because it lifts up the epiglottis for easier visualization of the larynx.

3. Select the appropriate size tube (see Table 17-1). The AHA generally recommends a cuffed tube for children 8 to 10 years of age or older. Infants and children less than those ages can use uncuffed tubes because of their "natural cuffs" at the level of the cricoid cartilage.

TABLE 17-1 Endotracheal Tube Sizes in Infants and Children Less Than 8 Years of Age

AGE	INTERNAL DIAMETER OF TUBE IN MM	SUCTION CATHETERS*
Premature infant	2.5–3.0 uncuffed	5–6 French
Newborn (term)	3.0–3.5 uncuffed	6–8 French
6 months	3.5–4.0 uncuffed	8 French
1 year	4.0–4.5 uncuffed	8 French
2 years	4.5–5.0 uncuffed	8 French
4 years	5.0–5.5 uncuffed	10 French
6 years	5.5 uncuffed	10 French
8 years	6.0 cuffed or uncuffed	10 French
10 years	6.5 cuffed or uncuffed	12 French
12 years	7.0 cuffed	12 French
Adolescent	7.0, 8.0 cuffed	12 French
Adult woman	7.5–8.0 cuffed	12 French
Adult man	8.0–8.5 cuffed	14 French

Source: American Heart Association, Pediatric Advanced Life Support, 1994.

*Endotracheal tube selection for a child should be based on the child's size, not age. Tubes one size larger and one size smaller should be allowed for individual variations.

4. Place the child's head in the "sniffing" position. If trauma is suspected, manually maintain a neutral position so that the head and neck are stabilized for each intubation attempt.

5. Hold the laryngoscope in the left hand, and insert it into the child's mouth from the right. Sweep the tongue to the left and move the blade into position. Because the airway is shorter and the glottis higher than an adult's, the cords will appear quickly.

6. Lift the mandible and tongue until the glottis can be seen. Remember to keep the wrist straight and to avoid pressure on the mouth or teeth if present. If the cords are not visualized, slowly withdraw the blade and watch for the larynx to drop into view.

7. Using the right hand, insert the tube into the mouth through the glottic opening until it passes through the cords. Do not insert the tube through the groove in the laryngoscope blade, which may block the view of the cords. Continue to hold the tube in place.

8. Do not let intubation attempts last more than 30 seconds. If intubation is unsuccessful, hyperventilate the patient with a bag-valve-mask device before any subsequent attempts.

9. Once intubation is successful, ventilate the patient with a bag-valve-mask device. Listen for breath sounds in the upper and lower lung fields and over the epigastrium. Breath sounds alone may not adequately represent success due to easy transmission of sounds in the child's small chest, especially in the infant. Also look for rise and fall of the chest as well as improvement in the child's or infant's color and/or heart rate.

10. After confirming placement of the tube, secure it to the face. Minimize movement of the head and neck so as not to dislodge the tube. Even after the tube has been secured, continue to manually stabilize it whenever possible.

11. Continue to reassess the child to ensure proper placement of the tube throughout transport.

Considerations

Several items are important to remember when working with the airway of an infant or child. First, a child has a greater proportion of soft tissue in the oropharynx as well as a larger tongue. Extra care should be used when inserting the laryngoscope so as not to cause any trauma. Also, the EMT–I should be careful to sweep the tongue out of the way as completely as possible. Secondly, the larynx is higher in the pediatric patient than in the adult, and the epiglottis is not as firm. Visualization of the cords prior to intubation may therefore be more difficult. Thirdly, the cricoid cartilage is the narrowest part of the upper airway, and the structures are more flexible than in an adult. These differences may make correct tube placement even more of a challenge. With all of these points in mind, the EMT–I should not be tempted to extend the intubation attempt more than 30 seconds.

The child's or infant's heart rate should be monitored during the intubation procedure. If the laryngoscope is moved around excessively while inserting the endotracheal tube, the vagal nerve may be stimulated, causing a marked decrease in the heart rate and a subsequent decrease in the blood pressure. Hypoxemia from prolonged intubation attempts also can decrease the heart rate. If the cardiac rate drops significantly, the EMT–I should stop the procedure and provide high-concentration oxygen using a bag-valve-mask device.

Suction equipment should be readily available and in good working order. The child's airway may become obstructed with vomitus, blood, increased saliva, or mucus. The EMT–I should use a pediatric suction catheter to clear away the obstruction as quickly as possible and provide hyperventilation with high-concentration oxygen before and after suctioning.

End-tidal carbon dioxide detector
The end-tidal carbon dioxide detector can be used in children and is most effective in verifying correct endotracheal tube placement in infants weighing more than 2 kg. It can, however, be misleading during the resuscitation phase of a pulseless arrest. The low reading in that situation is probably a result of low pulmonary blood flow, not placement of the tube in the esophagus.

Ventilatory adjuncts
Ventilatory adjuncts used to ensure breathing in pediatric patients include the devices listed in the following sections.

Bag-valve-mask ventilation
The proper use of the bag-valve-mask (BVM) device will assist greatly in the survival of the infant or child. The mask of the system must be tightly secured and sealed to the patient's face. If it is difficult to obtain or maintain a seal around the patient's mouth and nose, it may be beneficial to invert the mask on the infant's or child's face (see Fig. 17-6).

 List at least three techniques for bag-valve-mask ventilation in the infant or child.

The chin-lift maneuver should be performed when ventilating as long as cervical trauma is not suspected. The EMT–I should be careful not

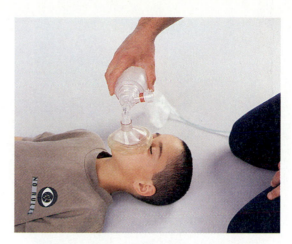

Fig. 17-6   In order to ensure a tight seal during BVM ventilations, the mask may be inverted on a child's face.

to push too hard on the soft tissue under the chin because this may move the tongue into an obstructing position.

The ventilation rate for infants and children is at least 20 breaths per minute. The EMT–I should be sure that the oxygen is attached to the BVM and is set to at least 15 L/min. It is best to use a BVM that provides at least 450 cc of volume and is not equipped with a "pop-off" valve on pediatric patients. The infant BVM only provides approximately 250 cc and should NOT be used because it cannot give enough tidal volume and provide a longer time for inspiration.

For infants and young children, the EMT–I should not use an adult BVM with the intention of just giving smaller puffs. The child in respiratory arrest presents a very stressful situation, and the EMT–I may lose sight of the goal to give small breaths. Larger breaths will cause the lungs to overinflate, and a pneumothorax may result.

When airway management is performed in older children, it may be necessary to use the adult BVM to provide a larger volume of ventilation. The EMT–I should be extremely careful not to force high volumes of oxygen into the patient's airway.

Bag-valve-mask ventilation must be done with two hands: one to hold the mask on the face and maintain the head-tilt/chin-lift maneuver and one to squeeze the bag (Fig. 17-7). When treating infants and toddlers, the EMT–I should support the mandible with the middle or ring finger. For older children, the fingertips of the third, fourth, and fifth fingers should be placed under the mandible to hold the jaw forward and extend the head (which accomplishes the jaw-thrust maneuver).

If one EMT–I is having difficulty ventilating the child, a two-person approach should be used. One EMT–I uses both hands to maintain the airway

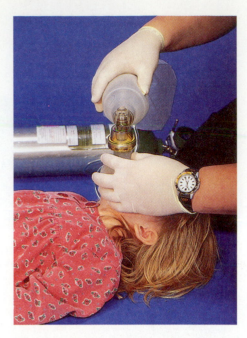

Fig. 17-7 BVM ventilations on a pediatric patient can be performed with one rescuer.

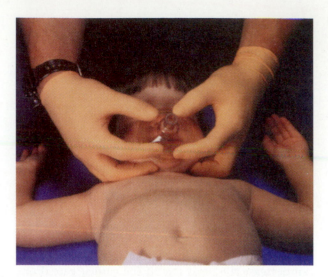

Fig. 17-8 With two-person BVM ventilations, one rescuer uses the airway and mask seal; the second rescuer delivers the ventilations.

maneuver and mask seal on the face, while the second EMT–I performs the ventilation (Fig. 17-8).

Maintenance of the head in a neutral, sniffing position without hyperextension is usually adequate for infants and toddlers. Hyperextension actually can occlude the infant's soft airway. Children more than 2 years of age do well with padding behind the head to displace the cervical spine anteriorly.

Obviously, if the EMT–I suspects a cervical spine injury, all airway maneuvers and ventilation should be done with the head in a neutral, in-line position. A trauma jaw-thrust or chin-lift without head-tilt can be used to maintain airway patency.

The goal of the BVM is to achieve effective ventilation. If this goal is not achieved, the EMT–I should do the following:

- Make sure the tongue is not obstructing the airway.
- Reposition the head. Using a folded towel under the infant's or child's shoulders may help maintain the sniffing position.
- Make sure the mask is snug against the patient's face.
- Lift the jaw.
- Suction the airway.
- Check the bag-valve-mask for damage.
- Provide an adequate source of oxygen.

The EMT–I should watch for gastric distention, which is very common during BVM ventilation. Appropriate suction should be readily available. If the infant or child is unresponsive, cricoid pressure (Sellick's maneuver) should be applied to minimize gastric inflation and passive regurgitation. This maneuver compresses the esophagus between the cricoid ring and the cervical spine. The second EMT–I should apply this pressure with one fingertip in infants and the thumb and index finger in children. Excessive pressure should not be used because this can cause tracheal compression and obstruction in infants. Lastly, it is critical to use a child BVM system depending on the size of the pediatric patient.

Although it is recognized that there may not always be an abundance of personnel at the scene, it is crucial to the child's ongoing survival to provide adequate oxygenation and ventilation. If the EMT–I must request additional personnel, he or she should do so without unnecessarily delaying transport of the pediatric patient.

Needle decompression

For those EMT-Is approved to perform the skill of needle decompression, it can be done on the infant or child if a tension pneumothorax is suspected. The same procedure is used as for the adult except that an 18- to 20-gauge over-the-needle catheter is used.

Communication with medical direction is essential for this procedure. In addition, routine skills reviews should be offered for those EMT-Is who do not have an opportunity to perform this skill regularly in the field.

Oxygen delivery devices

Oxygen can be administered to pediatric patients via the nasal cannula and oxygen masks.

Nasal cannula

The EMT–I should use the pediatric size nasal cannula and insert the two plastic prongs into the child's nares. A flow rate of between 2 to 4 L/min should be used. Higher rates irritate the nasopharynx and do not substantially improve the child's oxygenation. If more oxygen is needed, the EMT–I should switch to a face mask.

Oxygen masks

Children can use a simple partial rebreather or non-rebreather face mask, depending on the etiology of their illness or injury. The pediatric size should be used to provide a proper fit on the child's face and adequate oxygen concentration. Many children, however, do not tolerate the face mask because they feel restricted or suffocated. The EMT–I may administer oxygen via the "blow by" method by having the child or parent hold the mask in front of the child's face instead of directly on it.

Intravenous therapy

Intravenous (IV) access is of utmost importance in ill or injured children. The insertion of an IV line in a child is not an easy task even when the child appears to be cooperative. However, at times venous access is necessary in the pediatric patient for drug and fluid administration.

The sites for insertion should include the hands, the arms just at the elbow, or, if the neck is accessible, an external jugular vein. Alternatively, the area inside the ankle just above the medial malleolus, near the ankle bone on each side of the patient, can be used. Scalp vein access may be permitted in some systems. Many times, local protocols dictate which pediatric IV sites can be used in prehospital care.

There are several instances when the EMT–I should not take the time or aggravate the child to start an IV line. First and foremost are traumatic situations. If the child has sustained a traumatic injury and is hemodynamically compromised, the EMT–I should not waste time at the scene trying to get that line started. He or she may start the line in the ambulance once en route to the hospital. Most of the time, the EMT–I cannot catch up to the amount of blood the child is losing. Rather than delaying that child's access to definitive care, the EMT–I should provide good respiratory support and transport immediately.

Another instance when an IV line should not be started is the child with epiglottitis or some other form of severe respiratory distress. If an IV is attempted, the child usually will experience at least a fair amount of emotional distress. This crying and struggling can cause the child with epiglottitis to completely obstruct and the child in respiratory distress to get worse. In either case the EMT–I runs the risk of complete respiratory arrest if the child is too agitated. It may be safer to defer the IV line until the child is in a controlled setting in the emergency department. Be sure to refer to local protocols.

Intraosseous infusion

In cases in which the child is in severe shock or cardiac arrest, consideration should be given to the use of **intraosseous infusion** if the EMT–I is approved to initiate this therapy. This technique is accomplished by inserting a needle into the long bone of the leg. Infusion of IV fluids into the marrow cavity of the bone can circulate to the heart in 20 seconds or less. The amount of fluid resuscitation with intraosseous infusion is comparable to IV therapy. Intraosseous infusion should be withheld as a last resource of fluid replacement.

This technique was used in the early 1900s to administer fluid and blood. It fell out of favor in the 1950s once disposable IV catheters became available. However, within the past decade, it again has become popular and is most effective in children 6 years of age and under.

This procedure should be used only in children who are unresponsive and *only* after all other attempts at peripheral cannulation have failed (eg, situations such as cardiopulmonary arrest, shock from trauma, burns, sepsis, and so forth that lead to peripheral vascular collapse). Again, local protocol may mandate when an infusion can be attempted.

Medications and fluids can be given through this direct route. If a rapid fluid bolus or viscous drugs and/or solutions are to be given, they should be infused under pressure to overcome resistance. If drugs are given, they should be flushed with at least 5 cc of a sterile saline solution to make sure they reach the central circulation. Sterile technique is recommended during intraosseous infusion whenever possible.

To perform intraosseous infusion, the EMT–I should do the following:

1. Consult with medical direction prior to the procedure or follow local protocol.

2. Gather the necessary equipment: betadine wipes, disposable gloves, adhesive tape, gauze 4×4s, a 10-cc syringe, a specialized intraosseous needle or a Jamshidi-type bone marrow aspiration needle, a microdrip or pediatric infusion set, and the IV fluid ordered (such as lactated Ringer's solution or normal saline).

3. Wash hands if possible and apply gloves.

4. Identify the preferred site at the anteromedial surface of the tibia, one to two fingerbreadths below the tibial tuberosity (Fig. 17-9 A). The bone marrow cavity under this flat area is very large, and the potential for injury to adjoining tissues is minimal.

5. Cleanse the skin over the insertion site with Betadine.

6. Check the needle for proper alignment of bevels of outer needle and internal stylet.

7. Insert the needle perpendicular to the bone or angled away from the joint. Point it away from the epiphyseal point (Fig. 17-9 B).

8. Use a boring or twisting motion to advance the needle through the bone. A decrease in resis-

tance will be felt when entering the bone marrow cavity. If bone marrow is aspirated, irrigate the needle to prevent obstruction.

9. Remove the stylet (Fig. 17-9 C). The needle should remain upright without support.

10. Stabilize the needle. Connect the syringe filled with 10 cc of normal saline and slowly inject the fluid to verify placement. Note any increased resistance to injection, increase in circumference of the calf, or increased firmness of the tissue (Fig. 17-9 D).

11. If there is no infiltration, remove the syringe and connect the infusion set and IV bag. Apply tape to the needle and tubing and wrap a bulky dressing (4×4s) around the needle for support (Fig. 17-9 E).

12. If signs of infiltration are present, stop the infusion, remove the needle, and attempt the procedure again on the other leg.

13. Document the process in writing.

14. Reassess the patient, and provide an update to medical direction.

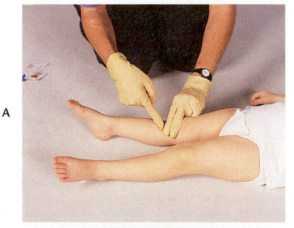
A

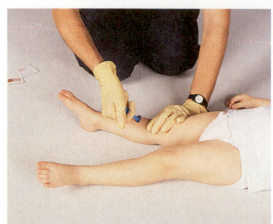
B

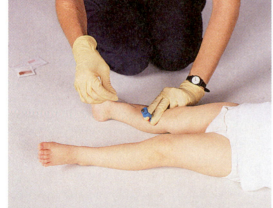
C

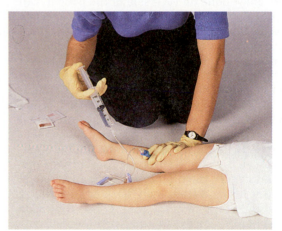
D

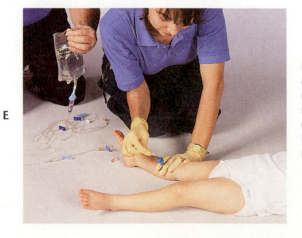
E

Fig. 17-9 **Intraosseous infusion. A, Identify and cleanse the area of injection. B, Insert the needle perpendicular to the bone with a boring motion. C, Remove the stylet. D, Inject 10 cc of normal saline and look for infiltration. E, Connect the infusion set and secure the needle in place.**

Note: Spinal needles (short, wide gauge needles with internal stylets) are not routinely recommended because they bend easily. They should be used only as a last resort. Regular hypodermic needles are NOT to be used.

Complications are uncommon but can be severe when they do occur, including tibial fracture, compartment syndrome, skin necrosis, and osteomyelitis. For the most part, this particular skill should be used only on critically ill infants and children until an alternate method of venous access can be obtained.

Fluid administration

Fluid resuscitation therapy is recommended at 20 mL/kg of an isotonic, crystalloid solution. This solution should be given as rapidly as possible (in less than 20 minutes). Many times these boluses are given through a 35- to 50-mL syringe to facilitate rapid administration. Ringer's lactate or normal saline can be used for this purpose. Large volumes of dextrose-containing solutions should not be used because the child may become hyperglycemic.

Frequent reassessments are necessary to determine the need for additional fluid boluses. If the signs of shock persist, another bolus of 20 mL/kg should be given. Additional boluses may be given depending on the patient's overall clinical picture according to medical direction. If the child begins to develop signs of fluid overload such as rales, the boluses should be stopped.

Medications

The drugs most commonly used in pediatric advanced life support are outlined in Table 17-2.

PEDIATRIC RESUSCITATION

In infants and children, cardiac arrest usually results from hypoxemia and acidosis caused by respiratory insufficiency or shock. These conditions interfere with normal function of the sinoatrial and atrioventricular nodes and slow conduction through the normal conduction pathways. This reduction leads to dysrhythmias such as sinus bradycardia, sinus node arrest with a slow junctional or ventricular escape, and asystole. Life-threatening rhythm disturbances are rarely a primary event except in those situations of congenital heart or other anomalies. The utmost attention must be given to establishing and maintaining a patent airway, effective ventilation, adequate oxygenation, and circulatory stabilization.

Figs. 17-10 and 17-11 represent the two most common situations encountered during pediatric resuscitations. These algorithms are recommended by the AHA.

Asystole

Asystole is characterized as a flat line on the electrocardiogram monitor. Occasionally P waves are seen. Clinically, there is no pulse, absent spontaneous respirations, and poor perfusion.

To treat the child with asystole, the EMT–I should do the following:

- Continue CPR.
- Ventilate with a bag-valve-mask device equipped with a reservoir and supplied with 10 to 15 L of oxygen.
- Perform endotracheal intubation using the appropriate tube.
- Establish an IV using normal saline (or lactated Ringer's solution).
- Administer epinephrine at an initial dose of 0.0 1 mg/kg (1:10,000) for the IV/intraosseous routes and 0.1 mg/kg (1:1,000) for the endotracheal route.
- Repeat epinephrine at a dose of 0.1 mg/kg (1:1,000) for the IV/intraosseous/endotracheal routes (doses up to 0.2 mg/kg of 1:1,000 may be effective) every 3 to 5 minutes.

Ventricular fibrillation

Ventricular fibrillation is a chaotic-looking rhythm with waveforms that vary in size and shape and no recognizable P waves, QRS complexes, or T waves. It rarely occurs in children unless there is the presence of congenital heart disease, acidosis, electrolyte imbalance (*eg*, calcium, potassium, magnesium, or glucose imbalance), hypothermia, or drug toxicity (*eg*, digitalis or tricyclic antidepressants).

To treat the child with ventricular fibrillation, the EMT–I should do the following:

- Continue CPR.
- Ventilate with a bag-valve-mask device equipped with a reservoir and supplied with 10 to 15 L of oxygen.
- Perform endotracheal intubation using the appropriate size tube.
- Establish an IV using normal saline (or lactated Ringer's solution).
- Defibrillate up to three times, starting with 2 J/kg (maximum of 200 J), then increasing the dose to 4 J/kg (maximum of 360 J) with subsequent shocks.
- Administer epinephrine at an initial dose of 0.01 mg/kg (1:10,000) for the IV/intraosseous routes and 0.1 mg/kg (1:1000) for the endotracheal route.
- Administer lidocaine, 1 mg/kg IV or intraosseous.
- Repeat defibrillation at 4 J/kg (maximum of 360 J) 30 to 60 seconds after the medication administration.
- Repeat epinephrine at a dose of 0.1 mg/kg (1:1,000) for the IV/intraosseous/endotracheal routes (doses up to 0.2 mg/kg of 1:1,000 may be effective).
- Repeat lidocaine, 1 mg/kg.
- Consider administration of bretylium, 5 mg/kg first dose, 10 mg/kg second dose IV.

TABLE 17-2 Most Commonly Used Drugs in Pediatric Advanced Life Support

DRUG	PEDIATRIC DOSAGE	REMARKS
Adenosine	0.1 to 0.2 mg/kg; maximum single dose: 12 mg	Give a rapid IV bolus.
Atropine sulfate	0.2 mg/kg/dose	Minimum dose is 0.1 mg. Maximum dose is 0.5 mg in a child and 1.0 mg in an adolescent.
Bretylium	5 mg/kg; may be increased to 10 mg/kg	Give rapidly through an IV line.
Calcium chloride 10%	20 mg/kg/dose	Give slowly.
Dopamine hydrochloride	2 to 20 μg/kg/min	Titrate to desired effect.
Epinephrine For bradycardia	IV/IO: 0.01 mL/kg (1: 10,000) ET: 0.1 mL/kg (1: 1000)	Be aware of effective dose of preservatives administered (if preservatives are present in **epinephrine** preparation) when high doses are used.
For asystolic or pulseless arrest	First dose: IV/IO: 0.01 mL/kg (1: 10,000) ET: 0.1 mL/kg (1: 1000) (Doses as high as 0.2 mL/kg may be effective.) Subsequent doses: IV/IO/ET: 0.1 mL/kg (1:1000) (Doses as high as 0.2 mL/kg may be effective.)	Be aware of effective dose of preservatives administered (if preservatives are present in **epinephrine** preparation) when high doses are used.
Epinephrine infusion	Initial dose: 0.1 μg/kg/min (Higher infusion dose is used if asystole is present.)	Titrate to desired effect (0.1 to 1.0 μg/kg/min).
Glucose	0.5-1.0 g/kg IV.	Use maximum concentration of 25% dextrose in water ($D_{25}W$) via a peripheral vein. If supplied as $D_{50}W$, dilute 1:1 with sterile water before administration. For infants, use $D_{10}W$ (dilute $D_{50}W$ 1:4 with sterile water).
Lidocaine	1 mg/kg/dose	—
Lidocaine infusion	20 to 50 μg/kg/min	—
Naloxone	If $\leq$ 5 years of age or up to 20 kg: give 0.1 mg/kg IV If > 5 years of age or > 20 kg: give 2 mg IV	Titrate to desired effect.
Sodium bicarbonate	1 mEq/kg/dose or 0.3 $\times$ kg $\times$ base deficit	Infuse slowly and only if ventilation is adequate.

Note: For endotracheal administration, dilute medication with normal saline to reach a volume of 3 to 5 mL. Follow the injection with several positive-pressure ventilations.

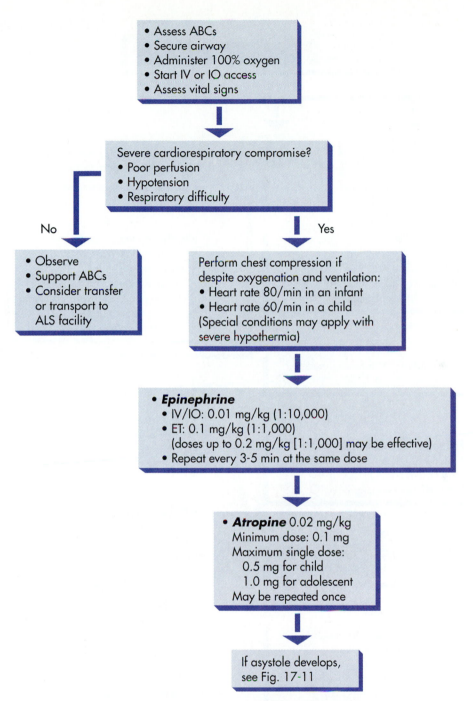

Fig. 17-10   Bradycardia decision tree.

• Repeat defibrillation at 4 J/kg (maximum of 360 J), 30 to 60 seconds after the medication administration.

Note: the EMT–I should open the airway and begin ventilations before defibrillating. However, the EMT–I should not delay defibrillation by attempts at IV insertion or intubation.

COMMON PEDIATRIC MEDICAL EMERGENCIES

There are several illnesses that are usually seen primarily in children. Some of these illnesses may be life-threatening and must be recognized and treated in an appropriate manner. Infections of the upper

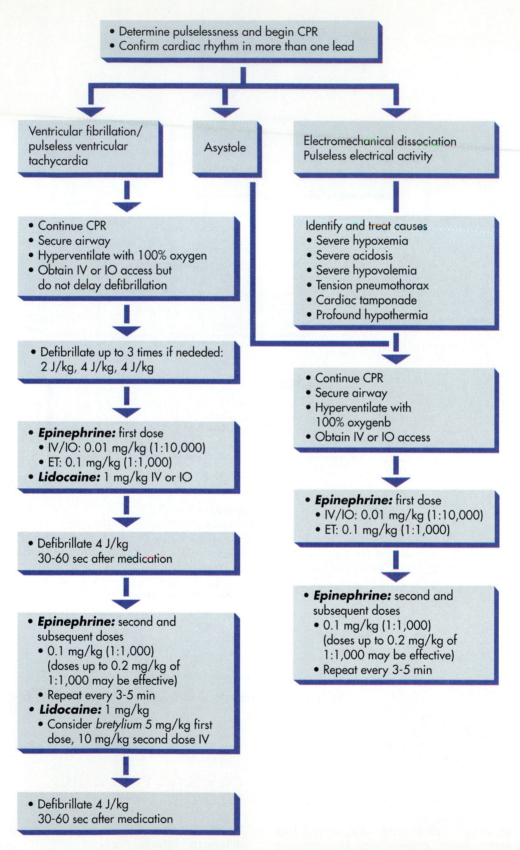

Fig. 17-11 Asytole and pulseless electrical activity (PEA) arrest decision tree.

airway include tonsillitis, croup, and the very rare yet dangerous epiglottitis. It is of utmost importance that the EMT–I is able to tell the difference between croup and epiglottitis.

For any of the respiratory illnesses, the EMT–I should note if there are any smokers around the child or residing in the house. Smoking can contribute to the severity of the illnesses.

 Recognize two characteristics of the following: croup, epiglottitis, asthma (reactive airway disease), and bronchiolitis.

Croup

Also known as *laryngotracheobronchitis*, **croup** is a respiratory illness that occurs in children between 3 months and 3 years of age. It is usually a viral infection that has a slow onset, usually after the child has had an upper respiratory infection and low fever. Inflammation of the larynx causes the primary symptoms.

Most commonly, the child will be hoarse with respiratory stridor and a characteristic "bark" in the form of a cough. The stridor is due to subglottic edema, and the barking cough is from edema of the vocal cords. If the lower airways are involved, wheezing will be heard.

The emergency frequently occurs during the middle of the night. The child wakes up with a barking cough and may show signs of respiratory distress. The amount of swelling usually will dictate the severity of the situation. The EMT–I must be aware, however, that the child is at risk of complete airway obstruction from the narrowed diameter of the trachea. The patient often prefers to lie down.

High-concentration oxygen should be administered (cool and humidified when possible), and the patient should be transported in a comfortable position. If the patient is lying down, the EMT–I should be alert for airway compromise. Monitor vital signs, the cardiac rhythm, and the pulse oximeter, if used. Many times the outside environment (if air is cool and humid) during transfer from the home to the ambulance may cause an improvement in the child's condition. The patient should be reassessed frequently to detect any changes or signs of airway obstruction.

Epiglottitis

Epiglottitis is an inflammation of the epiglottis, which most often occurs in children from 3 to 7 years of age. It is caused by bacteria and progresses rapidly. It is a true emergency because the child can progress to complete airway obstruction and respiratory arrest if the epiglottis swells over the opening of the trachea.

The child with epiglottitis will look very ill, will be quiet, and will be doing everything possible just to keep breathing. The child will sit upright and lean slightly forward on his or her hands with the neck extended forward (tripod position). The mouth is usually open with the tongue protruding. Swallowing is very painful so the child may be drooling. In addition, the child usually will show signs of respiratory distress and, in severe cases, hypoxia. A muffled voice and stridor also may be present.

Every patient who has indications of epiglottitis should be treated as having a life-threatening condition. No attempts should be made to visualize the airway. Under no circumstances should anything be placed in the patient's mouth. Manipulation of the child's airway can lead to complete obstruction and respiratory arrest. All efforts should be made to keep the child comfortable and as calm as possible. To properly care for these patients the EMT–I should not make them lie down. The parent should remain with the child at all times to alleviate fear and more importantly to keep the child from crying. If possible, the child should sit on the parent's lap. The EMT–I should handle the child gently. Rough handling and stress could lead to a total airway obstruction. High-concentration, humidified oxygen should be given via either a mask or blow-by method, depending on what the child will tolerate. Administration of oxygen should not be delayed, however, while waiting for humidification. The EMT–I should monitor the child's vital signs, cardiac rhythm, and pulse oximeter if doing so does not further agitate the child.

The EMT–I should be prepared to ventilate using positive pressure through a bag-valve-mask device. He or she should be able to force enough oxygen past the obstruction to buy some time until arriving at the hospital. Needle cricothyrotomy may be ordered as a last resort, but this procedure is difficult to perform on small children. Intubation only should be done by those EMT–Is highly experienced in the skill and in an environment where an emergency cricothyrotomy or tracheostomy can be performed if the intubation is not successful. The patient should be transported to the nearest appropriate facility as soon as possible.

The EMT–I should communicate with medical direction so that everyone at the receiving facility is prepared. Optimal treatment includes intubation and IV antibiotics once the child reaches the hospital.

Table 17-3 outlines the differences between croup and epiglottitis.

Asthma (reactive airway disease)

Commonly known as asthma, reactive airway disease is considered the most common chronic illness among children and the leading cause of school absences.

Children can have an acute asthma attack as well as status asthmaticus, exhibiting the same signs and symptoms as adults, including wheezing. Status asthmaticus is a life-threatening situation in which an asthma attack is severe, prolonged, and cannot be broken with traditional bronchodilators. The child should be transported rapidly in a position most comfortable for him or her. The EMT–I should monitor the airway, cardiac rhythm, and pulse oximeter and be prepared to intubate and provide ventilation.

Sometimes the attack can be so severe that there is no wheezing because the child is not able to move air adequately. As with adult patients with asthma or status asthmaticus, this condition should be considered life threatening. Any first case of asthma must be dealt with as if it were anaphylactic shock.

EMS may be requested because the child is having an episode of dyspnea and increased wheezing. Treatment is focused on opening the air passages to make the child breathe easier. The EMT–I should provide humidified oxygen (he or she should not wait for a humidifier if one is not immediately available) and monitor the child's vital signs, cardiac rhythm, and pulse oximeter. The EMT–I should communicate with medical direction, and follow local protocols concerning administration of drugs such as bronchodilators or epinephrine.

In severe cases, respiratory failure can occur. If the child has been struggling for a while, he or she finally may tire and stop breathing altogether. Equipment should be readily available to assist the child's ventilations and for intubation, if necessary. Circulatory support also may be necessary if the ventilatory support is not adequate.

When treating a child with asthma, the EMT–I should not be fooled by a cooperative, lethargic child who is not wheezing. This child's bronchioles may be so tight that he or she cannot move *any* air.

Bronchiolitis

Bronchiolitis is an infection of the lower respiratory tract, which is most often caused by a virus. It usually affects children between the ages of 6 and 18 months. Usually the child has a mild fever, cough, and runny nose, which progress to respiratory distress. Edema and increased mucus secretions obstruct the bronchioles, and wheezing is sometimes present. The child is usually most comfortable in a sitting or semisitting position. This condition is different from asthma because it is caused by a virus, and bronchospasms may not always respond to medications.

The EMT–I should provide high-concentration, humidified oxygen (again, he or she should not wait for a humidifier if it is not readily available), and transport the patient to the hospital for further evaluation. These patients often will benefit from vaporized or nebulized water. These patients also must be seen at a medical facility. The respiratory and cardiac status as well as vital signs and pulse oximeter should be monitored. The EMT–I should attempt to keep the child as calm as possible and maximize respiratory effect.

If respiratory distress increases, ventilatory support should be provided, including intubation if necessary. Medical direction should be contacted with an update. Sometimes epinephrine or an albuterol treatment through a nebulizer may decrease the respiratory symptoms.

TABLE 17-3 Differences Between Croup and Epiglottitis

CROUP	EPIGLOTTITIS
Usually caused by viral infection	Usually caused by bacterial infection
Usually occurs during late fall and early winter	No seasonal preference
Occurs in ages 3 months-3 years	Occurs in ages 3-7 years
Slow onset	Rapid onset
Patient will either lie down or sit up	Patient will sit upright in a tripod position
Barking cough present	No barking cough
No drooling	Pain on swallowing causing drooling
Temperature > 104° F	Temperature > 104° F

TABLE 17-4 Differences Between Asthma and Bronchiolitis

ASTHMA	BRONCHIOLITIS
Occurs at any age	Occurs between 6-18 months of age
Occurs in winter and spring	Can occur at any time
Response to allergy, exercise, or infection	Caused by a virus
Family history of asthma	Usually no history of asthma
Drugs reverse bronchospasm	Drugs may not always be effective

Table 17-4 lists the differences between asthma and bronchiolitis.

Pneumonia

Pneumonia in children usually presents with fever, poor eating habits, and irritability. Grunting respirations secondary to air trapping and expiratory obstruction should suggest pneumonia. Localized findings such as rales and decreased breath sounds are more common in children more than 1 year of age.

Shock

A child's circulatory system is different than an adult's system and may lose up to 20% of its blood volume before showing any change in the child's appearance.

The circulatory aspect of pediatric patients can best be evaluated by looking at the child's skin color and feeling the pulse. The skin of children is thinner than adults' skin. Therefore, changes in color or temperature are very obvious. Mottling of the skin or skin that appears to have two different colors is a very common finding in a child who has lost a significant amount of blood volume. Also, simultaneous palpation of the peripheral pulse and apical heart rate can provide clues regarding pediatric hypovolemia. The child who is in shock will have a rapid, thready peripheral pulse indicating that there is not an adequate blood volume circulating to the extremities.

The leading cause of shock in children across the world is gastroenteritis with dehydration. This infection along with diarrhea causes dehydration, and the severe loss of fluid can lead to hypovolemic shock.

Shock also can occur from partial-thickness and full-thickness burns, which damage the skin and allow fluid to escape through the burn surface (Fig. 17-12). That fluid often enters extravascular tissue. Nevertheless, it is not available to the circulating volume, and the child's blood pressure drops. Blood loss associated with trauma is also a cause of hypovolemic shock.

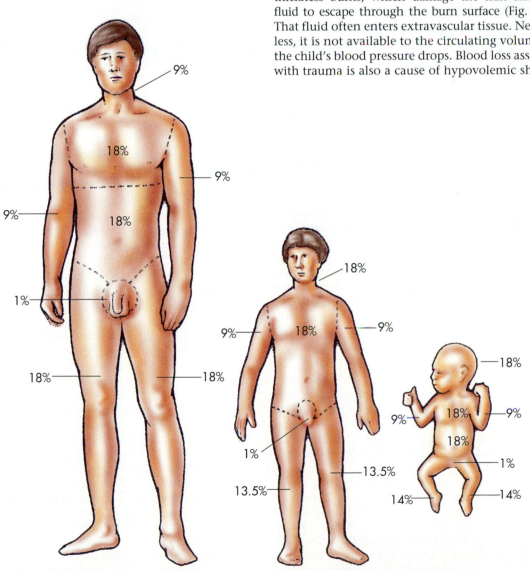

Fig. 17-12 The pediatric rule of nines can be used to estimate the percentage of the body that is burned.

Other reasons for shock in the child are sepsis and anaphylaxis. The child with meningitis or some other type of infection can develop sepsis (systemic infection), which can lead to septic shock.

Signs of shock include the following:

- Altered level of responsiveness (confusion to irritability to lethargy to coma—make a note if the child does not care if the parent leaves)

- Hyperventilation leading to respiratory failure

- Tachycardia

- Normotension progressing to hypotension

- Cool or cold, clammy skin

- Diminished peripheral pulses

- Prolonged capillary refill

- Oliguria (the EMT–I should ask if the child has urinated recently or how many diapers the child has wet within the last 24 hours)

- Acidosis

The treatment for shock in the pediatric patient is the same as that for the adult patient. If bleeding is present, it should be controlled with direct pressure. When appropriate, the patient should be placed in the Trendelenburg position or the shock position.

The EMT–I should be aware, however, that the infant or child can compensate for shock longer than the adult. The patient will maintain an adequate blood pressure and appear stable only to "crash" very quickly and become hypotensive. Therefore, the EMT–I should not be misled and have a false sense of security based on blood pressure.

Dehydration

Vomiting, diarrhea, fever, burns, and poor fluid intake can contribute to a loss of body fluids. These symptoms can lead to dehydration, which poses a threat to the infant and child. The subsequent decrease in cardiac output from a smaller circulating volume can lead to renal failure, shock, and death if not treated properly.

A fever in a child can cause diaphoresis and tachycardia. If a viral gastrointestinal disorder is present, the child may be nauseated or have vomiting and/or diarrhea. These symptoms may cause the child to refuse food and fluids, which further jeopardizes the body's fluid balance. This cycle continues until the child is lethargic and in danger of circulatory collapse.

Infants are particularly susceptible to this loss of fluid because a greater proportion of their bodies is

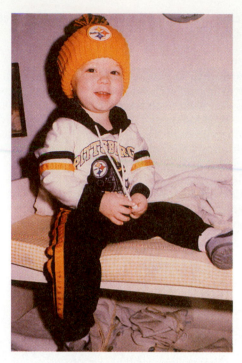

Fig. 17-13 An infant weighing 22 pounds is approximately 14 pounds of water.

composed of water. In addition, their fluid needs are higher. For example, 65% of an infant's total weight is water. If an infant weighs 10 kg (22 lbs), approximately 7 kg (14 lbs) are made up of water alone (Fig. 17-13).

 Identify the signs and symptoms of the infant or child with dehydration.

During the assessment, signs and symptoms of dehydration should be noted (Table 17-5). The dehydration can be mild, moderate, or severe depending on what clinical signs are found during the assessment. In fact, the EMT–I simply may discover signs and symptoms of mild dehydration as he or she assesses the child for another chief complaint (eg, the child who has had a febrile seizure).

The EMT–I should ask the parents/caregivers or child (if he or she is old enough and developmentally appropriate) specific questions about the child's history. How long has the child been ill? Was there any fever, vomiting, or diarrhea? If present, how high was the fever? How much or how often has the child vomited or had diarrhea? When did the child last have something to drink (by cup or bottle)? How many bottles has the infant taken within the past 24 hours? Is the child urinating or wetting his or her diaper in the usual manner? How many diapers have been wet with urine or diarrhea within the past 24 hours?

No special treatment is necessary if mild dehydration exists. It is important, however, to reassess the child in case the dehydration progresses.

TABLE 17-5	Dehydration Assessment		
CLINICAL FINDINGS	**MILD**	**MODERATE**	**SEVERE**
Heart rate	Normal	Increased	> 130/min
Respiratory rate	Normal	Increased	Tachypneic
Blood pressure	Normal	Normal	Systolic < 80
Peripheral pulses	Normal	Diminished	Absent
Capillary refill	Normal	2-3 seconds	> 2 seconds
Mental status	Alert	Irritable	Lethargic
Fontanelle	Flat	Depressed	Sunken
Turgor	Normal to slightly decreased	Decreased	Markedly decreased
Mucous membranes	Dry	Very dry; may see some tears	Parched; no tears
Temperature	Warm	Cool	Cool; clammy
Eyes	Normal	Darkened; sunken	Sunken; soft
Thirst	Increased	Intense	Intense if conscious

Modified from: Eichelberger MR, et al: *Pediatric emergencies,* Englewood Cliffs, 1992, Prentice-Hall.
Emergency Nurses Association, Emergency Nursing Pediatric Course, 1994

In moderate to severe cases of dehydration, high-concentration oxygen should be provided. The child's vital signs and cardiac status should be monitored, and ventilations assisted, if necessary. If the patient is hypovolemic, the EMT–I should start an IV of normal saline or lactated Ringer's solution, give a bolus of 20 mL/kg initially, and repeat this procedure in 5 minutes if the child's vital signs do not improve. Further boluses may be necessary to restore an adequate blood pressure and subsequent tissue perfusion. The EMT–I should prepare for immediate transport and maintain contact with medical direction. CPR may be required.

Seizures/Epilepsy

Seizures account for approximately 8% of pediatric prehospital transports. In many children seizures are a complication of a fever. In fact, approximately one out of every 20 children under the age of 7 years will have a seizure resulting from a fever. Seizures occur because of the rapid rise in temperature and not the final degree of the temperature.

Some children with epilepsy continue to have seizures on a regular basis despite aggressive medical therapy. The seizures interfere with the daily lives of the child and his or her family and subsequently constitute a chronic problem. Also, the growth and development of the child may be affected, and injuries often result, at which time EMS may become involved.

Assessment of infants and children experiencing seizures includes thorough initial and ongoing examinations. If no life-threatening instances are discovered, attention is then directed toward the seizure itself.

During the assessment of the child having a seizure, the EMT–I should make note of the following:

- Duration of the seizure
- Presence of any aura
- Level of responsiveness
- Part(s) of body involved
- Eye deviation and direction (if present)
- Postictal period (if present)
- Loss of bladder or bowel control (which can affect the older child's self-esteem)

The EMT–I should find out if the child has a history of seizures and under what circumstances they usually occur. He or she also should determine what precipitated this recent event, if more than one seizure occurred, what medications may have been taken, and so forth.

If a seizure is witnessed, the child gently should be assisted to a lying position with the head turned to the side. In addition, the area should be cleared of hazardous items that might cause injury during the seizure activity. The EMT–I should not insert anything into the mouth if the patient's teeth are clenched. A nasal airway is an appropriate alternative adjunct for this situation, and the airway should be maintained and suctioned ONLY as necessary.

Ventilations should be assisted with a bag-valve-mask device if hypoventilation or apnea occur for a prolonged period. Short periods of apnea occur with most tonic-clonic seizures, and respirations then return at the completion of the seizure. The EMT–I should use common sense to decide if the infant or child must be ventilated.

If the seizure is due to a fever, attempts to reduce the fever may be appropriate, such as removing clothing, sponging the infant or child with 4×4s moistened with tepid water only, keeping the patient compartment cool, and so forth.

CLINICAL NOTES

Caution: Sponging the infant or child in the pre-hospital setting is controversial. It usually works best after a fever-reducing medication has been given. If sponging is done prior to oral adminis-tration of a medication, the patient may shiver more, be uncomfortable, and have an increased metabolic rate, which actually may increase the fever. Medical direction should be consulted for a policy on this procedure.

When the seizure has subsided, the EMT–I should reassure the child and the family. If a post-ictal period occurs, the EMT–I should continue to maintain the airway as appropriate. For some seizures an IV line and administration of diazepam (Valium) or lorazepam (Ativan) may be required to stop the seizure activity. The EMT–I should follow local pro-tocols and maintain contact with medical direction whenever possible.

 Describe the treatment of an infant or child in status epilepticus.

Status epilepticus is a continuous seizure lasting more than 30 minutes or a series of seizures in which the patient does not regain responsiveness. If this con-dition occurs, immediate intervention is necessary. Complications include aspiration of blood or vomit, hypoxia resulting in brain damage, long bone and spinal fractures, and severe dehydration. The EMT–I should maintain the child's airway and monitor car-diac activity. IV glucose (25% to 50% depending on the size of the child) may be ordered to correct hypo-glycemia from the prolonged seizure activity.

Meningitis

Meningitis is defined as an inflammation of the membranes that surround the brain and spinal cord. It is caused by viruses, bacteria, or other microorgan-isms and may develop concurrently with viral ill-nesses such as mumps or chickenpox or a bacterial illness such as that seen with an ear infection. However, the child also may contract meningitis *without* any ongoing illness. The diagnosis is con-firmed only after the infant or child has a lumbar puncture, or "spinal tap."

Bacterial meningitis is much more serious than viral or aseptic meningitis. The most common forms of bacterial meningitis are hemophilus meningitis (caused by *Haemophilus influenzae*), pneumococcal meningitis (caused by *Streptococcal pneumoniae*), and

meningococcal meningitis (caused by *Neisseria meningitidis*). The first strain is much less common with the current *H. influenzae* type B vaccine rou-tinely given to children. Meningococcal meningitis is the most life-threatening strain of the three.

 Identify the signs and symptoms of the infant or child with meningitis.

In younger patients, signs and symptoms of meningitis may include:

- Fever
- Dehydration
- Disorientation or lethargy
- Bulging fontanelle
- Irritability (infant or child does not want to be touched or held)
- Loss of appetite
- Poor feeding (may be a sign in young infants)
- Vomiting
- Seizures
- Respiratory distress
- Cyanosis
- Rash

In the older child, in addition to the above signs and symptoms, the following may be present:

- Stiffness of the neck
- Kernig's sign (pain when extending the legs)
- Headache

As the bacteria or virus spreads, the child will become increasingly ill. In bacterial meningitis, cere-bral edema can occur, which can lead to increased intracranial pressure with brain stem herniation.

Permanent complications, which occur in approx-imately 30% of children with bacterial meningitis, include hearing loss (most common), seizure disor-ders, developmental and cognitive delay (mental retardation), hydrocephalus, motor impairment, paralysis, and ataxia. Approximately 5% to 15% of children with bacterial meningitis die, depending on the type of bacteria involved.

Some patients with meningococcal meningitis develop meningococcemia, which occurs when the *N. meningitidis* bacteria invade the bloodstream. Symptoms may include a sudden onset of chills, mus-cular and joint pain, sore throat, headache, petechiae (a perfectly round, purplish red spot caused by intra-dermal or submucous hemorrhage), and severe exhaustion. Profound shock occurs as the peripheral circulation collapses, and it is fatal if not treated aggressively. Infants and children who survive may be left permanently disfigured by the loss of skin and parts of their limbs damaged by the bacteria.

Treatment focuses on maintaining the child's respiratory and circulatory efforts. The EMT–I should monitor vital signs and cardiac status, provide high-concentration oxygen, and assist ventilations as necessary. He or she also should start an IV of lactated Ringer's solution and infuse fluid in boluses of 20 mL/kg as necessary to treat shock. The child should be made as comfortable as possible and transported immediately if meningitis is suspected. The EMT–I should notify medical direction and frequently reassess the child, watching closely for any seizure activity.

HELPFUL HINT
Meningitis is considered a true emergency in infants and children.

In a suspected case of meningitis, the EMT–I must protect himself or herself. The Centers for Disease Control and Prevention recommends using body substance isolation precautions. Because meningitis is spread by respiratory secretions (eg, mucus) and not droplet nuclei like tuberculosis, a specialized mask or respirator is not necessary. Any mask is appropriate as long as it provides a barrier that prevents contact with the patient's respiratory secretions.

If an exposure to bacterial (meningococcal) meningitis has occurred, the healthcare facility receiving the patient is required by law to notify emergency personnel involved in that patient's care. Prophylactic antibiotics usually are prescribed to prevent the spread of the disease. They should be taken exactly as prescribed, and the exposed individual should be monitored by a physician for development of meningitis symptoms.

HELPFUL HINT
SAFETY TIP: For the EMT–I's own protection, he or she should talk with personnel at the receiving facility after the call is completed. He or she should ask to be notified if the child is diagnosed with bacterial meningitis. In such a case, the EMT–I may be given medication to prevent contracting the disease.

Drowning and near drowning

Define drowning and near drowning.

In the United States, drowning is the third leading preventable cause of pediatric deaths. Distinction is made between **drowning**, which is death within 24 hours after a submersion accident, and **near drowning**, in which the infant or child survives at least 24 hours after a submersion incident, although death may eventually occur.

Most drowning events involving younger children occur in fresh water without proper adult supervision (eg, bathtubs, buckets, swimming pools, lakes, toilets, fish tanks). Because children under 3 years of age have such large, heavy heads, they cannot get out of

the water after falling head first into buckets, toilets, and so forth. In older children, drowning usually occurs after drug or alcohol use, swimming long distances, or boat accidents.

During the initial assessment, the EMT–I should focus on airway, breathing, and circulation. In many cases of drowning and near drowning, the child will be in cardiopulmonary arrest.

Treatment for these patients focuses on maintaining the respiratory and cardiac status. CPR should be initiated if appropriate. The EMT–I should remove wet clothing, wrap the child with blankets or towels, and use heat packs or other rewarming measures if the infant or child is hypothermic.

While the EMT–I is resuscitating the child, someone at the scene (eg, police officer, additional prehospital personnel, fire department personnel) should gather more information about the incident. How long was the child under the water? Was the child found in warm or cold water? Was the water shallow or deep? Were there signs of breathing or a pulse on rescue? Was CPR started? If so, how quickly was it started after the child was removed from the water? Is there any other medical history available such as medications, seizure history?

Resuscitation should be attempted on children who have been submerged in cold water for a long period of time. If the child is very cold and has a heart rate, invasive procedures such as intubation should not be performed, because stimulation of the vagus nerve may cause asystole. Instead, bag-valve-mask ventilation with high-concentration oxygen should be provided.

The patient should be rapidly transported to a receiving facility that ideally should be a pediatric trauma center or have the capability to provide intensive care services for pediatric patients.

Poisoning
Young children are at an extremely high risk for accidental poisonings because of their inquisitive nature. As the child grows older, poisoning may occur from drugs or alcohol as the child experiments with mind-altering substances. Poisoning is a preventable death.

Identify common poisons ingested by children.

Poison is defined as "any substance that produces harmful physiologic or psychologic effects." Children between the ages of 18 months to 3 years account for approximately 30% of all accidental ingestion of poisons. The most common types of poisons are as follows:

- Household products (eg, petroleum-based agents, cleaning agents, cosmetics, lawn and garden supplies)
- Medications (prescription and nonprescription)

- Toxic plants (*eg*, poinsettia plants during the holiday season)
- Contaminated foods (*eg*, potato salad left out all day at a summer picnic)

Between school age and adolescence, the most common poisons are:

- Alcohol
- Organic solvents (*eg*, hydrocarbons and fluorocarbons, which are present in gasoline, typewriter correction fluid, and airplane glue)
- Mind-altering drugs (*eg*, marijuana, hashish, LSD, PCP, mescaline)
- Narcotics (*eg*, heroin, morphine)
- Central nervous system depressants (*eg*, barbiturates)
- Central nervous system stimulants (*eg*, amphetamines, cocaine, crack)

Treatment for the prehospital patient depends on the type of poison ingested.

PEDIATRIC TRAUMA

Children will present with a particular injury pattern and physiologic response to trauma. These responses depend on the child's size, level of maturation, and overall development. However, basic life support and adequate assessments are still critical to the child's survival.

Prevention
The most frightening fact about pediatric trauma is that 20% to 40% of the deaths that occur are preventable. Many EMS and trauma systems are now focusing more on trauma prevention. Educational activities, for example, are directed toward children and their families and may include such things as helmet safety, bike rodeos, seat belt use, proper use of car seats, swimming pool safety, spinal injury prevention programs, antiviolence campaigns, and so forth.

Unique pediatric characteristics of trauma

 List the causes of pediatric trauma in order of the most common to the least common.

Blunt trauma continues to be the most common pediatric mechanism of injury. However, penetrating injuries have increased to almost 15% of all injuries. Causes of pediatric injuries are categorized from most to least common:

1. Falls (most frequent in children less than 5 years of age)
2. Vehicular-related trauma
3. Accidental injury
4. Sports-related injury
5. Assaults

Children may not show many external signs of injury. Therefore, it is important to expect multisystem injuries as opposed to single-system injuries until otherwise confirmed (which usually takes place once the child reaches the hospital).

The physical differences between children and adults include the following:

- The child is smaller than an adult and therefore prone to a wider range of injuries.
- A child has less body fat.
- The child's connective tissue is more elastic.
- The child's organs are much closer together. Therefore, more organs can be injured when energy is released during a traumatic situation.
- The child's skeleton is not completely calcified and has many active growth centers. This difference makes the skeleton more resistant to injury so that a severe injury may exist to the underlying organs without any broken bones. Children can withstand a higher level of energy without signs of external injury.
- The child has a larger surface area and can lose heat more quickly.

The child's future growth and development may be adversely affected by the trauma and subsequent injuries. The injuries may heal, but the child may be left with life-long physical, mental, and/or psychologic disabilities. In addition, the costs for rehabilitation and subsequent care for these children can be staggering.

The EMT–I directly influences not only the immediate survival of the child but also the long-term functioning of that child.

Assessment
Thorough initial and ongoing assessments are still performed on the pediatric patient, and it is even more critical for the EMT–I to recognize the potential for life-threatening injuries. Even if the child appears stable during assessment of the airway, breathing, and circulation, the EMT–I should go with his or her instincts if it is possible the child has sustained a substantial mechanism of injury. The EMT–I should initiate rapid transport to a pediatric trauma center if he or she believes the potential for decompensation exists.

If a life-threatening situation does not exist, the ongoing assessment should be continued. The EMT–I should pay close attention to anything that possibly could cause permanent damage such as injuries resulting in paralysis or paresthesias. In addition, any isolated extremity injury may require hospital evaluation to determine if the growth plate has been damaged.

The three most common causes of death in the infant and child are the same as in the adult: hypoxia, overwhelming central nervous system trauma, and massive hemorrhage. If the EMT–I is not quick to recognize these conditions or the possibility of these life-threatening conditions, he or she may contribute to the child's death or long-term disability.

Head trauma

Head injury is the most common cause of death in the pediatric patient, because children tend to land on their heads after a fall. Closed head injuries often result and may range from a momentary loss of responsiveness to coma to death. Adequate assessment, resuscitation, and transport to a facility designed to manage pediatric trauma are critical.

 List the most important intervention for a child with head trauma.

It is crucial to initially manage the airway and provide ventilation and supplementary oxygenation in an attempt to prevent further damage and sustain neurologic function. If the child is unresponsive, ventilation should occur immediately by either bag-valve-mask device or, optimally, endotracheal intubation. Ventilation helps to adequately oxygenate the child. **It is the most important intervention for the child with head trauma**.

Even if the child only briefly has lost responsiveness, it is important for that child to be evaluated. Cerebral edema, hematoma formation, and hypoperfusion still may occur and serious secondary injury must be ruled out.

Spinal trauma

The spine in the infant or child has not yet calcified, has more active growth centers, and is more flexible. Serious injury to the spinal cord can occur (eg, pinching, stretching, bruising, tearing) without any signs of external injury. In fact, there may not even be any changes seen on a radiograph once the child is evaluated at the hospital. If the child has any signs of deficit or if the mechanism of injury was significant, serious injury should be suspected and adequate precautions taken.

Causes of pediatric spinal trauma

Despite an increase in the use of car safety seats, the potential for injury to infants and young children still exists. Many parents buckle their infants into the seats and forget to secure the seats in the vehicles. If a motor vehicle collision occurs, the seat bounces around the inside compartment, which can result in injury to the child and/or other occupants of the vehicle.

Motor vehicles are also an origin of spinal trauma for older children. Many children, especially those between ages 4 and 10 years, ride completely unfastened despite laws requiring them to be secured in the car. Some parents simply do not adhere to the law and do not serve as good role models themselves. For example, some parents who own a minivan or station wagon permit children to ride unrestrained in the cargo area. During a collision, these unrestrained children become missiles and are susceptible to serious head, spinal, and other traumatic injury.

Children who do wear safety belts also may suffer spinal injury but this injury usually is not nearly as great as that suffered by unrestrained children. Use of a lap belt may cause injury to the abdomen or lumbar spine, so it is important for the EMT–I to examine the placement of the belt on the child. Is it high on the abdomen, or was it secured across the pelvis? Also, in vehicles equipped with shoulder harnesses in the front and back seats, the shoulder strap sometimes falls across the smaller child's neck or face, contributing to a possible cervical spine injury.

Children riding on dirt bikes, all-terrain vehicles, or as passengers on a motorcycle also may suffer spinal trauma. The EMT–I should observe the mechanism of injury, the vehicle involved, and what type of safety equipment may or may not have been used.

Lastly, warm weather tends to mean more children will be outside and will be prone to more injuries. Riding bicycles, skateboarding, playing kickball in the street, swimming, and so forth are all recreations during which serious injury may occur.

Initial assessment

Initial evaluation of the scene and mechanism of injury is crucial to performing a good assessment on any patient. When called to an incident involving possible pediatric spinal trauma, it is especially important for the EMT–I to notice what type of equipment, if any, was being used at the time of the incident. Has the equipment (eg, a bicycle) sustained any damage? Was the surface on which the child landed made of cement, grass, padded material, or dirt? If it was a bicycle accident, was the child wearing a helmet? If so, is the helmet still in place or was it knocked off the head upon impact? Was the helmet damaged? This information, if available, can tell the EMT–I a great deal about the injuries that may have occurred.

Particular attention should be paid to playgrounds and the equipment available to children. Many playgrounds now have cedar chips or some similar material on the ground under the equipment. This material provides a softer surface in the case of falls. It is important for the EMT–I to make note of this surface when evaluating the mechanism of injury and relay the information to personnel at the emergency department.

A thorough initial assessment with frequent reassessment is even more important in children. Infants and children can compensate for a serious injury longer than an adult because they usually are healthy before the trauma. However, they decompensate rapidly. Evaluation of the airway with special attention to the cervical spine in addition to assessment of breathing and circulation should be done first. Then the EMT–I should perform a quick neurologic examination and expose the patient to complete the initial assessment. Once any life-threatening injuries have been ruled out, the EMT–I then can begin the ongoing assessment.

Children between the ages of 12 and 17 years actually have bodies with the same anatomic ratios as adults. Children 7 years of age and younger, however, are significantly different in their anatomic configurations. The most notable difference is the size of the head.

Treatment

The indications for pediatric immobilization are based on the same criteria used for adults: evaluation of the mechanism of injury, one or more injuries suggesting some type of violent interaction, or specific signs and symptoms indicative of spinal trauma such as numbness, tingling, and so forth. However, mechanism of injury should be a key determination for immobilization even if the patient is asymptomatic. If the EMT–I believes the child may have been exposed to a force great enough to cause violent or sudden movement of the spine, the child needs to be properly immobilized.

 Describe the process for pediatric immobilization.

Once the possible existence of cervical and/or other spinal trauma has been identified, the EMT–I should begin treatment. The goal is to secure the child in a neutral, in-line position to a rigid board. Although this procedure may sound the same as that for an adult, the process used to achieve that goal is different for children.

To immobilize a pediatric patient, the EMT–I should do the following:

1. Ensure scene safety and quickly evaluate the mechanism of injury.

2. Approach the child and manually hold the head.

3. Bring the head into a neutral, in-line position. If any resistance is met or pain is elicited, stop any movement and immobilize the head in that position.

4. Perform an initial assessment to rule out any life-threatening injuries. If any are found, immediately begin treatment.

5. Apply a rigid cervical spine immobilization device to the neck ONLY IF IT FITS PROPERLY (Fig. 17-14 A). If a properly sized device is not available, use towels, washcloths, or other material to immobilize the head as best as possible (Fig. 17-14 B).

6. If no life-threatening injuries are found, continue with the ongoing assessment.

7. Perform any treatments necessary (eg, administer oxygen, immobilize fractures).

8. Logroll the child onto a rigid board and fasten the torso to the board (Fig. 17-14C).

9. Secure the torso as appropriate.

10. Fasten the head securely to the board (Fig. 17-14D). Manual immobilization can be discontinued at this time.

11. Secure the board to the stretcher and reassess the patient.

12. Prepare to transport and perform any other treatments as necessary.

Immobilization devices

Regardless of the immobilization equipment used, some padding may still be necessary depending on the size of the child. The EMT–I should use his or her best judgment to pad the open areas.

Child safety seats

If the child is small and is found in an infant safety seat, chances are that the thoracic and lumbar spine may have been protected. However, the cervical spine is susceptible to maximum flexion, especially if the seat is not in the backward position, as recommended for infants.

Other safety seats accommodate a child until approximately 4 years of age or 40 lbs. In these seats, the child actually extends beyond the margin of the seat and may be susceptible to all types of trauma. Also, if the child's head is above the back of the seat (more common in older models), the head may be hyperextended during a rear-end collision.

If the child is critically injured or if the EMT–I anticipates deterioration, the safety seat should NOT be used for immobilization. Instead, the child gently should be extricated from the seat onto a rigid board. Short backboards work well for this. The EMT–I should maintain manual stabilization of the head and move the child as a unit onto the board. The child then can be secured as discussed below.

No EMT–I can be an expert on each child safety seat, so in the event of a motor vehicle collision, he or she should do the following:

- When an infant or child is found in a safety seat, it can be used for immobilization only after a brief inspection. Has the car seat sustained any major structural damage as a result of the accident? In other words, can it still effectively support immobilization? Can it be secured appropriately in the ambulance? If the answer to either of these questions is no, do not use the seat for immobilization.

- If the seat includes a protection plate over the baby's chest, remove it so the patient's thoracic area is easily accessed (Fig. 17-15 A). This removal will permit adequate lung assessment and manual chest compressions if necessary. Usually the plate can be lifted and taped to the back of the seat. If that is not possible, the straps should be cut and the plate completely removed

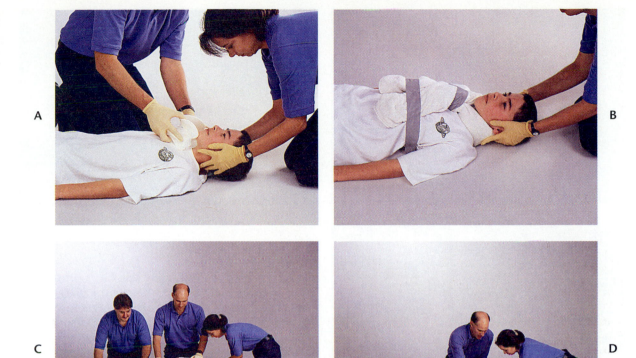

Fig. 17-14   Immobilizing a child patient. A, Apply a properly sized rigid cervical collar. B, If a collar is not available, provide immobilization with other materials. C, Logroll the child onto a rigid board and fasten the torso to the board. D, Securely fasten the child's head to the board.

from the seat. The child's torso then can be secured using cravats and padding.

- If a chest plate is not present, use the straps to secure the infant in place whenever possible. Additional padding and/or cravats between the straps and the child or tightening of the straps straps may be needed.

- Small blankets, towels, and the like should be used as padding for all open areas around the child's body so the child does not move. Padding also should be placed around the head and neck if a properly sized rigid cervical spine immobilization device is not available (Fig. 17-15 B).

- Once adequately immobilized, the patient and seat should be transferred to the ambulance. The seat then should be carefully secured to the stretcher or captain's seat so that it is not mobile during transport to the hospital (Fig. 17-15 C).

- Remember, only take the time to immobilize the infant or child in the safety seat if the patient is stable. Do not waste precious time if the patient is seriously injured.

Cervical spine immobilization devices

A rigid cervical spine immobilization device is recommended for any patient who is suspected to have sustained a cervical spine injury. In pediatric patients, however, the EMT–I should make sure the device chosen does not hyperextend the child's neck because of improper sizing. If the device is too large, it should not be used. If an appropriate-sized device is not available, the EMT–I should improvise as much as possible with padding to attempt to keep the neck immobilized. A cervical spine immobilization device alone is not adequate immobilization, therefore, manual stabilization must continue until the child is completely secured to a long backboard or equivalent device.

Backboards

A short or long backboard can be used for immobilization depending on the height of the child. If the short backboard is used to secure an infant, for example, it should be turned around so the head can be immobilized to the larger end.

Children have larger heads than adults and have less developed back muscles, which causes a natural flexion when the child is supine. The torso may need

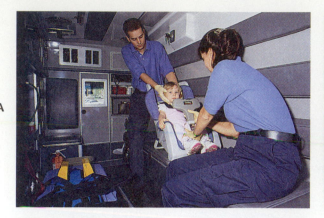

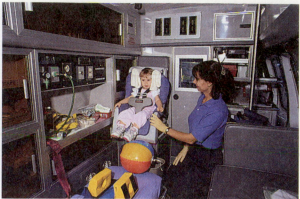

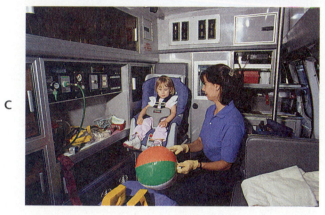

Fig. 17-15   A, If a child safety seat has a protection plate over the baby's chest, remove the plate to make the thoracic area accessible. B, Pad any open areas of the child seat so that the child cannot move, especially around the head and neck. C, Secure the safety seat in place for transport.

as much as 2 inches of padding to bring the spine into a neutral, in-line position. A flat blanket should be placed under the back from the upper margin of the pelvis and extended out to the left and right edgesof the board. All open areas then should be additionally padded.

When the child has been strapped to the backboard, the EMT–I will notice open areas between the straps and the edge of the board. Additional padding is also necessary along the outside of the torso and around both sides of the legs so that the board can be tilted without any movement of the child from side to side (Fig. 17-16).

For a smaller child, cravats should be used instead of straps. One area of importance is across the pelvis because young children have abdomens that extend past the iliac crest of the pelvis. Abdominal excursion is a necessary part of ventilation through approximately 7 years of age, and a strap could impede that process. Cravats also are advised instead of straps under the axillae. Big, wide straps can inhibit brachial circulation and actually cause more damage. If cravats are not available, tape may be used.

Vest Devices

Although in many parts of the country an adult vest device such as the Kendrick extrication device is used to immobilize children, this method is not recommended. Using this device in a manner other than that for which it was intended has not been proven

in the literature to be beneficial. For example, wrapping an adult vest device around the child like a papoose raises several concerns. One problem is that respiratory distress can occur if the thorax or abdomen is not permitted to expand adequately. Another concern is that in-line spinal immobilization is not achieved in many instances. More appropriate studies are needed before this method can be recommended.

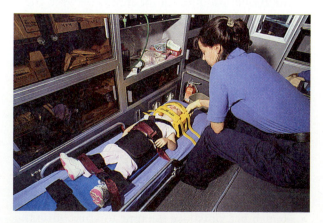

Fig. 17-16   When immobilizing a child on a backboard, padding may be necessary under the back, along the torso, and around both legs.

Helmets

Because children are now strongly encouraged to wear helmets during biking, skateboarding, and so on, chances are the EMT–I will be confronted with an injured child who is wearing a helmet. Should the EMT–I immobilize around the helmet or remove it as for adults?

According to the American College of Surgeons Committee on Trauma, helmet removal is recommended so that vital functions can be assessed and immobilization can be maintained. They make no distinction between adults and children. In fact, it may be even more critical to remove a helmet in children to prevent increased flexion of the child's head from the helmet when placed in the supine position (Fig. 17-17). Also, because cartilage in children may not be calcified, airway compromise can occur easily during hyperflexion.

Many children participate in sports in which a helmet is used in conjunction with other equipment (eg, football helmet plus shoulder pads). The EMT–I should work with the athletic trainers in the area. In some situations, the helmet and additional equipment such as shoulder pads may need to be removed as a unit.

Special considerations

When faced with a potential spinal injury in a child, the EMT–I should remember to rule out life-threatening injuries before turning his or her attention to full-body immobilization. Initial manual stabilization of the head and cervical spine should begin immediately during assessment of the airway. Further immobilization should not occur until adequate assessment and treatment have been completed. When immobilization can be performed, the best possible equipment available should be selected.

Chest and abdominal trauma

The child's rib cage is extremely resilient, and the chest can suffer major internal injury without any bony fractures. Rib fractures that do occur are associated with a high mortality.

The EMT–I should carefully observe for respiratory compromise and shock when treating a child with trauma to the chest and torso. He or she should evaluate the mechanism of injury and suspect injury even if the child appears to be fine. In addition, the child's cardiac rhythm should be monitored for signs of a cardiac contusion if present.

 List two signs of blunt trauma to the abdomen in the pediatric patient.

The EMT–I should assess for any signs of blunt trauma to the abdomen such as bruising (eg, from a lap belt in a motor vehicle); unstable pelvis; abdominal distension, rigidity, or tenderness; or signs of unexplained levels of shock. Children less than 8 years of age also tend to be "belly breathers,"

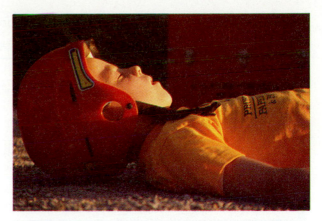

Fig. 17-17   Helmets should be removed in child patients.

therefore respiratory distress also may be a sign of abdominal trauma.

If the child is crying, it may be difficult to perform an abdominal examination. Guarding and distention can be missed if the child is upset. A crying child, however, is usually one who is hemodynamically intact. The EMT–I should become concerned if the child suddenly quiets down and allows him or her to assess the abdomen.

The ideal treatment for chest and abdomen trauma in the child is the same as for an adult: definitive care at the hospital. The EMT–I should provide high-concentration oxygen, monitor vitals, make the child as comfortable as possible, and prepare for rapid transport to an appropriate facility. The EMT–I should not waste time in the field if chest or abdominal trauma is suspected in the pediatric patient even if the child appears to be stable. This patient can decompensate rapidly.

Hypothermia

Children are susceptible to hypothermia due to their large body surface area in comparison with their weight. In addition, their compensatory mechanisms such as shivering are not well developed. Newborns in particular quickly can become hypothermic because they have little subcutaneous fat.

Hypothermia is defined as a core body temperature below 35° C (95° F). It often occurs in children as a result of prolonged exposure to cold temperatures. Leaving the child uncovered in a cool environment during examination and treatment also can lead to hypothermia. Other causes include metabolic disorders (eg, hypoglycemia), sepsis, and trauma or other brain disorders that interfere with the body's temperature regulating system. If alcohol and/or drugs have been ingested, the peripheral blood vessels dilate, and the body cannot conserve heat. Hypothermia often develops in such cases.

During the assessment, information about the incident should be obtained. How long was the child

TABLE 17-6	Signs and Symptoms of Hypothermia	
MILD	**MODERATE**	**SEVERE**
32-35° C	28-32° C	< 28° C
Slurred speech	Deteriorating responsiveness	Unresponsiveness
Mild uncoordination	Cyanosis	Dilated, fixed pupils
Shivering	Edema	Ventricular dysrhythmia
Decreased judgment	Muscle rigidity, no shivering Decreased respiratory rate, bradycardia	Respiratory arrest

Modified from: Eichelberger MR, et al: *Pediatric emergencies,* Englewood Cliffs, 1992, Prentice-Hall.

exposed to the cold, rain, or snow, etc.? Was the child submersed in water? What was the approximate temperature of the water? Is it known if the child ingested any alcohol or drugs? Does the child have a history of diabetes or an ongoing infection?

The EMT–I should look for specific signs and symptoms of hypothermia (Table 17-6). Types of hypothermia include mild, moderate, and severe depending on the temperature.

In addition, the EMT–I should look for areas of frostbite on the hands, fingers, feet, toes, ears, and nose. If the child complains of pain and a burning feeling, superficial frostbite probably has occurred. If there is no pain or feeling and the body part is blistered, a deeper injury may be present.

 Describe treatment for a child with hypothermia.

When treating the patient with hypothermia, the EMT–I should move him or her to a warmer environment as quickly as possible. If trauma is suspected, the child should be briefly immobilized before moving. All wet clothing should be removed and the child should be wrapped in blankets. Once the blankets become wet, new, dry blankets should be applied. The head should be covered, especially in young children, to minimize further heat loss. If the child is responsive, the EMT–I may give warm liquids by mouth. Under no circumstances should the EMT–I allow anyone to give the child any form of alcohol to increase warmth (some people mistakenly believe a "hot toddy" will help the rewarming process).

If the hypothermia is moderate to severe, the first priority is maintenance of the airway. The EMT–I should provide high-concentration oxygen by face mask or ventilate with a bag-valve-mask device if necessary. If there is no pulse, he or she should begin chest compressions. The EMT–I should transport the child rapidly and continue CPR until arrival at the hospital. Resuscitation should not be discontinued

until the child's temperature has returned to normal. At that time a decision can be made to stop or continue the resuscitation.

If a heart rate is present, the EMT–I should not provide any stimulation, including endotracheal intubation, CPR, or suctioning. The goal is to prevent ventricular fibrillation from occurring. In addition, the EMT–I should not waste time attempting to start an IV. The patient should be handled gently when moving to prevent any lethal dysrhythmias. The EMT–I should continue with basic life support and rapidly transport to the hospital.

Heat packs may be used as long as they do not directly touch the skin. They should be placed under the axillae and in the groin area over the blanket. If frostbite has occurred, those affected extremities should be wrapped in a blanket. The EMT–I should not aggressively rub the part or expose it to dry heat, which may cause tissue damage.

OTHER PEDIATRIC PROBLEMS

Child abuse or maltreatment

Child abuse, also called *nonaccidental trauma,* happens to more than 1 million children in the United States annually. It involves the maltreatment of children by their parents, guardians, or other individuals responsible for their care. Although the reporting of abuse has increased 31% from 1985 to 1990, it is still difficult to know how many cases actually are occurring each year, despite that reporting is mandatory by law in all 50 states.

Certain factors can place families and children at a greater risk to abuse or be abused. Table 17-7 shows some of these risk factors for child maltreatment.

Child abuse can be divided into the following four major types:

- Physical abuse—Any injury intentionally delivered to the child by a caregiver

TABLE 17-7	Risk Factors for Child Maltreatment	
CHILD	**FAMILY**
Prematurity	Alcohol dependency
Prenatal drug exposure	Drug dependency
Developmental disability	Childhood history of maltreatment
Physical disability	Belief in use of corporal punishment
Chronic illness	Rigid expectations regarding child's behavior
Product of multiple birth	Negative parental perceptions of child
	Single parent
	Social isolation
	Psychologic distress
	Low self-esteem
	Extreme poverty
	Acute and chronic stressors
	Unrealistic expectations of child

Source: *Emergency nursing pediatric course,* Emergency Nurses Association, 1993.

Indicators of Possible Abuse

1. Any obvious or suspected fractures in a child under 2 years of age
2. Injuries in various stages of healing, especially burns and bruises
3. More injuries than usually seen in other children of the same age
4. Injuries scattered on many areas of the body
5. Bruises or burns in patterns that suggest intentional infliction
6. Suspected increased intracranial pressure in an infant
7. Suspected intraabdominal trauma in a young child
8. Any injury that does not fit the description of the cause given
9. An accusation that the child injured himself or herself intentionally
10. Long-standing skin infections
11. Extreme malnutrition
12. Extreme lack of cleanliness
13. Inappropriate clothing for the situation
14. Child who withdraws from parent
15. Child who responds inappropriately to the situation (*eg,* quiet, distant, withdrawn)

- Sexual abuse—Any sexual activity between a child and an older child or adult
- Emotional or psychological abuse—Behaviors inflicted on the child that are degrading, terrorizing, isolating, or rejecting

- Neglect—Failure to meet the child's basic needs (*eg,* food, clothing, shelter, medical care, safety)

 List five indicators of child abuse or maltreatment.

As difficult as it may be, the most important role for the EMT–I in a suspected case of child abuse is to be nonjudgmental. The EMT–I must not accuse anyone of child abuse even though it may appear obvious to him or her. That type of approach may make the potential abuser angry and may even place the EMT–I in danger.

The EMT–I should focus on patient care yet be aware of the surroundings by objectively documenting where the child was found, the condition of the home, interactions with parents or family members, the condition of other children at the same location, and so forth. This information should be relayed to the physicians and nurses at the receiving facility. In some states, it is mandatory that EMTs report suspected child abuse or maltreatment. The EMT–I should consult confidentially with medical direction if he or she has any doubts.

CHILDREN WITH SPECIAL NEEDS

The EMT–I does not need to have a degree in special education to treat "special" children. When responding to a scene involving an ill or injured child who also has a hearing impairment, mental retardation, a tracheostomy, gastrostomy, cerebral palsy, or spina bifida, the EMT–I must think about how his or her assessment and treatment will change.

The term *special needs* indicates any condition with the potential to interfere with usual growth and development and can include physical disabilities, mental disabilities, chronic illnesses, or forms of technologic support. When specifically relating to children with special needs, the issues of growth, development, and education may surface. Therefore, the EMT–I's treatment of these unique patients can have a profound effect on their future well being.

Various disabilities may be encountered in the pediatric patient. Only a handful are discussed here, but many others exist. The EMT–I should incorporate this knowledge into his or her overall patient management.

 Recognize examples of cognitive and physical disabilities.

Cognitive disabilities

Cognitive disabilities involve some degree of impaired adaptation in learning, social adjustment, and/or maturation. They result from a variety of causes such as metabolic disorders, infections, intracranial hemorrhage, anoxia, inherited disorders, trauma, or other conditions that may damage the brain. The child usually is considered to have a learning disability, mental retardation, or some form of developmental delay.

In most circumstances, the actual physical examination is essentially unchanged. The most prominent differences will be in the child's level of understanding and ability to communicate. In addition, the EMT–I should direct questions in a positive light and focus on the child's *a*bilities instead of his or her *dis*abilities. The EMT–I should ask the parent or teacher what the child is able to do and what he or she understands.

Respect should be the key ingredient to any modality involving the child with a cognitive disability. Regardless of what action is taken, the EMT–I should explain it even if it seems that the child does not understand. It is possible that the patient may comprehend what the EMT–I is saying without registering any reaction. A short explanation of what the EMT–I is doing to the child also will go a long way to alleviate some of the fears on the part of the parents or caregiver.

Physical disabilities

Physical disabilities involve some type of limitation of mobility and are caused by birth anomalies, spinal cord injuries, infections, disease processes, and so forth. Examples include hearing or vision impairments, cerebral palsy, spina bifida, and spinal cord injuries.

During the assessment, it is important to determine, if possible, what type of disability was present prior to the emergency (*eg*, did the child previously have any paralysis of the lower extremities or is that a result of the present injury?).

Many children with physical disabilities use some type of adaptive device, such as a wheelchair, braces, crutches, or a combination of devices. Some children may use corrective splints at different times during the day or night. The EMT–I should ask the patient, parents, or caregivers to explain the device and use their knowledge to help assess and treat the child. Splints or braces also can serve as tools for immobilization if trauma is suspected. However, if circulation or breathing are impaired or major bleeding is present, these devices should be removed.

Chronic illnesses

Any disease, condition, or situation that extends for a prolonged period of time is considered chronic. Chronic illnesses include reactive airway disease (asthma), diabetes, epilepsy, terminal illnesses such as cancer or cystic fibrosis, children who are awaiting or who have had transplants, children with head or spinal cord injuries after rehabilitation, and children with congenital cardiac anomalies.

Technological aids
Tracheostomy

A tracheostomy is used as a temporary or permanent device. In some patients, it provides protection against secretions that may be aspirated. In other patients, it is necessary because of direct trauma to the airway or weakened respiratory muscles or after prolonged mechanical ventilation (Fig. 17-18).

Mucous plugs commonly obstruct the lumen of the tracheostomy tube because it is of such a small diameter. This obstruction may lead to cardiac arrest if the patency is not restored. Assessment should include a detailed inspection of the tracheostomy device and site. Is it patent? Are secretions present, and if so, what color and consistency are they? Is there any bleeding noted around the site?

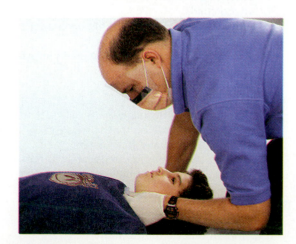

Fig. 17-18 Some patients may have a tracheostomy in place as a temporary or permanent device to aid in breathing.

Describe treatment of an obstructed tracheostomy in an infant or child.

The tracheostomy tube should be suctioned if it is occluded. Only approximately 4 to 5 seconds of suctioning are necessary because the tube is so short. If the EMT–I cannot remove the obstruction or cannot insert the suction catheter, he or she should remove the entire tube. He or she should suction the stoma, or opening in the neck, and insert a new tube if it is available and the EMT–I has been trained to do so. If another tracheostomy tube is not available, a standard infant endotracheal tube can be substituted.

If unable to ventilate through the stoma and the upper airway is patent, the EMT–I should manually occlude the stoma. Bag-valve-mask ventilation should be performed over the nose and face until orotracheal intubation can be done or a replacement tracheostomy tube becomes available.

In older children who are responsive, alternative methods of communication may be necessary. Some will use a communication board or simply write down their needs on a piece of paper. The EMT–I must be sure to ask what method is best for this particular patient.

Apnea monitors

Many premature infants are sent home with apnea monitors to warn parents and caregivers of any lapses in breathing. Some monitors also warn of bradycardia or tachycardia. An alarm sounds if the device does not detect a breath within a specific time interval or if there is a significant change in the infant's heart rate.

The EMT–I will most likely be called to the home to assist with CPR, to transport the infant back to the hospital, or simply to provide reassurance to frightened parents. If the infant does not need to be transported, the EMT–I should let the family know he or she is available in the future if the infant's condition changes.

Gastrostomy tube

A gastrostomy tube is used for children who cannot take food by mouth for an extended period of time. Various types of devices are used, and each is inserted and secured in a different way. The EMT–I should look at the insertion site for bleeding or to see if the tube has become dislodged. If the tube is secured within the stomach, he or she should be aware that more bleeding may occur internally. If there is any suspicion of internal bleeding, further evaluation is necessary at the hospital (Fig. 17-19).

Medications

Some children take many medications for their particular disability. The EMT–I should obtain this information from the parents or examine medication bottles if necessary.

The EMT–I should determine when the child last took each medication. In someone with a gastrointestinal illness, nausea and vomiting may preclude the patient from taking or absorbing the drugs, which may in turn precipitate other serious consequences.

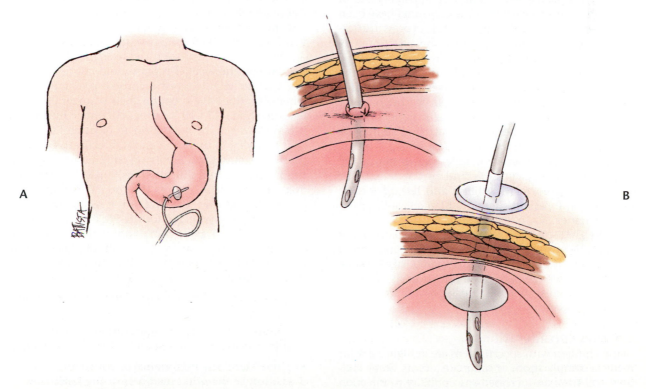

A   B

Fig. 17-19 Gastrostomy tubes may be secured (A) internally, or (B) externally.

During assessment of the patient, obvious medication side effects may include drowsiness, irritability, or puffiness such as that seen with steroids. These side effects should be noted in the EMT–I's documentation.

 Identify family issues encountered when working with children who have special needs.

Family issues

Dealing with a child with special needs can be stressful for the entire family. The family should be included during the EMT–I's assessment of the pediatric patient, because they have been forced to become experts regarding their child and his or her disability or special circumstance. The EMT–I should trust them when they say there is a change in their child's routine behavior. If they are providing treatment on the EMT–I's arrival (*eg*, suctioning their child or performing CPR), the EMT–I should either allow them to finish the procedure while he or she gathers more information or gently assume a primary role. They should be allowed to assist in providing treatment if they prefer to do so. If the family is overwhelmed or significantly stressed, the EMT–I may need to be more assertive. However, the EMT–I should not simply take over as the medical professional and push the family aside.

Frequent hospitalizations may be a big part of these families' lives; and as part of the emergency response team, the EMT–I might see many different emotions at play. The child may be unusually fearful if past experiences with medical personnel have been painful or unpleasant. Parents may express frustration with yet another trip to the hospital, or they may be complacent about it.

It is also important to consider the siblings of the child with special needs. Their lives have been disrupted by the amount of care their brother or sister requires, by the frequent hospitalizations, and by constant questions about why that child cannot do things other children are doing. If a sibling is at the scene, the EMT–I should include him or her in the treatment whenever possible and appropriate. He or she should listen to the sibling and let him or her help hold the patient's favorite blanket, doll, or toy as reassurance.

If the EMT–I notices that the family is particularly anxious, he or she should pass this information on to the staff in the emergency department. This is a time when social service personnel, nutritionists, or other medical specialists may be able to provide some assistance or guidance.

General considerations

Many children with special needs are at higher risk for medical complications or traumatic events. Some children will have an increased susceptibility to infection resulting from immunity-suppressing medications.

Guidelines for Disability Awareness

Use the word "disability" instead of handicapped.

Refer to the person first and the disability second, *eg*, the child with mental retardation instead of the retarded child.

The child with a disability instead of the disabled child.

Never refer to someone as "wheelchair bound" or "confined to a wheelchair," because a wheelchair actually makes the person more mobile.

Avoid negative descriptions whenever possible. Do not use "invalid," "afflicted with," or "suffers from." Do not refer to children with Down syndrome as "mongoloids" or to children with epilepsy as "epileptics." Do not call seizures "fits."

Do not use "normal" to describe people who do not have disabilities. Use "typical" or "people without disabilities."

Do not refer to a person's disability unless it is relevant.

Source: Adapted from *Talking About Disability: A Guide to Using Appropriate Language* published by COALITION for Tennesseans with Disabilities, Nashville, Tennessee.

Others may show signs of skin breakdown from the use of braces or splints. Yet another group may have physical impairments that can result in decreased reflexes, low muscle tone, altered sensation, or even paralysis, which can limit their protective mechanisms.

The EMT–I should look for a Medic Alert bracelet or necklace on these patients but should not rely on this solely as an indication of a chronic problem. Many parents do not have them for their younger child for fear the child will pull it off or actually be hurt by it. It may, however, be present on an older child.

It is crucial to involve medical direction as soon as possible in situations involving children with special needs. Early communication will help ensure adequate treatment as well as the proper patient destination. In addition, the staff at the receiving facility will be properly prepared for the EMT–I's arrival.

As the EMT–I gains more confidence in treating these types of patients, he or she should take part in educating other EMS personnel in the area by doing the following:

- Become more familiar with different types of disabilities.

- Incorporate the discussion of various disabilities into pediatric assessment and treatment modalities.

- Understand the importance of conveying information to the other members of the healthcare team.

- Use the parents as a resource for information and advocacy.

One way the EMT–I can take a proactive approach is to ask if the service area includes children at home with any type of disability, special education programs, or seasonal residential camps. If any of these are within the EMT–I's jurisdiction, he or she should take an active role. The EMT–I can visit the child's home, the educational program, or camp and make sure adequate information such as the correct telephone number for dispatch is available to summon EMS assistance. The EMT–I can meet the staff and educate them as to the skills he or she possesses and how he or she can work with them in an emergency. The EMT–I also can offer to provide CPR training as a community service and be available to work at the camp as an EMS provider or as part of a medical personnel team.

Most importantly, the EMT–I should interact with some of the children (*eg*, giving them tours of the ambulance, demonstrating how different pieces of equipment are used). This interaction will make them feel more comfortable in the EMT–I's environment should an emergency require EMS services, and it will certainly give the EMT–I an opportunity to get to know a piece of the child's world.

Remember that the child for whom the EMT–I is caring is a person first and a person with a disability second. For many families, it takes quite a bit of time to adjust to a chronic illness. In many cases, the mixed emotions about this "change in plans" surface at different times throughout the child's life, one of which may be the emergency situation in which the EMT–I is involved. The EMT–I's sensitivity and compassion toward the child and the family during this time can help everyone involved appreciate the unique characteristics of these special children.

SPECIAL CONSIDERATIONS

The EMT-I should remember to involve the parents, caregivers, or teachers throughout the call because it is often emotionally as well as physically traumatizing to the child and the family. In addition, if the illness or accident occurs in a crowded area such as a school or playground, other children or the patient's brothers or sisters may be in the area. They also may be frightened by the entire experience and may need some extra emotional support.

CASE HISTORY FOLLOW-UP

En route to the emergency department, the crew performs an ongoing assessment of EMT–I Ward's child. Audible wheezes are still present, and he continues to use his neck muscles to breathe. The pulse oximeter indicates an oxygen saturation of 89%. The crew contacts medical direction to advise them of the patient's status, his medication history, and their 5-minute ETA to the hospital. Because wheezes are still present, the on-line physician directs the crew to administer a second dose of albuterol by inhalation, but the drug has little effect on his respiratory status.

On arrival at the hospital, EMT–I Ward's son is quickly evaluated by the emergency department physician. An IV line is established, and a respiratory therapist begins to administer a bronchodilator via a nebulized updraft. Within minutes, the wheezes begin to clear and his color improves. Although he looks weary, EMT–I Ward knows her son is going to be OK.

EMT–I Ward is aware that an asthma attack can be life-threatening. She also knows that medications often are required to reverse reactive airway disease. She hopes her son will outgrow this illness. But until then, EMT–I Ward and her family must be prepared to manage this common childhood emergency.

SUMMARY

The EMT–I should try to speak to the child as much as possible to explain what is happening. If the patient is a young child, simple distraction from the activities at hand may be better than attempting to logically detail all of the actions. Diversionary tactics such as allowing the child to play with a toy or teddy bear can be quite helpful.

When faced with a potential spinal injury in a child, the EMT–I must rule out life-threatening injuries before turning his or her attention to full-body immobilization. Initial manual stabilization of the head and cervical spine should begin immediately, as the EMT–I assesses the airway. Further immobilization should not occur until adequate assessment and treatment have been completed. When immobilization can be performed, the EMT–I should select the best equipment available.

Pediatric illness or injury can be frightening to even the most experienced EMS provider. On those days when life is not too busy, the EMT–I should take the opportunity to review the equipment he or she would use to immobilize the pediatric patient. The EMT–I can practice pediatric assessment with his or her own children or children of other EMS or fire department members. This is great experience for the EMT–I as well as for the children. As they say, "Practice makes perfect." Once the EMT–I feels more confident with the process and the equipment, all of his or her concentration can be directed toward patient care.

The EMT–I must be adequately trained to deal with pediatric emergencies. He or she should concentrate on the differences between adults and infants or children. The assessment and treatment of these patients should be performed with those differences in mind. Special attention should be paid to the pediatric airway, because respiratory distress usually precedes cardiac dysrhythmias. Infants and children can compensate longer while in shock, yet deteriorate rapidly when their bodies can no longer maintain that compensation.

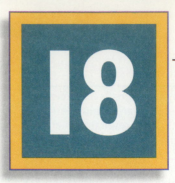

18 SUBSTANCE ABUSE AND BEHAVIORAL EMERGENCIES

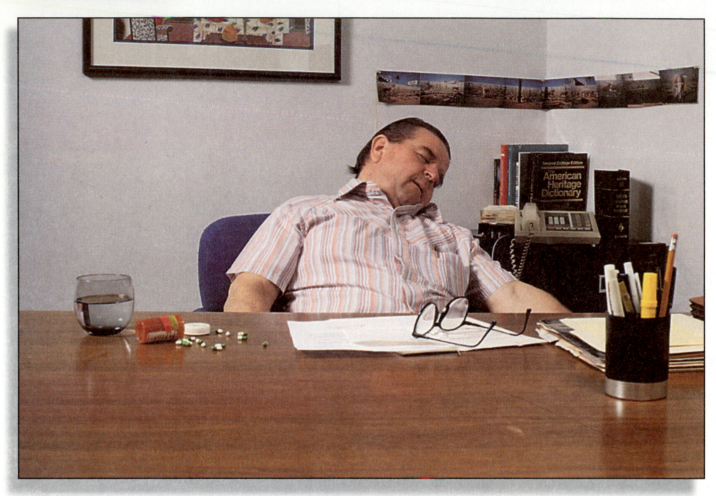

CASE HISTORY

EMT–Intermediates Keegan and Bravo are dispatched to 2135 Sunrise Drive at 5:17 PM for a "possible overdose, 17-year-old female." They arrive in 12 minutes and are directed to a second floor bedroom by the patient's mother.

Her mother says, "I came home from work and found her lying in bed. I couldn't wake her up, that's when I called 9-1-1."

EMT–I Bravo begins the initial assessment and treatment for the unresponsive teenager while EMT–I Keegan continues to ask the patient's mother questions and takes a quick look around the bedroom for clues to the patient's condition.

Case History, continued

"Has anything like this ever happened before?" EMT–I Keegan asks.

"No. Never," her mother responds.

"Does she have any medical conditions that require a doctor's care?" EMT–I Keegan asks.

"No."

"Is she a diabetic?"

"No."

"Is she allergic to anything?"

"Penicillin. But she isn't ill. She hasn't needed any medications."

EMT–I Bravo has placed the patient in the left lateral recumbent position and applied oxygen and the electrocardiogram monitor. He is preparing to start an intravenous lifeline of normal saline. EMT–I Keegan notes that the pulse oximetry shows 92% saturation.

EMT–I Keegan takes a look at the patient's dresser and notices two empty pill bottles, and then she sees a handwritten note next to them:

Dear Mommy and Daddy:

I'm sorry. I love you. Please don't be too mad at me. I can't tell you everything.

    Love,

    Susie

LEARNING OBJECTIVES

Upon completion of this chapter, the EMT–Intermediate should be able to:

- IDENTIFY four conditions that may mimic alcohol intoxication.
- DESCRIBE alcohol withdrawal syndrome.
- IDENTIFY five major classes of abused drugs.
- DESCRIBE the care given to patients suspected of alcohol or drug abuse.
- DEFINE the term *behavioral emergency.*
- DESCRIBE general methods to approach and treat persons with behavioral emergencies.
- DIFFERENTIATE between neurosis and psychosis.
- DESCRIBE three signs of depression.

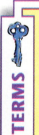

KEY TERMS

ALCOHOL ABUSE

ALCOHOLISM

ALCOHOL WITHDRAWAL SYNDROME

BEHAVIORAL EMERGENCY

DELIRIUM TREMENS

DEPRESSANTS

DISULFIRAM

HALLUCINOGENS

NARCOTICS

NEUROSIS

PSYCHOSIS

STIMULANT

SUBSTANCE ABUSE

Alcohol abuse

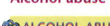 **ALCOHOL ABUSE:** Excessive alcohol consumption that leads to medical, behavioral, or social changes in an individual.

ALCOHOLISM: A dependence on alcohol.

Alcohol is a drug—it can be lethal. **Alcohol abuse** is the presence of medical, behavioral, or social problems related to excessive alcohol consumption. Alcohol abuse is not the same as **alcoholism,** which is a chronic condition characterized by dependence on alcohol as well as a pattern of abnormal behaviors. Alcohol abuse has no socioeconomic boundaries.

Similar percentages of alcohol-related problems are found in high-income areas as in lower-income areas.

STREET WISE

Alcohol and other drugs (especially marijuana and cocaine) also have been shown to play a significant role in homicide, suicide, child abuse, and unintentional trauma (such as falls or motor vehicle accidents). If the EMT–I has reason to suspect that the patient has been drinking or taking illicit drugs, these observations should be documented on the run report.

Alcohol tends to potentiate many drugs, especially sleeping pills and other depressants. Ingestion of alcohol in combination with other drugs can be fatal.

Patient assessment

Signs and symptoms of alcohol intoxication are often multiple and include:

- Odor of alcohol on the breath
- Unsteady gait
- Slurred, loud, and inappropriate speech
- Nausea, vomiting
- Flushed face
- Altered level of responsiveness
- Abnormal behavior, ranging from elation to violence
- Injuries, often from unexplained sources
    Additional signs seen with severe alcohol intoxication include:
- Hallucinations
- Hypotension
- Slow or labored respirations
- Marked dehydration
- Seizures
- Unresponsiveness or coma

Conditions that mimic alcohol intoxication

Identify four conditions that may mimic alcohol intoxication.

Other life-threatening illnesses can mimic alcohol intoxication. Even patients who have alcohol on the breath and appear intoxicated can have other, more serious problems. The EMT–I should consider the possibility of the following conditions in any patient who appears to be intoxicated:

- Drug abuse
- Brain tumor
- Hypoglycemia
- Meningitis
- Head injury
- Stroke

- Postictal state
- Diabetic ketoacidosis
- Hypoxia

STREET WISE

The EMT–I should not be fooled by the smell of alcohol on the breath. The patient may have been the victim of serious trauma or have a medical problem in addition to being intoxicated. The EMT–I should assume the patient is suffering from a serious medical problem and provide care accordingly, until proven otherwise.

HELPFUL HINT

Many medical problems can mimic alcohol intoxication. The most common masqueraders are hypoglycemia, diabetic ketoacidosis, and head injury. The EMT–I should always assume that the "apparently drunk" patient may have a concomitant medical problem.

Emergency care

To care for a patient with alcohol intoxication, the EMT–I should do the following:

- Maintain the airway and assist breathing if necessary.
- Be prepared to suction.
- Give high-concentration oxygen, if the patient permits.
- If trauma is suspected, stabilize and immobilize the cervical spine.
- Check for hypoglycemia using a fingerstick blood sugar.
- Attempt to build rapport and trust with the patient.
- Restrain the patient as necessary for his or her protection (as well as the EMT–I's safety).
- Summon police or other assistance when necessary if the patient is uncooperative, agitated, or combative. Remember, in this and all other types of cases, that the purpose of obtaining help from law enforcement is to protect both the EMT–I AND the patient.

STREET WISE

The EMT–I should consider the acutely agitated patient to be a danger to himself or herself and to others. This person may appear restless or angry and is potentially violent. The patient should be restrained as necessary. The EMT–I should document the reasons for restraints in the run report and involve law enforcement as per local protocols.

Severely intoxicated patients should be transported to the emergency department. It is possible that another illness may be present. A severely intoxicated patient is a danger to himself or herself as well as to others. These patients should be evaluated medically and observed for a period of time in the emergency department.

> ### HELPFUL HINT
> The amount of alcohol required to impair a person's mental or physical function varies widely from individual to individual. Chronic alcohol abusers are able to tolerate much higher blood alcohol levels than are less frequent drinkers. In terms of alcohol content, one beer equals one cocktail. Severe intoxication, by itself, also can be a medical emergency resulting in cardiac arrhythmias, shock, and death.

Alcohol withdrawal syndrome

> **ALCOHOL WITHDRAWAL SYNDROME:** Physical reactions a person experiences when he or she abruptly stops consuming alcohol.
> **DELIRIUM TREMENS:** A severe state of alcohol withdrawal consisting of delirium, hallucinations, and nervous system hyperactivity.

 Describe alcohol withdrawal syndrome.

When a patient abruptly stops drinking alcohol, especially after a prolonged period of intoxication, the body can experience **alcohol withdrawal syndrome.** These reactions include:

The shakes
The "shakes" occur within 24 hours of drinking cessation. The patient is shaky and tremulous and has a mild sleep disturbance. The eyes are bloodshot, and the blood pressure is elevated. Although these patients often are uncomfortable, this condition by itself is not dangerous. The EMT–I should care for these patients as described previously (see "Emergency Care") and transport to the hospital for further evaluation and care.

Withdrawal seizures
Withdrawal seizures such as grand mal (generalized) seizures may occur within 24 to 48 hours of drinking cessation. One third of these patients will progress to delirium tremens. The EMT–I should care for these patients as he or she would any patient with a seizure.

Delirium tremens
Delirium tremens is a severe state of delirium, hallucinations, and autonomic nervous sytem hyperactivity (fever, tachycardia, hypertension). Delirium tremens is a serious condition; up to 15% of patients die from associated problems.

Symptoms of alcohol withdrawal syndrome may begin from 12 to 48 hours after the last ingestion of alcohol. The patient should be restrained as necessary. The EMT–I should care for any related conditions and transport the patient to the hospital. The emergency department should be notified in advance that the EMT–I is transporting a violent patient. The EMT–I should involve law enforcement personnel per local protocols.

> ### CLINICAL NOTES
> Some patients with chronic alcohol abuse problems are on a medication called **disulfiram** (trade name, Antabuse). This drug causes a violent reaction in the body if the patient ingests even the smallest amount of alcohol. Antabuse is prescribed for the purpose of providing a significant deterrent to drinking.
>
> Other commonly prescribed drugs (not related to alcohol abuse) have a side effect that can cause an Antabuse-like reaction following alcohol ingestion in some patients. These drugs include:
> * Flagyl (metronidazole)—Commonly prescribed for vaginal and intestinal infections.
> * Antibiotics—Most of these drugs are given in the hospital and are therefore of little risk in the home and community setting.
> * Oral diabetic medications
> Antabuse or Antabuse-like reactions can be a threat to life. Patients have nausea, vomiting, palpitations, anxiety, hypotension, and flushing. Shock and cardiovascular collapse can develop.
>
> If the EMT–I suspects this type of reaction in a patient, he or she should administer oxygen, start a large-bore IV lifeline of normal saline, protect the airway, place the patient on the cardiac monitor, care for shock, and transport to the hospital immediately.

Drug abuse
Drugs are substances taken by mouth; injected into a muscle, the skin, a blood vessel, or a body cavity; or placed onto the skin (topical) to treat or prevent a disease or condition. Drugs may be ethical, manufactured by a legitimate pharmacologic company for the purpose of treating certain medical problems, or illicit, manufactured (usually illegally) solely for the purpose of abuse. Sometimes, ethical drugs (also known as *ethical pharmaceuticals)* are used for illicit purposes.

Drug misuse is the intentional or accidental use of a medication for a medical purpose other than the one intended, or in a dose different than that prescribed (eg, taking penicillin tablets left over from a previous sore throat for an ear infection). Failure to take prescribed medication is also a form of drug misuse. This misuse is called *poor patient compliance* and is common.

Drug abuse is the use of a drug for a nontherapeutic effect, especially one for which it was not prescribed or intended. The most common reason is to "get high." The exact meaning of this term differs from person to person. To some people, getting high means escaping reality. To others, it may mean inducing hallucinations. Often, the term *substance abuse* is used, instead of drug abuse, in order to include alcohol and marijuana. In this same category are various substances that are taken as drugs that were not "intended" to be used as such (eg, glue, gasoline, solvents).

Drug addiction is a condition characterized by an overwhelming desire to continue taking a drug. True addiction is both a psychologic and physical condition. The patient has both a physical need and a psychologic craving for the drug and its effect. Drug dependence is a psychologic craving for or reliance on a chemical agent, resulting from abuse or addiction. Drug dependence is a psychologic problem, not a physical one.

Drug withdrawal is a set of signs and symptoms that develop in a person following abrupt cessation of taking a drug. Most times, the individual has developed a dependence or addiction to the drug. The most dangerous drug withdrawal reactions occur in persons who are addicted, meaning they are both physically AND psychologically "hooked" on a particular substance. Classic examples include alcohol withdrawal seizures and delirium tremens. Psychologic withdrawal, although severe, often is not life-threatening.

Withdrawal syndromes also can result from the sudden stoppage of several prescription medications that are not considered "addictive" by most criteria. For example, if a person suddenly stops taking certain antihypertensive drugs, he or she can develop a rebound hypertensive emergency. Persons who abruptly stop using beta-blockers, a type of heart medicine, may develop a myocardial infarction.

Drug abuse is a significant problem in the United States and is a leading cause of trauma, heart attacks, and strokes. Illicit drugs are taken by various routes: inhalation, oral ingestion, or injection. Persons may take drugs illicitly to get high or as part of a suicide attempt.

CLINICAL NOTES

Drug abuse (especially the abuse of alcohol, marijuana, and cocaine) has been shown to play a significant role in homicide, suicide, and unintentional trauma (such as falls or motor vehicle accidents).

Drugs of abuse

 Identify five major classes of abused drugs.

There are five classes of drugs of abuse. The classes, representative agents, and common symptoms of intoxication are:

Stimulants

Stimulants (uppers) stimulate the central nervous system. Cocaine is the most widely used drug in this category. Other drugs include amphetamines (speed), caffeine, and thyroid medication. "Ice" is a highly concentrated form of amphetamine, which lasts 12 to 24 hours.

Symptoms of stimulant intoxication include hyperactivity, euphoria, tachycardia, hypertension, dilated pupils, diaphoresis, sleeplessness, seizures, and disorientation. Cocaine causes hypertensive crisis, seizure, myocardial infarction, and stroke.

Depressants

Depressants (downers) depress the central nervous system. Marijuana is the best known agent. Other depressants include barbiturates, sleeping pills, tranquilizers, and antidepressant pills.

Symptoms of depressant intoxication include sluggishness, poor coordination, slurred speech, decreased respiration or respiratory arrest, and impaired memory and judgment.

Hallucinogens

Hallucinogens induce a sense of euphoria and hallucinations. LSD is the best known agent. Other hallucinogens include mescaline, psilocybin, and PCP (angel dust). PCP may result in suicidal and extremely violent behavior. Many times, several people are required to restrain a violent patient under the influence of PCP.

Hallucinogen ingestion leads to hallucinations, unpredictable behavior, tachypnea, nausea, dilated pupils, and increased pulse and blood pressure.

Narcotics

Narcotics include heroin, morphine, methadone, Demerol (meperidine), Dilaudid (hydromorphone), Talwin (pentazocine), codeine, Vicodin (hydrocodone), and Darvon (propoxyphene).

Ingestion of these agents may result in drowsiness, coma, impaired coordination, sweating, respiratory depression, constricted pupils, shock, convulsions, and coma. Respiratory and cardiac arrest also are possible.

Volatile chemicals

Volatile chemicals include aerosols (spray paint, hair spray, industrial chemicals), glue, and gasoline.

Patients who inhale or otherwise ingest these compounds may have an altered level of responsiveness, swollen mucous membranes of the mouth and nose, increased pulse and respiratory rates, respiratory distress (particularly with gasoline inhalation, such as during siphoning), and nausea.

STREET WISE

Any drug, prescription or otherwise, may be abused. Nitroglycerin or amyl nitrate ("poppers") are used to treat heart pain. These agents also have become popular as street drugs because they cause a warm, flushed feeling, which is said to be especially good during sex. The anesthetic gas nitrous oxide ("laughing gas") is abused in a similar fashion.

Patient assessment

In addition to the signs and symptoms of substance abuse, the EMT–I should expect the patient's history to be unreliable. If possible, the EMT–I should determine what substances were taken, when they were taken, how they were taken, how much was taken, and if any care has been started.

The EMT–I also should attempt to assess if the patient is suicidal. He or she should ask, "Did you want to hurt yourself?" The answer should be recorded in the run report. This record is essential, particularly if the EMT–I needs to restrain the suicidal patient to prevent him or her from doing further harm.

The EMT–I should expect a mixed intoxication. Many ingestions, especially if a suicide attempt is involved, are a mixture of alcohol and other drugs.

The EMT–I must always expect the unexpected. Violent behavior is common in many patients who are on drugs.

Ineffective street treatments for drug withdrawal or overdose include ice immersion, placing an ice bag on the groin, intravenous (IV) milk, and IV saline (salt water). These treatments often are used by drug abusers in the hopes of avoiding having to call an ambulance. These findings in the history or physical examination may aid the EMT–I in suspecting drug abuse.

 Describe the care given to patients suspected of alcohol or drug abuse.

Emergency care

To care for patients with drug abuse-related problems, the EMT–I should do the following:

- Maintain the airway and assist breathing as necessary. Monitor these patients carefully for deterioration in their respiratory status.
- Give oxygen by nasal cannula, 3 to 4 L/min, or per local protocols.
- Watch for vomiting. Be prepared to suction.
- Notify law enforcement officials and the Poison Information Center as required by local protocols.
- Consult with the local Poison Information Center or emergency department physician to determine whether syrup of ipecac or activated charcoal should be given to induce vomiting. Many EMS physicians no longer prescribe ipecac in the prehospital setting or hospital. Activated charcoal or gastric lavage (usually in the hospital) are becoming the treatment of choice. Only give ipecac on the advice of the Poison Information Center or medical direction.
- Give 50% dextrose in water if indicated by fingerstick blood sugar results.
- Give naloxone if advised by medical direction or the Poison Information Center.
- Monitor the electrocardiogram.
- Place an IV lifeline.
- Monitor for shock and provide care as appropriate.

- Restrain the patient as necessary to prevent injury to himself or herself or others. Follow local protocols for holding a suicidal patient against his or her will.
- Do not try to be a hero. Get help from the police if necessary.
- Do not be judgmental.

BEHAVIORAL EMERGENCIES

 Define the term *behavioral emergency.*

A **behavioral emergency** is a situation in which the patient feels he or she has, in some way, lost control of his or her life. In some cases, the patient may not be aware of this loss of control. These patients tend to be more severely emotionally compromised and may in fact have serious psychiatric illness. These situations are challenging in all areas of medical practice, especially in the prehospital setting.

There are several potential causes for behavioral emergencies. Often outside influences or forces appear to the patient to be stronger than his or her ability to deal with them. Feeling "overwhelmed," the patient gives in to frustration, and an emergency develops.

Drugs, especially cocaine, can induce behavior problems, either acutely or as a chronic problem. Hallucinogens, such as LSD or PCP, may significantly distort reality, resulting in a behavioral emergency.

True psychiatric disorders, such as schizophrenia (a form of seriously disoriented thinking), also can result in behavioral emergencies. Often persons with chronic disease have acute worsening of their condition, which may be due to a lack of medications, a need for different medications, or a life event such as the death of a relative. In addition to psychiatric problems, several medical conditions can present as behavioral disorders.

Some patients who present with behavioral emergencies evoke strong personal feelings in the EMT–I. Regardless of personal attitudes, the EMT–I must remember that he or she is a professional and should keep thoughts and attitudes to himself or herself. Excellent patient care comes first.

Legal issues

Generally, the EMT–I should act in a calm manner but never jeopardize his or her own safety. Each state, and sometimes each locality, has specific regulations for handling of apparently behaviorally challenged individuals, including patients who exhibit self-destructive behavior. The EMT–I is responsible for following both state laws and local protocols regarding treatment of persons with mental illness, as well as those with temporarily impaired mental status (*eg*, alcohol intoxication, drug overdose). The EMT–I should be aware of local facilities and procedures for psychiatric evaluation and hospitalization, alcohol and drug detoxification, and crisis intervention.

Common prehospital situations
The general approach

 Describe general methods to approach and treat persons with behavioral emergencies.

Although people often experience emotional "ups and downs," a behavioral emergency occurs when the patient is unable to handle the situation emotionally. Often, the patient perceives the situation as threatening or dangerous to his or her well-being.

The reaction to crisis varies from individual to individual. Once someone feels that he or she has "lost control" or has lost his or her support system (eg, spouse, children, job), the world appears to "crash in." Some persons withdraw, whereas some become excessively active. The patient may become depressed or violent. When violent tendencies develop, these may be directed either at the patient, such as in a suicide attempt, or at others.

Management of behavioral emergencies first consists of maintaining scene and personal safety. If the scene is safe, the EMT–I's next task is to build good rapport with the patient. He or she should speak in a calm, even voice and exhibit a willingness to listen to the patient. The EMT–I should be honest because most people can easily detect a snow job! The EMT–I should describe every step that he or she intends to take with the patient. Any sudden moves should be avoided.

To minimize the chances of a violent situation developing in the unrestrained patient, the EMT–I should do the following:

- Have physical assistance nearby in the prehospital setting, such as a partner, additional personnel, or law enforcement.

- Maintain an open exit for the EMT–I and the patient. If there is an open exit for both, the patient will be calmer and the EMT–I will be safer. Do NOT attempt the initial contact with a person who has a behavioral emergency in the back of a closed ambulance compartment.

- Allow the patient to "ventilate" by expressing anger and frustration verbally instead of physically.

- Form an alliance with the patient and try to understand how he or she is feeling. The EMT–I does not have to agree with the patient. For example, if a patient says, "FBI agents are following me," the EMT–I might make a comment like, "That would bother me, how do you feel?"

- Avoid extended eye contact. Looking someone directly in the eye often is taken as a challenge or threat.

If the situation escalates, the EMT–I has two choices: regain control or leave the scene. If the EMT–I is trapped, he or she should try to keep talking to the patient until help arrives. Otherwise, the EMT–I should get away from the patient as quickly as possible and summon assistance.

Although an apparently calm patient sometimes rapidly becomes out of control, the EMT–I should avoid getting into a situation in which a patient may become violent unless the EMT–I is trained and has adequate backup immediately available.

It is impossible to list every single behavior that might be a warning of impending violence. The EMT–I needs to rely on his or her judgment, experience, and "gut feelings." Clues that a patient may develop violent behavior include:

Pacing back and forth; unable to keep one position for more than a couple of seconds—The EMT–I may ask the patient, once, to be seated. If this fails, and the EMT–I is uncomfortable, he or she should leave the scene.

Appearing to get more and more angry as the patient speaks—This behavior simply may go along with the patient venting to the EMT–I. If there is excessive body language, such as swinging arms, the EMT–I must make a choice. He or she may try and talk with the patient, stating, "I know you're upset, but you need to let yourself calm down just a bit." If talking to the patient does not work, or if the EMT–I feels uncomfortable, he or she should leave the scene.

Starting to act out, such as thrashing out with the arms, hitting a wall, throwing things—In this situation, the EMT–I may be the next target. There is no room for negotiation here; the EMT–I should get away from the patient as soon as possible. If the EMT–I notices any obvious weapons (eg, knives, guns, baseball bats), he or she should leave the scene immediately.

Bragging about how tough the patient is—The easiest way to deal with this sort of behavior is to agree with the patient, "I'm on your side, I'm not going to hurt you." If the patient begins implying that the EMT–I would make an easy target, "I could whip your butt with one hand," he or she can either agree with the patient ("I'm sure you could") and continue the interview, or leave the scene.

Any domestic violence-related situation, particularly in which the alleged perpetrator is still present—In this situation, the EMT–I should separate the involved parties as soon as possible, employing law enforcement assistance if necessary. It is unwise to enter a scene involving domestic violence without appropriate law enforcement backup on-scene and available.

Any patient suspected of being intoxicated or on drugs—The potential for violence varies from person to person, but the mere presence of substance abuse makes violent behavior more likely to occur.

The patient persistently complains about the EMS system, or the service he or she and the family has received in the past—Statistically speaking, unhappy patients are more likely to become violent, whether they are in the midst of a behavioral emergency or not.

Men are more likely than women to exhibit violent behavior—The EMT–I should not let his or her guard down, however, if dealing with a female patient. Similarly, he or she should not be fooled by a patient's age because persons of all ages can become violent.

Neurosis and psychosis

 NEUROSIS: An anxious reaction to a perceived fear.
PSYCHOSIS: A mental condition, whereby the patient has lost his or her sense of reality.

 Differentiate between neurosis and psychosis.

Neurosis is an abnormal anxiety reaction to a perceived fear. There is no basis in reality for that fear (*eg*, a fear of heights so strong that it prevents a person from going any higher than the first floor of any building). To some degree, just about everyone has some type of neurotic fear at one time or another and this fear does NOT mean that a person is mentally ill. Most people are able to cope with their fears. Again, a behavioral emergency only occurs when a person is UNABLE to cope. **Psychosis,** on the other hand, exists when the patient has no concept whatsoever of reality. The person truly believes his or her situation or condition is real. A person suffering from psychosis also often may hear voices.

In drug-induced psychosis, hallucinogens or stimulant agents cause the patient to lose touch with reality. Often, he or she develops hyperactive and often dangerous behavior. The best way to deal with hallucinations is the "talk-down" technique, which involves gently calming and reassuring the patient that everything is OK.

Depression

 Describe three signs of depression.

Depression is a common reaction to major life stresses. Several signs and symptoms may suggest that a person is depressed:

- An unkempt appearance—As though the patient doesn't care about anything.
- Speech that is different from usual—These persons may not speak or may reply in short, monotone phrases. They lack any spark or enthusiasm in their speech and actions.
- Frequent crying bouts—Often these appear to have no precipitant.
- Abnormally increased or decreased appetite—Significant weight gain or loss is common.
- Sleep disturbances—Often depressed persons fall asleep without a problem, only to wake within a

couple of hours. They are then unable to fall asleep again the rest of the night.

Depression may present as another disease. Elderly persons commonly appear to have organic illness (*eg*, cardiac or respiratory conditions) when, in reality, they are severely depressed.

The EMT–I's primary responsibility is to provide a safe and caring environment for these patients. The EMT–I should respect their feelings and communicate to them that he or she cares. Depending on community resources and local protocols, the EMT–I may be able to arrange for a mental health specialist or social worker to evaluate the patient. Otherwise, the EMT–I should transport the patient to the nearest appropriate facility for assistance.

Suicidal patients

Suicide is the intentional taking of one's own life. It is a significant cause of death in the United States, especially among young men (ages 15 to 35 years) and in the elderly (both sexes).

A suicide gesture is something done by a person that is intended to ask for help, rather than to take the person's life. The person performs the deed in a potentially reversible way, such as taking a few aspirin or a small handful of pills. Unfortunately, small amounts of certain medications can be very poisonous. The EMT–I should treat persons with suicidal gestures as poisoning patients and pay careful attention to the behavioral emergency. Sometimes, people intend to kill themselves, take pills, and then change their minds.

A suicide attempt occurs when the patient has a true desire to die. Often the person has planned the event; he or she may have purchased a gun, or driven far out of town, or gotten a double refill of his or her prescription medication.

Whether an action is an actual suicide attempt or a gesture, the EMT–I should not discount the patient's emotional state in any way. The EMT–I should not be afraid to directly ask the patient: "Were you trying to kill yourself," or "Did you want to die?" Many persons are not aware of what resources are available to them for help, but they know that people at the hospital do know. A suicide gesture is the patient's way of seeking help.

The following factors increase the risk that a person is suicidal:

- Male sex
- Age less than 19 or greater than 45 years
- Depression or feeling of hopelessness
- Previous suicide attempts or psychiatric care
- Excessive alcohol or drug use
- Loss of rational thinking
- A patient who is separated, widowed, or divorced
- An organized or well-thought-out attempt (*eg*, use of a firearm, a "life-threatening" presentation, leaving a suicide note)

- No good support system (eg, family, friends, job, religious affiliation)
- Stated intent to try again in the future to commit suicide
- A major life event (eg, recent divorce, buying a house, recent loss of job, death of spouse or other loved ones).

Many states require that a person who has threatened or attempted suicide be evaluated by a mental health professional. The EMT–I should follow local laws and protocols regarding transporting persons who do not wish to go to the hospital. Otherwise, the EMT–I should transport the patient to the hospital and provide as gentle and nonthreatening an environment as possible. The EMT–I should not make any judgmental comments, pro or con, regarding what the patient did, regardless of his or her own personal feelings. Professionalism is paramount, and the patient should always come first.

CASE HISTORY FOLLOW-UP

EMT–I Keegan sees that the bottles had contained 20 barbiturate and 30 acetaminophen tablets. "Do you know how many pills were left in these bottles?" she asks the patient's mother. "It will help us determine how many she may have taken."

"I had about five of the Seconal left. The bottle of Tylenol was nearly new. Only two or three pills would have been missing," her mother says.

"Do you know when she took them?" she asks.

"No. I got home from work about 5:00 and started dinner. She usually gets home around 3:45; but I found out from a neighbor that she hadn't gone to school today. She could have taken them any time."

EMT–I Bravo says, "Her pulse is 136 and strong, respirations are 32, and her blood pressure is 136/84. She's responding to a sternal rub with groaning and withdrawing from pain."

EMT–I Keegan calls medical direction for physician's orders and is instructed to "transport only."

It looks as though the patient has a good chance to recover. When EMT–I Keegan checks with the hospital 3 days later, however, they tell her that the patient had died the day before. She asks her service medical director about the case at the next continuing education program. "Why wouldn't she have made it if her vital signs weren't that bad?" she asks.

The medical director answers, "Well, acetaminophen is one of the safest drugs on the market, if it's used appropriately. However, taken with alcohol, or other drugs that affect the liver, or even in moderate overdoses, the effects can be lethal, as you saw here. Also, the effects of the poisoning are insidious. That is, they don't appear to be too bad, at first; but once the liver damage is done, the patient is doomed. Patients often appear to improve for a few days, and will look like they're out of the woods, for a while. We treated her aggressively here. We evacuated her stomach with a gastric lavage and administered mucomyst, an antidote, as well as mazicon. Her death was a tragedy."

SUMMARY

Alcohol abuse includes the medical, behavioral, or social problems related to alcohol consumption. Patients who are intoxicated exhibit inappropriate behavior and abnormal coordination. Severe intoxication may lead to hypotension, respiratory depression, seizures, and coma. The EMT–I should always be alert to life-threatening conditions that can mimic alcohol intoxication. Severely intoxicated persons should be transported to the hospital for evaluation and observation.

Abrupt cessation of alcohol can cause withdrawal symptoms including the shakes, seizures, or delirium tremens. Alcohol reactions to the drug Antabuse can be life threatening. These patients should be transported to the hospital as soon as possible.

Drug abuse is a common problem. There are five categories of drugs of abuse: stimulants, depressants, hallucinogens, narcotics, and volatile chemicals. The history in any drug abuse patient is usually unreliable. The EMT–I should attempt to determine whether the patient has tried to commit suicide. The EMT–I should also be certain to get assistance from law enforcement personnel, according to local protocols.

The airway should be watched carefully in any patient who has ingested drugs. These patients tend to develop respiratory depression quickly.

Behavioral emergencies involve situations in which the patient feels that he or she has, in some way, lost control of his or her life. The patient may or may not be violent. In many instances, medical problems or substance abuse may contribute to the patient's behavior. The EMT–I MUST be aware of local procedures for dealing with patients who have acute behavioral problems.

The cardinal principle in dealing with a behavioral emergency is to try to build good rapport with the patient. The EMT–I should always try to allow himself or herself an exit if the situation escalates. The EMT–I should never place himself or herself in a potentially violent situation without appropriate backup.

A

Abandonment: A form of negligence that occurs when the relationship between the EMT–I and the patient is terminated by the EMT–I without ensuring continuity of care for the patient.

Abbreviation: A shorter way of writing something.

Abruptio placenta: The premature detachment of the placenta.

Absorption: Substances passing into tissues, taking one substance into another.

Acid: A substance that increases the hydrogen ion concentration of water; a substance with a pH less than 7.0.

Active transport: The movement of a solute across a membrane from an area of lower concentration to an area of higher concentration.

Acute pulmonary edema: A quick excessive back-up of fluid in the lungs.

Adrenaline or epinephrine: A drug that stimulates the adrenal glands and narrows the blood vessels.

Adult respiratory distress syndrome (ARDS): Pulmonary insufficiency that occurs due to a number of bodily insults. Pathological findings include alveolar and interstitial edema due to leaking capillaries.

Adverse reactions: Undesirable side effects of a drug.

AEIOU-TIPS: A mnemonic for causes of coma: Acidosis-Alcohol, Epilepsy, Infection, Overdose, Uremia, Trauma, Insulin, Psychosis, Shock-Stroke.

Aerobic metabolism: Metabolism that occurs with oxygen.

Aerosol: A gas under pressure that contains a drug which is breathed in.

Afterload: The pressure the ventricular muscles must generate to overcome the higher pressure in the aorta.

Alcohol abuse: Excessive alcohol consumption that leads to medical, behavioral, or social changes in an individual.

Alcohol withdrawal syndrome: Physical reactions a person experiences when he or she abruptly stops consuming alcohol.

Alcoholism: A dependence on alcohol.

Ambient: Environmental or room air.

American Hospital Formulary Service: A source of drug information that contains concise information that is arranged according to drug classifications.

Amniotic sac: Protective membranous sac that insulates and protects the fetus during pregnancy.

Ampule: A glass container containing a drug; the bottle must be broken at the neck to retrieve the medication.

Anaerobic metabolism: Metabolism without oxygen.

Anaphylactic reaction: A severe allergic response to a foreign substance that the patient has had contact with before.

Anaphylaxis: Allergic reaction.

Anatomic figure: Diagram of a human body, with anterior and posterior views. Part of some run reports, it is used to mark and label patient's injuries or physical findings.

Anatomy: The study of structures and organs of the body.

B

Baroreceptors: Sensory nerve endings that adjust blood pressure as a result of vasodilation or vasoconstriction.

Base: A substance that decreases the concentration of hydrogen ions; a substance with a pH greater than 7.0.

Battery: Criminal offense of attempting to inflict bodily injury upon another.

Battle's sign: Ecchymosis or bruising behind the ears present with a basilar skull fracture; may be a late sign.

Behavioral emergency: A situation in which the patient feels he or she has, in some way, lost control of his or her life.

Biotelemetry: The process of transmitting physiologic data, such as an ECG, over distance, usually by radio.

Body substance isolation precautions: The use of protective equipment to minimize the chances of the EMT–I being exposed to contagious diseases.

Breath sounds: Sound of air passing in and out of the respiratory passageways as heard with a stethoscope.

Breech presentation: In childbirth, a delivery in which the baby's buttocks or feet present before the head.

Bronchiolitis: An infection of the lower respiratory tract, which is most often caused by a virus.

Bronchospasm: The tiny muscles layers surrounding the bronchioles spasm and narrow the lumen of the airways.

Broselow tape: A reference guide containing pediatric resuscitation information.

Bundle of His: Part of the cardiac conduction system in the ventricles.

Cardiac conduction system: The pathway through which electrical impulses travel in the heart.

Cardiac dysrhythmia: A disorder of cardiac rhythm.

Cardiac tamponade: The pericardial sac rapidly fills with fluid, such as blood, the heart is no longer able to adequately fill and the signs and symptoms of shock result.

Cardiogenic shock: Cardiac failure whereby the heart cannot sufficiently pump blood to the rest of the circulatory system.

Carina: Point at which the trachea divides (bifurcates, or separates into two sections) into the right and left mainstem bronchi.

Cartilage: Connective tissue found primarily in the joints that allows for movement.

Cation: An ion with a positive charge.

Caudal: Near the lower end of the torso.

Central nervous system: The portion of the nervous system comprised of the brain and the spinal cord.

Cerebrovascular accident (CVA): A stroke, is a condition that results from a disruption of circulation to the brain, causing ischemia and damage to brain tissue.

Cerebrospinal fluid: Clear fluid surrounding the brain and spinal cord that acts as a cushion.

Certification: Action by which an agency or association grants recognition to an individual who has met its qualifications.

Cervix: The interior, narrow portion of the uterus that opens into the vagina.

Chemical name: Drug name that gives the exact description of the chemical structure of the drug.

Cheyne-Stokes respirations: An abnormal pattern of breathing. There are periods of breathlessness and deep, fast breathing.

Chief complaint: Brief statement describing the reason for the patient's seeking medical attention.

Chronic obstructive pulmonary disease (COPD): A respiratory disease that causes decreased inspiratory and expiratory function.

Circulatory system: The body system composed of the heart, blood, and blood vessels that is responsible for the circulation of blood.

Coma: A state of unresponsiveness characterized by the absence of spontaneous eye movements and response to painful stimuli and vocalization.

Combining form: A word root followed by a vowel.
Examples of combining forms and combining vowels:
cardi + o + logy = cardiology (study of the heart)
neur + o + logy = neurology (study of the nervous system) (see Table 6-5)

Combining vowel: A vowel that is added to a root before a suffix.

Compendium of Drug Therapy: A source of drug information distributed to practicing physicians.

Congestive heart failure (CHF): An inability of the heart to pump blood caused by heart muscle damage.

Connective tissue: Binds other types of tissue together.

Consent: Agreement or approval.

Contractility: The extent and velocity (quickness) of muscle fiber shortening.

Contraindications: Conditions or instances for which a drug should not be used.

Controlled Substances Act: An act passed in 1970 that regulates the manufacture and distribution of drugs whose use may result in dependency.

Contusion: Bruising below the dermis caused by blunt trauma.

Costovertebral angle: Angle formed where the lowest rib meets the spinal column.

Cranial: In or near the head.

Cricoid cartilage: The narrowest part of the child's upper airway.

Cricothyroid membrane: Membrane situated between the cricoid and thyroid cartilages of the larynx.

Croup: A respiratory illness that occurs in children between 3 months and 3 years of age; also called laryngotracheobronchitis.

Cumulative effect: Increasing by steps with an eventual total that may go past the expected result.

Cushing reflex: When increased intracranial pressure causes a slowing pulse rate, deep or erratic respirations, and increasing blood pressure.

Cyanosis: Bluish color to the skin, associated with hypoxia.

D **Decerebrate posturing:** The patient presents with stiff and extended extremities and retracted head.

Decoder: A device that block out radio traffic that is not directed at the specific base station.

Decorticate posturing: The patient presents with arms flexed, fists clenched, and legs extended.

Dedicated land lines: Telephone lines with continuous direct connection from one geographical location to another.

Defibrillation: An electrical shock delivered to the heart in order to restore an effective rhythm.

Definitive care: In-hospital care that resolves the patient's illness or injury after a definitive diagnosis has been established.

Delirium tremens: A severe state of alcohol withdrawal consisting of delirium, hallucinations, and nervous system hyperactivity.

Demographic information: Includes patient's name, address, age, phone number, parent's name if patient a minor.

Depressants: Depress the central nervous system.

Detailed assessment: A continuation of the patient assessment process in which in-depth information is obtained concerning the patient and his or her condition.

Diabetes mellitus: A disease whereby an insufficient amount of insulin is produced to regulate blood sugar levels in the body.

Diabetic ketoacidosis: A metabolic condition consisting of hyperglycemia, dehydration, and the accumulation of abnormal compounds, called ketones and ketoacids, in the body; also called diabetic coma.

Diaphoresis: Profuse sweating.

Diaphragm: A wide muscular partition separating the thoracic, or chest, cavity from the abnormal cavity. It is attached to the lumbar vertebrae, the lower ribs, and the sternum or breastbone. It slants upward, higher in front than in the rear, and is dome-shaped when relaxed. Three major openings in the diaphragm allow passage of the esophagus, the aorta, the veins, the nerves, and the lymphatic and thoracic ducts.

Diastole: The relaxation of the heart.

Diffusion: A passive process of molecules moving from an area of higher concentration to an area of lesser concentration.

Digitally: Intubation using the fingers.

Distal: Farthest from that point.

Distribution: Moves the drug from the bloodstream into the tissues and fluids of the body.

Disulfiram: A drug that causes violent reactions in the body if the patient ingests even the smallest amount of alcohol; also called Antabuse.

Do Not Resuscitate order (DNR): A physician's order indicating that a patient is not to be resuscitated in the event of a cardiac arrest.

Documentation: Process used to record patient information.

Dorsum: Back of.

Drowning: Death within 24 hours after a submersion accident.

Drug: A substance taken into the body to affect change to one or more body functions, often to prevent or treat a disease or condition.

Drug action: The cellular change produced by a drug.

Drug allergy: Allergy to a drug shown by reactions ranging from a mild rash to severe allergic reaction and shock.

Drug effect: Degree of a drug's physiologic change.

Drug Enforcement Agency (DEA): Established in 1970, deals with controlled substances only and enforces laws against manufacture, sale, and use of illegal drugs.

Drug tolerance: When the body becomes accustomed to a particular drug over a period of time.

Drug toxicity: Results from overdosage, ingestion of a drug intended for external use, or buildup of the drug in the blood due to impaired metabolism or excretion.

Duty to Act: The EMT–I has an obligation to provide care.

Dyspnea: Shortness of breath or difficulty in breathing.

Dysrhythmias: Disturbances in the normal rhythm of the heart.

Eclampsia: A condition whereby a pregnant female experiences seizures in addition to preeclampsia; usually occurs during the third trimester of pregnancy.

Ectopic pregnancy: The implantation of a fertilized egg outside of the uterus; usually occurs in the fallopian tube.

Electrocardiogram: A record of the electrical activity within the heart.

Electrolytes: Salts that when dissolved in a solvent break up into ions that are capable of conducting an electrical current.

Elixir: Drug dissolved in alcohol with flavoring added.

Emergency Medical Dispatcher (EMD): A specially trained person who receives calls for emergency assistance and ensures proper EMS response.

Emergency Medical Services (EMS) System: An organized approach to providing emergency care to the sick and injured.

Emergency Medical Technician (EMT): A person trained according to criteria established by the Department of Transportation in the care of the acutely sick or injured person.

Emphysema: A form of COPD. Lung tissue damage with loss of elastic recoil of the lungs.

EMS system: An organized approach to providing emergency care to the sick and injured.

EMT–Basic: The primary level of EMT–Basic training; requires completion of a minimum 110 hour EMT–B training program meeting Department of Transportation (DOT) standards.

EMT–Intermediate: EMT who has completed training beyond the EMT–B level; the degree of training and skills practiced varies widely between states and EMS systems.

EMT-Paramedic: EMT who has advanced training in patient assessment, medical emergencies, pharmacology, trauma, obstetrics, rescue, behavioral emergencies, and other EMS activities.

Emulsion: Drug combined with water and oil. Must be thoroughly shaken to disperse the medication evenly.

Encoder: A device that blocks out radio traffic that is not directed at the specific base station.

Endocrine system: The body system comprised of ductless glands that are responsible for hormone production.

Endotracheal: Within or through the trachea.

Endotracheal intubation: The insertion of an open-ended tube into the trachea.

Enhanced 9-1-1: Emergency phone number that includes a visual system that displays the caller's phone number and address.

Enteric-coated tablet: A compressed dry form of a drug coated to withstand the stomach acidity and dissolve in the intestines.

Epiglottitis: An inflammation of the epiglottis, which most often occurs in children from 3 to 7 years of age.

Epinephrine: A drug that stimulates the adrenal glands and narrows the blood vessels; also called adrenalin.

Erythrocytes: Red blood cells.

Ethics: The discipline dealing with what is good and bad.

Eupnea: Normal inhalation and exhalation.

Excretion: The elimination of waste products from the body.

Expressed consent: Given when the patient provides verbal or written consent for the EMT–I to examine, care for, and transport the patient to an appropriate medical facility.

Extracellular fluid: Fluid found outside of the cell membranes.

Facilitated diffusion: Transports molecules of a substance across a cell membrane that would otherwise be impermeable to the substance.

FACTS: A mnemonic for historical information that should be obtained about a seizure patient.

Fallopian tubes: A pair of muscular tubes that extend from the uterus into the pelvic cavity.

False imprisonment: Intentional and unjustifiable detention of a person against his will.

Federal Communications Commission (FCC): The federal agency established to control and regulate all radio communications in the United States.

Federal Food, Drug, and Cosmetic Act: Required that the safety of a drug must be proven before it could be distributed to the public.

Federal Trade Commission: Regulates drug advertising.

Fetus: An unborn child.

Fibrosis: Abnormal formation of scar tissue in the connective tissue framework of the lungs following inflammation or pneumonia and in pulmonary tuberculosis.

Fick principle: For oxygen to be delivered to the body's cells, four components must be in place:
1) Inspiration of adequate oxygen in the atmospheric air.
2) On-loading of oxygen to the red blood cells at the lungs.
3) Delivery of the red blood cells to the tissue cells.
4) Off-loading of oxygen from the red blood cells to the tissue cells.

Fight or flight: A sympathetic stimulation to prepare the body when in a dangerous situation.

FIO₂: Percentage of oxygen in inspired air.

First responder: Trained person who provides initial care until other EMS providers arrive on the scene.

Flexion: The act of bending or being bent.

Fluid extract: An alcohol solution of a drug from a vegetable source. The most concentrated of all fluid preparations.

Focused history and physical examination: An in-depth examination to determine the severity and cause of the patient's condition. It includes both a hand's-on examination and a gathering of the patient's history.

Fontanelles: Soft spots on the top of an infant's head.

Food and Drug Administration: Established to review drug applications and petitions for food additives; inspect factories where drugs, cosmetics, and foods are made; and to remove unsafe drugs from the market

Frontal: Vertical line dividing the body into a front and back portion.

Frostbite: The formation of ice crystals within the tissues.

Gag reflex: Retching or striving to vomit; it is a normal reflex triggered by touching of the soft palate or the throat.

Gastrointestinal bleeding: Refers to hemorrhage anywhere in the gastrointestinal (GI) tract.

Gastrointestinal system: The body system responsible for digestion.

Generic name: The nonproprietary designation of a drug.

Glasgow Coma Scale: A numerical scale used for neurologic assessment in a critical patient.

Glottis: The slitlike opening between the vocal cords.

Good Samaritan Laws: Laws that may provide immunity from prosecution or civil suit for people who render care at the scene of an emergency.

Grand mal seizure: Generalized major motor seizure.

Gross negligence: The willful and reckless giving of care that causes injury to the patient.

Half life: Time required by the body, tissue, or organ to metabolize or inactivate half the substance taken in.

Hallucinogens: Induce a sense of euphoria and hallucinations.

Harrison Narcotic Act of 1914: The first federal legislation designed to stop drug addiction or dependence.

HBV: Abbreviation for hepatitis B virus.

Heat cramps: Cramps or pains in the muscles which occur due to heat exposure.

Heat exhaustion: More severe loss of fluid and salt than occurs in heat cramps, usually following exertion in a hot, humid environment.

Heat stroke: A failure of the body's temperature regulation mechanisms; also called sun stroke.

Hematocrit: The volume percentage of red blood cells in whole blood.

Hematoma: Swelling caused by leaking blood vessels below the dermis.

Hemiplegia: A condition in which one side of the body is paralyzed.

Hemoglobin: A protein that bonds oxygen to red blood cells.

Hepatitis B virus (HBV): A virus that causes an inflammation of the liver.

Histamine: Released into the body during anaphylactic shock; may cause airway compromise and vasodilation.

History of present illness/injury: Events or complaints associated with the patient's complaint.

HIV: Abbreviation for human immunodeficiency virus.

Hypercarbia: Excessive partial pressure of carbon dioxide in the blood.

Hyperglycemia: The elevation of the blood sugar level above normal.

Hypersensitivity: Allergy to a drug shown by reactions ranging from a mild rash to severe allergic reaction and shock; also called drug allergy.

Hypertensive: The condition of having high blood pressure.

Hypertensive crisis: A sudden increase in blood pressure that leads to problems with in the nervous system, the kidneys, or the heart.

Hypertonic solution: A solution that has an osmotic pressure greater than that of normal body fluid.

Hyperventilation: A respiratory rate greater than the required for normal body function.

Hypoglycemia: An abnormally low blood sugar level.

Hypoperfusion: Fluid passing through an organ or part of the body that does not have properly oxygenated blood.

Hypoperfusion syndrome: Shock.

Hypotensive: The condition of having low blood pressure.

Hypotonic solution: A solution that has an osmotic pressure less than that of normal body fluid.

Hypoventilation: A reduced rate or depth of breathing, often resulting in an abnormal rise of carbon dioxide.

Hypovolemic shock: A form of shock caused by the loss of blood or fluid volume from the body.

Hypoxemia: Insufficient oxygenation of the blood.

Hypoxia: Reduced oxygen supply to the cells.

Idiosyncratic reactions: An abnormal or unexpected reaction to a drug peculiar to a certain patient. This is not technically an allergy.

Immune system: The body system that protects the body from foreign materials.

Implied consent: The EMT–I assumes that a patient who is severely ill or injured would want care if he or she were able to respond.

Indications: Disease states or instances for which a drug is prescribed.

Inferior: Below or lower, on the body.

Informed consent: The patient consents to care only after receiving all the information necessary to understand his or her condition, the risks and benefits of care, and the risks and benefits of refusal of care.

Inhalation: Administration of drugs, water vapors, or gases by inspiration of the substance(s) into the lungs.

Initial assessment: A quick evaluation of the patient to determine immediate life-threatening emergencies.

Integumentary system: The body system comprised of the skin and its appendixes.

Interstitial fluid: Fluid found outside of the blood vessels in the spaces between the body's cells.

Intracellular fluid: Found within individual cells.

Intracranial pressure: Pressure within the skull.

Intramuscular: Small quantities of a drug are injected into a muscle.

Intraosseous: Within or into a bone.

Intraosseous infusion: Infusion of IV fluids into the marrow cavity of the bone.

Intrapulmonary shunting: The circulation of blood to non-ventilated alveoli. This results in the blood having the same oxygen content as systemic venous blood.

Intravascular fluid: Fluid found within the vascular system; comprises the fluid portion of blood; plasma.

Intravenous: A sterile solution or drug that is injected into the body by venipuncture.

Intravenous cannulation: The placement of a catheter into a vein.

Intubation: Passing a tube into an opening of the body.

Ipsilateral: On the same side of the body.

Ischemia: A lack of oxygen to an organ.

Isotonic solution: A solution that has the same osmotic pressure as bodily fluids.

Joints: Occur where two or more bones meet or articulate.

Kinematics: The process of predicting injury patterns that may result from the forces and motions of energy.

Kussmaul: Rapid and deep respirations usually found in patients with diabetes or others with imbalances of the acid content in their bodies.

Kyphoscoliosis: Lateral curvature of the spine, can interfere with normal breathing.

Large-bore catheter: Catheter with a large interior diameter (14-16 gauge).

Lateral: To the side.

Leukocytes: White blood cells.

Libel: The injury of a person's character, name, or reputation by false and malicious writings.

Licensure: Process by which a governmental agency grants permission to an individual to engage in a given occupation upon finding that the applicant has attained the minimal degree of competency necessary.

Lidocaine: An antidysrhythmic drug.

Liniment: An oily liquid used on the skin.

Local effect: Limited to the area where it is administered.

Lymphatic system: The body system comprised of capillaries, thin vessels, valves, ducts, nodes, and organs that allows for the transport of lymph through the body.

Mandible: The large bone forming the lower jaw.

Mast cell: A specialized type of white blood cell.

Maxilla: One of a pair of large bones that form the upper jaw.

Medial: A plane that passes near the midline of the body.

Medical control: Supervision and management of an EMS system and the field performance of EMTs.

Medical direction: Medical supervision of an EMS system and the field performance of EMTs.

Meningitis: An inflammation of the membranes that surround the brain and spinal cord.

Menstrual cycle: Each month the uterus is stimulated by hormones to develop a thickened inner lining or endometrium. If an egg is fertilized it is implanted in the uterus and nourished by this lining and pregnancy begins. If no egg is fertilized, the uterus sheds the lining, which is composed of cells and blood.

Metabolic acidosis: A condition in which the level of bicarbonate is low in relation to the levels of carbonic acid.

Metabolic alkalosis: A condition in which the level of bicarbonate is high in relation to the level of carbonic acid.

Metabolism: The sum of all chemical processes that take place in the body as they relate to the movement of nutrients in the blood after digestion, resulting in growth, energy, release of wastes, and other body functions.

Metric system: A decimal system of weights and measures based on the meter and the kilogram.

Midsagittal: A vertical line dividing the body into right and left halves.

Milliequivalent: The concentration of electrolytes in a certain volume of solution based on the number of available ionic charges.

Minute volume: The tidal volume multiplied by the respiratory rate.

Miscarriage: A sudden and unexpected loss of pregnancy; also called spontaneous abortion.

Mucous membrane: A thin layer of connective tissue lining many of the body cavities that air passes through, usually contains small, mucus-secreting glands. Mucus is a thick, slippery secretion that functions as a lubricant and protects various surfaces.

Multi-system trauma: Serious injury occurs to two or more major systems of the body; a rapid, accurate initial assessment is needed to recognize and treat hypoxia and shock.

Muscular system: The body system composed of contractile tissue that allows for movement.

Myocardial infarction (MI): The death of heart muscle caused by a lack of oxygen.

Narcotic Act: Passed in 1956 and amended the Harrison Act, and increased the penalties for the laws's violation. This act also made the possession of heroin and marijuana illegal.

Narcotics: A substance that dulls senses and relieves pain in moderate doses.

Narrative: Portion of the run report that is written out longhand.

Nasal septum: In the nose, the wall dividing the nostrils. It is made up of bone and cartilage covered by mucous membrane.

Near drowning: The patient survives at least 24 hours after a submersion accident, although death may eventually occur.

Neck vein distention: A bulging outward of the veins in the neck.

Needle: Sharp stainless steel hollow tube that is used to penetrate the skin and blood vessel.

Negligence: Professional conduct which falls below the standard of care; also called medical liability.

Nervous system: The body system that controls the body's functions.

Neurogenic shock: A form of shock in which the nervous system is no longer able to control the diameter of the blood vessels.

Neurosis: An anxious reaction to a perceived fear.

Nitroglycerin: A tablet or spray commonly prescribed to cardiac patients; acts to dilate blood vessels to increase oxygen flow to the myocardium.

Normotension: The condition of having normal blood pressure.

Occiput: The back portion of the head.

Official name: The drug name that is listed in one of the official publications.

OPQRST: Acronym for assessing the complaint, signs, and symptoms of a patient (Onset, Provocation, Quality, Radiation, Severity, Time).

Ordinary negligence: Acts or omissions that occur in the attempt to deliver proper care.

Orotracheal: Through the mouth.

Orthostatic hypotension: A condition in which a patient's blood pressure suddenly drops upon standing up.

Oscilloscope: Television-like screen that displays an electrical current, such as the impulse that travels through the heart's conduction system.

Osmosis: The movement of water across a semipermeable membrane.

Ovaries: A walnut-sized pair of glands located on each side of the uterus in the upper pelvic cavity.

Oxygenation: The process of combining or treating with oxygen.

Palpitation: A sensation of pounding or racing of the heart.

Paraplegia: A condition in which the lower extremities become paralyzed.

Parasympathetic division: Part of the nervous system that originates in the brain and sends messages to affect organs by the cranial nerves. It affects the heart, stomach, and gastrointestinal tract; also called the cholinergic division.

Parasympathetic nervous system: Division of the autonomic nervous system responsible for slowing the heart rate, intestinal activity, respiratory rate, and pupillary responses.

Parenteral drugs: Drugs that are received by the body by other means then the digestive tract.

Paresthesia: A condition in which the patient complains of tingling or numbness in the arms or legs.

Past medical history: Significant past medical illnesses or traumatic injury that the patient has experienced.

Patent: Wide open.

Patent airway: An open, unblocked airway.

PCO$_2$: Abbreviation for partial pressure of carbon dioxide.

Perfusion: The process by which oxygenated blood is delivered to the body's tissue and wastes are removed from the tissue.

Perineum: The external female genital region between the urinary opening (urethra) and the anus or rectal opening.

Peripheral nervous system: The portion of the nervous system comprised of cranial nerves, the spinal nerves, and the autonomic nervous system.

Permeability: The degree to which a substance is allowed to pass through a cell membrane.

Pertinent negative: The absence of a sign or symptom or lack of a response to treatment that helps substantiate or identify a patient's condition. A patient experiencing angina often responds to the administration of nitroglycerin with a cessation of chest pain; the failure of nitroglycerin to relieve chest pain leads the EMT–I to suspect that the patient's chest pain is due to some other condition.

Pertinent positive: The presence of a sign or symptom or response to treatment that helps substantiate or identify a patient's condition. A patient suspected of having a heart attack typically experiences chest pain and accompanying symptoms such as shortness of breath and nausea. The presence of these symptoms helps support that the patient may be having a heart attack.

pH: Potential of hydrogen and is measurement of hydrogen ion concentration.

Pharmacokinetics: The movement of the drugs through the body; including absorption, distribution, metabolism, and excretion.

Pharmacology: The study of drugs and their effects and actions on the body.

Phonation: Process of generating sounds or speech with the vocal cords.

Physicians' Desk Reference (PDR): Widely used reference for drug information.

Physiology: The study of the functions and processes undertaken by the body.

Placenta: A disk-shaped spongy organ that develops in the uterus during pregnancy. The placenta exchanges oxygen and nourishment from the mother to baby and transfers waste products from the baby to the mother's bloodstream via blood vessels in the umbilical cord.

Placenta previa: An abnormal positioning of the placenta in the uterus.

Plasma: The fluid or water portion of the blood.

Platelets: Formed elements suspended in plasma that are essential to blood clotting.

Pneumatic antishock garment (PASG): An inflatable garment sometimes used on patients with severely low blood pressure.

Pneumonia: Inflammation of the lungs, commonly caused by bacteria.

PO$_2$: Abbreviation for partial pressure of oxygen.

Posterior: Toward the back of the body.

Postictal state: A period following a seizure lasting approximately 30 minutes, whereby the suffer gradually returns to a normal state.

Potentiation: One drug prolongs or multiplies the effect of another drug.

Pre-arrival instructions: Instructions for initial care of the patient, often provided by the emergency medical dispatcher, to a person who calls for EMS assistance.

Preeclampsia: During pregnancy, hypertension and excess fluid retention.

Prefilled syringe: A syringe and drug solution packaged together, to be used to deliver a single dose.

Prefix: A sequence of letters that comes before the word root and often describes a variation of the norm.

Preload: The passive stretching force exerted on the ventricular muscle at the end of diastole.

Pressure of gases: To understand how oxygen and carbon dioxide are carried in the blood, it is helpful to understand about partial pressures of gases. Usually, gases are found as mixtures of several gases together, like the air we breathe. Dalton's law of partial pressure states that the pressure exerted by a mixture of gases is equal to the sum of the partial pressures of each, and each gas acts as if it were present alone. The symbol used to designate partial pressure is the capital P preceding the chemical symbol for the gas. Some references still use the older symbol, a capital P and small a (Pa) to denote partial pressure. In air, the pressure of 760 mm Hg is the sum of the partial pressures of oxygen, nitrogen, carbon dioxide, water vapor, and trace gases. The partial pressure of each gas is directly related to its concentration in the total mixture. Atmospheric air contains 21% oxygen, 0.03% carbon dioxide, 78% nitrogen and 0.97% other gases. The partial pressure of each is determined by multiplying its percentage by the sum (760 mm Hg). Atmospheric PO_2 = 21% × 760 = 159.6 mm Hg (rounded off to 160 mm Hg).

Professional: A person who has certain special skills and knowledge in a specific area and conforms to the standards of conduct and performance in that area. The EMT–I does not need to be paid in order to be a professional.

Prolapsed cord: During childbirth, a delivery in which the umbilical cord presents during delivery.

Protocols: A set of written policies and procedures. Written instructions listing guidelines for the care of patients with specific conditions, illnesses, or injuries.

Proximal: Nearest the origin of a structure.

Psychogenic shock: Simple fainting. The blood vessels dilate, allowing blood to pool.

Psychosis: A mental condition, whereby the patient has lost his or her sense of reality.

Public Health Service: Inspects and licenses establishments that manufacture drugs.

Pulmonary edema: An excessive backup of fluids in the lungs.

Pulmonary embolism: The blockage of a pulmonary artery by foreign matter.

Pulse oximeter: A device used to determine the percent of hemoglobin bound to oxygen in the blood.

Pulse pressure: Obtained by subtracting the diastolic pressure from the systolic pressure.

Pulseless electrical activity (PEA): A condition where there is a rhythm noted on the monitor that should result in adequate perfusion, but the patient is pulseless and apneic.

Pupillary reactivity: The reactivity of a patient's pupils to light.

Pure Food and Drug Act: Enacted in 1906; prohibits the manufacture and trafficking of mislabeled, poisonous, or harmful food and drugs.

Q

Quadriplegia: A condition in which all four extremities become paralyzed.

Quality improvement: An evaluation of services provided and the results achieved as compared with accepted standards.

Raccoon eyes: Bilateral ecchymosis or bruising around the eye present with a basilar skull fracture; may be a late sign.

Rales: A crackling or bubbling sound in the lungs.

Rapid transport: Delivering the patient with multi-system trauma to definitive care without unnecessary delay; the EMT–Intermediate should spend no longer than 10 minutes in the field unless extenuating circumstances occur (entrapment, dangerous or hazardous environment, etc.).

Rapid trauma assessment: A quick and thorough hands-on examination of the trauma patient to evaluate his or her condition.

Reciprocity: Mutual exchange of privileges or licenses by two certifying agencies.

Red blood cells: Round disks, concave on two sides, and approximately 7.5 thousandths of a millimeter in diameter. The mature red blood cell contains no nucleus. Hemoglobin, a protein in red blood cells, is the most prevalent of the special blood pigments that transport oxygen from the lungs to the body cells, where it picks up carbon dioxide for transport back to the lungs to be expired. The red cells are formed in the bone marrow. After an average life of 120 days, during which they incur substantial damage, they are broken down and removed by the spleen.

Regurgitation: A passive, backward flow of gastric contents from the stomach into the oropharynx.

Repeater system: Devices that receive transmissions from relatively low-wattage transmitters on one frequency and retransmit them at a higher power on another frequency, increasing the range of the transmissions.

Reproductive system: The body system responsible for sexual reproduction.

Research: The scientific study, investigation, and experimentation in order to establish facts and determine their significance.

Respiratory acidosis: An abnormal condition with high blood levels of carbon dioxide.

Respiratory alkalosis: occurs with low blood levels of carbon dioxide and large amounts of alkali in the blood.

Respiratory system: The body system that allows for the exchange of oxygen and carbon dioxide in blood.

Response to treatment: The patient's response or lack of response to the care that was rendered.

Retractions: The inward movement of the soft tissues of the chest, commonly the suprasternal notch and the intercostal spaces. Usually associated with respiratory compromise or airway obstruction.

Rh factor: An antigen factor considered during blood typing.

Rhonchi: A coarse gurgling sound in the lungs during the process of breathing.

Rigidity: A condition characterized by hardness and stiffness.

Rule of nines: A system used to estimate the percentage of body surface involved in a burn injury.

Run critiques: Sessions where providers and medical control physicians (typically in a group setting) review run reports and/or case histories to identify positive and negative aspects of care and documentation provided by EMT–Is in given cases.

Sagittal: A vertical line dividing the body into right and left portions.

SAMPLE history: An acronym for obtaining a patient's history (Signs and Symptoms, Allergies, Medications, Past medical history, Last oral intake, and events leading to present event).

Scene size-up: The immediate evaluation of an emergency scene for the safety of the crew, patient, and bystanders.

Sclera: The whites of the eyes.

Sclerotic: Hardening or thickening of tissues.

Scope of practice: Description of what assessment and treatment skills an EMT–I may legally perform.

Seizure: A sudden, intense episode of heightened electrical activity in the brain.

Semipermeable: Cell membranes that allow only certain substances to pass through them.

Septic shock: A form of shock caused by an infection resulting in a massive vasodilation of the circulatory system.

Serous membrane: A two-layer epithelial membrane that lines body cavities and covers the surfaces of organs.

Shock: The body's response to poor perfusion.

Side effect: Any effect of a drug that is unintended.

Sinoatrial node: Point of origin of a cardiac electrical impulse, located high in the right atrium.

Skeletal system: The framework of the body comprised of bones that allows for protection and movement of the body.

Skin: The tough, supple membrane that covers the entire surface of the body.

Slander: The utterance of false statements that defame and damage another's reputation.

Snoring breathing: Noisy, raspy breathing, usually with the mouth open.

Solutes: A substance dissolved in a solution.

Solvent: A dissolving substance, usually a liquid.

Special sensory system: The system of the body responsible for the five senses.

Spinal shock: A complete transection of the spinal cord that causes the patient to lose sensation and voluntary movement below the injury.

Spontaneous abortion: A sudden and unexpected loss of pregnancy; also called miscarriage.

Spontaneous pneumothorax: A sudden accumulation of air in the pleural space.

Standard of care: The degree of medical care and skill that is expected of a reasonably competent EMT–I acting in the same or similar circumstance.

Standing orders: EMT–I field interventions that are completed before contacting medical control.

Status asthmaticus: A severe prolonged asthma attack that does not respond to standard medications.

Status epilepticus: A series of seizures without an interval of wakefulness between them.

Stimulant: Stimulate the central nervous system.

Stridor: A high-pitched noise heard on inspiration.

Stroke: A condition that results from a disruption of circulation to the brain, causing ischemia and damage to brain tissue; also called CVA.

Stroke volume: The amount of blood pumped into the cardiovascular system as a result of one heart contraction.

Stylet: A bendable plastic coated wire.

Subcutaneous: Under the skin.

Subcutaneous emphysema: Presence of air beneath the skin (in the subcutaneous tissues), giving it a characteristic crackling sensation on palpation.

Subcutaneous injections: Injections that are given into the fatty layer of tissue below the skin.

Sublingual: Under the tongue.

Suffix: A sequence of letters that occurs at the end of the word; it often describes a condition of or act performed on the word root.

Superior: Above or in a higher position.

Supine hypotensive syndrome: When in a supine position, a restriction of the flow of blood to the placenta due to the fetus compressing the inferior vena cava.

Suppository: One or more drugs mixed in a firm base that dissolves gradually at body temperature.

Suspension: Finely ground drugs that are dissolved in a liquid, such as water.

Sympathetic division: A part of the nervous system that is primary effect is to increase the heart rate, bronchiole dilation, and increased metabolism and strength; also called the adrenergic division.

Sympathetic nervous system: Division of the autonomic nervous system that is responsible for constriction of blood vessels, elevation of blood pressure and heart rate, and a feeling of nervousness in a stressful situation.

Syncope: A transient state of unresponsiveness due to inadequate perfusion of the brain from which the patient has recovered.

Synergism: Two drugs working together.

Systemic effect: Pertaining to the whole body rather than one of its parts.

Systole: Each contraction of the heart.

Tendons: White fibrous tissue that attaches muscles to bones.

Therapeutic effect: A drug's desired effect and the reason the drug is prescribed.

Thrombolytics: "Clot-busting drugs" that chemically dissolve the blockage in blood vessels.

T.K.O. rate: "To keep open" rate of infusing the IV solution. It is also referred to as KVO (keep vein open). It is equal to approximately 8 to 15 gtts per minute.

Tort: The breach of a legal duty or obligation resulting in an injury, either physical, mental, or financial.

Tort law: Law that covers a private or public wrong or injury that occurs due to a breach, or break, of a legal duty or obligation.

Tracheal tugging: Where the Adam's apple appears to be pulled upward on inspiration. It occurs in the presence of airway obstruction.

Tracheal lumen: Cavity or channel within the trachea.

Trade name: The brand of the drug that is registered by the US Patent Office.

Transceivers: The radio component that serves as both a transmitter and receiver.

Transdermal: Through the skin.

Transient ischemic attack (TIA): A stroke-like neurologic deficit that completely resolves within minutes to hours; also called a mini-stroke.

Transverse: A horizontal line dividing the body into an upper and lower portion.

Trauma center: Hospital providing emergency and specialized intensive care to critically ill and injured patients; has a well-rehearsed in-house team that can place the trauma patient suffering with hemorrhage in the operating room within 10 to 15 minutes after arrival.

Trunking: Allows multiple agencies or systems to share frequencies.

Umbilical cord: The attachment between the fetus and the placenta.

United States Pharmacopeia: A reference for drug information.

Urinary system: The body system responsible for the removal of waste products from the body in the form of urine.

Uterine rupture: Rupture of the uterus during pregnancy, has a high mortality rate for both mother and fetus. Occurs most commonly after the onset of labor.

Uterus: A hollow, muscular organ shaped like an inverted pear located in the pelvic cavity between the urinary bladder and the rectum.

Vagina: The birth canal or passageway between the uterus and the external genitalia or perineum.

Ventilation: Breathing; moving air in and out of the lungs.

Vials: Glass or plastic medication containers that have a self-sealing rubber stopper on the top, from which multiple doses may be drawn.

Visual acuity examination: A brief exam to determine how accurately the patient is seeing.

W

Wheezes: A high-pitched squeal in the lungs during the process of breathing.

The White Paper: A 1966 report published by the National Academy of Sciences entitled Accidental Death and Disability: The Neglected Disease of Modern Society. This report was responsible for emphasizing the need for organized out-of-hospital patient care.

Wide open rate: No restriction of fluid flow from the IV bag to the patient.

Word root: The foundation of a word; establishes the basic meaning of a word.

All photographs by Tom Page unless otherwise noted. All line drawings by Kimberly Battista unless otherwise noted.

Chapter 2

Fig. 2-1: Reprinted with permission from Page JO: The Paramedics, Morristown, NJ, 1979, Backdraft Publications.

Fig. 2-2: Reprinted with permission from the National Broadcasting Corporation from Page JO: The Paramedics, Morristown, NJ, 1979, Backdraft Publications.

Fig. 2-8: Vincent Knaus from Stoy W: Mosby's EMT–Basic Textbook, St. Louis, 1995, Mosby–Year Book.

Chapter 3

Fig. 3-1: Courtesy of the Virginia Department of Health, Office of EMS, Richmond.

Fig. 3-4: Prehospital Trauma Life Support Committee of the National Association of Emergency Medical Technicians, in cooperation with the Committee on Trauma of the American College of Surgeons: PHTLS: Basic and Advanced Prehospital Trauma Life Support, ed 3, St. Louis, 1994, Mosby–Year Book.

Chapter 4

Figs. 4-1, 4-3: Fox Photography.

Fig. 4-4: James Silvernail from Sanders M: Mosby's Paramedic Textbook, St. Louis, 1994, Mosby–Year Book.

Chapter 5

Chapter opener, Figs. 5-1, 5-3, 5-4: Courtesy of EMS Data Systems, Inc. Phoenix, Arizona from Stoy W: Mosby's EMT–Basic Textbook, St. Louis, 1994, Mosby–Year Book.

Chapter 6

Chapter opener: Duckwall Productions.

Figs. 6-3, 6-4: Seeley R: Anatomy and Physiology, ed 3, St. Louis, 1995, Mosby–Year Book.

Chapter 7

Fig. 7-1: From Thibodeau GA and Patton KT: Anatomy and Physiology, ed 3, St. Louis, 1996, Mosby–Year Book.

Fig. 7-2: Christine Oleksyk (art), Pat Watson (photo) from Seeley R: Essentials of Anatomy and Physiology, ed 2, St. Louis, 1996, Mosby.

Figs. 7-3, 7-21: Christine Oleksyk from Seeley R: Anatomy and Physiology, ed 3, St. Louis, 1995, Mosby–Year Book.

Fig. 7-4: Joan M. Beck from Thibodeau GA and Patton KT: Anatomy and Physiology, ed 3, St. Louis, 1996, Mosby–Year Book.

Figs. 7-5, 7-40: Joan M. Beck from Thibodeau GA and Patton KT: Structure and Function of the Body, ed 3, St. Louis, 1992, Mosby–Year Book.

Figs. 7-6, 7-7: Nadine Sokol from Seeley R: Anatomy and Physiology, ed 3, St. Louis, 1995, Mosby–Year Book.

Fig. 7-8: David J. Mascaro from Thibodeau GA and Patton KT: Anatomy and Physiology, ed 3, St. Louis, 1996, Mosby–Year Book.

Fig. 7-9: John V. Hagen from Seeley, R: Essentials of Anatomy and Physiology, ed 2, St. Louis, 1996, Mosby–Year Book.

Figs. 7-10, 7-15, 7-17, 7-18, 7-20, 7-24, 7-28, 7-29, 7-37: Duckwall Productions.

Fig. 7-11: Courtesy of Vidic B and Suarez FR: from Thibodeau GA and Patton KT: Anatomy and Physiology, ed 3, St. Louis, 1996, Mosby–Year Book.

Figs. 7-12, 7-13: David J. Mascaro & Associates from Seeley R: Essentials of Anatomy and Physiology, ed 2, St. Louis, 1996, Mosby–Year Book.

Fig. 7-14: Seeley R: Essentials of Anatomy and Physiology, ed 2, St. Louis, 1996, Mosby–Year Book.

Figs. 7-16, 7-32, 7-33, 7-34: Barbara Cousins from Seeley R: Anatomy and Physiology, ed 3, St. Louis, 1995, Mosby–Year Book.

Fig. 7-19: Rusty Jones from Seeley R: Essentials of Anatomy and Physiology, ed 2, St. Louis, 1996, Mosby–Year Book.

Fig. 7-22: Ernest W. Beck from Thibodeau GA and Patton KT: Anatomy and Physiology, ed 3, St. Louis, 1996, Mosby–Year Book.

Fig. 7-23: Kimberly Battista from Stoy W: Mosby's EMT–Basic Textbook, St. Louis, 1995, Mosby–Year Book.

Fig. 7-25: Network Graphics from Thibodeau GA and Patton KT: Anatomy and Physiology, ed 3, St. Louis, 1996, Mosby–Year Book.

Fig. 7-26: Ronald J. Ervin from Seeley R: Anatomy and Physiology, ed 3, St. Louis, 1995, Mosby–Year Book.

Fig. 7-27: Barbara Cousins from Thibodeau GA and Patton KT: Anatomy and Physiology, ed 3, St. Louis, 1996, Mosby–Year Book.

Fig. 7-30: Barbara Stackhouse from Thibodeau GA and Patton KT: Structure and Function of the Body, ed 3, St. Louis, 1992, Mosby–Year Book.

countries. From First Aid: Responding to Emergencies, St. Louis, 1991, Mosby–Year Book.

Fig. 9-42: Courtesy of Life Support Products, Inc., Irvine, CA from Sanders M: Mosby's Paramedic Textbook, St. Louis, 1994, Mosby–Year Book.

Figs. 9-48, 9-49 A, B, 9-51: From Sanders: Mosby's Paramedic Textbook, St. Louis, 1994, Mosby–Year Book.

Fig. 9-50: Courtesy of Brunswick Biomedical Technologies, Inc., Wareham, MA from Sanders M: Mosby's Paramedic Textbook, St. Louis, 1994, Mosby–Year Book.

Fig. 9-52: Courtesy of Respironics, Inc., Monroeville, PA from Sanders: Mosby's Paramedic Textbook, St. Louis, 1994, Mosby–Year Book.

Fig. 9-59 C: Kimberly Battista from Cummins and Graves: ACLS Scenarios: Core Concepts for Case-Based Learning, St. Louis, 1996, Mosby–Year Book.

Figs. 9-59 F, 9-59 I: Courtesy Michael Gorback, MD from Sanders M: Mosby's Paramedic Textbook, St. Louis, 1994, Mosby–Year Book.

Fig. 9-61: Duckwall Productions.

Chapter 10

Fig. 10-1: Stacy Lund from Stoy W: Mosby's EMT–Basic Textbook, St. Louis, 1994, Mosby–Year Book.

Fig. 10-5: Kimberly Battista from Stoy W: Mosby's EMT–Basic Textbook, St. Louis, 1994, Mosby–Year Book.

Fig. 10-10: Rolin Graphics from Thibodeau GA and Patton KT: The Human Body in Health and Disease, St. Louis, 1992, Mosby–Year Book.

Fig. 10-11: Bill Ober, inset Joan M. Beck from Thibodeau GA and Patton KT: Anatomy and Physiology, St. Louis, 1996, Mosby–Year Book.

Fig. 10-12: From Sanders M: Mosby's Paramedic Textbook, St. Louis, 1994, Mosby–Year Book.

Fig. 10-13: From NAEMT: Prehospital Trauma Life Support, ed 3, St. Louis, 1994, Mosby–Year Book.

Fig. 10-15: Yvonne Wylie Walston from Thibodeau GA and Patton KT: Anatomy and Physiology, St. Louis, 1996, Mosby–Year Book.

Fig. 10-16 A: Barbara Cousins from Thibodeau GA and Patton KT: Anatomy and Physiology, ed 3, St. Louis, 1996, Mosby–Year Book.

Figs. 10-16 B, 10-18: Rolin Graphics from Thibodeau GA and Patton KT: Anatomy and Physiology, ed 3, St. Louis, 1996, Mosby–Year Book.

Fig. 10-17: Christine Oleksyk from Thibodeau GA and Patton KT: Anatomy and Physiology, ed 3, St. Louis, 1996, Mosby–Year Book.

Fig. 10-19: Barbara Cousins from Sanders M: Mosby's Paramedic Textbook, St. Louis 1994, Mosby–Year Book.

Fig. 10-20: David Phillips/Visuals Unlimited from Seeley R: Essentials of Anatomy and Physiology, ed 2, St. Louis, 1996, Mosby–Year Book.

Fig. 10-21: Molly Babick/John Daugherty from Thibodeau GA and Patton KT: Anatomy and Physiology, ed 3, St. Louis, 1996, Mosby–Year Book.

Fig. 10-22: Seeley R: Anatomy and Physiology, ed 3, St. Louis, 1995, Mosby–Year Book.

Figs. 10-26, 10-27: From Sanders M: Mosby's Paramedic Textbook, St. Louis 1994, Mosby–Year Book.

Figs. 10-28, 10-32: Christine Oleksyk from Seeley R: Anatomy and Physiology, ed 3, St. Louis, 1995, Mosby–Year Book.

Fig. 10-29: Modified from Seeley R: Anatomy and Physiology, ed 3, St. Louis, 1995, Mosby–Year Book.

Figs. 10-33, 10-35, 10-36: Sanders M: Mosby's Paramedic Textbook, St. Louis, 1994, Mosby–Year Book.

Fig. 10-43: Courtesy of Jobst Institute, Inc., Toledo, Ohio from Sanders M: Mosby's Paramedic Textbook, St. Louis, 1994, Mosby–Year Book.

Figs. 10-44 A-D: Vincent Knaus from Stoy W: Mosby's EMT–Basic Textbook, St. Louis, 1996, Mosby–Year Book.

Table 10-1: Seeley R: Anatomy and Physiology, ed 3, St. Louis, 1995, Mosby–Year Book.

Table 10-2: Sanders M: Mosby's Paramedic Textbook, St. Louis, 1994, Mosby–Year Book.

Chapter 11

Fig. 11-9: E.W. Beck from Thibodeau GA and Patton KT: The Human Body in Health and Disease, St. Louis, 1992, Mosby–Year Book.

Figs. 11-14 I, 11-18: Mark J. Weiber from Sanders M: Mosby's Paramedic Textbook, St. Louis, 1994, Mosby–Year Book.

Chapter 12

Figs. 12-1, 12-4, 12-7: From Sanders M: Mosby's Paramedic Textbook, St. Louis, 1994, Mosby-Year Book.

Figs. 12-10 A, B: Vincent Knaus from Stoy W: Mosby's EMT–Basic Textbook, St. Louis, 1996, Mosby–Year Book.

Chapter 13

Figs. 13-1, 13-30, 13-31, 13-32 A, B, 13-33: From Sanders M: Mosby's Paramedic Textbook, St. Louis, 1994, Mosby.

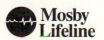